MEDICAL INSTRUMENTATION

ACCESSIBILITY AND USABILITY CONSIDERATIONS

MEDICAL INSTRUMENTATION

ACCESSIBILITY AND USABILITY CONSIDERATIONS

EDITED BY

JACK M. WINTERS
MOLLY FOLLETTE STORY

CRC Press
Taylor & Francis Group
Boca Raton London New York

CRC Press is an imprint of the
Taylor & Francis Group, an informa business

CRC Press
Taylor & Francis Group
6000 Broken Sound Parkway NW, Suite 300
Boca Raton, FL 33487-2742

Printed in the United States of America on acid-free paper
10 9 8 7 6 5 4 3 2 1

International Standard Book Number-10: 0-8493-7165-1 (Hardcover)
International Standard Book Number-13: 978-0-8493-7165-3 (Hardcover)

Visit the Taylor & Francis Web site at
http://www.taylorandfrancis.com

and the CRC Press Web site at
http://www.crcpress.com

Table of Contents

PART V Outputs of the Workshop: Key Knowledge Gaps, Barriers, Recommendations

List of Contributors

- Carla J. Alvarado, Ph.D., C.I.C., is a research scientist with the Center for Quality and Productivity Improvement at the University of Wisconsin–Madison. She received her B.S. degree from Miami University, Oxford, Ohio, and her M.S. in preventive medicine–epidemiology and Ph.D. in industrial engineering–human factors from the University of Wisconsin–Madison. She is board certified in infection control.
- Thomas J. Armstrong, Ph.D., is a professor of industrial and operations engineering and of biomedical engineering at the University of Michigan. He directs the University of Michigan Center for Ergonomics. He is a fellow of the American Industrial Hygiene Association, the Human Factors and Ergonomics Society, and the American Institute for Medical and Biological Engineering.
- David Baquis is an accessibility specialist with the U.S. Access Board, which is an independent federal agency devoted to accessible design. In that capacity he develops technical assistance materials, delivers presentations nationwide, and responds to public inquiries. He specializes in the electronic and information technology standard for Section 508 of the Rehabilitation Act. He was recently appointed as a designated federal official for accessible voting systems standards.
- Kris Barnekow, Ph.D., O.T.R., is assistant professor of occupational therapy at the College of Health Sciences, University of Wisconsin–Milwaukee, and performs research on the relationship of individuals to their environments by monitoring physiological effects of social contexts.
- Marilyn Sue Bogner, Ph.D., is president and chief scientist of the Institute for the Study of Medical Error in Bethesda, Maryland. In that capacity, she directs and conducts research using her systems approach to identify factors that contribute to error. She was previously employed by U.S. government agencies, where she addressed the contribution of medical device design to user error, examined user error issues in military equipment, and studied crosscutting issues in health services.
- Judy Brewer, Ph.D., is director of the Web Accessibility Initiative (WAI) at the World Wide Web Consortium (W3C). She is W3C's chief liaison on accessibility policy and standardization internationally, promoting awareness and implementation of Web accessibility and ensuring effective dialog among industry, the disability community, accessibility researchers, and government. She holds a research appointment at MIT's Computer Science and Artificial Intelligence Laboratory (CSAIL).
- Sean Campbell, B.B.E., is a graduate student in biomedical engineering who has been associated with the Rehabilitation Engineering and Research Center (RERC) on Accessible Medical Instrumentation. His bachelor's degree is from Marquette University.
- Pascale Carayon, Ph.D., is Procter & Gamble Bascom Professor in Total Quality in the Department of Industrial and Systems Engineering and the director of the Center for Quality and Productivity Improvement at the University of

Wisconsin–Madison. She received her engineering diploma from the Ecole Centrale de Paris, France, in 1984 and her Ph.D. in industrial engineering from the University of Wisconsin–Madison in 1988.

- Jay Crowley, M.S., is currently senior advisor for patient safety in the U.S. Food and Drug Administration's (FDA) Medical Product Safety Network (MedSun), where he focuses on developing new methods and tools for identifying, understanding and resolving hazards associated with the use of medical devices. He holds degrees in risk analysis and mechanical engineering.
- R. Sarma Danturthi, Ph.D., is a senior biomedical engineer with the RERC on Accessible Medical Instrumentation, at Marquette University. His doctoral degree is from the University of Tennessee.
- John D. Enderle, Ph.D., is Biomedical Engineering Program director and professor of electrical and computer engineering at the University of Connecticut. Enderle is the current editor-in-chief of the EMB Magazine and editor of the NSF Book Series on *NSF Engineering Senior Design Projects to Aid Persons with Disabilities,* published annually since 1989. He also directs a national student design competition for the RERC on Accessible Medical Instrumentation.
- Robert F. Erlandson, Ph.D., is professor of electrical and computer engineering and director of the Enabling Technologies Laboratory at Wayne State University in Detroit, Michigan. Before joining Wayne State University in 1976 he worked at Bell Telephone Laboratories.
- Xin (Tyre) Feng, M.S., is a doctoral student in biomedical engineering at Marquette University. His research interests include neurorehabilitation, accessible medical instrumentation, personalized interfaces for therapy and access. While obtaining his master's degree from Tsinghua University in Beijing, China, he was involved in telehealth and health informatics research.
- Daryle Gardner-Bonneau, Ph.D., is the principal of Bonneau and Associates, a human factors consultancy in Portage, Michigan. She is active in several national and international ergonomic standards committees. Her consulting focuses on addressing the needs of older adults and people with disabilities in the design of a variety of products.
- Alfred S. ("Al") Gilman, Ph.D., has been a technical leader in the development of the global positioning system (GPS) and the VHSIC hardware description language (VHDL, IEEE Std. 1076) used to design computer chips. Based in Arlington, Viriginia, he has been a classroom teacher and built human factors instruments and innovative computer interfaces. He consults for the Trace Center and the RERC on Telecommunications Access. He chairs the Protocols and Formats Working Group in the Web Accessibility Initiative (WAI) of the World Wide Web Consortium (W3C).
- John W. Gosbee, M.D., M.S., is director of patient safety information systems at the Department of Veterans Affairs (VA) National Center for Patient Safety in Ann Arbor, Michigan. A human factors engineering and health care specialist, he has consulted with health care organizations, industry, and professional societies to develop and implement human factors engineering methods for national and local patient safety management processes.
- Anne-Sophie Grenier is a graduate student in the Department of Industrial and Systems Engineering and works as a research assistant at the Center for Quality

and Productivity Improvement at the University of Wisconsin–Madison. She received her engineer diploma from the ENSIACET school of engineering in Toulouse, France, in 2004.

- Ira Janowitz, P.T., M.S., is a senior ergonomics consultant and a faculty member of the Ergonomics Graduate Training Program at the University of California–San Francisco and University of California–Berkeley. His degrees are in industrial engineering, management, and physical therapy.
- Michael L. Jones, Ph.D., is vice president for research and technology at Shepherd Center and codirector of the Rehabilitation Engineering Research Center on Mobile Wireless Technologies, a joint research program of Georgia Tech and Shepherd Center. He also serves as board chairman of Side by Side Clubhouse, a program supporting people with acquired brain injuries in their return to community living.
- June Issaacson Kailes, M.S.W., is director of dissemination activities at the RERC on Accessible Medical Instrumentation. She is an adjunct associate professor and associate director of the Center for Disability Issues and the Health Professions at Western University of Health Sciences, and a consultant and a disability rights advocate who consults for and trains businesses, universities, state associations, government entities, centers for independent living, and other not-for-profit organizations.
- Ron Kaye, M.S., is a human factors specialist with the FDA's Center for Devices and Radiological Health (CDRH). His work focuses on safety of medical equipment with respect to use issues including research on device use–safety issues, participation in standards and guidance development, and outreach to professional communities and medical device users. He has a master's degree in applied psychology and has worked in human factors for 20 years.
- Melissa R. Lemke, M.S., received her B.S. and M.S. degrees in biomedical engineering at North Carolina State University and Marquette University, respectively. She is currently the director of operations and a rehabilitation engineer with the RERC-AMI, and her fields of interest include disability research, rehabilitation engineering, and accessible and universal design.
- Christie MacDonald, M.P.P, is a research associate at the RERC on Accessible Medical Instrumentation. She is senior policy analyst at the Center for Disability Issues and the Health Professions at Western University of Health Sciences. She previously served as project manager and analyst for Berkeley Policy Associates (BPA) in Oakland, California, a private social policy research–consulting firm.
- Steven Mendelsohn, J.D., is an attorney, author, and advocate who specializes in disability and civil rights issues. For the past 15 years, his work has focused on assistive technology funding and the role of technology as a tool for the achievement of full participation in society by people with disabilities. He is the author of numerous books and articles, and has spoken and trained widely on technology funding and systems change issues.
- Rochelle Mendonca, M.S., is a researcher with the Rehabilitation Research Design and Disability Center at the University of Wisconsin–Milwaukee. She has studied the usability of the MED-AUDIT and directs current reliability and validity investigations.
- Gerald E. Miller, Ph.D., is chairperson of the Department of Biomedical Engineering at Virginia Commonwealth University, Richmond, VA.

- James L. Mueller, M.A., is an industrial designer who has worked in the field of design for people with disabilities since 1974 as an assistive technology provider, researcher, universal design consultant, and workplace accommodation specialist and instructor. He serves on the staff or advisory boards of several Rehabilitation Engineering Research Centers and chairs the Industrial Designers Society of America's Special Interest Section on Universal Design.
- John W. Peifer, M.A., is the research director of the Biomedical Interactive Technology Center at the Georgia Institute of Technology and the co-director of the Mobile Wireless Rehabilitation Engineering Research Center sponsored by the National Institute on Disability and Rehabilitation Research.
- Brenda Premo, M.B.A., is director of training activities at the RERC on Accessible Medical Instrumentation, and is the founding Director of the Center for Disability Issues and the Health Professions at Western University of Health Sciences. She was Director of the California State Department of Rehabilitation and was deputy director of its Independent Living Section from 1991 until Governor Wilson appointed her director in 1994. She was appointed by President Reagan to serve on the National Council on Disability in 1986.
- Robert G. Radwin, Ph.D., is a professor and founding chair of the Department of Biomedical Engineering at the University of Wisconsin–Madison. His research is concerned with measuring, quantifying and understanding human physiological and biomechanical capacities to do productive, quality, and healthful work.
- David Rempel, M.D., M.P.H., is a professor of medicine at the University of California at San Francisco, a professor of bioengineering at the University of California at Berkeley, and director of the Ergonomics Graduate Training Program at UC-Berkeley. He is a Fellow in the Human Factors and Ergonomics Society and the American College of Occupational and Environmental Medicine.
- Curtis Richards is a Senior Policy Fellow with the Institute for Educational Leadership, a Washington, DC-based think tank. He also maintains a public policy consulting firm known as The Advocrat Group. Richards previously served as Deputy Assistant Secretary of the Office of Special Education and Rehabilitative Services in the U.S. Department of Education and as an Assistant Director for the California State Department of Rehabilitation.
- Kathy Longenecker Rust, M.S., O.T.R., is Research Coordinator, Rehabilitation Research Design & Disability (R2D2) Center, University of Wisconsin–Milwaukee. Ms. Rust oversees key components of the ATOMS Project (Assistive Technology Outcomes Measurement System) and has co-authored seminal publications regarding the inclusion of assistive technology when measuring outcomes related to health and disability. She also has led the compilation and instructional activities of the R2D2 Center library of assistive technology assessments.
- Todd Schwanke, M.S.E., A.T.P., is a rehabilitation engineer and technical specialist for the Rehabilitation Research Design and Disability (R2D2) Center at the University of Wisconsin–Milwaukee. He also oversees the technical linkage between the OTFACT software and the MED-AUDIT taxonomies being developed by the RERC on Accessible Medical Instrumentation.
- Erin Schwier, O.T.D., O.T.R./L., is a research associate with the RERC on Accessible Medical Instrumentation, and a Senior Policy Fellow at the Center

for Disability Issues and the Health Professions at Western University of Health Sciences. She also works as a clinical practitioner of occupational therapy for acute rehabilitation at Scripps Green Hospital in San Diego, California, as well as for local school districts for special education services.

- Katherine D. Seelman, Ph.D., is associate dean and professor of rehabilitation science and technology, School of Health and Rehabilitation Sciences, University of Pittsburgh. She served as the director of the National Institute on Disability and Rehabilitation Research for seven years under President Bill Clinton. Seelman's research interests involve science, technology, and disability policy and disability studies.
- Pawan Shroff, M.S., completed a master's degree in biomedical engineering in 2005 at Marquette University, working on a project funded by the RERC on Accessible Medical Instrumentation.
- Stephanie Siegler, B.S., is a graduate student in the department of occupational therapy, University of Wisconsin–Milwaukee. Her work focuses on universal design audits and assessment instrumentation.
- Roger O. Smith, Ph.D., O.T., F.A.O.T.A., is professor of occupational therapy in the College of Health Sciences and director of the Rehabilitation Research Design and Disability Center at the University of Wisconsin–Milwaukee. He researches measurement methods related to disability and technology and has published and presented widely on this subject. He was the author of the OTFACT software sponsored by the American Occupational Therapy Association to measure the impact of occupational therapy interventions.
- Molly Follette Story, M.S., is president of Human Spectrum Design, L.L.C. and codirector of the RERC on Accessible Medical Instrumentation. From 1994 to 2004, she was coordinator of research at the Center for Universal Design at North Carolina State University and twice served as its interim executive director. She is also a Ph.D. student in ergonomics at University of California–Berkeley.
- Binh Q. Tran, Ph.D. is associate professor and chairperson of the biomedical engineering department at Catholic University of America. His research focus is to develop innovative solutions for delivery of health care services at a distance to people with disabilities and those living with chronic illnesses.
- Linda van Roosmalen, Ph.D., is an industrial design engineer conducting research and development at the University of Pittsburgh. She is task leader on the University of Pittsburgh RERC on Telerehabilitation. Her interests are in product safety, product usability, and universal design.
- Michael E. Wiklund, M.S., is president of Wiklund Research & Design, Inc. (in Concord, Massachusetts), a human factors consulting firm that specializes in medical technology development and evaluation. He is a certified human factors professional, member of AAMI's Human Factors Committee, co-author of *Designing Usability Into Medical Devices*, and an adjunct associate professor at Tufts University.
- Stephen B. Wilcox, Ph.D., is a principal in and the founder of Design Science, a 16-person, Philadelphia-based consulting firm that provides services for making products and information intuitive and easy to use. With nearly 20 years of experience in product development, he has worked with many leading manufacturers,

and has taught courses on human factors in the design departments of the University of the Arts and of Carnegie Mellon University.

- Jack M. Winters, Ph.D., is professor of biomedical engineering and John P. Raynor Distinguished Chair at Marquette University and director of the RERC on Accessible Medical Instrumentation. Since receiving a Ph.D. in bioengineering from the University of California, Berkeley and San Francisco, he has been a biomedical engineering faculty member for 20 years, twice serving as department chair. His areas of research include movement biomechanics, neurorehabilitation, telerehabilitation, and accessible medical instrumentation.
- Jill M. Winters, Ph.D., R.N., is an associate professor and the director of the Office of Nursing Research and Scholarship in the College of Nursing at Marquette University. Her research primarily has focused on use of technologies in health care, as well as health promotion activities for persons with cardiac disease.
- Thomas Y. Yen, Ph.D., is an assistant scientist in the Department of Biomedical Engineering and the Trace Research and Development Center at the University of Wisconsin–Madison. His research interests include human factors, ergonomics, biomechanics, user interface design, and rehabilitation engineering with a strong focus on developing innovative instrumentation and methodologies for measuring human capabilities.

Preface

This book is motivated by the recognition that as we move forward into the 21st century, we have an opportunity and responsibility to make medical instrumentation as accessible and usable as possible for all persons, including older adults and people with disabilities. To do so requires an evolutionary process on many levels: good science in understanding human–technology interfaces for a diversity of devices and people; educational materials and design guidelines that can help train current and future product designers and engineers in accessible design principles and processes; multidisciplinary teams passionate about social policy change that can make access to such technology a priority, and so on. It is intended to capture current knowledge and thought in the areas most relevant to this aim and to serve as a resource that will help push this process forward.

Written by leaders in the areas of human factors engineering and accessibility, this book is loosely tied to a workshop titled "Accessible Interfaces for Medical Instrumentation: Draft Guidelines and Future Directions," which was sponsored by the RERC on Accessible Medical Instrumentation (funded by the National Institute on Disability and Rehabilitation Research of the U.S. Department of Education) and the Office of Science and Engineering Laboratories of the U.S. Food and Drug Administration (FDA). It was held at FDA facilities in Rockville, Maryland, over two days in October 2005. Key goals for this workshop were to generate ideas and draft priorities for user–device interface design guidelines that may broaden device accessibility and improve patient safety, to identify and discuss current trends in user–device interfaces, and to anticipate emerging accessibility and safety issues for such interfaces in the future.

The book is divided into five parts. Part 1 addresses the extent of the problem. The first three chapters identify access barriers to medical devices by individuals with disabilities, both in the role of medical patient (Chapters 1 and 2) and health care provider (Chapter 3). The extent of the problem is especially documented through the national survey described in Chapter 2, where for many medical device product lines it was found that over 50% of participants had difficulties accessing and using the devices. Chapters 4 and 5 target policy issues, with a special focus on existing infrastructure, including both product acquisition and reimbursement (Chapter 4) and tax incentives (Chapter 5).

Part 2 of the book addresses tools for usability and accessibility analysis of medical instrumentation. Chapter 6 provides a foundation in the principles of universal design, as applied to medical devices. The methodology of ethnographic research, which studies device use in a larger context, is developed in Chapter 7, with a focus on inclusive design of home-based medical products. Chapter 8, written by a group of engineering educators, distinguishes between universal design and accessible design, and provides a range of strategies for incorporating such universal and accessible design into engineering curricula. Integration of assistive technology and universal design assessments is the theme of Chapter 9, especially as related to measurement approaches. Chapter 10 and Chapter 11 target ergonomic analysis tools, with Chapter 10 focusing on methods of sensor-based performance measurement, and Chapter 11 on analysis of hand operation of medical devices. Chapter 12 to Chapter 14 target usability and accessibility task analysis using advanced video-based analysis protocols. Chapter 14 applies tools and methodology from Chapter 12, Chapter 13, and Chapter 22 to the biomechanical study of medical device accessibility.

Part 3 of the book builds on Part 2, only with a focus on considerations for design guidelines. In Chapters 15 and 16, leaders in standards development provide insightful reviews of standards in the areas of accessibility and human factors, especially as related to medical devices. Chapter 17 provides an important perspective from human factors experts at the FDA on how accessibility analysis can enter into the medical device evaluation process. A key motivation in Chapters 15 to 17 was the recognition that many of the intended users of products will have disabilities, often with a larger proportion than in the population as a whole. Chapter 18 addresses this head-on and describes methods for having users with a diversity of abilities, both actual subjects and virtual personas, affect usability analysis. Chapter 19 addresses a different perspective of how the many practical implementation issues impact the development and use of guidelines. Chapters 20 and 21 discuss issues especially applicable to home care technologies, specifically the importance of addressing use error by designing with home care providers in mind (Chapter 20) and using an innovative problem-solving method for generating creative alternative solutions that address conflicting needs (Chapter 21). Chapter 22 reports on progress in developing a tool for measuring device accessibility, which includes embedded questions that are directly related to existing accessibility guidelines. Finally, Chapter 23, from a leader in the area of Web-based accessibility guidelines, provides a perspective on medical device accessibility that addresses not only the trend towards Internet-enabled medical devices but also the possibilities for transferring insights from web accessibility to any type of medical device interface.

Part 4 of the book views emerging trends and future technologies for medical device interfaces. This section starts in Chapter 24 with a perspective by a past director of the National Institute on Disability and Rehabilitation Research (NIDRR) that provides a vision on what is needed and is possible in the context of technology innovation that targets improving consumer access to medical devices, and the important roles for sociotechnical studies facilitating such change. The remaining chapters in Part 4 focus on technology trends and innovation that could impact on medical device interfaces, potentially in paradigm-shifting ways. Chapter 25 addresses key technical and social challenges associated with universal access, noting that realization of the potential for increased access to medical devices requires not only consideration of the universally designed and/or personalized interface, but also innovative solutions that address the barriers of distance and cost. This is followed in Chapter 26 with an insightful analysis of emerging technological and market trends, and how these could bear on new generations of medical device interfaces. Chapter 27 then builds on the vision of the two previous chapters by explicitly addressing possibilities for personalized interfaces, focusing especially on rehabilitation and medical monitoring products for home-based use. Chapter 28 then reports on a specific attempt to implement the vision of the previous chapters, namely through a simulation environment that demonstrates the possibilities for personalized interfaces through use of the new User Interface Socket/Universal Remote Console national standard. Each of the chapters in this section hints at telerehabilitation applications, and Chapter 29 addresses interface design from the perspective of a researcher with the Rehabilitation Engineering Research Center (RERC) on Telerehabilitation. Similarly, Chapter 30, written by researchers at the RERC on Mobile Wireless Technologies, explores the natural ties between certain medical instrumentation interfaces and wireless and mobile medical devices.

Part 5 of the book constitutes the final report of the Workshop on Accessible Interfaces for Medical Instrumentation, the culmination of the work of five breakout themes involving more than 60 participants. The results include a summary of prioritized vision statements for the year 2010, key barriers and challenges to be overcome, knowledge gaps and action items to be addressed, and overriding recommendations generated by workshop participants. It also includes a synthesis by the organizers and invited commentary by several of the participants.

The book closes with a glossary of terms because of the diverse, multidisciplinary nature of the contributors to this book and the participants at the workshop. These have provided a unique opportunity to bring together a diverse melting pot of expertise and perspectives, especially including some of the leading human factors engineering and accessibility professionals in the U.S. However, during the process of coming together, it became clear that terminology differs among fields, and the same words and phrases can have very different meanings in different contexts. For example, in the medical professions, the term "caregiver" refers to a health care provider such as a doctor, practicing nurse, or medical assistant but in the disability field, it can describe a personal attendant, friend or family member who provides care to an individual, often in the home. In the disability community, the term health care "access" may refer to the ability to get to and use medical equipment or a health care facility, but among people without disabilities the term may refer to the benefits available, the ability to reach health care providers, to make an appointment, or to successfully connect to the internet to get health information. The challenges, and presuppositions, differ. Such differences in meaning can make communication difficult, which is counter-productive to the goals of this book. For this reason, a glossary of terms is provided as an appendix at the back of the book in hope of achieving effective communication among all stakeholders.

Finally, a book about accessibility should also be accessible. For this reason, this book is available, by request to the publishers, in an alternative soft-copy format at the same price. While not included with the chapters, long descriptions of all figures are also available by contacting the editors directly or by going to http://www.rerc-ami.org/ami/book/figs. Finally, the font used for the text in this book is slightly larger than is common for many similar books, and the larger physical size of the book helps facilitate hands-free reading of a given page. Please contact the editors for any additional accommodations, and we will do our best. Access is important, whether it be to the content within this book or to effective use of a medical device!

Acknowledgments

This book would not be a reality without the existence of the Rehabilitation Engineering Research Center on Accessible Medical Instrumentation (RERC-AMI), which is funded by a grant, #H133E020729 from the National Institute on Disability and Rehabilitation Research (NIDRR) of the U.S. Department of Education. The editors would like to thank NIDRR for its support and, even more significantly, for having the vision to recognize this as an important area worthy of investment. We especially recognize the previous and present NIDRR program officers for the grant, William Peterson and Robert Jaeger, respectively, for their enthusiastic participation in this project. It is important to state that all opinions expressed within this book are those of the contributing authors and not of NIDRR or the Department of Education.

We also thank the U.S. Food and Drug Administration (FDA) for hosting a workshop that was convened in parallel with development of this book. We particularly thank the Office of Science and Engineering Laboratories (OSEL), under the Center for Devices and Radiological Health (CDRH) of the FDA, for their significant assistance with the workshop, particularly the visionary leadership of Dr. Larry Kessler and the remarkable organizational and hosting skills of Donald Marlowe.

Finally, the editors express their deep appreciation to the dedicated authors of the chapters of this book, some of whom were working overtime and/or outside their comfort zones in addressing issues not central to their usual focal area. We also acknowledge the assistance of the staff of CRC Press and of RERC-AMI staff member Melissa Lemke in helping bring this together.

Jack M. Winters

Molly Follette Story

Part I

Background: The Problem, Existing Infrastructure, and Possible Solutions

1 The Patient's Perspective on Access to Medical Equipment

June Isaacson Kailes

CONTENTS

1.1 INTRODUCTION

> It takes a village to get me on and off an exam table, which means I don't go to preventive care appointments [1].

This chapter describes common access barriers to health care for people with disabilities, with specific focus on medical equipment access. It overlays a "human face" on the barriers by providing examples from the reality of individuals who regularly deal with healthcare systems. These experiences often go undocumented and, thus, underreported.

1.1.1 Health Care Access

The term "access" refers to the ability of individuals or groups to receive needed services from the health care system. This may include availability of a particular service, awareness by individuals that the service exists and how to obtain it, and ability to get the service in a reasonable amount of time. Health care access for people with disabilities and activity limitations includes additional layers of equipment, physical, communication, and program access necessary to benefit from quality health care.

For people with disabilities, equipment access represents one of the fundamental barriers to receiving health care and health-promoting services. Many people have vivid memories of medical procedures and the instructions they received, such as, "Just hop up, look here, read this, listen up, don't breathe, and stay still!" These directions can be amusing or uncomfortable for many, but they can be difficult to impossible for people with a variety of functional activity limitations.

In addition to barriers resulting from facility design, attitudinal, and competency barriers, many people experience lack of access because of inaccessible diagnostic, therapeutic, procedural, rehabilitation, and exercise equipment, such as examination and treatment tables and chairs, weight scales, x-ray equipment, glucometers, blood pressure cuffs, treadmills, and exercise machines.

1.2 WHO ARE PEOPLE WITH DISABILITIES?

The 2000 U.S. Census found that people with disabilities represented 19.3% of the 257.2 million people aged 5 and older in the civilian noninstitutionalized population, or nearly 1 person in 5 [2]. In addition, the Government Accountability Office has estimated that at least 1.8 million individuals with disabilities are being served in institutional settings, including 1.6 million in nursing facilities [3].

1.2.1 Functional Limitations Increase with Age

The 2000 Census showed that disability rates rise significantly with age. The data showed that 54% of people over the age of 65 reported having a disability compared to 19% of people under the age of 65. The Census Bureau predicts that if current trends continue, Americans 65 years and older will constitute 20% of the total population by the year 2030, compared with about 12% in 1997 [4].

Most people, if they live long enough, will age into disability. As time alters our bodies, activity and functional limitations become natural occurrences. Arthritis, the leading cause of disability among adults, affected 70 million people in 2001, including 60% of people age 65 and older [5]. If current rates of arthritis prevalence remain unchanged, the number of persons over age 65 living with arthritis will double by 2030. Obesity among adult Americans is also increasing [6]. In addition to often being disabling itself, obesity contributes to other potentially debilitating conditions, including diabetes, arthritis, high blood pressure, and asthma [2].

Preparing to accommodate people with disabilities often translates into being better equipped to serve all people. Medical, technology, legal, and social advances keep more people with disabilities, chronic conditions, and activity limitations alive, healthy, productive, and functioning independently in their communities. If the age-specific prevalence of major chronic conditions remains unchanged, the absolute number of people in the U.S. with functional limitations will rise by more than 300% by 2049 [2]. Increasing numbers of people will live with multiple coexisting, chronic, and disabling conditions. This trend will continue to increase the number of people who will benefit from and require equipment access. Given the arriving age wave of the "baby boom" generation, people who live with disabilities today are truly "canaries in the [health care] mine," who are more sensitive to barriers in the system.

1.2.2 Taking the Broad View of Disability

Disability is not a condition that affects the "special" or the "unfortunate few." Disability is just one variation on the diversity of being human, and it is a common and natural occurrence within the human experience. The notion that people either have a disability or do not have a disability perpetuates misperceptions about the nature of disability and activity limitations. Activity limitations exist along continuums of gradation (partial to total) and duration (temporary to permanent) that affect almost everyone at some point in their lives.

In health care, given these continuums of activity limitation, the number of people who benefit from equipment, physical, communication, and program access is a significant percentage of the patient population. Traditional narrow definitions of disability are not appropriate. If the value that everyone should be accommodated and treated in health care is not infused into planning, then not everyone will be served. By adopting a broad disability definition, one that includes the wide spectrum of people with varying abilities and activity limitations, no one gets left behind [2].

For the remainder of this chapter, this broad group of people is referred to as people with activity limitations.

1.3 THE HEALTH CARE HASSLE FACTOR

For many people with disabilities, maneuvering through the complex health care system is a dense minefield full of access, safety, competency, and attitudinal barriers. A common impact of existing medical equipment, physical, communication, and program access barriers is that people with disabilities feel defeated by the experience of a continual "hassle factor." This experience often culminates in the "four F" experiences — frustration, fatigue, fear, and failure. For some people, the effort of seeking health care is just too exhausting or degrading. This leads to people postponing or avoiding care, which results in lack of care, delayed diagnosis, and worsening conditions that begin a downward spiral of deteriorating health and that eventually requires more extensive and expensive treatments. These barriers diminish opportunities for longer, healthier productive lives for people with disabilities and compromise the quality of those lives.

The following comments illustrate safety issues and the common "four F" experiences [7]:

> My primary physician and several specialists I respect all practice at a major university medical center fairly close to my home. Recently, though, when I requested a gynecology referral there, I was told that I would not be seen unless I could bring my own assistants to help me get on the examining table. This is a huge world-renowned hospital. This is the era of ADA. Still I am treated as though I don't belong with the other women who seek services in OB/GYN unless I can make my disability issues go away. This news makes me weary. I know it means once again that I can't simply pursue what I need as an ordinary citizen. I can't be just a woman who needs a pelvic exam; I must be a trailblazer. I must make the many bits of legal information and persuasive arguments it will take to get me into that clinic.
>
> **— Female power wheelchair user with post-polio [8]**

> I have avoided [gynecology] exams. I'm a 31-year-old woman, and I have not had a pelvic exam — ever — because of all the different complications and fears, for multiple reasons. ... Here I am, a woman who's a researcher in sociology and health, and I'm a real health advocate for others and myself — and this is my secret shame.
>
> **— Female power wheelchair user with muscular dystrophy [9]**

> Shortly after my spinal cord injury, while in a rehab program, I was being transferred to a hospital bed from my wheelchair by an LVN [licensed vocational nurse]. During the transfer, she slipped and I fell, hitting my head on a metal rail of the bed, rebreaking my neck!*

1.4 HEALTHCARE BARRIERS FOR PEOPLE WITH ACTIVITY LIMITATIONS

People with disabilities as a group have a higher need for short- and long-term health services than people without disabilities. In 1989, individuals with no activity limitations reported having approximately four contacts with physicians per year; individuals who had some activity limitation reported twice this amount; individuals unable to perform major life activities (i.e., bathing, dressing, getting

* Ed Tessier, personal communication, 09/27/05.

around, toileting, eating, walking, climbing stairs) reported five times as many; and for people needing help with instrumental activities of daily living (shopping, transportation, money management, etc), the number was seven times as high [10].

> People with disabilities are more likely to have early deaths, chronic conditions, and preventable secondary conditions and to make more emergency room visits, at the same time as they have less health insurance coverage and less overall use of the health care system (as indicated by numbers of pap tests, mammography and oral health exams). One indicator of the health disparities experienced by people with disabilities is that the rate of diabetes among people with disabilities is 300% higher than the general population [11].

Secondary and multiple disabling conditions often cause individuals with disabilities to delay routine care and to seek medical attention only for more serious problems. In addition, lack of access to health care may cause individuals to withdraw and isolate themselves from society and loved ones [12].

There are huge gaps between adequate, equitable, safe, disability-literate, and competent care and the reality of the current health care experience for people with activity limitations. They deal with many more health care barriers than people without activity limitations. Inadequate attention to ensuring Americans with Disabilities Act compliance is a major contributor to many of the documented health disparities experienced by people with disabilities.

1.4.1 Health Care Compliance with Americans with Disabilities Act

Many disability rights advocates have spent years working to maximize compliance with the Americans with Disabilities Act of 1990 (ADA). The positive payoffs in our built environment are apparent (accessible hotels, airports, paths, parking, doors, restrooms, etc.) and significantly contribute to helping people with disabilities live independently and participate Productively in their communities.

The intent of the ADA is that people with disabilities receive health care that is equally as effective as care provided to people without disabilities. But ADA implementation in health care lags far behind implementation in other industries such as hospitality, entertainment, and retail.

When health care providers are unable to get an accurate weight or perform an appropriate examination because patients cannot use a traditional scale or cannot get onto or are not assisted in getting onto diagnostic, therapeutic, or procedural equipment, then patients may receive unequal health care. Patients may be undiagnosed or misdiagnosed because of lack of sufficient assessment, and patients may miss the benefit of early detection and treatment. When health care providers are unable or unwilling to adapt their techniques to perform procedures that accommodate people with a variety of limitations, people do not receive medical and preventive care that is adequate or equitable with care provided to others.

Many health care providers do not understand the intent of the ADA with respect to the practical aspects of choosing an accommodation. They do not understand why and how providing accommodations can advance the goal of effective health care. People with disabilities often do not get the kinds of health services they need. For example, some postpone or avoid checkups because the health care providers' office staffs don't accommodate their needs. Many health care staffs are not trained or available to help with transfers to equipment and positioning. Many staffs lack disability-specific experience, expertise, and training.

For example, providing health care services to women who need mammograms illustrates many accommodation, safety, and equipment access barriers.

> Women with disabilities often have less access to breast health services than any other group of women. Overall, women who are not disabled receive mammograms 11% more [frequently] than women with considerable limitations. Even if women with disabilities schedule mammograms or clinical breast exams, many cannot receive either service when they arrive because of inaccessible health care facilities and medical equipment [13].

1.4.2 Attitudinal Barriers

For people with disabilities the biggest barrier, often beyond access barriers, is attitudes. Negative health care provider attitudes and misconceptions about people with disabilities contribute to wide disparities in the services they receive [14].

People with disabilities report hearing from health care providers a variety of responses that reflect negative misconceptions and biases.

> We can't treat you here; this is an ambulatory clinic, which means you have to be able to walk. You are wheelchair-bound.
>
> **— Told to a woman about to start chemotherapy [9]**

> I was so frustrated at having to tell the people in the emergency room, "I can't get up on the gurney; I can't stand up to do this; you're going to have get someone to help me get on this examination table" ... and they just look at you like, "Hey, what's the problem?"
>
> **— Female power wheelchair user with post-polio [9]**

As the following examples highlight, when a patient requests a specific accommodation, some health care institutions either resist providing it or take ineffective or inappropriate action.

> Two women, who visited the clinic for women with disabilities ... reported being treated in an unsafe, demeaning, and painful manner when they sought services from another provider in their area. One woman with cerebral palsy was lifted onto an examination table by an untrained security guard. The other woman, who has multiple sclerosis, was held under the arms in a standing position by two staff members in order to reach an inaccessible mammogram machine [14].

> At the urologist ... there is a cutout in the table. The cutout alone makes transferring a little bit difficult but ... it was covered with one of those papers and I didn't know it was there. So I was asked if I could manage the transfer, and the table was low enough, and I said, "Sure, no problem," and they left the room. And I went to transfer, stuck my hand in the hole, and ended up on the ground because I didn't know there was a hole there and nobody thought to [tell me] ..."
>
> **— Female manual wheelchair user with spinal cord injury [9]**

> The people who are taking the mammograms will grab for your (wheelchair control) joystick, and you have your breasts between the things, and they don't realize how fast the chair can go. So you have to be very assertive and say, "Do not touch my joystick, please!"
>
> **— Female power wheelchair user with muscular dystrophy [9]**

> During a routine physical, Lois's doctor suggested it was time for her to get a baseline mammogram. When she called her hospital to arrange it and mentioned that she was paraplegic, they asked Lois if she could stand. Lois said no, she used a wheelchair. "Then we can't do it," they said. When Lois called her doctor's office to ask for guidance, she discovered her doctor had just been taken in to have heart surgery. Because the breast exam in that doctor's office revealed no problem, Lois decided to wait. Later, she had to be hospitalized for treatment of a decubitus ulcer. During the pre-surgical exam, a lump was discovered in her breast. Under doctor's orders, a mammogram was performed in the same hospital that refused to serve her before. Sadly, the lump, already palpable in size, was malignant and she had a mastectomy. Had her cancer been diagnosed earlier, her treatment options may have been different [14].

People with significant difficulty walking receive significantly fewer screening and preventive services such as mammograms and pap smears [15]. Less than 1% of people with arthritis receive public health interventions, such as community-based exercise programs, that could improve or maintain their function [5,15].

> If you always do what you always did, you always get what you always got.
>
> — **Anonymous**

Attitudes about equipment access must also change. If we believe we can improve the design of equipment and incorporate safety, accessibility, and universal design principles (see Chapter 6 of this book), then it will happen and patients with and without disabilities as well as health care professionals will benefit.

1.5 MEDICAL EQUIPMENT ACCESS

There are multiple reasons for the aforementioned disparities, and lack of accessible medical equipment is one major factor. When diagnostic, therapeutic, and procedural equipment is not safe and accessible, individuals with disabilities are denied access to health care, health promoting exercise, rehabilitation, and potentially life-saving procedures.

A 2005 survey of approximately 400 Californians with disabilities found exam tables were inaccessible to 69% of wheelchair users and 46% of cane, crutch, and walker users [1]. The height of exam tables was the most commonly reported complaint. The survey respondents who used wheelchairs reported the following:

- 69% had difficulty using exam tables.
- 60% had difficulty being weighed due to inaccessible scales.
- 45% had difficulty using x-ray equipment, such as mammography equipment.
- 43% had difficulty using exam chairs.

In addition, 33% of all people with mobility disabilities experienced barriers accessing examination rooms.

The Rehabilitation Engineering Research Center on Accessible Medical Instrumentation (RERC-AMI) conducted a nationwide survey of 408 participants with a variety of disabilities. Survey participants ranked examination tables, radiology equipment, exercise and rehabilitation equipment, and weight scales as the top four categories of medical devices that were most difficult to use [16; Chapter 2 of this book]. The most prominent theme in describing these difficulties involved safety issues. The next most prevalent categories of difficulty were positioning and comfort, transferability, lack of clear and understandable visual displays and markings, and difficulties conducting activities requiring fine motor movements [16; Chapter 2 of this book].

The usability, safety, and accessibility of medical equipment play a significant, but until recently overlooked, effect on the quality and delivery of health care services for people with activity limitations. People with mobility limitations have difficulty getting onto and positioning themselves on equipment. The nature of difficulties include equipment (such as exam tables, medical chairs, weight scales, diagnostic and radiological equipment, and exercise equipment) being too high or too low, too narrow, too long or too short, too hard, and unsafe.

1.5.1 EXAMINATION TABLES

Other exam table difficulties reported on the survey [16; Chapter 2 of this book] and in the focus groups [9] were how hard it was to get onto tables, with nothing to hold onto; and fear of being able to stay on the table alone (given difficulties with coordination, spasticity, and pain) during what can be a long wait for the health care provider to return.

> Often [technicians] will jack you up on a table and then leave the room, so you're there not knowing how long, and you can't independently move because there's nothing to grab on. There's no rail or no hand grab alongside these things at all, so you can't independently adjust yourself on the tables, and there's a lot of sharp edges.
>
> **— Male manual wheelchair user with spinal cord injury [9]**

> The table is so hard and my back — I have scoliosis so it hurts … They leave me there [and say], "Wait a minute, hold your breath," and I'm cold because my body is 10° lower than anybody. I ask for more blankets. They say, "Oh, it's just going to take a few minutes." They're seeing that I am completely in pain and I'm shaking, and they want me to hold it, to be steady, and to take the x-ray. … It's so scary when he leaves me in the position that … they put me sideways with the pillows there and the plate under me, and leave. And [he says], "Hold your breath!" … I just feel like I'm going to crash right there and then just praying all the time, holding onto nothing. It's very traumatic.
>
> **— Female power wheelchair user with paralysis [9]**

> I literally chose my doctors because of those tables, so that it would be easier for them to examine me.
>
> **— Female power wheelchair user with cerebral palsy [9]**

People also reported having difficulty with the small step provided for climbing up on the table, which also had nothing to hold on to, and with stirrups, which were hard to use. Some people commented that the paper, usually spread out across the table surface, was slippery and could make getting onto and off the table more difficult; but people with visual limitations said the paper made it easier for them to see where to sit, if it contrasted with the color of the table surface; and people who were deaf reported that they sometimes used the paper to communicate by written notes with a health care provider.

1.5.2 Medical Chairs

Medical chairs are difficult for some people to get onto and off, because of the height, size, and shape of the base of the chair. When the base of the chair extends beyond the side of the seat, it prevents wheelchair users, for example, from maneuvering close enough to safely transfer to the chair. Armrests are also critical. When they are missing or too low, they are not available to help people get on or off the chair, and when they are too high, they can interfere with body movements. Medical chairs are also uncomfortable for some people to sit in for any length of time.

> The assumption for all of these chairs is that you have to have a standard shaped body. The designs weed out so many people that it seems there should be an adjustment that accommodates unique body shapes … different shaped backs, whether it is curvature, scoliosis, or whatever…
>
> **— Female leg brace user with spina bifida [9]**

> I think it would be helpful if the leg part of it [medical chair] was adjustable … When [the chair] is at a particular angle, not only are [my legs] falling off but they are basically constantly [in] spasms. So having it adjustable, where I can say, "Hey, for me let them be more bent," or "Let them be straighter" — that would be better, rather than having to fit my body to the chair.
>
> **— Female manual wheelchair user with spinal cord injury [9]**

Another comment about medical chairs was that depending on the shape of the footrest, people's feet sometimes get tangled in them, or their feet are not adequately supported.

1.5.3 Weight Scales

Survey respondents and focus group participants reported that standard scales may be unstable, and they may provide nothing to hold on to (see Chapter 2 of this book). Most scale displays are not usable by people with visual limitations. It was common for wheelchair users to report that they do not know their weight because they have not been weighed in many years. They described health professionals who often asked them to guess or estimate their own weight.

> I've not been on a wheelchair scale since rehab, over 22 years [ago]. ... My HMO has one, but apparently it's in a storage room down by emergency somewhere, and nobody has ever seen it.
>
> **— Male manual wheelchair user with spinal cord injury [9]**

> There have been long periods of years when I have not been weighed. I have been weighed more on laundry scales than on actual human scales. ... I actually prefer that because I have a great big wheelchair.
>
> **— Female with muscular dystrophy and heavy [9]**

> I have never been weighed at my doctor, ever. ... I was once at the doctor's with my boyfriend, who is six-foot-five and is perfectly able to hold me, but the scale doesn't have a maximum to carry both of us on the scale at the same time.
>
> **— Female manual wheelchair user with spinal cord injury [9]**

1.5.4 Exercise Equipment

People with visual limitations have difficulty using equipment with visual displays such as touch screens and visual prompts, common on many forms of exercise equipment. This makes using bikes, treadmills, and other equipment frustrating, difficult, and sometimes impossible. The following experiences are common:

> To fully participate in a fitness facility, I either need to hire (and then train) a personal trainer or memorize, by repeated trips with a sighted guide, the equipment that I am able to use without assistance and where it is located. Of course, that only works until the personal trainer and equipment is moved around. I know of no gym or fitness center that has incorporated cardio equipment with audio or Braille information into its fleet of equipment choices. The more electronic and digital exercise equipment becomes, the more impossible it is for blind people to use. It is almost impossible for someone with significant vision loss to participate at a gym or fitness center without a sighted guide. Navigating the crowded landscape (crowded with people and equipment), locating the equipment you want to use, being able to set up the equipment for yourself, i.e., set time and speed on treadmills or exercise bikes or set weight machines for position and amount of weight, or find free weights, dressing rooms, etc., are all partially or totally inaccessible.*

1.5.5 Communication between Healthcare Provider and Patient

Communication between health care provider and patient is critical but often problematic, especially for people with visual, hearing, and intellectual disabilities. Providers may not bother to explain procedures and expectations of patients beforehand, which can cause problems. People with hearing disability may have particular difficulty receiving directions from technicians ("Don't breathe," "Turn on your left side," etc.).

* Anita Aaron, Executive Director of the Rose Resnick Lighthouse in San Francisco, personal e-mail 2005.

> I was just lying there and it was my first time and so I'm lying there and I have no idea. I'm just lying there and I was breathing and kind of looking around, and the nurse was like, "No, don't breathe!" And I said, "Well, why didn't you tell me in the first place?" I go in and she's, like, rushing me; and then they shove me in there and there's no explanation. … "Now you have to do it again," she says. It's her fault and not mine.
>
> **— Deaf male on having an MRI [9]**

1.6 SUMMARY

For people with disabilities and activity limitations, the work of the RERC-AMI is serious business. Equipment design plays a critical role in improving access to safe, competent, quality care for everybody. It is about getting it right in areas that are essential to health and independence. It is about giving many people with activity limitations tools and services they need to keep going and be productive, and to prevent the world from unnecessarily closing in and becoming confining. It is about translating the words and mantras such as "health-care services that are available and accessible to all" into reality.

As this chapter reports, the experiences of people with disabilities, advocates, and health-care providers demonstrate specific equipment access problems. However, anecdotal data does not carry much weight. Without respected data these stories are minimized, devalued, and viewed as coming only from people with opinions.

The RERC-AMI's focus is to convert these stories into critical data that contribute to developing guidelines to improve the usability and accessibility equipment access for a broad spectrum of health care users. By converting these stories into meaningful data, and converting data to systems change, the words will not remain empty promises.

ACKNOWLEDGMENT

This work is supported by the RERC-AMI, funded by the National Institute on Disability and Rehabilitation Research, U.S. Department of Education Grant #H133E020729. All opinions expressed are those of the author.

REFERENCES

1. Markwalder, A., Disability Rights Advocates (2005). *A CALL TO ACTION: A Guide for Managed Care Plans Serving Californians with Disabilities*. Oakland, CA: DRA
2. Reis, J.P., Breslin, M.L., Iezzoni, L., Kirschner, K. (2004). *It Takes More Than Ramps to Solve the Crisis of Healthcare for People with Disabilities*. Chicago, IL: Rehabilitation Institute of Chicago, p. 30.
3. U.S. Department of Health and Human Services (2005). The Surgeon General's Call to Action to Improve the Health and Wellness of Persons with Disabilities. U.S. Department of Health and Human Services, Office of the Surgeon General, Washington, D.C. www.surgeongeneral.gov and at http://www.hhs.gov/od.
4. U.S. Census (1997). Disabilities Affect One-Fifth of All Americans: Proportion Could Increase in Coming Decades, Census Brief 97-5, Washington, D.C.
5. Centers for Disease Control and Prevention (2003). Public health and aging: projected prevalence of self-reported arthritis or chronic joint symptoms among persons aged > 65 years — U.S., 2005–2030. *Morb. Mort. Wkly. Rep.*, 52(21): 489.
6. Mokdad, A.H., Ford, E.S., Bowman, B.A., Dietz, W.H., Vinicor, F., Bales, V.S., Marks, J.S. (2003). Prevalence of obesity, diabetes, and obesity-related health risk factors, 2001. *J. Am. Med. Assoc.*, 289(1): 76–79.
7. Story, M.F., Winters, J.W.M., Premo, B., Kailes, J.I., Schwier, E., and Winters, J.M. (2005). Focus groups on accessibility of medical instrumentation. *Proc. RESNA 2005 Annu. Conf.*, Atlanta, GA.

8. Gill, C.J. (1993, May–June). When is a Woman Not a Woman, *The Disability Rag ReSource*, pp. 26-29.
9. Rehabilitation Engineering Research Center on Accessible Medical Instrumentation (RERC-AMI) R1.1 Focus Groups, March 21–23, 2005.
10. LaPlante, M.P. (1993). Disability, Health Insurance Coverage, and Utilization of Acute Health Services in the U.S. U.S. Department of Health and Human Services, Washington, D.C.
11. U.S. Department of Health and Human Services. (2001). *Healthy People 2010*, 2nd ed. Office of Disease Prevention and Health Promotion, Washington, D.C.
12. Burgdorf R.L. (1991). Equal access to public accommodations. In West, J., Ed., *Americans with Disabilities Act: From Policy to Practice*. Milbank Memorial Fund, New York, pp. 183–213.
13. National Women's Health Information Center (n.d.). Barriers to Health Care Access. Retrieved from Internet on July 26, 2002, at http://www.4woman.gov.
14. Krotoski, D.M., Nosek, M.A. and Turk, M.A. (editors). (1996). *Women with Physical Disabilities: Achieving and Maintaining Health and Well-Being*. P.H Brookes Pub. Co., Baltimore, MD.
15. Iezzoni, L.I., McCarthy, E.P., Davis, R.B., and Siebens, H. (2000). Mobility impairments and use of screening and preventive services. *Am. J. Public Health* 90, 955–961.
16. Winters, J.W.M, Story, M.F., Barnekow, K., Kailes, J.I., Premo, B., Schwier, E., and Winters, J.M. (2005). Accessibility of medical instrumentation: a national healthcare consumer survey. *Proc. RESNA 2005 Annu. Conf.*, Atlanta, GA.

2 Results of a National Survey on Accessibility of Medical Instrumentation for Consumers

Jill M. Winters, Molly Follette Story, Kris Barnekow, June Isaacson Kailes, Brenda Premo, Erin Schwier, Sarma Danturthi, and Jack M. Winters

CONTENTS

ABSTRACT

Health care consumers with disabilities often lack adequate access to diagnostic, therapeutic, and procedural health care devices and assistive technologies. In order to better understand accessibility and usability issues of these devices and technologies, a Web-based national consumer survey was developed, and it was completed by 408 individuals. Respondents ranked examination tables, radiology equipment, exercise and rehabilitation equipment, and weight scales as the top four most difficult categories of medical devices to use. The most prominent themes in the narrative data describing these difficulties were safety issues, positioning and comfort, patient transfer issues, visual displays and markings, and activities requiring fine motor movements.

2.1 INTRODUCTION

From 1994 to 1995, the Centers for Disease Control estimated that approximately 54 million Americans had one or more types of disability [1]. In 1999, the National Institute on Disability and Rehabilitation Research proclaimed that "Persons with disabilities must have access to, and satisfaction with, an integrated continuum of health care services, including primary care and health maintenance services, specialty care, medical rehabilitation, long-term care, and health promotion programs" (p. 68594) [2]. Nevertheless, for a variety of reasons, many persons with disabilities do not have access to adequate health care. For many years, persons with disabilities have encountered barriers to engaging in diagnostic and preventive health care activities, and adequate access to primary health care, hospital care, and long-term care services [3,4]. The disparity of health care services available for persons with disabilities may reflect the variability, extent, and nature of health services required [5] and the greater need for short- and long-term health services, health care reimbursement issues, and lack of accessible medical devices. Although the Americans with Disabilities Act of 1990 stipulated that access to medical care and public accommodations be provided for all, many medical devices commercially available today fall short of this requirement.

The most obvious barriers for persons with disabilities trying to obtain satisfactory health care services relate to issues of physical access to health care facilities, issues that extend well beyond stairs and doorways. Early research in this area has focused on breast and reproductive health in women [6], and significant accessibility issues have been identified related to breast and cervical cancer screening [7,8]. Nosek [6] found that inaccessible mammography equipment made it less likely for women with disabilities to receive breast screening. Examination tables that do not accommodate women with disabilities have resulted in many undetected or untreated gynecologic problems in this population [9,10]. Cheng et al. [8] found that ambulatory patients had 5.32 times greater odds of having a cervical smear test and 3.24 greater odds of getting a mammography exam, when compared to their nonambulatory counterparts with multiple sclerosis [8].

The health-related benefits of physical activity are well accepted. However, according to the Healthy People 2010 report and public health objectives, people with disabilities are 20% less likely to engage in any leisure-time activity than those without disabilities (36% vs. 56%) [11]. Issues such as exercise equipment that is not adaptive and accessible has been cited as a dominant contributing factor to this disparity [12,13]. Although there is a growing body of evidence illustrating the disparity of health care services available for persons with disabilities, little is known about the nature and extent of barriers to accessing medical devices and technologies in relation to levels of ability and disability, as well as medical diagnoses. Therefore, the Rehabilitation Engineering Research Center on Accessible Medical Instrumentation (RERC-AMI) planned a national consumer survey to provide a more thorough understanding of the types of medical devices that were most difficult for persons with disabilities to use or access and to gain a better understanding of the nature of the barriers that make these devices difficult to use.

2.2 METHODS

2.2.1 Survey Development

Prior to undertaking the national consumer survey, members of the research team recognized the need to develop a comprehensive survey to elicit detailed information about respondents that would complete the survey, as well as information about their experiences with medical devices.

The initial instrument was developed by members of the research team. Demographic data were selected to mirror the types of data collected in the National Health Interview Survey [14,15]. After compiling an instrument the research team believed was comprehensive, while attempting to limit the burden to respondents, a Delphi technique [16] was employed to improve the instrument and provide preliminary evidence of content validity. During this process, feedback relative to content, layout, and degree of burden was solicited from a number of nationally respected key informants and experts with disabilities, most of which were employed in disability-related fields. Several rounds of the Delphi technique were completed until consensus was achieved. As a result, a Web-based survey was launched, with confidence that the instrument was user friendly and comprehensive, and presented minimal burden for participants. The Web version of the survey provided a great deal of versatility, allowing respondents to select font style, size, and color, background color, and was compatible with most screen readers. The survey was also available to participants as a Microsoft Word form, as standard and large print PDF documents, by means of telephone survey using either voice or TTY technology and via a face-to-face interview.

2.2.2 Design

In mid-2004, the national survey was launched. The study incorporated an exploratory, cross-sectional survey design. A diverse sample of individuals with a wide range of disabilities and medical diagnoses was targeted for participation. Eligibility criteria included being at least 18 years of age, providing self-report of at least one disability, ability to understand English, and experience with medical devices. Persons with cognitive disabilities were excluded.

2.2.3 Procedure

Disability-related list-serves and Web sites, flyers, posters, personal contacts at independent and assisted living facilities, and personal contacts at disability-related conferences and meetings were used as primary methods of recruitment. Completion of the survey took approximately 30 to 45 minutes, and it could be completed in one or multiple sessions.

Fifteen categories of medical devices were specified in the survey in an attempt to include the vast array currently in use. Categories included examination tables and chairs, dental equipment, monitoring devices, exercise equipment, and a variety of devices used for cardiac, pulmonary, orthopedic, and neurological rehabilitation. Also included were equipment used for vision and hearing testing, radiology procedures, cardiac stress testing, pulmonary function testing, medication administration, oxygen delivery, and determining patient weights. A final category of "other" was included, allowing participants to share experiences that they believed did not fit the categories provided.

The survey was divided into two parts — (1) a demographic and functional ability questionnaire and (2) the usability and accessibility instrument. Content validity was established prior to and following the Delphi procedure, with a final content validity index of 3.47 (0 to 4 scale). Survey items were either forced-choice or open-ended in nature.

2.2.4 Data Analysis

Quantitative data were analyzed using descriptive statistics. Valid sample sizes were used when data were analyzed for the usability and accessibility of specific classifications of medical devices; that is, calculations were based on the number of individuals with experience using the specified devices. Content analysis, using constant comparative techniques, was employed for analyzing the narrative data [17]. Two investigators coded all narrative data independently. The resultant themes or categories were discussed and consensus was achieved. At least 10% of respondent comments were required to support consideration as a final category in the classification scheme. The resultant categories will be presented in rank order of frequency of occurrence for a variety of disabilities.

2.3 RESULTS

2.3.1 Demographic Data

On the survey Web site, 457 individuals created accounts or completed the survey in an alternative format. Of these prospective subjects, 408 participants provided usable data. At least one individual from each of the 50 states completed the survey. Participants were asked to respond as to whether they were 18 to 24, 25 to 44, 45 to 64, or 65 years or older. All categories were represented, with the majority of participants being between the ages of 25 and 64 (86.0%). The majority of respondents were female (66.1%), Caucasian (90.2%), had at least a bachelor's degree (57.3%), worked full (36.0%) or part time (20.9%), and used at least one form of assistive technology (98.0%) (see Table 2.1). The most commonly used assistive technologies included eyeglasses, manual wheelchairs, power wheelchairs, and canes/crutches/walker.

Individuals with a wide variety of sensory and physical disabilities, as well as medical diagnoses, completed the survey (see Table 2.2). Disability types were separated as to whether they represented

TABLE 2.1
Demographic Characteristics of Sample

Characteristic	Prevalence (%)
Sex	
Male	33.9
Female	66.1
Age	
18–24	6.8
25–44	39.5
45–64	46.5
65–74	4.8
75 and older	2.5
Race	
Caucasian	90.2
African American	3.9
Native American	2.0
Other	3.9
Education	
High school equivalency or less	20.8
Vocation/trade/associate degree	21.2
Bachelor's degree	29.8
Graduate or professional degree	27.5
Other	0.7
Employment	
None	43.1
Part-time	20.9
Full-time	36.0
Use of assistive technology	
Eyeglasses	65.0
Manual wheelchair	45.1
Power wheelchair	44.4
Cane, crutches, walker	36.8
Hearing aid	8.1
Other	17.9

TABLE 2.2
Types and Incidence of Impairments

Type of Impairment	N	Percentage
Visual impairment	130	31.9
Hearing impairment	62	15.2
Speech impairment	30	7.4
Mobility impairment		
Orthopedic impairment	156	38.2
Back pain	132	32.4
Chronic pain	119	29.2
Arthritis and rheumatism	103	25.2
Paralysis	92	22.5
Spinal cord injury	87	21.3
Multiple sclerosis	36	8.8
Muscular dystrophy	31	7.6
Cerebral palsy	30	7.4
Loss of limb	20	4.9
Parkinson's disease	2	0.5
Myasthenia gravis	1	0.2
Cardiopulmonary		
Cardiac disease	32	7.8
Hypertension	95	23.2
Pulmonary disease	59	14.4

more visual, hearing, speech, mobility, or cardiopulmonary impairments. The sample had significant representation of persons in all these categories, with 31.9% indicating they had a visual impairment, 15.2% indicating they had a hearing impairment, and 7.4% indicating they had a speech impairment. Mobility impairments, particularly ambulatory (74.5%), were also highly represented. Nearly 90% of respondents indicated limitations in stooping, crouching, or kneeling activities, as well as standing or being on their feet for up to 60 min (88.9%). Carrying and lifting up to 10 lb (75.4%) and difficulties with transferring to chairs, beds, and examination tables (58.7 to 82.4%) were identified as significant problems for this sample. Fine motor movements of the fingers and hands (31.4%), as well as ability to sense temperatures and shapes (27.7% and 25.2%, respectively), were significantly limited as well.

2.3.2 Ranked Categories of Medical Device

After completing the demographic and functional ability sections of the survey, participants were asked to indicate their level of experience with each of the 15 categories of equipment, ranging from "no experience" (0) to "extensive experience" (4). If experience with devices was indicated, they were asked to rate the degree of difficulty or discomfort they experienced when attempting to use or access the identified items, using a scale of "none" (0) to "impossible to use" (4). When all types of disabilities and diagnoses were analyzed together, the top four categories of medical equipment rated as at least moderately difficult to use were exam tables (75.0%), radiology equipment (68.0%), rehabilitation and exercise equipment (55.3%), and weight scales (53.1%) (see Table 2.3). When each category of disability or diagnosis (n = 39) was examined separately, examination tables were identified as the most difficult type of equipment by all categories of disability or diagnosis by all but four categories, and those categories ranked them as the second most difficult. These four categories included hearing impairment, speech impairment, cerebrovascular disease, and latex sensitivity.

TABLE 2.3
Rated Degree of Difficulty When Attempting to Use or Access Medical Devices

Type of Device	Mean ± SD	None n (%*)	Little n (%*)	Moderate n (%*)	Extreme n (%*)	Impossible n (%*)
Exam tables	2.14 ± 1.09	30 (10.0)	45 (15.0)	103 (34.3)	97 (32.3)	25 (8.3)
Radiology	1.89 ± 1.10	41 (15.4)	44 (16.5)	92 (34.6)	80 (30.1)	9 (3.4)
Exercise and rehab	1.62 ± 1.16	45 (21.6)	48 (23.1)	67 (32.2)	37 (17.8)	11 (5.3)
Weight scales	1.64 ± 1.40	71 (31.4)	35 (15.5)	53 (23.5)	39 (9.6)	28 (6.9)
Mobility aids	1.39 ± 1.01	62 (24.9)	62 (24.9)	93 (37.3)	31 (12.4)	1 (0.4)
Exam chairs	1.49 ± 1.11	63 (23.5)	72 (26.9)	81 (30.2)	44 (16.4)	8 (3.0)
Communication aids	1.22 ± 1.09	76 (40.2)	35 (18.5)	43 (22.8)	31 (16.4)	4 (2.1)
Medication administration	1.30 ± 1.18	51 (33.1)	40 (26.0)	35 (22.7)	22 (14.3)	6 (3.9)
Dental	1.16 ± 1.10	89 (36.9)	60 (24.9)	62 (25.7)	25 (10.4)	5 (2.1)
Eye examination	1.16 ± 1.12	90 (37.0)	63 (25.9)	58 (23.9)	25 (10.3)	7 (2.9)
Cardiac stress testing	1.17 ± 1.37	42 (44.7)	21 (22.3)	16 (17.0)	3 (3.2)	12 (12.8)
Oxygen delivery	0.87 ± 1.09	48 (50.5)	20 (21.1)	19 (20.0)	7 (7.4)	1 (1.1)
Monitoring	0.91 ± 1.15	102 (52.3)	39 (20.0)	27 (13.8)	23 (11.8)	4 (2.1)
Pulmonary function testing	0.92 ± 1.16	52 (50.0)	26 (25.0)	11 (10.6)	12 (11.5)	3 (2.9)
Hearing testing	0.44 ± 0.83	108 (72.0)	25 (16.7)	12 (8.0)	3 (2.0)	2 (1.3)

Note: Values are mean ± SD (range, 0 to 4) or number endorsing (percentage).

*Percentages shown as valid percent, i.e., percentage of individuals who indicated having had experience with specified devices and rated their degree of difficulty when attempting to use or access the device.

In order to better understand the barriers to using specific categories of devices, data were examined by disability type for each device category. These impairment categories included visual, hearing, speech, mobility, cardiopulmonary, and "other" (see Table 2.4). Each will be discussed separately. For the purposes of this study, it is important to note that respondents self-identified themselves to the individual disability and medical diagnosis categories, and no formal evaluation or confirmation was completed.

2.3.2.1 Visual Impairments

Visual impairment is a term used to describe many degrees of vision loss, including low vision, legally blind, and totally blind. Visual impairments are a very prevalent problem. Based on the National Health Interview survey, approximately 20.4 million Americans aged 18 and older (10%) have some form of visual impairment, even when wearing glasses or contact lenses [14]. *Low vision* is generally defined as an uncorrectable condition that interferes with a person's ability to perform everyday activities, or as having 20/70 vision in the best eye, with a correction. The term *legally blind* is used for individuals whose central visual acuity does not exceed 20/200 in the better eye with corrective lenses or whose visual field is less than an angle of 20°. *Total blindness* is the term that is used to denote the complete absence of vision and light perception.

One hundred thirty survey respondents indicated they had a visual impairment. Of these individuals, 103 noted that they wore eyeglasses, and 87 specified that they had difficulty reading a newspaper or book. The top four categories of medical devices that were ranked as at least moderately difficult to use, in rank order, were examination tables (68.2%), weight scales (61.9%), radiology equipment (59.8%), and exercise and rehabilitation equipment (58.1%). Another category of medical device that more than 50% of respondents with visual impairments indicated at least moderately difficult to use was examination chairs (52.0%).

TABLE 2.4
Top Four Categories of Medical Devices That Were Ranked As at Least Moderately Difficult to Use or Access, by Type of Disability

Type of Device	Visual Impairment (rank/valid %)	Hearing Impairment (rank/valid %)	Speech Impairment (rank/valid %)	Mobility Impairment (rank/valid %)	Cardiopulmonary Impairment (rank/valid %)
Exam tables	1 (68.2%)	2 (66.7%)	2 (82.6%)	1 (78.1–90.0%)	1 (72.4–82.0%)
Radiology	3 (59.8%)	1 (67.4%)	1 (84.2%)	2 (56.3–89.5%)	2 (65.4–81.0%)
Exercise and rehabilitation	4 (58.1%)			3 (58.6–72.7%)	3 (55.6–67.6%)
Weight scales	2 (61.9%)				
Exam chairs			3 (71.4%)	4 (33.3–87.0%)	4 (57.7–60.9%)
Communication aids		3 (59.0%)	4 (69.2%)		
Dental equipment		4 (46.2%)			
Medication admin.					
Mobility aids					
Eye examination					
Cardiac stress testing					
Oxygen delivery					

*Percentages shown as valid percent, i.e., percentage of those having experience with identified devices that rated the devices as at least moderately difficult to use. The ranges shown represent the lowest and highest values for the categories of impairment included in that group (see Table 2.2).

2.3.2.2 Hearing Impairments

Hearing impairments can vary widely from mild hearing loss to profound deafness. Overall, approximately 18% of Americans aged 18 and older have some form of hearing impairment [15]. *Hard of hearing* is a term that is used to describe those who have mild to moderate hearing loss. *Mild hearing loss* is the term that is generally used to describe those individuals who are able to hear everything except very high-pitched sounds, whereas *moderate hearing loss* is the term used with individuals who are unable to hear a conversation without amplification. The term *deaf* includes people with severe to profound hearing loss, who cannot hear anything except the loudest sounds, e.g., a jet airplane.

Sixty-two survey respondents indicated they had a hearing impairment. Of these individuals, 33 indicated they used a hearing aid, 3 had cochlear implants, and 60 indicated they had difficulty hearing a normal conversation. The top four categories of medical devices that were ranked as at least moderately difficult to use, in rank order, were radiology equipment (67.4%), examination tables (66.7%), communication aids (59.0%), and dental equipment (46.2%). It should be noted that only four of these individuals identified hearing impairment as their only disability.

2.3.2.3 Speech Impairments

Speech and language impairments refer to one or more disorders affecting voice, articulation, rhythm, and the receptive and expressive processes of language. These impairments limit the quality, accuracy, intelligibility, or fluency of producing the sounds that result in spoken language. The terms *speech* and *language impairments* do not apply to individuals who speak with a foreign accent or to limitations resulting from a physical or hearing impairment, psychological disability, or an acquired brain impairment. Stuttering, a common speech impairment, affects more than three million Americans [18]. Other speech impairments with relatively high prevalence rates include articulation or phonological disorders, with prevalence rates ranging from 8 to 9% [18].

Thirty respondents indicated they had speech impairment. Although only 30 respondents identified themselves as having speech impairment, 60 individuals indicated they had difficulty speaking so others could understand them. This disparity may be the result of disruptions in speech resulting from hearing impairments or a brain injury. Only the 30 who indicated they had speech impairment were included in the analysis. The top four categories of medical devices that were ranked as at least moderately difficult to use, in rank order, were radiology equipment (84.2%), examination tables (82.6%), examination chairs (71.4%), and communication aids (69.2%). Other categories of medical devices that a minimum of 50% of these respondents indicated were at least moderately difficult to use were dental equipment (57.1%) and rehabilitation and exercise equipment (50.0%).

2.3.2.4 Mobility Impairments

Mobility impairment is a term used to describe many disabling conditions that affect movement and ambulation. Common disabling conditions that result in mobility impairments include, but are not limited to, chronic pain, arthritis, cerebral palsy, multiple sclerosis, muscular dystrophy, spinal cord injury (e.g., paraplegia, quadriplegia), orthopedic injuries, and stroke. Mobility impairments may be caused by accidents or other traumatic events, or they may result from chronic diseases or conditions arising at birth. These impairments may occur before, during, or after birth. They can occur anytime during the course of one's life. The National Health Interview Survey found that 15% of adults had great difficulty with at least one of nine physical activities without help or the use of assistive equipment [15]. Examples of these activities include climbing 10 steps without resting, sitting for 2 h, stooping, bending, kneeling, or reaching over the head. In addition, nearly 27% of adults in the U.S. have chronic joint symptoms, 21.6% have been diagnosed with arthritis [15], nearly 1% are paralyzed, and 13.9% experience limitations in activity [19]. This limitation in activity increases to 34.4% by age 65 [19].

The types of mobility impairments noted by respondents in this survey included orthopedic ailments (n = 156), back pain (n = 132), chronic pain (n = 119), arthritis, and rheumatism (n = 103), paralysis (n = 92), spinal cord injury (n = 87), multiple sclerosis (n = 36), muscular dystrophy (n = 31), cerebral palsy (n = 30), loss of limb (n = 20), Parkinson's disease (n = 2), and myasthenia gravis (n = 1) (see Table 2.5). When respondents were asked to identify specific mobility and activity impairments related to upper extremity movement, significant numbers reported difficulty reaching (n = 197), grasping (n = 178), pinching (n = 129), twisting their wrist (n = 98), and pushing buttons (n = 69). Upper extremity impairments resulted in difficulty lifting or carrying 10 lb, (n = 266), using hands and fingers (n = 159), and using a manual wheelchair to go a city block (n = 111) and using manual wheelchair to go 10 ft (n = 64). Specific lower extremity mobility impairments included standing or being on feet for an hour (n = 313), stooping, crouching, or kneeling (n = 310), walking up a flight of stairs (n = 253) and walking less than 10 ft (n = 221). A number of activities of daily living were significantly impaired as a result of mobility issues including getting in or out of a bed or chair (n = 221), transferring from chair to chair (n = 196), taking a bath or shower (n = 190), dressing (n = 180), eating or feeding oneself (n = 100), preparing meals (n = 233), and doing light housework (n = 240). When queried about use of assistive devices related to mobility impairments, responses included use of canes, crutches, or walker (n = 150), manual wheelchair (n = 184), power wheelchair (n = 181), brace (n = 13), shower or bath chair (n = 12), Hoyer or power lift (n = 10), reacher (n = 5), and grab bars (n = 3). The assistive devices with fewer than 20 respondents were the result of participants adding these under "other" devices. Participants were not asked specifically about these devices.

All respondents who self-identified as having mobility impairments identified examination tables as the most difficult type of device to use (78.9 to 90.0%). Other categories of medical devices that

TABLE 2.5
Specific Mobility Impairments

Type of Impairment	n	Percentage
Upper extremity		
Lifting or carrying 10 lb	266	65.2
Reaching	197	48.3
Grasping	178	43.6
Using hands and fingers	159	39.0
Pinching	129	31.6
Using a manual wheelchair to go a city block	111	27.2
Twisting wrist	98	24.0
Pushing buttons	69	16.9
Using manual wheelchair to go 10 ft	64	15.7
Lower extremity		
Standing or being on feet for an hour	313	76.7
Stooping, crouching, or kneeling	310	76.0
Walking up a flight of stairs	253	62.0
Walking less than 10 ft	221	54.2
Activities of daily living		
Doing light housework	240	58.8
Preparing meals	233	57.1
Getting in or out of a bed or chair	221	54.2
Transferring from chair to chair	196	48.0
Taking a bath or shower	190	46.6
Dressing	180	44.1
Eating or feeding oneself	100	24.5

were ranked as at least moderately difficult to use, in rank order, were radiology equipment (56.3 to 89.5%), exercise and rehabilitation equipment (58.6 to 72.7%), examination chairs (33.3 to 87%), weight scales (50.0 to 70.0%), and mobility aids (35.3 to 75.0%). None of the categories of mobility impairments appeared significantly different than the group as a whole.

2.3.2.5 Cardiopulmonary Impairments

Cardiopulmonary impairment is a term used to describe individuals with pathophysiologic conditions that limit an individual's ability to circulate oxygenated blood to the tissues, resulting in activity intolerance, orthopnea, and dyspnea. Specific conditions that might contribute to cardiopulmonary impairments include, but are not limited to, coronary artery disease, history of myocardial infarction, heart failure, cardiac arrhythmias, hypertension, asthma, chronic bronchitis, emphysema, cystic fibrosis, and lung cancer. In the U.S., more than 11% of noninstitutionalized adults have diagnosed heart disease [20], nearly 30% of adults at least 20 years of age have hypertension [19], 1.5% of noninstitutionalized adults have emphysema [20], and 10.4% of adults aged 18 and older have asthma [19]. The prevalence of cardiopulmonary impairment is difficult to estimate globally, but these few examples of cardiopulmonary disease provide an underestimation of the overall impact of cardiopulmonary disorders.

Thirty-two respondents indicated they had a heart disease, 95 had hypertension, and 59 had pulmonary disease. Eleven respondents indicated they had cancer, but site involved was not identified. Therefore, they were not included in this analysis. The top four categories of medical devices that were ranked as at least moderately difficult to use, in rank order, were examination tables (72.4 to 82.0%), radiology equipment (65.4 to 81.0%), exercise and rehabilitation devices (55.6 to 67.6%), and examination chairs (57.7 to 60.9%). Other categories of medical devices that the majority of respondents indicated were at least moderately difficult to use were mobility aids (55.0 to 56.4%) and weight scales (42.9 to 58.6%).

2.3.2.6 "Other" Impairments

The category of "other" impairments includes those disabilities or diagnoses that were not subsumed under the previous major headings. Sixty-nine individuals self-identified as being depressed and 45 indicated they suffered from frequent anxiety. The four categories of medical devices that were ranked by these two groups as at least moderately difficult to use, in rank order, were examination tables (85.0 to 89.7%), radiology equipment (74.5 to 85.3%), examination chairs (66.0 to 77.1%), and exercise and rehabilitation devices (63.6 to 68.0%). These individuals had other concomitant disabilities and are represented in these other impairment categories as well.

A medical diagnosis that does not directly link with the aforementioned impairments is diabetes mellitus. Approximately 6.6% of noninstitutionalized adults have been diagnosed with diabetes mellitus. In our sample, 58 respondents (14.2%) indicated they had diabetes mellitus. The four categories of medical devices that were rated as at least moderately difficult to use, in rank order, were examination tables (81.3%), exercise and rehabilitation devices (67.9%), radiology equipment (66.7%), and weight scales (60.6%). Other categories of medical devices that the majority of respondents with diabetes mellitus indicated were at least moderately difficult to use were medication administration devices (60.0%), mobility aids (56.4%), examination chairs (55.8%), and monitoring equipment (50.0%).

Eleven individuals with cancer completed the survey. Involved organ systems were not identified. The four categories of medical devices that were rated as at least moderately difficult to use, in rank order, were examination tables (90.0%), mobility aids (88.9%), radiology equipment (70.0%), and pulmonary function testing (66.7%). Similar to other categories, other types of devices that the majority of respondents with cancer found at least moderately difficult to use included medication administration devices (66.7%), exercise and rehabilitation equipment (62.5%), eye examination equipment (60.0%), weight scales (57.1%), oxygen equipment (50.0%), and monitoring equipment (50.0%).

The last category comprised 33 individuals with latex sensitivities. The four categories of medical devices that were rated as at least moderately difficult to use, in rank order, were radiology equipment (90.5%), examination tables (78.6%), mobility aids (63.2%), and weight scales (60.0%). Other types of devices that the majority of these respondents found at least moderately difficult to use included exercise and rehabilitation equipment (59.1%), examination chairs (59.1%), dental equipment (59.1%), cardiac stress testing equipment (58.3%), and eye examination devices (54.5%).

2.3.3 Narrative Themes of Difficulty with Using Medical Devices

After the degree of difficulty for using specified equipment was identified by respondents, descriptions of difficulties and suggestions for improving devices were solicited. Safety issues were identified as the most prominent theme in the narrative data for all categories of equipment. The next most prevalent categories, in rank order, were physical positioning and comfort, patient transfer issues, visual displays and markings, and activities requiring fine motor movements. The following sections will provide representative examples of comments about a few types of equipment under each category identified in the narrative data.

2.3.3.1 Safety Issues

Safety issues were identified for all categories of medical devices. Two of the most prevalent safety issues were potential physical harm and inability to determine values or markings that could result in wrong dosing or making decisions about treatment based on erroneous data. The issue of safety was consistently prominent across disability types and medical diagnoses. Subject #90, who identified herself as having diabetes, as well as hearing, mobility, and cardiovascular impairments, commented that exam tables were "Too tall so I need assistance. Even if they have a step it is difficult to use. I fear falling off of table when trying to get on them. Tables are too narrow, so my bad arm dangles off the side ...." When asked about difficulties related to using radiology equipment, subject #9, who identified himself as having visual and mobility impairments commented, "If I have to get onto an [X-ray] table, I may have to be lifted, and these tables are notoriously cold and slippery, great for falling off." When commenting on exercise and rehabilitation equipment, subject #261, who identified himself as having visual, mobility, and cardiovascular impairments, commented that "Equipment needs to be designed so someone paralyzed on 1/2 a body (little use of leg and arm) can get on and off; can keep paralyzed arm and leg on the equipment; railings on both sides. [Treadmill] that is not dangerous for someone with limited use of 1 arm and 1 leg ... i.e., a place to put my useless arm ... to help me exercise my entire body, though left side is weak ..."

2.3.3.2 Physical Positioning and Comfort

The second most prevalent theme in the narrative data related to physical positioning and comfort. Subject #25 identified herself as having chronic pain with mobility and cardiopulmonary impairments, and when commenting on use of examination tables she remarked, "... I aggravate my symptoms of pain and spasm even with help the table is not adjustable and is not [comfortable] enough ..." Comments about radiology equipment that were shared by two women with mobility impairments included, "Tables are difficult to get onto. Certain films are hard to get because my body parts cannot turn to adjust to the angles needed to get the shot" (subject #411), and "Rigidity of table makes it difficult/painful to [lie] on or stay [still]. During standing x-rays (lungs) there is no supportive device to assist ..." (subject #434).

2.3.3.3 Patient Transfer Issues

The next most prevalent theme in the narrative data was related to patient transfer issues. Subject #76, a woman with diabetes, frequent depression, morbid obesity, as well as visual, mobility, and cardiopulmonary impairments, shared the following comments about transferring on to examination tables. "I am heavy. I do not trust the pull out step pad. [Often] step stools are not available and the table is too high to get on from the floor. There has to be something to hold on to for stability, a rail, a walker, etc ... They are often too narrow and too close to the wall." Subject #43, a woman with chronic pain, as well as mobility and cardiopulmonary impairments, shared that her difficulties with examination tables stemmed from "Getting on and off — especially stepping on little step, turning around, and sitting ... I just need to be able to get to them without tripping or FALLING into them." Subject #61, a woman with mobility impairment commented about her difficulties using weight scales, and stated that she "Can't get up on a regular scale [due] to the closeness of the center part and how small the foot area is." Subject #411, a woman with a mobility impairment commented " 'Regular' scales are not wide enough for me to obtain secure balance; wheelchair scales are difficult because you need to get out of them first (to weigh the chair) before weighing you sitting in your chair."

2.3.3.4 Visual Displays and Markings

Visual displays and markings that could not be interpreted provided difficulties for individuals with visual impairments for a variety of categories of devices. Subject #44, a woman with diabetes, as well as visual and mobility impairments, provided the following comments about insulin pumps, "...cannot read display to control functions, count beeps but afraid [I] will make a mistake, cannot determine between error alarms." Subject #334, a woman with chronic pain, visual, mobility, and cardiopulmonary impairments shared her views of the difficulties faced when trying to use exercise and rehabilitation equipment in the following comments, "Everything these days are monitor or digital in starting machines [i.e.,] treadmills, bikes, ultra sounds, stimulators and other equipment.

This makes it really difficult for someone with very limited vision. I enjoy working in a rehab setting and yet this was one of the issues that came up for me. Another was free weights or pulley systems are not modified in Braille or large print. This would help senior as well as [the] visually impaired/blind work and use equipment. I used [TENS] units too and this was also difficult to put on the right level. I did it by feel but sometimes this was painful."

2.3.3.5 Activities Requiring Fine Motor Movement

The final major category identified in the narrative data that was evident by a significant portion of the sample across multiple device categories was difficulties using or accessing devices that require fine motor movement. Several individuals indicated they had experienced difficulties with medication administration devices or packaging. Subject #360, a woman with chronic pain and mobility impairment commented, "For self-administered injections: measuring and mixing the medication was difficult due to unsteady hands." Similarly, subject #184, a woman with frequent depression, diabetes, morbid obesity, visual, mobility, and cardiopulmonary impairments commented, "... Syringes and safety needles hard for arthritic fingers." Subject #357, a woman with latex sensitivity, mobility and cardiopulmonary impairments shared comments about her difficulties with using communication devices including, "Can no longer type for long periods, like to fill out this questionnaire! [Also] can't hold phone to head for long calls, can't easily use on–off switch on top of [XYZ brand] cell phone, requires finger strength." Likewise, subject #160, a woman with chronic pain, mobility, and cardiopulmonary impairments commented that, "Key pads on cell phones are small and difficult to use, and ear pieces are sometimes difficult to [strategically] place over [your] ear while talking into the mouth piece so people can hear you."

2.4 DISCUSSION

These data provide strong evidence of repeated patterns of barriers to using medical devices across disabilities and diagnoses. The high percentage of participants who repeatedly rated categories of medical devices as at least moderately difficult to use, coupled with the five categories of difficulties identified in the narrative data when using common medical devices, demand attention. It is very alarming to see the serious threats to safety for individuals with disabilities when attempting to use common, essential medical devices. Consistent comments that conveyed a lack of access to health care and threats to the quality and adequacy of health care provided for persons with disabilities is alarming. The American Disabilities Act (ADA) of 1990 stipulated that access to medical care and public accommodations be provided for all, yet these findings provide evidence that many medical devices and technologies impede compliance with these regulations. The ADA not only required architectural environments to accommodate persons with disabilities, but they also mandated that persons with disabilities have the right to access the same health care services as all Americans, including diagnostic tests, treatment, and rehabilitation. Narrative comments from survey participants indicated that patients who have disabilities often are not referred for testing or treatment that otherwise would represent standard practice for a given diagnosis, or have chosen not to partake in potential testing or treatment options because previous experiences have left them with the impression that accessible devices or technologies were not available.

Few studies have examined accessibility issues of medical devices for persons with disabilities. This study was the first large-scale investigation attempting to examine the landscape of accessibility and usability of medical devices and technologies, across a vast array of abilities, disabilities, and medical diagnoses. This study provided findings that are consistent with, and more extensive than, earlier studies. As noted in previous studies [6,7,9,10,21], examination tables and stirrups for gynecological evaluation present significant barriers for women with disabilities seeking medical care for reproductive health issues. Similarly, participants in this national survey reinforced findings from earlier studies [7,8] that persons with mobility impairments experienced significant barriers to taking advantage of breast and cervical cancer screening. Difficult transfer issues from wheelchairs to examination chairs [22] and lack of fitness equipment for persons with disabilities [12,13] were reported in earlier studies, and they were reinforced in this national survey. However, findings from this study identified that there are difficulties experienced across all categories of medical devices when persons with disabilities are attempting to meet their health care needs. Clearly, the categories of medical devices that respondents rated highly as being at least moderately difficult to use are essential types of equipment for meeting basic health care needs. These critical barriers to essential services ultimately will diminish the quality of health care available to individuals with disabilities, and they have the potential to negatively impact overall quality of life in these populations.

Although this national study has provided a great deal of data, its limitations must be considered when interpreting the findings. Compared to national demographics, this sample was predominantly Caucasian and more highly educated than the general or disability population at large. This may be related to the fact that the majority of participants completed the web-based version; however, alternative forms and methods for completion were available and proactively supported. Nonetheless, less than 10% of surveys were completed in an alternative format. When considering these limitations, it seems reasonable to assume that physical barriers to access are unlikely to be a function of education or ethnicity. It is conceivable that some communication barriers may be related to some of these issues. Therefore, findings from different racial and educational groups were compared and no differences were noted.

Another important consideration is that these findings represent comments only from respondents who reported having had experience with devices. Because many respondents have not had experience with many categories of devices, the moderate or higher levels of difficulty may be underestimations, as many individuals may not have been referred for services with devices, or they may have chosen not to engage in activities if they believed they would be unable to use them appropriately and safely. It is known that experiences with medical technologies increase with age, and the sample in this study may have an underrepresented elderly population. This fact is significant in that unlike the elder cohort, most young or middle-aged adults in the role of patients might not be expected to have direct experience with as many types of devices, e.g., medical monitoring equipment.

In an effort to be more inclusive and gain greater insights into some of these issues, this national consumer survey is being followed up with a health care practitioner survey that includes both providers with disabilities and providers without disabilities who have had extensive experience serving patients with disabilities. The rationale for this follow-up study is that practitioners may be able to better identify issues that consumers may not be aware of and that are unique to providing care. Health care providers also may have a broader range of experience with more varied devices, and they may be in a better position to compare barriers across devices and disabilities. A manufacturer survey also is planned to gain insight into how accessibility issues are considered when medical devices are designed.

The investigators are aware that some commercially available medical devices may provide more accessible features than some that respondents have had experience using. However, it is unclear why they are not used more extensively. Possible explanations to be considered include issues such as cost, space required, and familiarity with available devices.

These findings serve as an information resource. Findings from the collective efforts of the national consumer, health care provider, and manufacturer surveys, along with follow-up focus group data, will be used by the RERC-AMI to refine, redesign, or develop new devices that will be more universally accessible to all individuals, irrespective of disability or diagnosis. Concerted efforts need to be implemented to produce affordable, accessible medical devices for all, without regard to level of ability or disability.

Clearly, transformational change will require fundamental change in policy and practice guidelines that will encourage health care agencies to purchase and utilize the most accessible devices available for all individuals, regardless of level of ability or disability. Without policy mandating their use, the status quo will persist and this population will continue to find accessible, high-quality health care to be challenging, at best.

ACKNOWLEDGMENT

This work is supported by the RERC-AMI, funded by the National Institute on Disability and Rehabilitation Research, U.S. Department of Education Grant #H133E020729. All opinions expressed are those of the authors.

REFERENCES

1. CDC, Prevalence of disabilities and associated health conditions among adults — U.S., 1999, *MMWR,* 50, 120, 2001.
2. National Institute on Disability and Rehabilitation Research, Correction for final long-range plan for fiscal years 1999–2003, Department of Education, Washington, D.C., 1999.
3. Lishner, D.M. et al., Access to primary health care among persons with disabilities in rural areas: a summary of the literature, *J Rural Health,* 12, 45, 1996.
4. DeJong, G., Primary care for persons with disabilities: an overview of the problem, *Am J Phys Med Rehabil,* 76, S2, 1997.
5. Sofaer, S. et al., Meeting the Challenge of Serving People with Disabilities: A Resource Guide for Assessing the Performance of Managed Care Organizations, Center for Health Outcomes Improvement Research, Center for Health Policy Research, U.S. Dept. of Health and Human Services, Washington, DC, 1998.
6. Nosek, M.A., The John Stanley Coulter lecture. Overcoming the odds: the health of women with physical disabilities in the U.S., *Arch Phys Med Rehabil,* 81, 135, 2000.
7. Nosek, M.A. and Howland, C.A., Breast and cervical cancer screening among women with physical disabilities, *Arch Phys Med Rehabil,* 78, S39, 1997.
8. Cheng, E. et al., Mobility impairments and use of preventive services in women with multiple sclerosis: observational study, *Br Med J,* 323, 968, 2001.
9. Schopp, L.H. et al., Removing service barriers for women with physical disabilities: promoting accessibility in the gynecologic care setting, *J Midwifery Womens Health,* 47, 74, 2002.
10. Society for the Advancement of Women's Health Research, Gynecological Cancer Screening for Women with Disabilities, *Women's Health Research News,* Summer, 8, 1998.
11. U.S. Department of Health and Human Services, *Healthy People 2010: Understanding and Improving Health*, 2nd ed., Washington, D.C., 2000.
12. Rimmer, J.H. et al., Physical activity participation among persons with disabilities: barriers and facilitators, *Am J Prev Med,* 26, 419, 2004.
13. Nary, D.E., Forehlich, K., and White, G.W., Accessibility of fitness facilities for persons with physical disabilities using wheelchairs, *Top Spinal Cord Inj Rehabil,* 6, 87, 2000.
14 Lucas, J.W., Schiller, J.S. and Benson, V., Summary Health Statistics for U.S. Adults: National Health Interview Survey, 2001, *Vital Health Stat 10,* 1, 2004.
15. Lethbridge-Cejku, M. and Vickerie, J., Summary Health Statistics for U.S. Adults: National Health Interview Survey, 2003, in *Vital Health Statistics* , National Center for Health Statistics, 2005.
16. Winters, J.M.W. et al., A Delphi study to develop a national survey of accessibility of medical instrumentation, presented at *RESNA's 27th International Conference*, Orlando, FL, 2004.
17. Joffe, H. and Yardley, L., Content and thematic analysis, in *Research Methods for Clinical and Health Psychology*, Marks, D.F. and Yardley, L., Eds., Sage, Thousand Oaks, CA, 2004, p. 56.
18. National Institute on Deafness and other Communication Disorders, Statistics on voice, speech, and language, National Institutes of Health, 2005. http://www.nidcd.nih.gov/health/statistics/vsl.asp.
19. CDC, Health Data for All Ages, National Center for Disease Statistics, 2005. http://www.cdc.gov/nchs/health_data_for_all_ages.htm.

20. CDC, Fast Stats A to Z, National Center for Disease Statistics, 2005. http://www.cdc.gov/nchs/fastats/Default.htm.
21. Becker, H., Stuifbergen, A., and Tinkle, M., Reproductive health care experiences of women with physical disabilities: a qualitative study, *Arch Phys Med Rehabil,* 78, S26, 1997.
22. McClain, L. et al., A qualitative assessment of wheelchair users' experience with ADA compliance, physical barriers, and secondary health conditions, *Top Spinal Cord Inj Rehabil,* 6, 99, 2000.

3 Emerging Human Factors and Ergonomics Issues for Health Care Professionals

Molly Follette Story

CONTENTS

ABSTRACT

This chapter discusses some of the recognized and emerging human factors and ergonomics issues for health care professionals. Two known major issues, and the subjects of numerous studies, are medical errors and physical injuries, particularly injuries related to patient handling. Other issues are increasing in importance as the demographics of health care professionals and the nature of medical care both change. One of these emerging issues is disability among and aging of individuals employed in health care professions, and another is medical care that is increasingly frequently being administered in the home. These changes introduce new ergonomics challenges for health care professionals.

3.1 INTRODUCTION

The challenges associated with providing good ergonomic solutions for health care professionals are numerous, diverse, and complex, and are the focus of this chapter.

Derived from two Greek words, *ergon* for "work" and *nomos* for "laws," the classical definition of *ergonomics* is the "science of work," and the primary concerns of ergonomists are worker health, safety, and productivity in the workplace. Consistent with this approach, in the field of health care, medical professionals have been the focus of most ergonomic studies conducted to date. Patients are experiencing discomfort and difficulties using medical instrumentation, as described in Chapter 2 of this book, but the productivity and comfort (and dignity) of the patient have received little attention. The primary concern of the health care industry for the recipients of health care — that is, patients — is their safety.

In its publication, *Do It by Design,* the U.S. Food and Drug Administration (FDA) suggested the following:

> Good user interface design is critical to safe and effective equipment operation, installation, and maintenance. Human factors should be considered early in the design process, and systematic analysis and hands-on testing should be conducted throughout development stages and involve participants from the end-user population. It is not simply a matter of "fine tuning." Thorough attention to design will result in safer, more usable devices and, correspondingly, fewer accidents, reduced training costs, fewer liability problems, and less trial-and-error during device development [1].

Two major ergonomics issues for health care professionals, and the subjects of numerous studies, are medical errors and physical injuries. Other issues have received less attention but are increasing in importance as the demographics of health care professionals and the nature of medical care both change. One of these emerging issues is disability among, and aging of, individuals employed in health care professions, and another is medical care that is increasingly frequently being administered in the home.

3.2 MEDICAL ERRORS

Medical errors are an issue of considerable concern in the U.S. In the landmark book, *To Err is Human* [2], the Institute of Medicine estimated that the total national cost (including lost income or decreased household production and the costs of disability and associated health care) of preventable adverse events (that is, medical errors that result in injury) is between $17 billion and $29 billion, with health care costs representing more than half of this total. The Harvard Medical Practice Study conducted in New York in 1984 [3,4] found that adverse events occurred in 3.7% of hospitalizations, that 13.6% of the adverse events led to death, and that 58% of the adverse events resulted from preventable medical errors. Extrapolating these rates to the 36.6 million hospital admissions in the U.S. in 2003 [5], these rates imply that more than 100,000 people die each year as a result of medical errors, more people than died in 2003 as a result of diabetes mellitus (73,965), influenza and pneumonia (64,847), Alzheimer's disease (63,343), motor vehicle accidents (44,059), or all other types of accidents (61,636) [6].

Importantly, medical errors occur not only in hospitals but also in physicians' offices, outpatient clinics, urgent care centers, long-term care facilities, pharmacies, and the home. However, very little data exist on the extent of the problem outside of hospitals [7]. The Institute of Medicine report pointed out that it is likely that many errors occur outside the hospital [2], but it is difficult to know their quantity and nature.

Although medical errors are recognized as being very important, some health care providers believe that the medical liability system in the U.S. discourages error reporting and learning from errors, which hinders improvement [8]. The fragmented nature of the health care system in the U.S. also contributes to inconsistent reporting of problems.

3.2.1 Medication Errors

The Institute of Medicine report [2] found that more Americans die each year from medication errors (7000 that occur either in or out of the hospital) than from workplace injuries (6000). Medication-related errors occur frequently in hospitals but also in other locations, such as medical clinics, pharmacies, long-term care facilities, and the home. These errors do not always result in harm, but if they do they can be very expensive, both directly and in terms of actions that must be taken in remediation. Not all of these costs can be measured, including medical patients' loss of trust in the health care system and reduced satisfaction on the part of both patients and health care professionals [2].

3.2.2 Equipment- Related Errors

Equipment-related errors are harder to identify and may not be reported. These types of errors may be corrected (at least once) so that harm to the patient is avoided or reduced, and the provider may not recognize any reason to report an incident. Providers may also fear malpractice claims and so may avoid reporting an incident if they fear negative consequences.

In a 2005 presentation, Peter Carstensen, Human Factors Team Leader in the U.S. FDA's Division of Device User Programs, reported that the FDA receives some 100,000 reports each year, more than one-third of which involve use error, a number he described as "the tip of the iceberg." He also commented that 44% of medical device recalls were identified as being related to design problems, and that use error is often linked to device design. In addition, he said, more than one third of medical device incident reports involved use error, and more than half of device recalls related to design problems involved the user interface [9]. The clear implication is that improved design of medical devices and their interfaces may reduce errors.

3.3 PHYSICAL INJURIES

Another health care ergonomics issue that has attracted a lot of attention is physical injuries. Health care workers are at relatively high risk of musculoskeletal injury. According to the U.S. Department of Labor, in 2003 hospitals reported the second-highest rate of nonfatal occupational injuries in the private sector with an incidence rate of 7.9 per 100 full-time equivalent (FTE) workers, compared to a rate of 4.7 per 100 FTE for all industries combined [10]. In addition, the incidence rate for all ambulatory health care services was 3.0 per 100 but more specifically, for workers in physicians' offices the rate was 2.3 per 100, for medical and diagnostic laboratories it was 2.7 per 100, for outpatient care centers it was 4.3 per 100, and for other ambulatory health care services the injury rate was 8.8 per 100 FTE workers [10].

3.3.1 Patient- Handling Injuries

A major source of musculoskeletal injuries in health care workers is patient handling. Patient-handling injuries, especially back and shoulder overexertion problems, commonly occur in medical facilities when patients need to be moved, especially when being transferred from one support surface to another (e.g., wheelchair to table, gurney to bed), held in position (e.g., during a medical examination or procedure), or repositioned (e.g., raised up in bed or rolled over on a table). Patient handling may be performed by nurses, nurse aides, lift teams, hospital transport teams, or long-term care attendants. Medical staff may perform patient-handling tasks several times a day, resulting in a large number of musculoskeletal injuries. In one study of nurses, 38% of questionnaire respondents reported having experienced occupation-related back pain severe enough to require leave from work. Of those with back pain, 20% reported having made at least one job transfer to decrease the amount of lifting or moving patients required, 12% more were considering requesting such a transfer, and another 12% were considering leaving the nursing profession because of job-related back pain [11,12].

It is important to recognize that similar to medical errors in hospitals, the number of injuries that occur outside of hospitals is likely higher than inside because the number of visits to outpatient settings is much higher. In contrast to the 36.6 million hospital admissions in the U.S. in 2003 [5], in 2002 hospital outpatient departments received an estimated 83.3 million visits [13], and physician offices received 890 million visits (an overall rate of 314.4 visits per 100 persons) [14]. The injury rates are harder to obtain but no less important.

Although it is commonly believed that behavior modification and training in body mechanics and lifting techniques will prevent job-related injuries, 35 years of research suggest otherwise [15], and much of the research may not be generalizable to nurses. Most research on lifting has been conducted on male subjects lifting boxes vertically from the floor, which was used in creation of the NIOSH guidelines that limit the maximum lift to a 23-kg (51-lb) stable object with good handles [16]. However, in health care settings lifting is often performed by females, who move humans (who do not have "handles" and whose weight distribution is not uniform or static or even predictable), typically in a lateral direction between surfaces (which may involve awkward postures, torso bending, and twisting), using a variety of techniques [15]. Also, whereas NIOSH's guidelines reduce the weight limit for females to 20.7 kg (46 lb), medical patients frequently weigh three or more times this amount.

Back injuries cost employers a substantial amount of money, for workers' compensation, medical treatment, and vocational rehabilitation. Estimates in 1990 of the total cost of low back pain in the U.S. ranged from $50 billion to $100 billion per year [17]. The average costs of health care-worker-related musculoskeletal injuries per 100,000 work hours were observed to exceed $160,000 [18]. On a national basis, the average cost per claim is estimated to be $24,000, and if surgery is involved, at least $40,000 per injury. Indirect costs are much harder to quantify, and include decreased employee morale, continual employee hiring and training, use of replacement workers, overtime, medical management, incident reporting and other paperwork, increased costs of workers' compensation insurance, and increased costs of employee health care [19]. Insufficient or inappropriate patient handling may cause physical and psychological harm to patients as well.

3.3.1.1 Bariatric Patients

Almost 35% of the adult population (20 years old or older) of the U.S. is classified as overweight, with a body mass index (BMI) of 25 to 29.9 kg/m^2, and 20% is classified as obese, with a BMI of 30 kg/m^2 or higher. Higher body weights are associated with increased risk of morbidity from hypertension, dyslipidemia, type 2 diabetes, coronary heart disease, stroke, gall bladder disease, osteoarthritis, sleep apnea and respiratory problems, and endometrial, breast, prostate, and colon cancers; higher weights are also associated with increases in all-cause mortality [20].

The growing percentage of patients who are overweight or obese puts added demands on the health care system and increases the physical stresses on health care workers, who must provide appropriate care for these patients and also avoid injuring themselves.

3.3.1.2 Nursing Shortage in the U.S.

The health care professions are experiencing a shortage of workers, particularly nurses. Since the 1980s, many nurses have changed positions or even left the nursing profession because of overexertion injuries [12]. A number of factors are contributing to this situation:

- An aging population — The aging of the population, led by the Baby Boom generation, will put more demands on the health care system.
- Fewer workers — Generations subsequent to the Baby Boomers are smaller, providing a smaller number of workers in many professions, including health care.

- An aging workforce — The average age of nurses is now 44 and, especially due to the physical demands of the profession, many of those individuals will retire in the next 10 to 15 years.
- A mismatch on diversity — The demographics of the nursing workforce does not match the diversity of the population at large. Correcting this disparity should be a priority in the coming years.
- More options for women — Many women have chosen professions other than nursing in the past few decades, and men have not made up the difference.
- The generation gap — The generation of recent graduates is not attracted to the nursing profession because they perceive it to be highly structured and stressful.
- Work environment — Increases in the workloads of nurses without compensatory increases in associated support systems have led to nurse disillusionment and dissatisfaction.
- Consumer activism — In recent years, health care consumers have become more active in their own care, due in part to increased patient empowerment, wider publicity of the incidence of medical errors, and a backlash against managed care.
- A ballooning health care system — The nursing profession has experienced expansion of the health care system caused by competition, regulation, and changes in financing programs, but not an increase in its ability to affect change [21].

Improved ergonomic solutions must be developed to help stem, and eventually reverse, the shortage of nurses.

3.3.1.3 Safe Patient- Handling Policies

In 1993 England instituted a policy, the Manual Handling Operations Regulations 1992 [22], which dealt specifically with the manual handling of loads, defined to include "any person or any animal," which implicitly pertains to handling of patients by medical staff. These regulations resulted in a significant decrease in job-related injuries, but they have also been complicated to comply with in practice, sometimes leading to patients not being moved at all to avoid injury to health care workers [23].

Many organizations and institutions in the U.S. are also advocating for safe patient-handling policies in health care [17,24], and several states have been working to pass legislation. In 2004, California's Senate and Assembly passed a safe patient-handling bill, but it was vetoed by Governor Arnold Schwarzenegger later that year; legislation was reintroduced in February 2005. Massachusetts introduced a safe patient-handling bill in December 2004 that is pending. Ohio passed a bill to create interest-free loans to nursing homes for implementing no-manual-lift programs. New York passed two bills in April 2005 to study safe patient-handling programs and develop a report of best practices. Washington state's safe patient-handling bill was stalled in committee in February 2005, and reintroduction is planned [25].

In June 2005, the state of Texas successfully passed the first safe patient-handling law (SB 1525) in the U.S. The legislation, which took effect January 1, 2006, requires hospitals and nursing homes to adopt policies and procedures for safe handling of patients that "...control the risk of injury to patients and nurses associated with the lifting, transferring, repositioning, or movement of a patient." It discourages but does not prohibit manual moving and lifting of patients [25, 26]. However, the Veterans Health Administration's Patient Safety Center of Inquiry recommends that successful implementation of any safe patient-handling policy depends on having in place an infrastructure to support it, including provision of sufficient quantities of appropriate technological solutions (e.g., lifts, transfer aids, sliding aids, and standing aids) [27].

Another approach to reducing the physical demands on medical personnel is using lift teams that are responsible for total body transfers. Lift teams are typically designated staff members who are working within the medical facility and are available on an on-call basis. Studies of the usefulness of lift teams in acute care settings have found that the use of lift teams that used proper equipment resulted in reduced rates of injury, fewer lost work days, and fewer duty modifications associated with patient handling [28]; nurses reported high satisfaction with the lift team, and the total number of restricted (light-duty) days was reduced by 361% [29].

3.4 DISABLED AND AGING HEALTH CARE PROVIDERS

Whereas the ergonomics-related issues of medical errors and musculoskeletal injuries are receiving a substantial amount of attention from a wide range of organizations and institutions, other issues are emerging that merit attention as well. One issue is the growing number of health care providers who have disabilities, including disabilities that occur as a result of accidents or injuries or normal human aging.

3.4.1 Disabled Health Care Providers

Some health care providers are injured on the job. As mentioned in the preceding text, health care workers are at high risk of musculoskeletal injuries, particularly to the back [10]; some specialists (such as nurse anesthetists) are at higher risk for repetitive stress injuries such as carpal tunnel syndrome [30]. Some health care providers are bariatric themselves, and studies have found that overweight nurses have significantly higher risk of back pain [31].

Nurses have been studied extensively and a number of problems have been identified [12,32–40]. Interestingly, this author was not able to find any studies of musculoskeletal injuries or repetitive stress injuries among physicians — but that doesn't mean problems don't exist. For example, anecdotally, surgeons have been known to complain of back and neck discomfort or pain in the upper extremities during long procedures and, presumably, some may be changing duty or professions as a result.

Few health care professionals have significant disabilities, and few people with disabilities enter the field (see Chapter 1 of this book). Federal legislation, such as Section 504 of the Rehabilitation Act and the Americans with Disabilities Act, requires equal access to facilities, programs, and activities that receive federal funding. However, medical educational institutions have concerns about, for example, the abilities of nursing students with manual dexterity limitations to draw up medications in syringes, give injections, and perform various clinical procedures such as catheterization and tracheotomy suctioning; the abilities of students with hearing impairments to hear call bells, intravenous pump monitors, and calls for help from patients; and the abilities of students with short stature to reach equipment controls and medications in storage. Although legal judgments have been mixed, as a general rule, the courts have ruled that students with disabilities need to be able to perform all of the essential functions of the educational program, with or without accommodations. Working within these constraints, some individuals with disabilities have been successful in obtaining the needed education and licensure to work in medical specialties that match their capabilities [41]. Medical instrumentation that accommodates a wider range of operator abilities might increase the number of people with disabilities who can succeed in health care professions or continue practicing after acquiring a disability.

3.4.2 Aging Health Care Providers

The American population is growing. The 13.2% growth in population between the 1990 census and the 2000 census, from 248.7 million to 281.4 million, was the largest in U.S. history [42]. The American population is also aging. In that same decade, the median age increased from 32.9 to 35.3, reflecting a 4% decrease in people 18 to 24 years old and a 28% increase in people aged 35 to 64. The largest increase was 49% in the population aged 45 to 54, who belong to the Baby Boom generation; the smallest growth was in the group of people aged 65 and over, which increased at a slower rate than the overall population for the first time in the history of the census, due to the relatively low birth rate in the late 1920s and early 1930s [43].

That same Baby Boom generation, however, will continue to age, and will put extra demands on the health care system as they do. In 2003, the U.S. Department of Health and Human Services estimated that if current patterns continue, the demand for physicians will increase from 2.8 per thousand population in 2000 to 3.1 in 2020, and the demand for registered nurses will increase from 7.0 to 7.5 per thousand population. In 2000, physicians spent approximately 32% of their patient care hours providing services to people age 65 and older, which is expected to increase to 39% by 2020 [44].

At the same time, the health workforce is aging. In fact, there is concern that many medical workers will be retiring at about the same time as the demand for their professional services increases. Unfortunately, whereas the number of people in the 65-and-over age group will increase, the proportion of people in the 18-to-30 age group will decline, which will limit the number of new workers available to enter health care professions [44].

In the preface to the book, *Designing for an Aging Population,* editor Wendy A. Rogers stated that, "There is a good deal of evidence to suggest that individuals over age 65 experience declines in sensory, perceptual, motor, and cognitive abilities that may interfere with their ability to interact with systems ranging from doorknobs to microwave ovens to computers" [45]. Because the aging process varies considerably among individuals, some people will experience functional declines at a younger age. There are more than 100 types of arthritis and most people over the age of 50 show some signs of having it, but some people are affected at a younger age [46]. Many people experience increasing presbyopia after the age of 40 [47], or declining hearing abilities that occurs gradually with age. Hearing impairments may also be accelerated by noise-induced hearing loss from occupational sources, or from attending noisy concerts or clubs, or from using firearms or loud power tools or even recreational vehicles, or from listening to music through headphones or cellular telephones through headsets with the volume set too high [48].

When you consider age-related reduced capabilities in the context of using medical equipment, the ergonomic requirements of that equipment must be carefully considered. Of particular concern is introducing new instrumentation to older health care workers, who may be resistant to learning new ways of operating.

3.5 HEALTH CARE IN THE HOME

Another emerging ergonomics issue is that health care is increasingly moving into the home. In recent years the aging of the population, shortages in the numbers of some health care workers, and the growing costs of in-patient medical care have dramatically increased the demand for home health care.

Particularly to contain costs, in recent years patients have been leaving the hospital sooner and more health care is being conducted on an outpatient basis. At the same time, advances in medicine are helping people to live longer, sometimes with disabilities that may be difficult for them to manage independently. These two trends have driven enormous growth in the home health care industry. Home care is generally preferred and is particularly beneficial for people with chronic conditions or other long-term care needs [49].

One issue of concern with home health care is that, particularly as more types of equipment enter the home, the equipment user may be the patient, a family member, or a personal attendant or caregiver, and often this user does not have a background in medicine. Frequently, the medical devices used in the home were not designed for nonprofessionals. A number of issues exist, such as concern for use, maintenance, and regimen adherence. Although training can be helpful, to ensure the safety of the patient and the device operator, the device itself should be as easy to use and as forgiving of error as possible.

3.6 ATTITUDINAL BARRIERS

3.6.1 Attitudes about Disability

The *disability model* regards disability as a normal part of life, not as a deviance or defect [50]. Because most people will experience some amount of disability, either temporarily or permanently, at some point in their lives, this attitude is sensible. In contrast, the traditional *medical model* of disability suggests that someone who has a disability has a defect or sickness that should be cured or treated through medical intervention [50]. A related model is the *rehabilitation model* of disability, which regards the disability as a deficiency that should be fixed or ameliorated by a rehabilitation or similar professional [50].

In the latter two models of disability, the health care provider is considered to be the expert, and the patient is expected to be a largely passive recipient of services. Indeed, this is often the case with all patients, including those who do not have disabilities. However, these attitudes may not be appropriate or beneficial for optimal health care if the patient does not accept or share responsibility for his or her own care. Even when patients do accept responsibility for their own care, some health care providers do not respect the patient's personal knowledge and life experiences, even if that includes living with a disability [51].

In 1998, the National Institute on Disability and Rehabilitation Research (NIDRR) published in its long-range plan a new paradigm of disability:

> … Disability is a product of an interaction between characteristics (e.g., conditions or impairments, functional status, or personal and social qualities) of the individual and characteristics of the natural, built, cultural, and social environments. The construct of disability is located on a continuum from enablement to disablement. Personal characteristics, as well as environmental ones, may be enabling or disabling, and the relative degree fluctuates, depending on condition, time, and setting. Disability is a contextual variable, dynamic over time and circumstance. Environments may be physically accessible or inaccessible, culturally inclusive or exclusive, accommodating or unaccommodating, and supportive or unsupportive [52].

This definition of disability has significant implications for designers of the built environment and objects within the environment, including medical devices. The attitudes of all individuals involved in the health care system, from patient to primary care staff to administrator, can make a tremendous difference in management of patient care and quality of outcomes.

3.6.2 Attitudes about Health Care Providers

Leape [53, 54] suggested that the medical industry has a number of barriers to change, including the complexity of health care, the culture of "shame and blame," distorted concepts of professionalism, little organizational control, and little organizational commitment to safety. Of particular concern is the deeply embedded culture of shaming and blaming:

> … The consequence of a faulty paradigm: If practitioners are well educated, technically well trained, and taught to be conscientious and careful, they will not make mistakes. It follows from this paradigm that errors occur only if the individual was not careful and didn't try hard enough. He or she should be ashamed, blamed, and punished [53, 54].

This pervasive attitude — that the health care professional is the expert and must provide the needed care no matter what the obstacles — may contribute to the problem by obfuscating some of the factors that contribute to errors, such as the design of medical devices.

3.7 THE ROLE OF THE FDA

The role of the FDA's Center for Devices and Radiological Health (FDA-CDRH) is to "... regulate medical devices to assure their safety and effectiveness" [55]. The FDA requires that companies use a human factors design process when developing medical devices [56]. Title 21 of the Code of Federal Regulations (21CFR) addresses food and drugs, and its Section 820 addresses design controls. Subsection 820.30 implicitly mentions that human factors techniques or data are needed in the design process:

c. "Each manufacturer shall establish and maintain procedures to ensure that the design requirements relating to a device are appropriate and address the intended use of the device, including the needs of the users and patient. ...
f. "Each manufacturer shall establish and maintain procedures for verifying the design input. Design verification shall confirm that the design output meets the design input requirements. ...
g. "Design validation shall ensure that devices conform to defined user needs and intended uses, and shall include testing of production units under actual or simulated use conditions" [57].

Given the diversity of the human population and the aforementioned issues, medical device manufacturers should be concerned about satisfying the ergonomic needs of a diversity of potential health care workers and patients.

3.8 CONCLUSIONS

As medical devices become increasingly complex in the coming years (e.g., laparoscopic surgery equipment), human factors and ergonomics issues will become only more important. Device designers and manufacturers will need to utilize good human factors design processes to maximize patient safety and optimize quality of medical care for all patients while protecting the health and safety of health care workers.

To solve the problems of medical errors and physical injuries, it is important to scrutinize the medical devices involved and consider the possibility that the equipment is at fault, not the user. To address the needs of the growing numbers of disabled and aging health care providers and of laypeople providing health care within the home, medical devices need to be designed to accommodate the needs of a wide range of potential health care providers and patients. Medical device designs that do so may:

- Reduce errors and injuries (and associated malpractice claims)
- Accommodate both disabled and aging health care providers
- Accommodate both disabled and aging medical patients

ACKNOWLEDGMENT

This work is supported by the Rehabilitation Engineering Research Center on Accessible Medical Instrumentation, funded by the NIDRR, U.S. Department of Education Grant #H133E020729. All opinions expressed are those of the author.

REFERENCES

1. Aziz, K.J. Backinger, C.L., Beers, E.T., Lowery, A., Sykes, S.M., Thomas, A., Trautman, K.A. *Do It By Design: An Introduction to Human Factors in Medical Devices*, Public Health Service (P.H.S.) U.S. Department of Health and Human Services, Food and Drug Administration, Center for Devices and Radiological Health, Ed., Washington, D.C., 1996.

2. Institute of Medicine, *To Err is Human: Building a Safer Health System*, Washington, D.C.: National Academy Press, 2000, p. 287.
3. Brennan, T.A. et al., Incidence of adverse events and negligence in hospitalized patients: results of the Harvard Medical Practice Study I. *New England Journal of Medicine*, 1991, **324**(6), 370–6.
4. Localio, A.R. Lawthers, A.G., Brennan, T.A., Laird, N.M., Hebert, L.E., Peterson, L.M., Newhouse, J.P., Weiler, P.C., Hiatt, H.H. Relation between malpractice claims and adverse events due to negligence: results of the Harvard Medical Practice Study III. *New England Journal of Medicine*, 1991, **325**(4), 245–51.
5. Health Forum, *AHA Hospital Statistics: 2005 Edition*, American Hospital Association, Chicago, IL.
6. Hoyert, D.L., Kung, H.-C., and Smith, B.L., Deaths: preliminary data for 2003, in *National Vital Statistics Reports*, C.f.D.C.A. Prevention, Ed., 2005.
7. Agency for Healthcare Research and Quality, Medical Errors: The Scope of the Problem, Fact sheet 2000, cited August 11, 2005, available from http://www.ahrq.gov/ qual/errback.htm.
8. Leape, L.L. et al., The nature of adverse events in hospitalized patients: results of the Harvard Medical Practice Study II. *New England Journal of Medicine*, 1991, **324**(6), 377–84.
9. Carstensen, P., Human factors and patient safety: FDA role and experience, in *Human Factors, Ergonomics, and Patient Safety for Medical Devices*, Association for the Advancement of Medical Instrumentation, Washington, D.C., 2005.
10. Bureau of Labor Statistics, U.S. Department of Labor, Workplace Injuries and Illnesses in 2003, Washington, D.C., 2005.
11. American Nurses Association, Preventing Back Injuries: Safe Patient Handling and Movement, in *Occupational Health and Safety Series*, Silver Spring, MD, 2002.
12. Owen, B.D., The magnitude of low-back problems in nursing, *Western Journal of Nursing Research*, **11**, 234–42, April 1989.
13. Hing, E. and Middleton, K., National hospital ambulatory medical care survey: 2002 outpatient department summary, in *Advance Data From Vital and Health Statistics*, U.S. Department of Health and Human Services, Ed., 2004, National Center for Health Statistics, Centers for Disease Control and Prevention, Hyattsville, MD, p. 35.
14. Woodell, D.A. and D.K. Cherry, National ambulatory medical care survey: 2002 summary, in *Advance Data From Vital and Health Statistics*, U.S. Department of Health and Human Services, Ed., 2004, National Center for Health Statistics, Centers for Disease Control and Prevention, Hyattsville, MD, p. 44.
15. Patient Safety Center of Inquiry, Veterans Health Administration and Department of Defense, *Patient Care Ergonomics Resource Guide: Safe Patient Handling and Movement*, 2001, Tampa, FL.
16. Waters, T.R., Putz-Anderson, V., and Garg, A., *Applications Manual for the Revised NIOSH Lifting Equation*, 1994, U.S. Department of Health and Human Services, Centers for Disease Control and Prevention, National Institute for Occupational Safety and Health, Cincinnati, OH.
17. National Institute for Occupational Safety and Health, National Occupational Research Agenda (NORA), Priority Research Areas: Low Back Disorders, 1996, U.S. Department of Health and Human Services, Centers for Disease Control and Prevention, Cincinnati, OH.
18. Siddarthan, K., Nelson, A., and Weisenborn, G., A business case for patient care ergonomic interventions, *Nursing Administration Quarterly*, 2005, **29**(1), 63–71.
19. Premier, Inc., Preventing Back Injuries in Patient Care, 2005. Available from http://www.premierinc.com/all/safety/resources/back_injury/.
20. U.S. Department of Health and Human Services, National Institute of Occupational Health, National Heart, Lung, and Blood Institute, *Clinical Guidelines on the Identification, Evaluation, and Treatment of Overweight and Obesity in Adults*, Rockville, MD, 1998.
21. Kimball, B., Health care's human crisis — Rx for an evolving profession, *Online Journal of Issues in Nursing*, May 31, 2004 available from http://www.nursingworld.org/ojin/topic24/tpc24_1.htm.
22. Health and Safety Executive, *Manual Handling Operations Regulations 1992*, London. 1992.
23. Griffith, R. and Stevens, M., Manual handling and the lawfulness of no-lift policies, *Nursing Standard*, **18**(21), 39–43, 2004.
24. American Nurses Association, Position Statement on Elimination of Manual Patient Handling to Prevent Work-Related Musculoskeletal Disorders, 2003, Silver Spring, MD, p. 6.
25. Hudson, M.A., Texas passes first law for safe patient handling in America: landmark legislation protects healthcare workers and patients from injury related to manual patient handling, *Journal of Long-Term Effects of Medical Implants*, **15**(5), 559–566, 2005.

26. Texas Nurses Association, Texas Enacts Safe Patient Handling Law, 2005, available from: http://www.texasnurses.org/safepatienthandling.htm.
27. Nelson, A.L., Ed., *Patient Care Ergonomics Resource Guide: Safe Patient Handling and Movement*. 2003, Veterans Health Administration and Department of Defense, Tampa, FL.
28. Charney, W., Reducing back injury in nursing: a case study using mechanical equipment and a hospital transport team as a lift team, *Journal of Healthcare Safety, Compliance and Infection Control*, **4**, 117–120, 2000.
29. Meittunen, E.J. et al., The effect of focusing ergonomic risk factors on a patient transfer team to reduce incidents among nurses associated with patient care, *Journal of Healthcare Safety, Compliance and Infection Control*, **3**, 305–312, 1999.
30. Diaz, J.H., Carpal tunnel syndrome in female nurse anesthetists vs. operating room nurses: prevalence, laterality, and impact of handedness, *Anesthesia and Analgesia*, **93**(4), 975–980, 2001.
31. Coggan, C. et al., Prevalence of back pain among nurses, *New Zealand Medical Journal*, **107**(983), 306–308, 1994.
32. Bewick, N. and Gardner, D, Manual handling injuries in health care workers, *International Journal of Occupational Safety and Ergonomics*, **6**, 209–221, 2000.
33. Engkvist, I.-L. et al., Back injuries among nursing personnel: identification of work conditions with cluster analysis, *Safety Science*, **37**, 1–18, 2001.
34. Garg, A., Owen, B.D., and Beller, D., A biomechnical and ergonomic evaluation of patient transferring tasks: bed to wheelchair and wheelchair to bed, *Ergonomics*, **34**, 289–312, 1991.
35. Garg, A., Owen, B.D., and Beller, D., A biomechnical and ergonomic evaluation of patient transferring tasks: wheelchair to shower chair and shower chair to wheelchair, *Ergonomics*, **34**, 407–419, 1991.
36. Hignett, S., Work-related back pain in nurses, *Journal of Advanced Nursing*, **23**(6), 1238–1246, 1996.
37. Marras, W.S. et al., A comprehensive analysis of low-back disorder risk and spinal loading during the transferring and repositioning of patients using different techniques, *Ergonomics*, **42**(7), 904–926, 1999.
38. Nelson, A.L., Fragala, G., and Menzel, N., Myths and facts about back injuries in nursing, *American Journal of Nursing*, **103**, 32–40, 2003.
39. Retsas, A. and Pinikahana, J., Manual handling activities and injuries among nurses: an Australian hospital study, *Journal of Advanced Nursing*, **31**, 875–883, 2000.
40. Smedley, J. et al., Manual handling activities and risk of low back pain in nurses, *Occupational and Environmental Medicine*, **52**, 160–165, 1995.
41. Maheady, D.C., *Nursing Students with Disabilities: Change the Course*, Exceptional Parent Press, River Edge, NJ, 2003.
42. U.S. Census Bureau, *Population Change and Distribution*, in *Census 2000 Brief*, U.S. Department of Commerce, Ed., Economics and Statistics Administration, Washington, D.C., 2001.
43. U.S. Department of Commerce, Nation's Median Age Highest Ever, But 65-and-Over Population's Growth Lags, Census 2000 Shows, Economics and Statistics Administration, Bureau of the Census, Washington, D.C., 2001.
44. U.S. Department of Health and Human Services, Changing Demographics: Implications for Physicians, Nurses, and Other Health Workers, Health Resources and Services Administration, Bureau of Health Professions, National Center for Health Workforce Analysis: Washington, D.C., 2003.
45. Rogers, W.A., Ed., *Designing for an Aging Population*, 1997, Human Factors and Ergonomics Society, Santa Monica, CA, p. 396.
46. DynoMed, What is Arthritis? Learn About the Disease that Afflicts One Out of Seven Americans, all about Arthritis.com, available from http://www.allaboutarthritis.com/AllAboutArthritis/layoutTemplates/displayobjcontent/what_is_arthritis.htm.
47. Lee, J. and Bailey, G., Presbyopia, available from: http://www.allaboutvision.com/conditions/presbyopia. htm.
48. Hain, T.C., Hearing Loss, 2002, available from http://www.american-hearing.org/name/hearing_loss.html.
49. Meurer, L.N., New models of health care in the home and in the work site, *American Family Physician*, **56**(2), 384–386, 389, 1997.
50. Kaplan, D., The Definition of Disability, no date, available from http://www.accessiblesociety.org/topics/demographics-identity/dkaplanpaper.htm.

51. Maisels, L. et al., Access to Health Care for People with Disabilities in Massachusetts: Key Results of a Focus Group Study, 2000, Boston University School of Public Health, Boston, MA. p. 9.
52. U.S. Department of Education, Office of Special Education and Rehabilitative Services, National Institute on Disability and Rehabilitation Research, Long-Range Plan: 1999–2004, GPO, Washington, D.C., 2000, pp. 8, 9.
53. Leape, L.L., Human factors meets health care: the ultimate challenge*, Ergonomics in Design*, 2004, **12**(3), 6–12.
54. Leape, L.L., Error in medicine, *Journal of the American Medical Association*, 1994, **272**, 1851–1857.
55. U.S. Food and Drug Administration, Is My Product Regulated by FDA's Center for Devices and Radiological Health? 1998. available from: http://www.fda.gov/cdrh/ devadvice/31.html.
56. U.S. Department of Health and Human Services, Food and Drug Administration (F.D.A.) Center for Devices and Radiological Health. FDA's Human Factors Program: Promoting Safety in Medical Device Use, 2003, available from http://www.fda.gov/cdrh/humanfactors/.
57. *Code of Federal Regulations,* Title 21, Volume 8, Chapter I, Subchapter H, Part 820, Subpart C, Section 820.30, Food and Drug Administration (F.D.A.). U.S. Department of Health and Human Services, Ed., 2005.

4 Toward a New Health Care Policy: Accessible Medical Equipment and Instrumentation

June Isaacson Kailes, Brenda Premo, and Curtis Richards

CONTENTS

ABSTRACT

This chapter addresses the policy considerations, framework, and actions necessary to embed accessible medical equipment and instrumentation into health care policy and practice. For this to become commonplace in the health care system, advocates need to engage and build public–private partnerships at all levels of government and across service, education, and research systems.

4.1 INTRODUCTION

In a report to the American public issued in July 2005, the U.S. Surgeon General declared that, "The health and wellness of persons with disabilities today is a matter of public health concern" [1, p. 21]. The challenges of this public health concern cut across all aspects of health care and service delivery for persons with disabilities, including, among other things, a health care and health promotion service system that is limited in access or availability to persons with disabilities [1, p. 21].

The Surgeon General called for "a concerted action" to improve access to health and wellness services by persons with disabilities through "public–private partnerships" spanning all levels of government and "all service, education and research systems" [1, p. v]. The "Surgeon General's Call to Action to Improve the Health and Wellness of Persons with Disabilities" is based on American disability public policy and "the need to promote accessible, comprehensive health care that enables persons with disabilities to have a full life in the community with integrated services, consistent with the president's New Freedom Initiative. Persons with disabilities must have accessible, available and appropriate health care and wellness promotion services" [1, p. v].

As can be seen through its various chapters, this book helps better define an important piece of that "concerted action"; that is, how to improve access to health care for persons with disabilities through accessible medical equipment and instrumentation. This particular chapter addresses the policy considerations, framework, and actions necessary to embed accessible medical equipment and instrumentation into health care policy and practice.

As described in Chapter 1 and Chapter 2 of this book, equipment access represents one of the fundamental barriers to receiving health care and health-promoting services for persons with disabilities and activity limitations. It is not enough, though, to simply design medical equipment and instrumentation that is universally usable. To have maximum impact, policy must also address how instrumentation is selected (purchased), installed (arranged in its environmental context), used, introduced to its users (training), and regulated. Medical-instrumentation-related policy barriers to health care service delivery and employment must also be addressed.

A new health care policy agenda that addresses accessible medical equipment and instrumentation, after all, could play an important role in advancing the Surgeon General's principle that "good health is necessary for persons with disabilities to secure the freedom to work, learn and engage actively in their families and their communities" [1, p. 25].

4.1.1 Using Common Language

From the outset, it is important to be clear about language and terminology. All too often, public policy discussions are filled with jargon, acronyms, and words with specialized meaning. As policy attempts to cross disciplines and systems, a common understanding of language and terminology becomes essential. The glossary (which follows Chapter 31 of this book) offers some basic definitions around the subject matter of this book, whereas this chapter clarifies some specific words and phrases relevant to the policy context.

4.1.1.1 Policy and Public Policy

The word "policy" is used broadly and loosely and can be grounded in formal and informal means. For example, political scientist Andrew Dobelstein offers a broad definition: "A public policy is an action (and in some cases, inaction), usually undertaken by government, directed at a particular goal, and legitimated by the commitment of public resources" [2, p. 25]. As defined by one national technical assistance center, "policy" means "a principle, plan, or course of action established in statute, regulation, or proclamation by an elected chief executive or a federal, state, or local governing body" [3]. This is a common perception of — and a practical approach to — what the word policy means; that is, policy is embedded in the legalese of executive orders, laws, and implementing regulations.

Actions may be taken by any unit of government, or several units of government acting together. Statutes enacted by Congress or state legislatures and decisions made by courts are public policies, as are administrative rules and regulations and the actions of chief executives and their staffs.

Typically, governmental units must act together to produce a public policy as when the legislature passes a law that an executive must approve. However, sometimes governmental units act alone, as when administrative agencies change regulations [2, p. 25].

Policy can be developed from the top down or the bottom up. The top–down approach says that Congress enacts a statute, or the president issues an edict, or a federal agency imposes a set of standards and regulations that trickle through state and local governmental agencies and providers. In contrast, the bottom–up approach has policy starting at the local and state level until it becomes compelling enough to become developed, refined, and adopted into state or federal executive edict or law. The Americans with Disabilities Act Accessibility Guidelines (ADAAG) enacted by Congress and the president in 1996 (implementing regulations adopted by the U.S. Access Board and the Department of Justice and with cases interpreted by the courts over the last 15 years) is a good example of current public policy. Today, it can be viewed as exemplifying the top-down approach, yet it was created only after a number of bottom–up strategies were tried, including several state-level laws, many court cases, and a politically organized disability community.

Policy making can also take place in private nonprofit and for-profit sectors. When, for example, an entrepreneur chooses to invest in the development and production of accessible exam tables or easy-to-use diabetes testing equipment, policy is made and influenced as he or she sees a market for the equipment and begins to persuade potential buyers. Or, when an accrediting agency sees the importance of and administers a survey that includes an examination of physical, program, communication, and medical equipment accessibility, policy is made and influenced. "Private sector policy-making is public policy when it engages public problems," as Dobelstein [2] put it. "Knitting together the strands of public- and private-sector decisions and actions adds another level of complexity to the policy-making process" [2, p. 26]. Policy development around accessible medical equipment and instrumentation fits this description, as it involves a number of top–down and bottom–up approaches as well as public and private sector decision centers.

Policy making usually begins when a problem is identified and suggestions are made regarding its solution. From there, the rest of the policy-making process may become quite murky. As alluded to earlier, there are many different policy decision centers, each of which can involve a number of diverse policy-making actions. Policy makers differ widely as well. The activities involved in passing a law and the individual policy makers who are involved in making a law, for example, are quite different from the activities that produce regulations to implement the law and the people who develop regulations. Likewise, information gathered and used for policy analysis can vary widely. All policy analysis needs information that will lead to a decision, but the kind of information that the policy analyst uses depends upon the point in the policy process at which analysis is expected, and policy makers may or may not use the information in making their final decisions [2, p. 25].

However, as another political scientist, Deborah Stone, points out, both policy and thinking about policy are "produced in political communities" [4]. This is a point that cannot be underscored enough, for the political environments of policy making must always be kept in mind. In this case, policy around accessible medical equipment and instrumentation will need to take into account the political influence of the grassroots disability community, the organized disability advocacy groups, disability policy and technology researchers, appointees with disabilities or others responsible for disability-related programs in federal government, to name a few.

The essence of policy making in political communities boils down to a struggle over ideas. "Ideas are a medium of exchange and a mode of influence even more powerful than money and votes and guns," Stone asserts. "Shared meanings motivate people to action and meld individual striving into collective action. Ideas are at the center of all political conflict. Policy making, in turn, is a constant struggle over the criteria for classification, the boundaries of categories, and the definition of ideals that guide the way people behave" [4, p. 7].

4.1.1.2 Access Terminology

In the context of health care policy and what is known as *disability public policy*, access means different things. As a new health-care policy emerges that better addresses the needs of people with disabilities, it is important to understand the usages of the term *access*. The following definitions are offered to assist in understanding the usages in the context of this chapter. Similar definitions can be found in the glossary of this book, which follows Chapter 31.

Accessibility means "the degree to which an environment (physical, social, or attitudinal) makes appropriate accommodations to eliminate barriers or other impediments to equality of access to facilities, services, and the like, for persons with disabilities" [1, p. 36].

In the context of the Americans with Disabilities Act (ADA), compliance with access requirements involves not only attention to physical access but also attention to program, communication, and medical equipment access.

- *Physical access* involves removing physical barriers to allow people to get to, enter, and use the facilities, including accessible paths of travel from public transportation drop off points, parking lots, curb cuts, ramps, doorways, hallways, restrooms, drinking fountains, examination and treatment rooms, dressing rooms, etc.
- *Program access* involves programs, services, or activities that, when viewed as a whole, are accessible to and usable by people with disabilities. Overall program accessibility is achieved in a number of ways, such as altering existing facilities or constructing new ones and by means of nonstructural options, such as acquisition or redesign of equipment, assignment of personnel to assist individuals with disabilities, and provision of services at alternate accessible sites, to name a few.
- *Communication access* involves providing content in formats that are understandable and usable by people who are not fluent in the language, or with reduced or no ability to speak, see, and hear, or who have limitations in learning and understanding.
- *Medical equipment access* involves access to medical equipment that is usable by people with disabilities and activity limitations including accessible weight scales, exam tables, exam chairs, and other equipment facilitating access to routine care, preventive care, diagnostic tests, and necessary treatments.

Access to health care for persons with disabilities and activity limitations has two distinct meanings or "prongs." The first prong refers to the ability of individuals to seek services from a robust provider network that includes knowledgeable primary care physicians and specialists, and adequate coverage by health plans. Equally important, the second prong means that health care settings must be architecturally accessible, and providers must have the capacity to accommodate patients with a variety of disabilities. Accommodations can include, for example, providing effective communication such as through sign language interpreters for people with hearing loss and who are deaf, and materials in alternative formats for people with vision and other sensory and learning disabilities [5,6].

As can be seen from these definitions and those in the glossary, access to health care is analogous to peeling an onion with intricate quality and access layers. First, people with disabilities have to get to the door, then through the door, through the waiting and reception area, into an exam room and onto the examination equipment, and then interact with a clinically disability-competent health care provider.

In essence, as a package, these access-related definitions construct a new focus of attention, away from the individual with a disability *per se* to the environment within which that individual maneuvers and receives health care services. An adjustable mammogram machine that raises and lowers so a woman can be examined while seated in her wheelchair represents one example of reasonable equipment access, as opposed to a woman with paraplegia needing to be lifted from her wheelchair and held for the duration of the exam with her breasts placed in the mammogram machine. As is the case with many other innovations that had their origins in helping to accommodate people with disabilities, such as curb cuts, lowered counters, larger restroom stalls, phones with larger buttons and numbers and volume controls, etc., equipment access is inevitably sought after and used by others, including people of diverse ages and health conditions for whom it is uncomfortable or impossible to use equipment that is poorly designed.

4.2 UNDERSTANDING THE DISABILITY POLICY CONTEXT

Akin to the cognitive steps of the rational model of decision making, policy making can be viewed as what political scientist Deborah Stone describes as "a production model, where policy is created in a fairly orderly sequence of stages almost as if on an assembly line" [4, p. 7]. Under this model, government becomes a rational decision maker. An issue finds its way onto the public agenda and gets defined; it moves through the legislative and executive branches of government where alternative solutions are proposed, analyzed, legitimized, selected, and refined; a solution is implemented by the executive agencies and constantly challenged and revised by interested actors, oftentimes through the judicial system; occasionally, it provides a means of evaluating and revising implemented solutions [4, p. 7].

4.2.1 Disability Public Policy

The Americans with Disabilities Act of 1990 (ADA) [7] articulated a new framework of national disability public policy. A piece of civil rights legislation that prohibits discrimination based on disability, the ADA essentially establishes national public policy toward people with disabilities with the goals of assuring equality of opportunity, full participation in all aspects of society, independent living, and economic self sufficiency [8]. Underlying policy assumptions and objectives drive each of these major themes. For example:

- Disability is viewed as a natural part of the human experience; it is not something to be ashamed of or feared. People with disabilities are not broken or damaged goods in need of being fixed.
- Individualization is a major underpinning of disability policy. Decisions about someone with a disability are to be based on the individual strengths, resources, priorities, concerns, abilities, and capabilities of each person, rather than on stereotypes, assumptions, and misperceptions. Person-centered planning is embedded in disability public policy.
- Equal opportunity in a disability context means that programs and services must be accessible to and usable by people with disabilities, including the required provision of auxiliary aides, services, and accommodations necessary for equally effective health care. Additionally, programs and services are supposed to be available to people with disabilities in the most integrated setting possible, considering the person's unique needs and circumstances.
- The full participation tenet encompasses the long-developed disability concepts of individual and family empowerment, self-determination, self-advocacy, informed choice, and active participation of people with disabilities, and often their families, in the decision-making processes.

The ADA sets the national standard for defining a disability. That is, the ADA defines a person with a disability as (1) a person with a physical or mental impairment that substantially limits one or more major life activity, or (2) a person with a record of such a physical or mental impairment, or (3) a person who is regarded as having such impairment [7]. Examples of a major life activity, as set forth in the first portion of the ADA definition, include activities such as caring for oneself, performing manual tasks, walking, seeing, hearing, speaking, breathing, learning, or working.

Throughout the 1990s, Congress systematically wrote and rewrote other major pieces of disability program legislation with the intent of making them consistent with the values and principles of the ADA, particularly in the critical areas of education, employment, and independent living. As mentioned earlier in this chapter, this new disability public policy framework did not spring out of thin air. It has a rich and lengthy history that developed at local and state levels before being woven into federal legislation and regulations, and it has been tested, retested and shaped by numerous regulatory decisions and court interpretations. Through this body of disability public policy, Congress clearly intends to create federal programs and tools to achieve the promises and goals of the ADA. Collectively, these federal statutes establish new national policies toward people with disabilities and expectations and standards for programs and services for people with disabilities [9].

4.2.2 Applicability to Health Care Arena

The ADA and a companion statute, Section 504 of the Rehabilitation Act [10], already require that people with disabilities can receive equally effective health care as the general public. This new national policy, grounded in federal statutes and regulations described earlier, is then extended and implemented throughout federal government agencies through executive orders, budget proposals, and administrative actions, such as President Bush's New Freedom Initiative [11] and the Surgeon General's Call to Action [1]. For example, after establishing an overarching principle of good health for persons with disabilities, the Surgeon General established broad policy goals, including that health care providers have the knowledge and tools to screen, diagnose, and treat persons with disabilities. To achieve those goals, he offered a set of strategies, several of which address the policy objectives of this chapter; that is, to establish and promote policy around accessible medical equipment and instrumentation in the public and private sectors. The relevant strategies suggested by the Surgeon General include:

- Educate health care providers in an ongoing manner about state-of-the-art health services and supports that should be available to patients with disabilities.
- Promote development and use of medical equipment and devices that allow universal access to all recommended screening and diagnostic tests and treatments for all patients.
- Promote the development of research to enhance the evidence base for best practices in clinical service delivery for persons with disabilities.
- Bring inventors, clinicians, and industry together through more effective incubator and development programs to collaborate efficiently and effectively to enhance research and development of assistive technology for all types of disabilities.
- Promote and disseminate the adoption of new treatments, models of care, and adaptive or assistive technologies [1, pp. 22–24].

So the public policy framework around accessible medical equipment and instrumentation exists in statute, executive edict, and health policy proclamations. The next level policy question, in keeping with a sequential model of policy development, is how to implement this policy challenge.

4.2.3 Developing More Specific Policy

To make these broad policy statements and goals reality in the daily lives of people with disabilities seeking health care and wellness services, some further detailed policy guidance, rules and regulations, applied research initiatives, design and purchasing standards, and incentives and sanctions need to be developed at all levels of public and private sectors.

Medical instrumentation is designed and manufactured by an industry that differs significantly from the mass-market product industry in several fundamental ways, including:

- *Unique regulatory process:* Products must go through a process that provides reasonable assurance that a device is safe and effective for its intended use (e.g., in the U.S. through the Food and Drug Administration's Center for Devices and Radiological Health). This includes both premarket approval and postmarket reporting processes.
- *Unique reimbursement (third-party payment) infrastructure:* Third-party payment policies and procedures dramatically influence product development. For example, decisions of the U.S. Centers for Medicare and Medicaid Services (CMS) regarding what devices are reimbursable and at what price are influential (as they apply to 79 million Americans), and often private insurers follow CMS's lead.
- *Multiple types of "consumer" decision makers exist:* A device may be "sold" directly to an end user, but depending on the technology, the sale will more likely have to be made through a certain health professional (e.g., provider, practitioner, or manager).

The overarching policy guidance to further develop accessible medical equipment and instrumentation should be similar to the following: People with disabilities can receive equally effective health care through the implementation of policies and practices that facilitate the design and integration of accessible medical equipment and instrumentation that is accessible to and usable by people with disabilities as patients and as health care professionals.

The goal is that it become standard practice that medical equipment, devices, and instruments are designed to:

- Be universally usable, for practical and financial reasons
- Maximize the number of people who can use the devices and reduce the need for peripheral add-ons and assistive technologies (see Chapter 6 of this book)
- Be more accommodating of human variability in age, size, shape, mobility, dexterity, and visual, hearing, speech, and cognitive abilities, including language skills and learning styles (see Chapter 1 and Chapter 18 of this book)

The medical device industry recognizes that it is impractical and expensive to have multiple devices to suit the needs of all disability groups, or a multitude of assistive technologies that could be connected to the device, so striving for broad accessibility and usability of all equipment is the logical approach.

4.3 USING POLICY INSTRUMENTS FOR IMPLEMENTATION

As mentioned in the preceding text, converting this vision into reality requires changes on multiple levels — public and private at the federal, state and local levels, as well as all levels of service, research, and education systems. The question now is what it will take to make this happen. What are the pressure points and the incentives that will cause the swell that creates the waves of change that cause this to become embedded in health care policy and practice? This section offers some concrete suggestions, strategies, and outcomes to answer these questions.

Currently, accessible medical equipment and instrumentation is not even on the public agenda. It is not on the radar screen for Congress or the president, state legislatures or governors, the media, or even major disability rights advocacy organizations. The fact that the National Institute on Disability and Rehabilitation Research (NIDRR) had the foresight to fund a Rehabilitation Engineering and Research Center on the subject (Accessible Medical Instrumentation) is a powerful step toward getting the subject on the public agenda. The Surgeon General's goals and strategies help raise additional visibility and public awareness of the issue, whereas this book — supported by NIDRR — attempts to better define the subject matter. Equipment manufacturers are just beginning to explore the feasibility of accessible medical equipment and instrumentation, and the health care industry is in the embryonic stages of understanding the need for it. Because it is not yet prominent on the public agenda, there is a lack of regulation and standards for design and enforcement. Many different standards and new technologies are emerging that contribute to design and production of accessible medical equipment and instrumentation, but they are not yet recognized as applicable.

The means of addressing policy problems are often called *policy instruments* or *policy solutions*. These may more appropriately be thought of as "strategies for structuring relationships and coordinating behavior to achieve collective purposes," as Stone suggests. Because common goals cannot be based on governing every action or decision of individuals and organizations, policy needs to be based on broad structures and rules that will have a multiplier effect, shaping people's behavior without continuous and specific directions [4, p. 208].

A set of key policy instruments or strategies represent the broad structures that can create Stone's multiplier effect, which include, but are not necessarily limited to, rights, rules, powers, and inducements; these instruments will need to be addressed across policy-making and policy-influencing units such as federal and state executive, legislative, and administrative agencies, the judicial system, education and research institutions, advocacy groups and labor unions, and private sector organizations. Policy instruments are means of getting people to do what they otherwise might not do.

4.3.1 Rights

Rights are strategies that allow individuals or groups or organizations to invoke government power on their behalf. Rights describe those relationships between people or between people and organizations that government will uphold [4, p. 209]. This policy instrument is well known to the disability community. As discussed earlier, the American disability public policy is embedded in several pieces of federal legislation, many of which have companion state statutes. Children and youth with disabilities have the *right* to a "free appropriate public education" under the Individuals with Disabilities Education Act; people of all ages with disabilities have the *right* to nondiscrimination and equal access in employment, public and private sector services, transportation, and recreation under the Americans with Disabilities Act; the *right* to equal access to housing under the Fair Housing Act Amendments; the *right* to equal treatment in air travel under the Air Carrier's Access Act; and so on. All of these civil rights statutes carry administrative and legal remedies and sanctions for violations of these rights.

Under the ADA and Section 504 of the Rehabilitation Act, people with disabilities clearly already have basic rights to equal access and effective treatment in health care. When these rights are violated, people with disabilities have filed administrative complaints as well as pursued legal action through the judicial system, an important element in policy making and influencing.

The Department of Justice (DOJ) issues quarterly status reports tracking its enforcement of the ADA and Section 504 of the Rehabilitation Act. In *It Takes More Than Ramps to Solve the Crisis of Healthcare for People with Disabilities* [12], the Disability Rights Education and Defense Fund (DREDF) reviewed the DOJ quarterly status reports from April of 1994 through March of 2003. In those reports, DREDF found 114 health care-related cases; of those, 35 cases involved architectural access to medical offices and facilities, and an additional three cases concerned access to diagnostic equipment and examination tables [13].

In one of the most important private actions, to date, Metzler v. Kaiser Permanente of California, 2001, an agreement settled a class-action lawsuit filed against Kaiser Permanente, on behalf of all its California members with disabilities. The lawsuit argued that Kaiser discriminated against patients with disabilities by providing inferior medical care. Some of the terms of the settlement agreement include:

- Removal of architectural barriers
- Installation of accessible medical equipment, including wheelchair accessible scales
- Review of Kaiser Permanente's policies, procedures, and programs to improve access to quality health care for people with disabilities
- Development of a mechanism for responding to ongoing input from Kaiser Permanente members with disabilities
- Development of a training program to educate Kaiser Permanente's health care professionals about treating people with disabilities
- Conduction of outreach to Kaiser Permanente's patients with disabilities to inform them of improved access features
- Development of a complaint-handling system to meet the needs of people with disabilities [13]

Similarly, in November 2005, the DOJ reached a landmark settlement agreement with the Washington Hospital Center in Washington, D.C., that can serve as a model for other hospitals to address the need for access to medical services and, in particular, the need for accessible medical equipment and instrumentation. The agreement includes inpatient room renovation, outpatient barrier removal, survey and purchase of accessible medical equipment, policy review and development, training, new publications, and much more [14].

Although these cases are an indication that the rights of people with disabilities in the health care arena are gaining increasing standing, there is still a great deal more clarity needed around what accessibility really means for this population in the context of health care, especially when it comes to medical equipment, devices, and instruments.

Congress could begin by conducting oversight hearings concerning health care access for individuals with disabilities in which the experiences of people with disabilities can be brought to light, such as a young man with autism being examined by his neurologist for 2 years through a closed door due to fear of his erratic behavior [15] or a middle-aged man receiving a prostate exam in his wheelchair because the exam tables were inaccessible [5]. A clear outcome of such oversight hearings could easily become Congressional adoption of a medical instrumentation accessibility code (MIAC), which could guarantee the rights of people with disabilities to accessible medical equipment, devices, and instrumentation. This piece of public policy could also charge the Access Board with developing implementation standards and the Department of Justice with enforcement; it could also provide funding for research and development, health care provider training, ongoing technical assistance, or design and innovation incentives. This sort of policy development can also occur — beforehand, simultaneously, or afterward — at the state legislative level.

Congress is not likely to act, however, unless there is some groundswell of research, education, support, and advocacy to demonstrate the need for these rights. Certainly, the legal complaints and lawsuits have begun to build some of that groundswell, as do the research efforts funded by NIDRR and the public awareness sponsored by the Surgeon General. Yet, most disability rights advocacy organizations do not yet recognize the importance of accessible medical equipment and instrumentation. As key stakeholders, disability advocates themselves need to be oriented, trained, and empowered to pursue this next step in securing disability rights. If they were, they could begin to educate members of Congress, and their staff, to set the stage for a fundamental shift in public health care policy.

4.3.2 Rules

Rules are commands to act or not act in certain ways, and "more broadly, they are classifications of people and situations that determine permissions and entitlements." Rules are usually backed up by sanctions, and *inducements* are based on rules for handing out rewards or punishments [4, p. 209]. Disability public policy, starting with the statutorily established rights, is rife with rules, regulations, standards, and guidelines in an attempt to define desired behavior.

In the case of accessible medical equipment and instrumentation, the National Council on Disability (NCD) could advise Congress and the Administration of the issue and suggest that Congress give authority to the Access Board to promulgate rules, or standards, focused on ensuring that the industry design, develop, manufacture, and market products to be accessible to and usable by individuals with disabilities and that health care providers receiving any form of government assistance must purchase accessible equipment, devices, and instruments. The Access Board's standards would spell out what makes medical instrumentation products accessible for such items as diagnostic, therapeutic, and procedural equipment, including examination and treatment tables and chairs, weight scales, x-ray equipment, glucometers, blood pressure cuffs, treadmills, and exercise machines. Within the design process there needs to be a core set of access standards, but these are not yet complete. There should be a policy that designers must include, within their standard protocols, a requirement that the equipment, device, or instrument be accessible to and usable by the maximum possible range of potential users, i.e., patients as well as employees. These standards would then be adopted by and enforced by the Department of Justice.

The Access Board would be a logical venue for the development of these standards, which would build on the MIAC and be known as the Medical Instrumentation Accessibility Code Standards (MIACS). The Access Board has a long history of developing accessibility standards, including access standards for public accommodations under the ADA, the Section 508 of the Rehabilitation Act information and electronic technology standards, and the Section 255 of the Telecommunications Act accessibility standards. In the past, the Access Board has taken two approaches to requiring accessible technology: design production requirements and purchasing requirements. Procurement requirements are modeled by the Section 508 standards, while production requirements are modeled by the 255 standards.

The MIACS could be built on the best of both worlds by requiring medical instrument manufacturers to make sure their products are accessible, regardless of who purchased them and requiring medical instrument vendors to sell accessible products, regardless of who produced them, and requiring federal agencies that purchase medical equipment and instrumentation products to ensure that those products conformed to the MIACS.

One potential approach to rule making follows. The Access Board could develop standards that establish what equipment must be able to do, as opposed to specifying exactly how access is achieved, which will likely vary among different types of products. Structured as performance requirements, the standards could detail the characteristics and capabilities of the equipment interfaces necessary for access for the largest possible number of users. The products covered under such a set of rules would likely be quite varied and ever-changing through technological innovations. The standards would have to address product and equipment interfaces, including input, output, operating controls and mechanisms, as well as product information and documentation.

As is its common practice in the development of rules and regulations, the Access Board would need to establish an advisory committee to make recommendations on what the guidelines should contain. The Medical Instrumentation Access Advisory Committee (MIAAC) might include:

- Medical device manufacturers
- Health care service providers
- Disability groups
- Relevant government agencies, such as the FDA
- Standards settings organizations such as (see also Chapter 15 of this book):
  - Association for the Advancement of Medical Instrumentation (AAMI), which sponsors many equipment-specific standards committees that are developing design standards for everything from sterilization equipment to dialysis machines to infusion pumps

- International Standards Organization/International Electrotechnical Commission (ISO/IEC) Working Group on Accessibility
- International Telecommunications Union
- Institute for Electrical and Electronic Engineers (IEEE)
- European Committee for Standardization
- Consumer Electronics Association
- World Wide Web Consortium (W3C)

The MIAAC would generate a report on which the Access Board would base its proposed guidelines; the Access Board would then complete the rule making process.

4.3.3 Powers

Powers describes strategies that seek to alter the content of decisions by shifting the process of decision making to different people. These strategies include changing the membership or size of decision-making bodies and shifting decision-making authority from one part of government to another. "These strategies are usually promoted as efficient mechanisms for producing 'better' decisions, but they are fundamentally ways of restructuring political power — hence the name 'powers'" [4, p. 209].

This policy-making strategy has several viable possibilities when applied to accessible medical equipment and instrumentation. Currently, the power to impact policy lies with the medical device industry to design and manufacture accessible equipment and instrumentation, and with the Food and Drug Administration, which has a level of responsibility for approving equipment. The power for enforcement is shared between the U.S. Department of Health and Human Services and the Department of Justice. The latter has the stronger track record in ADA and Section 504 compliance enforcement.

If Congress were to enact a MIAAC, the structure of that law could shift the locus of power to people with disabilities themselves and to federal agencies better suited to craft the standards, enforce them, and provide technical assistance for compliance.

Planning for and not with people with disabilities reflects an old paradigm: "a lot about us without us." People with disabilities need to be involved in all aspects of this policy development, not in token ways, such as in advisory capacities, but in significant and meaningful ways. In other words, "nothing about us without us!" It is important to include qualified people with disabilities who understand and can think through issues from a cross-disability perspective, and in the research and practice processes as investigators, contributors, collaborators, and managers. *Cross-disability* means, given the complexity and diversity of disabilities and the low prevalence of many conditions, the focus should be on functional limitations across disabilities and not on discrete diagnostic groups. For example, people with cerebral palsy have some characteristics in common, but variations in abilities and limitations manifested in vastly different ways are more common. There are common functional limitations that need attention across disability groups. Being diligent in seeking qualified people with disabilities, and taking advantage of the wealth, depth, and breadth of information and knowledge available from the disability community, yields positive payoffs.

Unfortunately, the history of including people with disabilities has been, in large part, one of paternalism. Entire professions of "experts" have emerged who have taken control over basic life decisions away from people with disabilities. However, experience repeatedly demonstrates that, given the proper tools, people with many different types of disabilities can devise creative approaches to eradicate barriers that have stumped the so-called experts. For example, the newer, more popular, and functional lightweight "sports" wheelchairs that are now widely used were designed by innovative wheelchair users, not the established wheelchair industry [16]. Including people with disabilities can yield a multitude of innovative recommendations that serve the mutual interests of manufacturers and their customers. People with disabilities and activity limitations can be excellent problem solvers.

If disability community advocates become educated on the need for and importance of accessible medical equipment and instrumentation, they could work to persuade Congress to enact a MIAC that was built on the "nothing about us without us" approach, which would not only include tapping people with disabilities to help guide policy and standards development, but also for research, education and training, ongoing technical assistance, and enforcement activities.

Assigning the standards development and technical assistance to the Access Board would be an important step toward achieving this policy strategy. Another key strategy could be to get the Department of Health and Human Services and the Department of Justice to work collaboratively on an initiative to improve health care access for people with disabilities, including through the availability and use of accessible medical equipment, devices, and instruments. Such an initiative could address both after-the-fact complaint resolution and proactive technical assistance to the field.

4.3.4 Inducements

Inducements are instruments used to change people's behavior with rewards and punishments, or incentives and sanctions [4, p. 209]. This strategy is very popular in American policy making. Federal, state, and local tax codes are overflowing with tax breaks for business and industry to perform certain desired activities, including staying in a particular location, investing in research and development, and producing certain kinds of goods and products. In fact, disability public policy contains a number of tax incentives such as for small businesses to offset the cost of modifying facilities to assure physical access, as well as for training and hiring people with disabilities.

Although a passionate debate rages about the value and effectiveness of tax policy interacting with disability policy stimulated by the underutilization of many of the disability-related tax breaks, tax incentives are a policy strategy that could prove beneficial in stimulating research, design, manufacture, marketing, and purchase of accessible medical equipment and instrumentation. It is likely that other forms of rewards could serve a similar purpose, such as cost sharing, depreciation, low interest revolving loan funds, and research grants, to name a few.

Incentives developed to stimulate the industry should, at a minimum:

- Reward experimentation and innovation
- Incorporate universal design principles
- Assist health care providers who purchase accessible medical equipment and instrumentation products

Similarly, most of the civil rights laws addressing disability public policy offer administrative and legal procedures, remedies, and penalties. In fact, over the last few years, Congress has considered multiple proposals to restrict some of those remedies and penalties, such as the ADA Notification Act and the repeal of parents' rights to be reimbursed for attorneys fees if they win a court case under the Individuals with Disabilities Education Act.

Any accessible medical equipment and instrumentation statute would need to carry due process procedures, administrative and legal remedies, sanctions, and penalties comparable to those for violations of the Americans with Disabilities Act.

4.4 ADDITIONAL PRESSURE POINTS

4.4.1 Private Sector Strategies

An excellent example of the "multiplier effect" as it relates to accessible medical equipment and instrumentation is currently unfolding in the health care system in Southern California. One of the state's health maintenance organizations, the Inland Empire Health Plan (IEHP), made a policy decision to find out how many physicians in its plan have accessible medical equipment. IEHP developed and conducted a survey of its 1500 providers about the availability of accessible exam tables. IEHP has also undertaken an extensive facility review for physical accessibility and has begun to incorporate physical accessibility symbols in its membership directories to inform its patients of which facilities have accessible features. Although its survey and review process did not look at all types of accessible medical equipment and instrumentation, it does represent a significant step and is beginning to influence the rest of the industry.

Private accreditation and licensing agencies are uniquely positioned to play a significant role in improving health care service delivery and access for individuals with disabilities, which can include embedding accessible medical equipment and instrumentation into the fabric of the health care service delivery system. Two key agencies play central roles through accreditation and related services in improving the safety and quality of health care provided to the public. The major accreditation body for hospitals and care facilities is the Joint Commission on Accreditation of Healthcare Organizations (JCAHO), which evaluates and accredits more than 16,000 health care organizations and programs in the U.S. The Commission on Accreditation of Rehabilitation Facilities (CARF) reviews and accredits rehabilitation and human services providers. Currently, more than 38,000 services have CARF accreditation. CARF recently merged with the Continuing Care Accreditation Commission (CCAC), an agency that accredits aging services, including continuing care retirement communities.

Under the ADA and other applicable laws and regulation, hospitals have the responsibility to provide access to health care. JCAHO lists, in its 2001 accreditation manual, three types of specific actions or steps hospitals are expected to have taken to meet ADA requirements, all of which relate to communication access; it makes one oblique reference to physical access. In that context, the manual offers the following example: "Furnishings and equipment reflect patients' characteristics related to age, level of disability, and therapeutic needs" [17].

CARF, on the other hand, requires a written accessibility plan that must address architectural, environmental, attitudinal, financial, employment, communication, transportation, and other barriers identified by stakeholders. The standards manual states, "When a barrier is identified, a report is written that addresses the actions planned to remove the barrier. This report includes a realistic time line for removal of the barrier" [18]. This declaration does not specify who is accountable for writing the barrier removal report or for overseeing that the actions are carried out.

It is not enough simply to circulate standards manuals and check off items on a survey form during the accreditation process. Accreditation agencies must assert their leadership if this new vision of access for patients and employees with disabilities is to be realized within the health care systems they accredit. JCAHO and CARF must find new ways to monitor compliance with the standards, reward best practices, solicit user feedback, and incorporate that information into the ongoing accreditation effort [13, pp. 26–27].

The accrediting bodies have begun to address access to health care for people with disabilities, but there is much more they can do. For example, in the CARF process an organization can be accredited and not be accessible. In order for an institution to receive the highest level of accreditation, the accrediting bodies need to incorporate other access issues into their organizational assessments, such as purchase and installation of ceiling or portable lifts to assist patients to transfer onto examination tables; purchase of wheelchair-accessible examination tables, scales, gurneys, and beds; information about in-house resources that staff members can call on to address problems or issues that arise; and ongoing ethical and legal issues. CARF and JCAHO should also provide ongoing technical assistance to institutions seeking accreditation, either themselves or by contracting with qualified disability organizations.

A third, and very powerful, example of the private sector demonstrating leadership in helping shape this new policy agenda around accessible medical equipment again comes from California. In the midst of a process of the state considering a major expansion of managed care to the Medicaid population of beneficiaries with disabilities and chronic illnesses, the private, nonprofit California Healthcare Foundation (CHCF) sponsored a project to develop contract standards for managed care organizations that addresses all aspects of access to care, including medical equipment and instrumentation. The CHCF process models the policy outcome of involving people with disabilities and their representatives throughout the process as well as building consensus among diverse groups of advocates, health plans, and state agency experts [19].

4.4.2 Complaints and Litigation

Settlement of administrative complaints and lawsuits are also a potent influence on public policy making; some even go so far as to assert that judges make policy themselves with their rulings. A growing body of settlement agreements and court actions around accessible medical equipment and instrumentation helps reinforce the need for a more universal policy.

The following three summaries of Dept. of Justice (DOJ)-resolved cases mentioned earlier involve discrimination based on the failure of a medical provider to offer appropriate services to a person with a disability because either an examination table or diagnostic equipment was inaccessible.

- A Virginia medical center allegedly refused to treat a woman who used a wheelchair during her scheduled appointment because they said they could not lift her on to the examining table. The medical center completed a survey of current examination tables and developed a capital budget and a timeline to purchase motorized examination tables. It also provided training to staff members on ADA requirements.
- A Washington, D.C., radiology practice allegedly failed to provide adequate assistance to a woman who used a wheelchair to help her transfer from her wheelchair to an examination table. The practice purchased an additional height-adjustable examination table and designated three lead medical assistants as ADA patient advocates to help patients with mobility disabilities receive services as quickly and efficiently as possible.
- A Washington, D.C., hospital allegedly failed to offer reasonable accommodations to a woman who used a wheelchair by providing assistance to help her transfer from her wheelchair to an examination table for a gynecological examination in its obstetrics and gynecology clinic. The hospital agreed to pay the plaintiff $15,000. Additionally, they paid the U.S. a civil penalty in the amount of $10,000, and according to a DOJ official, they agreed to undertake a facility-wide review of related accommodation and accessibility problems [13].

Information obtained through a Freedom of Information Act request reveals that the Office of Civil Rights at the U.S. Department of Health and Human Services (OCR at HHS) has received several complaints addressing accessible medical equipment and instrumentation, the most relevant of which are summarized as follows, without the details of the involved organizations.

- *A university medical system (1992):* The complainant, an individual with paraplegia, used a wheelchair. She attempted to visit a mobile cancer detection van operated by the system, but the van lacked any lifting apparatus that would have made it wheelchair-accessible. The complainant discussed the problem with the medical system, and was told to visit the nonmobile medical center, where the same services would be provided, also free of charge. The investigation proceeded under Section 504 of the Rehabilitation Act of 1973, and OCR at HHS found that the mobile van was in compliance with Section 504.
- *A state department of health and mental hygiene (1999):* A state resident with tetraplegia was enrolled by the state into its Medicaid managed care organization (MCO). The complainant, whose various disabilities necessitated a physically accessible doctor's office and an adjustable examination table, alleged that she was unable to find a doctor who could meet her needs within the MCO to which she had been assigned. The complainant's doctor recommended her for a specific subprogram within state's Medicaid program, through which the complainant was able to access a physician who could meet

her needs. The complainant indicated to OCR at HHS that she was satisfied with the resolution of her complaint, and OCR at HHS found no violation of Section 504.

- *A private imaging company (2001):* The complainant, a breast cancer survivor and an amputee who used a wheelchair, scheduled an appointment at a mobile MRI bus parked on the premises of her local hospital. When she arrived for the appointment, she learned that the MRI bus was not accessible by wheelchair: the ramp leading onto the bus involved two steps, and the interior of the bus was too narrow to accommodate a wheelchair. OCR at HHS investigated the MRI bus, and determined that it was out of compliance with Section 504. However, the MRI bus was a particularly small business with only two employees, and physical alteration of the bus would have been both extremely difficult and prohibitively expensive. Therefore, OCR at HHS found that the MRI bus was permitted to refer individuals with disabilities to other providers, rather than provide accessible services itself.
- *A nursing facility (2002):* The complainant, a morbidly obese man, alleged that he was discriminated by the nursing facility when staff issued a discharge/transfer notice on the basis that the staff could no longer meet the complainant's needs. Specifically, the facility's doctors and nurses were concerned for the complainant's safety (should complainant fall and need to be lifted back into his bed) as well as the safety of the facility's employees (the complainant weighed nearly 500 lb). However, once the facility received notice that the complainant had filed the complaint, it took the following actions: rescinded the discharge/transfer notice, purchased a bed equipped with a scale to accommodate the complainant, placed the complainant on a 1500-calorie diet, and established an exercise regimen for the complainant. Based on these policy modifications, OCR at HHS found that the facility had resolved any alleged violations of Section 504 [13].

4.4.3 Organized Labor

Another potential pressure point for impacting policy around accessible medical equipment and instrumentation is from the vantage point of employees with disabilities and the organizations that represent them in contract negotiations and in political spheres. There are both a worker safety and an employment discrimination context here. Back injuries from lifting people with disabilities on and off of inaccessible equipment could be prevented. Likewise, employees with disabilities, who have the right to nondiscrimination in the workplace so long as they can perform the essential functions of the position with or without a reasonable accommodation, may be able to perform more safely and effectively with equipment that is accessible to and usable by them.

4.5 CONCLUSION

As described here and in the first three chapters of this book, equipment access represents one of the fundamental barriers to receiving health care and health promotion services for people with disabilities and activity limitations. A new health care policy agenda that addresses accessible medical equipment and instrumentation is clearly needed to achieve the Surgeon General's concerted action for people with disabilities to have accessible, available, and appropriate health care and wellness promotion services.

It is time for a new piece of disability public policy; that is, the enactment of a Medical Instrumentation Accessibility Code with accompanying standards, potentially developed by the U.S. Access Board, in conjunction with a brain trust of industry experts and knowledgeable people with disabilities. Disability community advocates need to better understand the issues around accessible medical equipment and instrumentation and begin to put the subject on the public agenda. Beyond design, manufacture, and purchase of such equipment, there is a strong need for ongoing education, training, and technical assistance that needs to be part of the policy initiative.

A wide variety of policy-making strategies need to be employed independently, simultaneously, and collectively at the federal, state, and local levels and across government and private sectors. As Stone points out, an understanding of the underlying theories about how to change and coordinate individual and organizational behavior toward collective goals demonstrates that "no policy strategy is ever purely one type" [4, p. 210] and "the process of choosing and implementing the means of policy is political and continuous" [4, p. 209]. Politics and policy go hand in hand, and public policy is about communities trying to achieve progress together. For accessible medical equipment and instrumentation to become commonplace in the health care system, the disability community needs to become engaged and build public–private partnerships at all levels of government and across all service, education, and research systems.

ACKNOWLEDGMENT

This work is supported by the Rehabilitation Engineering Research Center on Accessible Medical Instrumentation, funded by the NIDRR, U.S. Department of Education Grant #H133E020729. All opinions expressed are those of the authors.

REFERENCES

1. Carmona, R., The Surgeon General's Call to Action to Improve the Health and Wellness of Persons with Disabilities 2005, U.S. Department of Health and Human Services, Office of the Surgeon General, Rockville, MD, 2005.
2. Dobelstein, A.W., *Social Welfare: Policy and Analysis*, Nelson-Hall Publications, Chicago, IL, 1990.
3. National Collaborative on Workforce and Disability for Youth, Washington, D.C., www.NCWD-Youth.info, retrieved November 2005.
4. Stone, D.A., *Policy, Paradox and Political Reason*, Scott, Foresman, and Company, Glenview, IL, 1988.
5. Premo, B., Kailes, J.I., Schwier, E., and Richards, C., Adults With Disabilities in Medi-Cal: The Beneficiary Perspective, Medi-Cal Policy Institute, California Health Care Foundation, Oakland, CA, September 2003.
6. Chimento, L., Forbes, M., Sander, A., Kailes, J.I., Premo, B., Richards, C., and Perrone, C., Medical Beneficiaries with Disabilities: Comparing Managed Care with Fee-for-Service Systems, California Health Care Foundation Issue Brief, Oakland, CA, August, 2005.
7. Americans with Disabilities Act of 1990, Public Law 101-226, July 26, 1990. Title 42 of U.S.C. 12101 et seq.
8. Silverstein, R., Emerging Disability Policy Framework: A Guidepost for Analyzing Public Policy, *Iowa Law Review*, Vol. 35, No. 5, August 2000.
9. Richards, C., The Disability Policy Lens, unpublished paper prepared for the National Collaborative on Workforce and Disability for Youth, Washington, D.C., 2003.
10. Section 504 of the Rehabilitation Act (29 U.S.C. 794d), as amended by the Workforce Investment Act of 1998 (P.L. 105-220), August 7, 1998.
11. New Freedom Initiative, February 1, 2001. Available online at http://www.whitehouse.gov/news/freedominitiative/freedominitiative.html.
12. Reis, J.P., Breslin, M.L., Iezzoni, L., and Kirschner, K., It Takes More Than Ramps to Solve the Crisis of Healthcare for People With Disabilities, Rehabilitation Institute of Chicago, Disability Rights Education and Defense Fund, Berkeley, CA, 2004.
13. Brill, R.E., Esq., A Review of Legal Research on Accessible Medical Equipment, unpublished memorandum conducted for this publication, Disability Rights Education and Defense Fund, Berkeley, CA, 2005.
14. Levine, S., Suit Wins Changes for Disabled at Hospital, *Washington Post.* November 3, 2005. p. 1309.
15. Parent testimonial during an interview for the Joseph P. Kennedy Public Policy Fellowship Program, Washington, D.C., November 2005.

16. Kaplan, D., DeWitt, J., and Steyaert, M., Laying the Foundation: A Report of the First Year of the Blue Ribbon Panel on National Telecommunications Policy, World Institute on Disability, Oakland, CA, 1992.
17. Joint Commission on Accreditation of Healthcare Organizations, Comprehensive Accreditation Manual for Hospitals: The Official Handbook, 2001.
18. Commission on Accreditation of Rehabilitation Facilities, Medical Rehabilitation Standards Manual, 2002.
19. Center for Disability Issues and the Health Professions, Center for Health Care Strategies, The Lewin Group, Performance Standards for Medi-Cal Managed Care Organizations Serving People with Disabilities and Chronic Conditions, California Health Care Foundation. November, 2005.

5 Role of Tax Law in the Development and Use of Accessible Medical Instrumentation

Steven Mendelsohn

CONTENTS

ABSTRACT

Combined with other laws and strategies, the U.S. tax law can contribute to the accessibility of the medical system in many ways. This chapter introduces some of the major areas in which tax law can play this role most effectively: for individual health care consumers, for private sector health care providers, for medical instrumentation manufacturers and designers, for nonprofit medical facilities, and for health insurance carriers.

5.1 INTRODUCTION

Discussions of medical technology often focus on diagnosis and treatment of disease and, indeed, our age continues to witness unparalleled breakthroughs that promise the prolongation of life and vast improvements in its quality. Lately, increasing attention has also been focused on the key role of the health care delivery system in assuring that new breakthroughs become available to the general public. Economics and technology both play an important role in these considerations of what may be called the health care infrastructure.

As important as medical research and treatment may be, their impact is reduced if people do not have access to the variety of equipment and devices needed for medical diagnosis, treatment, and monitoring. Many reasons have been identified as to why various subgroups of our population may face access barriers or be underserved medically. Economics, geography, consumer awareness, insurance practices, medical professional assumptions, and others all play a role. But for Americans with disabilities yet another, less often discussed and little understood set of variables are also at work.

Unless people with disabilities have full access to the growing array of medical diagnostic and treatment devices and resources that we group under the broad heading of medical instrumentation, their health status, both in connection with and unrelated to their disabilities, cannot be optimal. Access to today's medical technology is at least as important to people with disabilities as it is to the population at large.

When we think of people with disabilities facing barriers to health care, we typically think of economic or social factors. Although variables ranging from low income to limited insurance coverage do play important roles, another key set of variables relate to the design of medical equipment and facilities. Concern exists that much of today's medical equipment and instrumentation is designed in ways that make its use by and on behalf of people with various disabilities more difficult, more costly, or impossible.

The Americans with Disabilities Act of 1990 (ADA) has familiarized us with many of the issues surrounding access to the physical environment. It has brought about heightened attention to the role of architectural barriers (e.g., stairs without ramps or elevators) that prevent people with physical or mobility disabilities from entering or moving about in buildings housing medical facilities. It has brought about heightened attention to the need for effective communication between health care providers and patients and their families. But the ADA has not, and by its existing jurisdiction and terms likely cannot, exert direct influence on the design of the instruments, modalities, and procedures through which our health care is delivered and our health status assessed.

Until the day when equal access to medical instrumentation comes to be regarded as a civil right, the absence of laws explicitly compelling such access requires that a variety of other approaches also be adopted to ensure equitable access. Accordingly, it is the purpose of this chapter to analyze the applicability and to propose strategies for bringing to bear one of the mechanisms with the greatest potential for leveraging the development and dissemination of accessible medical instrumentation (AMI). No less than in so many other policy areas, that lever is the tax law.

At an accelerating pace in recent years, the tax system is becoming a principal instrument for the achievement of a growing array of public policy and economic goals throughout our society. From health care and education to energy exploration and manufacturing promotion, tax law has become the vehicle of choice for shifting the cost-benefit equation and influencing personal and organizational decision making in numerous spheres. If, as we believe it can, this lever can be used to provide incentives and reward the development and deployment of AMI, such opportunities should be vigorously pursued.

In order for the tax law to be marshaled in the service of equal access to health care, two issues must be addressed. First is the question of why AMI is so badly needed in our society and, second, the question of how the tax system can be effective in helping to bring about accessibility and why the tax system is an appropriate vehicle for the achievement of this goal. We begin with a brief discussion of the powerful rationale and pressing need for such equality.

5.2 EMERGING RECOGNITION OF THE PROBLEM

In July 2005, marking the 15th anniversary of enactment of the ADA, the U.S. Surgeon General issued a landmark report, "The Surgeon General's Call to Action to Improve the Health and Wellness of Persons with Disabilities" [1]. The report underscores the fact that people with disabilities face unique barriers to obtaining and using health care. Among the four goals articulated by the Surgeon General for helping people with disabilities to live healthy lives, two are particularly noteworthy here. These are, providing health care professionals with tools needed to screen, diagnose, and treat the whole person with a disability with dignity; and increasing "accessible health care and support services to promote independence for people with disabilities" [1].

As the National Institute on Disability and Rehabilitation Research (NIDRR) described the problem in its statement of the priority for the Rehabilitation Engineering Research Center on Accessible Medical Instrumentation (RERC-AMI): "This center must research, develop, and evaluate methods and technologies to increase the usability and accessibility of diagnostic, therapeutic, and procedural health care equipment for people with disabilities. This includes developing methods and technologies that are usable and accessible for patients and health care providers with disabilities" [2].

This broad definition of "diagnostic, therapeutic, and procedural health care equipment" covers a large proportion of the activities and interactions occurring within the health care system. In today's increasingly specialized, complex, test-driven, and technology-driven health care environment, few diagnostic procedures or treatment modalities remain that are not mediated by or evaluated through the use of some form of medical instrumentation. Health care practitioners and facilities are not reimbursed by insurers for the time they spend talking to patients or for the advice they give, but for the tests they conduct and the treatments they administer. One need only review one's own experience with the health care system to realize how pervasive medical equipment and instruments have become, and to understand how little treatment and care would be available if this equipment were inaccessible.

5.3 EXTENT OF THE PROBLEM

There are estimated to be over 50 million Americans with disabilities. Inasmuch as an estimated 40 to 45 million Americans have no health insurance, it is likely that some portion of the population with disabilities face barriers to health care resulting from lack of insurance coverage. But any and all of America's citizens with disabilities, insured or not, may face barriers to health care resulting from inaccessibility of equipment or information. If equipment is not available to facilitate safe transfer between a wheelchair and an examination table, if a suitably trained sign-language interpreter is not present to communicate the treatment options available or to explain to the patient when to hold breath and when to exhale, if accessible documentation or other effective communication strategies are not available to convey the contents of an informed consent form, if the test strip on a home test kit cannot be manipulated or its change of color cannot be seen by the intended user, if monitoring equipment cannot be read or operated independently — in short, if any of the myriad devices involved in health care cannot be used by the practitioner, patient, or nonprofessional caregiver, the effect may be little different than it would be if the test or treatment in question were deliberately withheld.

Parallel research by the RERC on AMI has shed light on the prevalence and seriousness of this problem (see Chapter 2 of this book). Based on this and other research, there are strong reasons for believing that the consequences of inaccessibility may be widespread and severe, both in public health and economic terms.

From the health standpoint, consequences are likely to be of two sorts. First, diagnostic and screening measures, including some performed at facilities and others performed at home, may not occur. Second, treatment compliance may be reduced by the inability of the patient to monitor key indicators, even to open medicine bottles or to read or understand usage instructions.

Additionally, accessibility-related considerations of relative time, cost, and difficulty may result in the alteration of diagnostic recommendations or treatment protocols from what would normally be used for the conditions or cases in question. If a certain test requires two extra staff members to lift a patient into an apparatus, the cost-benefit equation of ordering the test is inevitably changed.

The economic consequences of equipment inaccessibility likewise appear to fall into two categories. First, there are the heightened costs associated with improvising methods for the performance of certain tests or procedures, or the costs of finding alternative methods. Second, there are the all too familiar cost consequences to insurers, consumers, and society of delayed diagnosis or treatment.

No data have been found on the aggregate economic impact of delay or underutilization of medical care due to the inaccessibility of instrumentation. Extrapolating from what we know about the economic and human costs of delayed treatment generally, one has no difficulty concluding that all major sources for such delay or underutilization should be identified and avoided wherever possible.

5.4 ROLE OF TAX POLICY

Given the increasingly central role of technology-mediated interactions in the health care and insurance reimbursement systems of our country, it is fair to say that today, as a practical matter, access to health care means access to medical instrumentation. Whether any lack of access derives from economic causes or instrumentation inaccessibility, the results may often be the same. Fortunately, as intractable as economic barriers may often seem, we believe that means exist, including through use of the tax code, to greatly increase awareness about, research in, and availability of accessible medical instrumentation for facility-based and home-based use.

Even when accessible instrumentation exists, lack of knowledge on the part of practitioners or restrictive reimbursement practices of insurers may also serve to limit its availability in ways that lead to the same adverse results. For example, if the seven Principles of Universal Design ([10], see Chapter 6) were more widely incorporated into mainstream medical instrumentation, especially in the design of devices intended for consumer or home use, such situations could be made less frequent. Accordingly, two related goals of tax policy in this area should be to make utilization of existing accessibility strategies as feasible as possible and to encourage the creation and utilization of new products and designs that incorporate accessibility. Tax law can contribute to these goals, and it can make the development and use of AMI advantageous to all key decision makers and all parties in the health care system. But for the tax system to perform these critical functions, certain key definitions must be clarified. * Less tax on this equipment to encourage production.

5.5 DEFINITIONAL ISSUES

With the tax law, no less than with other strategies for encouraging or discouraging particular actions or practices, individuals and organizations need clear standards and definitions in order to do what is asked of them. For this reason, the brief history of accessibility shows that articulation, dissemination, and implementation of accessibility requirements has always depended on the creation of standards that relevant target audiences, most notably architects and building planners up to now, can use. Implementation of the building accessibility and barrier removal requirements of the ADA, for example, has depended on and evolved through the ADA Accessibility Guidelines (ADAAG), a major periodic revision of which is currently under review by the U.S. Department of Justice (DOJ) [3].

Within the tax area the need for definitions and standards is no less than in any other. In fact, the existence or nonexistence of clear guidelines bearing upon certain disability-related provisions of the tax code goes a long way toward explaining their apparent underutilization and limited impact [4].

Because previously adopted, accessibility-related provisions of the Internal Revenue Code (IRC) and of other laws will prove to be of value in designing provisions to stimulate accessibility in the medical instrumentation field, some review of the role of disability-related definitions in the tax code may prove useful here. At the outset, it is worth noting that major tax law changes often leave it to the Internal Revenue Service (IRS) to define key terms by implementing regulations. As the task of articulating and operationalizing accessibility standards for medical instrumentation will be complex and detailed, and because many of the key terms and concepts involved will be unfamiliar to many members of Congress who must enact any new law, to the IRS officials who must enforce them, and to the health care practitioners, tax professionals and medical consumers who must apply them, considerable clarity will be needed in the law. This is so in order to ensure a full understanding of the scope of the problem, to increase the likelihood that well-intentioned solutions will prove effective, and to preserve coherence and integrity in the enforcement of the law. For these reasons, this chapter will recommend procedures for developing guidelines to implement legal changes in the AMI area.

In this connection, two key concepts are most in need of definition. These are medical instrumentation and accessibility.

5.5.1 Medical Instrumentation

5.5.1.1 What is Medical Instrumentation?

Medical instrumentation is not a legal term. It exists in no statute and is a term of art. Nevertheless, consensus should not be hard to develop around what is and is not medical, based on the function a device serves or the intention it fulfills.

Concepts such as durable medical equipment (DME), medical necessity, and prosthetics or orthotics are widely understood, though not uniformly defined. Various payers and providers may define some of these terms differently, but what is important for this discussion is that none of these terms are nearly so broad as medical instrumentation. The existence of "durable" medical equipment, for example, presupposes the existence of other kinds of medical equipment that, because not expected to last for as long or for other reasons, are not deemed durable. But they are still medical, sometimes as equipment, sometimes as supplies.

Likewise, the existence of "medical necessity" as a criterion for the use or availability of a given item of equipment, and in particular for its coverage by insurance, may serve to distinguish between items that insurers will or will not cover, or between goods and services that various laws require or do not require to be covered, but no one would equate medical necessity with medical purpose or health-related function. Put another way, we need not trouble ourselves over the definition or applicability of concepts such as medical necessity, because no one would seriously dispute that items or services may have a medical nature or a health impact, even if not sufficiently "necessary" as to warrant insurance reimbursement or legally required provision.

In this light, a practical and workable definition of medical instrumentation for use by the tax system may prove easier to devise than it first appears. Properly understood, then, the definition of medical instrumentation must hinge not on any inherent or predetermined design feature, not on whether any insurance policy covers it, not on whether the item or procedure is subject to FDA review or testing, and not on whether its authorized providers are restricted by any professional licensure or certification requirements. Ultimately, consistent with the NIDRR priority quoted earlier, medical instrumentation can only be defined by the function and use of a device in the diagnosis, treatment or management of illness or in the assessment and preservation of health.

If we were talking about mandating accessibility, this definition of the scope of instrumentation might be too broad. But as we are talking only about tax-based incentives to voluntary actions, there is no danger that anyone will be forced to modify or redesign any devices or equipment who does not choose to, and no danger that instrumentation will have to be designed or modified in ways that their constituencies deem inappropriate.

Indeed, the greater danger arising from such a broad definition of medical instrumentation would be the claim that something is medical instrumentation when it in fact has some other purpose. This problem can readily be addressed by reference to how and by whom the product or device is marketed and used. No one could seriously argue that a violin is medical instrumentation because music therapy is a recognized treatment modality in certain circumstances. If violins were routinely marketed as therapeutic devices, it might be different, but even then, it would be quite reasonable to limit the tax benefit to those violins manufactured and marketed as therapeutic devices. Concerns about misuse of the "medical" in medical instrumentation are therefore largely without merit, hypothetical, and little different from similar concerns that have been encountered and resolved over the last three generations of income and excise tax administration.

5.5.1.2 What Is Instrumentation?

It is possible that defining the term *instrumentation* will prove more challenging than identifying what instrumentation is medical. The term instrumentation has no recognized legal meaning either. Once again, it is a term of art. Nonetheless, definitional problems are likely to arise only if an attempt is made to restrict the concept to capital goods, items that have a given useful life, devices that cost more than a certain amount, or items with some other predetermined features. Utilization of an expansive definition, once again focusing on context and purpose of use, should suffice to avoid most problems.

One additional measure will be needed to ensure a definition that is responsive to the scope of the problem. Delivery vehicles and packaging, such as the boxes in which bandages are sold or the bottles or other containers in which medicines are dispensed, will need to be included within the range of items encouraged by the tax law to be made more accessible. A subsequent technical paper will propose statutory language for presentation to Congress covering all pertinent definitional and substantive issues. In anticipation of that further effort, let us propose the following definition of medical instrumentation:

> Medical instrumentation includes but is not limited to any furniture, measuring device, device that comes in contact with or is designed to be manipulated, monitored or read by health care professionals, layperson caregivers or end-user patients themselves as part of the provision or the receipt of medical services, interventions or care, and any user-controlled software designed or required to be installed and used in connection with any such technology, or any process or control system with which patients or caregivers must interact in order for medical services, medical information, or treatment results to be achieved, measured or communicated. This definition includes scanning devices into which people must fit, tables on which they must lie, test strips that they must apply and monitor, probes they must insert, gauges they must read, collection devices they must manipulate and any software, keypads, or control panels they must use to operate such devices or to access the information generated by such devices. Such definition shall also include any packaging, protective or storage containers, and mediums or materials that must be opened, closed or otherwise manipulated or used in order to utilize the instrumentation, maintain the instrumentation, obtain, utilize, store or communicate information generated from use of the instrumentation.

Given the changes currently occurring in health care and the law surrounding it, it may be useful to augment this tentative definition with the following: "This definition also includes all notices, package inserts, informed consent forms, and other documents and formal communications required by law to be provided, signed or maintained as an incident of the provision of medical services and care."

* tax benefits for barrier removal

5.5.2 Accessibility

If "accessible" medical instrumentation is to be encouraged through the tax law, then *accessibility,* too, must be defined. Numerous accessibility standards exist in various settings. These include standards for the accessibility of electronic and information technology (E&IT) [5], for the accessibility of Web sites [6], and of course, perhaps most widely known, for the accessibility of buildings and facilities under the ADA [3]. None of these standards has any direct role in the tax system. That is to say, compliance or noncompliance with them, though sometimes useful as evidence of intention, does not by itself trigger the granting or withholding of any tax benefit.

But we do have other accessibility standards that trigger the availability of tax benefits, when complied with. Two disability-related provisions of the Internal Revenue Code (IRC) illustrate the different ways accessibility definitions have been approached under the tax law. Under the architectural and transportation barrier removal deduction [7], businesses are entitled to a tax deduction of up to $15,000 per year for the costs of removing architectural and transportation barriers to the "elderly and handicapped." But it is not left up to the business to decide what is defined as a barrier or what constitutes successful barrier removal. The regulations implementing the statute include detailed lists of specifications, drawn from other federal laws, in regard to such physical features as sidewalks, doorways, restrooms, water fountains, and pay phones. Barrier removal expenses will qualify for the deduction if they are carried out in conformity with these design guidelines.

Use of such guidelines also largely avoids any disputes over intent. By contrast, the approach taken under another tax statute, the disabled access credit (DAC) [8], is somewhat different. This provision applies only to small businesses, as defined under the law. It authorizes a tax credit of 50% of the first $10,000 per year, over an initial outlay of $250, of what are termed *eligible access expenditures*. These expenditures are broadly defined as those incurred in order for the small business to comply with the ADA, and they include expenses for the "acquisition or modification of equipment."

The DAC statute, which was enacted in 1990 just months after passage of the ADA, directed the IRS to develop regulations to implement its provisions, but this has not been done. As a result, one must look to case law for the definitional standards that determine compliance. On examining the relatively few cases that have been decided under the provision [9], the criteria that emerge as decisive in evaluating claims for the credit are the function of the item or service purchased, the intention underlying the expenditure, and the possibility of violating the ADA if the item is not provided. Thus, under the DAC there is no official or uniform standard of accessibility, and small businesses are likely left somewhat confused as to when they can safely claim the credit.

Medical instrumentation is, of course, quite variable, and different products, devices, and settings may raise very different issues. An additional problem that needs to be confronted in articulating a definition of accessibility for medical instrumentation is the range of contexts in which the definition would have to be used. For example, with the DAC, where a business is buying or modifying a device or instrument for the use of its employees or customers with disabilities, the device or instrument, by definition, exists. Its features and functions can be assessed and verified. But the medical instrumentation provisions must cover a wider range of settings. In order to be effective, these definitions will have to provide tax benefits not only to the practitioners or health care facilities that buy and use the instrumentation, not only to the consumers and families who purchase the devices for use at home, but also to manufacturers and designers who create or attempt to create the items. As such, the tax benefit will need to be available to encourage accessible design research, meaning that the tax benefit will sometimes have to be granted before a device exists in the marketplace, perhaps on occasion even when, despite best efforts, no effective product is ever created. In such a case, intention, along with results, has to be taken into account. Fortunately, as will be shown later in our discussion of the research tax credit, ample precedent and methodology exists within the annals of tax administration for dealing with such situations in which intent and motive become key variables.

The procedural approach recommended for this accessibility standards-setting effort involves the delegation of authority by Congress to an appropriate entity charged with responsibility to develop detailed guidelines. This entity should take as a point of departure the Principles of Universal Design developed at the North Carolina State University's Center for Universal Design [10].

The best organizational model for such a standards-setting effort is the Section 508 electronic and information technology (E&IT) accessibility guidelines developed, under the auspices of the Architectural and Transportation Barriers Compliance Board (The Access Board), by the Electronic and Information Technology Access Advisory Committee (EITAAC), an ad hoc consumer–industry–government panel created to put flesh and bones on to the accessibility requirements of the law [11]. Ideally, these guidelines would be developed in close conjunction with all relevant federal health agencies, including the FDA and the Centers for Medicare and Medicaid Services (CMS), and would be subject to adoption by the IRS.

Pending that elaboration, it may be useful to provide a tentative definition of accessibility of AMI for tax law purposes. Accessibility does not mean that consumers should be enabled to perform do-it-yourself brain surgery. It does mean that an instrument is inaccessible where its use for its intended and customary health-related purposes, in its intended environments, by or on behalf of persons ordinarily expected to use or benefit from it, is rendered impossible by reason of the presence or absence of features or characteristics that render the instrumentation inaccessible to or unusable by persons with disabilities. As a practical matter, this means that where vision is required for instrumentation's use, alternatives, such as audio or tactile, should be available to facilitate the necessary input and output. It means that where grasping ability or strength are required to access or use instrumentation, clear standards need to exist as to the maximum amount of pressure, strength, or dexterity that should be required. And it means that where transfer, such as between wheelchair and examining table, is required, either an appropriate height-adjustable table should be used or other suitable lift equipment should be on hand.

All these specifications and more can be operationalized for tax law and other purposes. Many already have been in a variety of standards-setting contexts. It remains to refine and apply these standards to the medical instrumentation setting.

One major effort to operationalize such definitions and standards is underway currently. As the result of a settlement in a class action lawsuit brought under California state law, the Kaiser Permanente organization is engaged in a multiyear effort to achieve accessibility of its facilities and services to its members with disabilities. A follow-up paper will include details on the standards and methods growing out of this effort.

5.6 THE MARKETPLACE

5.6.1 The Commercial Marketplace

A recent item published in a Massachusetts General Hospital newsletter indicated that increasing obesity in the American population is creating problems for the use of MRI machines and other scanning and diagnostic equipment [12]. Increasing numbers of people cannot fit in or on the apparatuses, and various devices cannot operate under the weight of some of the patients who need to use them.

The marketplace is already responding to this problem. Because larger apertures, stronger tables, and other obesity-sensitive modifications are needed, the buyers, sellers, and designers of medical-testing equipment are working together to meet the need. But when it comes to the comparable needs of people with disabilities for specialized or modified design to meet their medical access concerns, history gives little reason for confidence that the marketplace will do the same job. Why the marketplace provides a solution in the one case but not in the other is a subject well beyond the scope of this chapter. Yet, regardless of its causes, it is this very disparity, this failure of the market to accommodate to the needs of medical consumers and practitioners with disabilities, that gives rise to the need for legal measures.

Laws to compel accessibility as a matter of civil rights, including laws requiring health care facilities to treat people with disabilities nondiscriminatorily, continue to play an important role, but for a variety of reasons it seems unlikely that the goals of AMI can be well served or significantly advanced through primary reliance on mandates. When we ask what kinds of laws are best suited to reduce the unintended but pervasive discrimination and the serious harm resulting from inaccessibility, the weight of evidence, logic, and contemporary sensibilities strongly falls on the side of laws that encourage and reward industry, practitioners, and consumers for doing what we believe to be the right thing. Few bodies of law are more effective or more frequently relied upon to create incentives and disincentives than the tax law.

With this in mind, let us examine what the tax law currently offers consumers and users, sellers, and creators of AMI, and let us discuss possible modifications in the law that could contribute significantly to the supply, quality, and affordability of such resources.

5.6.2 The Tax Marketplace

Before turning to the discussion of existing provisions and recommended amendments, though, let us pause to note that the marketplace for tax law, that is, the context in which taxes are discussed and legislated, the parts of our lives where tax law is used to influence actions and decisions, has itself undergone dramatic change in recent years. Unless we have a sense of these changes, both major opportunities and serious risks associated with tax-oriented advocacy may be overlooked.

* The role of tax policy

5.6.2.1 Harnessing the System

As noted in the introduction to this chapter, tax policy has never played so central a role in overall economic development policy as it does now. Indeed, the current federal administration appears to believe that tax cuts are the key to economic growth, almost without regard to what other measures might be available. In such an atmosphere, it is not surprising that attention should turn to tax policy as an important tool for advancing a variety of agendas, including the cause of AMI.

We also come to this discussion with our nation poised on the brink of potentially massive changes in the ways in which we levy and collect taxes. The administration has identified overhaul of the tax code as one of the president's key second term domestic goals. Under these circumstances, it becomes even more timely to turn our attention to the question of how tax system reforms can be designed to include greater access to equal and adequate medical services and care.

It is easy to advocate for any sort of outlandish tax proposal. One can find many examples of recommendations and proposals that people with disabilities should be entitled to automatic tax benefits of this or that amount, for one or another purpose, or based solely on their disabled status. Until recently, tax proposals of this or any sort were subject to scoring, meaning that their net revenue implications for the federal treasury (the amount they would cost compared to the amount they would bring in or save) over a fixed number of years had to be estimated, as best the Congressional Budget Office (CBO) and sometimes the Office of Management and Budget (OMB) could make such forecasts. Tax proposals are still subject to scoring, but a related requirement no longer seems to hold much sway.

Until 4 years ago, proposals, particularly tax-cut proposals, had to be revenue-neutral. This means that if they would result in decreases in federal revenue, methods and timeframes for offsetting those losses had to be identified. These could involve increases in other revenue sources, decreases in spending, sometimes changes in accounting techniques, or a combination of these and other methods. But in the early days of the current administration, large proposed tax cuts, such as those adopted in 2001, came to be justified on the grounds that they would create jobs and lead in the long run to economic growth. With that long-term expectation in mind, revenue neutrality and the need to identify offsets for revenue losses to the treasury were set aside.

Today, no one seriously attempts to impose revenue neutrality on proposed tax cuts or on the repeal of taxes. But other, new justifications, carrying with them new possibilities, have been introduced into tax policy debates. More and more, the justification for large or permanent tax cuts is predicated upon moral as much as economic grounds. It is increasingly believed that it is morally wrong to tax wealth, because to do so is to punish its creators, stifle incentive, or unjustly deprive its rightful inheritors. It is largely on this basis that one recent study concludes advocates for repeal of the inheritance tax were able to convince millions of Americans who would never be touched by it, and whose own taxes would have to absorb the shortfall resulting from its elimination, that repeal of the inheritance tax was a matter of morality and justice [13].

Whatever one may think of the merit of such arguments, they surely open the way for the making of other kinds of moral or justice arguments as well. In such a climate as today's, and in so much more emotional a tax environment, ethical and equity arguments of all kinds can perhaps be advanced with less embarrassment and more plausibility than in the past. This does not mean that the hard-core practical and economic benefits of AMI can or should be overlooked. On the contrary, these benefits should be probed and emphasized. But at the same time, arguments of justice, going beyond simple tax justice, may have a place in tax law deliberations today that they did not have even a few short years ago.

Discussions of tax policy can now take into account considerations that would have been unwise to raise in the past. That may open opportunities for new kinds of advocacy on behalf of accessibility.

None of this means that traditional approaches to structuring and understanding the tax law or arguments of cost benefit can be overlooked or abandoned. Nor does it suggest that traditional arguments of cost benefit can be overlooked. And it does not mean that one can safely or credibly engage in tax debates without rigorous analysis or without all possible information. But it does mean that emotional arguments once considered disreputable or naive may have found a place at the table.

All the proposals offered in the next section of this chapter are grounded in the demonstrable and unassailable advantages to our nation of achieving health parity for Americans with and without disabilities. But they are grounded, too, in an equity and ethical framework that goes beyond the economic, national security, or other practical benefits of accessibility. All the proposals advanced here will use existing features of the tax law as precedents and all recommendations will use concepts and techniques that are already well understood by Congress and familiar to tax professionals in the accounting community and in the IRS. In this way, a baseline of shared experience and common understanding can be established from which serious and informed debate can proceed. The issues surrounding accessibility may be new and strange to many in the tax and policy-making arena, but the language in which those issues are discussed will be reassuringly familiar.

5.6.2.2 The Beneficiaries of Tax Reform

An understanding of the tax marketplace also requires that we have some sense both of who needs to be convinced of the merits of our cause, and of who needs to be affected if the goals of reform are to be achieved.

Because our recommendations will address the groups who need to be affected and who most need to be convinced, let us address some key assumptions. For tax law to have a major impact on the accessibility of medical instrumentation, it needs to increase supply, stimulate demand, and lower costs. To achieve any one, or even two of these goals without the third will result in very limited success, perhaps in failure.

Reforms need to reach various groups. They need to encourage industry to develop and market accessible products. They must encourage private sector users of medical instrumentation such as hospitals, doctors, and skilled nursing facilities to purchase, use, recommend, and distribute accessible instrumentation. They need to find some way to make the purchase, use and dissemination of accessible instrumentation financially attractive to not-for-profit and public sector users of medical instrumentation who do not themselves pay taxes. They must give insurance companies reasons to provide AMI when it is available and to seek more of it when it is not, and finally, the tax law must make it possible for consumers who purchase medical instrumentation for use at home to obtain accessible instrumentation more often, more conveniently, and at equal or lesser cost to inaccessible versions.

5.7 OPPORTUNITIES AND BARRIERS UNDER CURRENT LAW

5.7.1 Health Care Consumers

Consumers are critical to the accessibility equation. Because many items of medical instrumentation used in the home will not be covered by insurance, consumer purchasing power is likely to play a pivotal role in many sectors of the instrumentation market. Moreover, to the extent accessible devices can be made more available and affordable, demand for such instrumentation can be expected to increase in ways to which other participants in the health care system will be obliged to respond. Let us examine existing provisions that could form the basis for this consumer's own accessibility.

Even for people who have health insurance, out-of-pocket costs for medical care, including deductibles, copayments, exclusions, and costs for noncovered items, are likely to rise steadily in the coming years. Accessible instrumentation, where available, is likely to be paid for with a disproportionately large amount of consumers' own funds.

5.7.1.1 The Medical Expense Deduction

5.7.1.1.1 Current Law

Under current law, individuals and families can deduct the costs of medical expenses under two major provisions. First, most medical equipment needed for the diagnosis, monitoring, treatment, or mitigation (including functional mitigation or amelioration through use of such assistive technology (AT) as wheelchairs, hearing aids, augmentative communications devices, or optical character recognition software) would qualify for the medical expense deduction [4].

But the medical expense deduction is very limited in its applicability and in the number of people it can benefit. In the first place, the medical expense deduction is an itemized deduction available on individuals' and families' personal returns. As such, similar to other itemized deductions, it is available only to those who itemize. A variety of considerations determine whether taxpayers choose to itemize or to claim the standard deduction, but less than 40% of taxpayers do itemize, according to recent statistics. This means that any benefits associated with the deductibility of medical expenses, including the deductibility of the costs of accessible medical equipment, are rendered unavailable to these more than 60% of taxpayers who do not itemize.

A related barrier to the use of the medical expense deduction to meet the costs of home-based medical instrumentation is that the medical expense deduction was designed to help offset catastrophic costs only. This is why it is available only for qualifying medical expenses that exceed 7.5% of the individual's or family's adjusted gross income (AGI). Of course, the lower a person's income, and hence the lower their AGI, the sooner will the 7.5% threshold be reached. But the irony here is that for people with low incomes who experience high medical costs, it is all too likely that the available medical expense deduction will exceed the tax they owe. In such a case, they will lose part of the value of their deduction, because itemized deductions cannot be used to reduce taxes below zero, and cannot even be used to offset Social Security or Medicare tax on wages.

A related fact of note here is that the medical expense deduction in no way responds to the probability that accessible medical equipment, if available, is likely to be more expensive than its inaccessible counterparts. Indeed, far from responding to this fact, current patterns of tax administration in the medical expense sphere may actually make it somewhat more difficult to deduct the extra costs related to accessibility. This occurs when those extra costs, rather than being for the device itself, are for research, travel or training necessary to obtain or learn to use accessible devices. Numerous technicalities surrounding the medical-expense-related deductibility of telephone usage, transportation, and lodgings away from home, or other contingent expenses, not to mention training and follow-up assistance, make it hard for the individual taxpayer to feel confident that all legitimate costs associated with getting and utilizing accessible versions of medical equipment will be entitled to medical deductions without challenge.

A final limitation on the existing law arises in situations where the costs of AMI, while substantial, do not amount to more than 7.5% of AGI, or where those costs combined with other deductions do not rise to the level that would permit itemization at all. In those cases too, the value of medical instrumentation deductibility is lost.

5.7.1.1.2 Potential Solutions

Within the framework of the existing medical expense deduction provisions, no strategy exists for enhancing the availability of accessible medical instrumentation or for lowering its costs to the end user. Fundamental changes in the approach to tax-system subsidization of medical expenses are definitely in order, but it is unlikely that any of these strategies would target medical instrumentation in isolation from medical treatment, let alone that accessible medical instrumentation would or could be singled out from standard instrumentation for special tax treatment.

Various suggestions have been made over the years to treat certain add-on costs of living with a disability differently from other medical or work expenses. These proposals usually focus either on creation of a new deduction or on the creation of a disability tax credit. If done as a new deduction, the proposed deduction would be of the above-the-line variety, meaning that it would be available whether or not taxpayers with disabilities were in a position to itemize. As a tax credit, the benefit would also offset taxes without regard to itemization. Some proposals for this credit call for it to be a refundable credit, such as the earned income tax credit (EITC), meaning that even if its value exceeded the individual's tax liability, the government would pay the individual or family its entire value.

Whatever the merit or feasibility of proposals such as these, they have implications going far beyond medical instrumentation and, hence, are outside the scope of this chapter. As they relate to the broad range of add-on and access costs incurred by people with disabilities in all areas of life, they are worthy of further refinement and discussion. However, care should be taken that the benefits of any tax-favored treatment for accessibility are not limited to consumers with disabilities as defined by the ADA or under any particular law. Such a limitation would inevitably and destructively shift the focus of every dispute away from accessibility to a jurisdictional inquiry based on whether the consumer qualified as an individual with a disability. The goals of broadly encouraging accessibility would not be served by such a focus.

Another more insidious potential problem with special treatment for add-on medical instrumentation–accessibility costs is that such treatment could actually hinder the growth of universal design (UD). Given the lack of consensus around accounting standards for distinguishing the basic from the add-on accessibility cost components of universally–designed devices, vendors and consumers might find it more effective, even if sometimes more expensive, to focus on assistive technology (AT)–based rather than universally designed devices.

Tax preparers and examiners should be trained to understand the nature and role of accessible medical instrumentation, so that the extra costs of such equipment will not give rise to unnecessary questions about the legitimacy of or necessity for the deductions claimed. But even if such training is provided, and even if the full potential of the existing medical expense deduction is more widely understood and more fully realized, the medical expense deduction as currently constituted holds little opportunity for helping to lower the cost of accessible medical instrumentation for consumers with disabilities and their families.

5.7.1.2 Health Savings Accounts

5.7.1.2.1 Current Law

As added to the law by the Medicare Modernization Act of 2003, [14], health savings accounts (HSAs) actually do not have much to do with Medicare at all. Applicable to private insurance, HSAs help subsidize the purchase of health insurance policies with large deductibles. They do this by allowing tax deferral of substantial amounts of money that can then be used tax-free to meet those deductibles, and they further allow the individual to keep much of this money if it remains unspent after a sufficient period of time.

The logic is twofold — first, tax deferral of funds needed to pay deductibles will encourage people to purchase lower premium, higher-deductible health insurance coverage; second, the opportunity to keep what they do not spend will encourage consumers to be frugal in the expenditure of health care funds.

From the standpoint of its potential to contribute to the accessibility of medical instrumentation, the problem with the HSA approach is that it links the benefits of the HSA too closely to what insurers will pay for. That is to say, it creates no incentive for insurers to pay for accessibility. If anything, it creates a safety valve to dissipate demands that they do so. At the same time, although it helps policyholders to pay for all their out-of-pocket deductibles, it does nothing in particular to help them pay for accessibility or to bring the price of accessibility down.

For HSAs to be effective in subsidizing the costs of accessible medical instrumentation or stimulating its availability, attention will have to be directed to broadening the coverage of these devices and instruments under existing insurance policies. For example, many anecdotal reports have been received of insurers paying for standard versions of diabetes testing and monitoring equipment but refusing to pay for talking glucometers for blind individuals. Various reasons are reported for these refusals: because the insurers have contracts with only one supplier that does not provide the accessible devices, because of per-item cost caps, or because the insurers contend that the add-on accessibility feature is a convenience item rather than a medical necessity.

5.7.1.2.2 Potential Solution

Except for encouraging insurers to offer high-deductible, lower-cost policies that interface with the HSA, nothing about the HSA lends itself to influencing what insurers do or what their policies cover. Accordingly, there is no reason to believe that the HSA can be used to leverage any broadening of coverage so far as AMI is concerned. Hence, the HSA holds out little prospect of generating added sales volume or consumer demand in this area.

In order for the HSA concept (which is likely to be extended, through cash-and-counseling and life-account programs, to many Medicaid recipients in the near future) to be effective in stimulating demand for accessible versions of medical instrumentation, insurers would have to be required to pay for accessible versions or accessibility add-ons if they pay for the basic inaccessible item. This could be accomplished, among other means, through changes in the rules governing the taxation of insurers, which are beyond the scope of this chapter. Such changes, embodying as they do an element of coercion, are unlikely to gain political traction in the current legal environment and would not likely be very effective if enacted.

But the improbability of compelling insurers to do anything does not mean that HSA reform plays no potential role here. At the very least, the sums that taxpayers are permitted to defer (or eventually exclude) from taxation through HSAs should be increased by the add-on costs of access in those situations in which the insurer pays for the inaccessible version of some device. This means that if a health plan would pay for a standard blood pressure gauge but refused to pay for an accessible, speech-output one where needed, any added cost to the consumer resulting from this refusal should be added to the amount that the consumer can put into the HSA.

5.7.1.3 Employment

5.7.1.3.1 Current Law

People who work for a living are entitled to an itemized deduction for certain employee business expenses, if such expenses exceed 2% of their AGI [14]. Expenses covered by this deduction would include those required but not paid for by the employer or by a union, such as union dues, uniforms, uncompensated business travel, professional organization memberships, etc.

A broader version of this provision applies to workers who incur impairment-related work expenses (IRWE) [15] in order to work. Such expenses are available as an itemized deduction to employees with disabilities but are not subject to the 2% threshold. Although medical instrumentation is ordinarily considered inherently personal in nature, and as such not deductible under a business or employment rationale even if used for work, there are some occasions when the nature and use of medical instrumentation would qualify it for the IRWE deduction. As the law presently exists, these occasions are likely to be very limited, however.

If any item of instrumentation, whether deemed medical or not, is used both at home and in the workplace, its costs can be allocated between personal and business components. Various formulas have been used for dividing the cost between the two categories. If that is done, then the deductibility of the IRWE part would not depend upon the deductibility of the personal/medical component. The taxpayer would still need to itemize, but the IRWE deduction would be available even if one's medical expenses did not reach the 7.5% of AGI threshold necessary for their deductibility. Under these circumstances, though the costs of accessible devices would likely be deductible to the same extent as any other IRWE costs, nothing in the law particularly encourages or especially rewards the purchase or use of accessible items.

5.7.1.3.2 Potential Solution

There is no plausible way for the IRWE deduction, even if clarified and enhanced, to do much either to reduce the consumer's costs of accessible technology or, by reducing that cost, to stimulate awareness and demand for such technology. However, if various business tax credits (such as the disabled access credit discussed in subsection 5.5.2) were made available to employed persons themselves, typically on the theory that they are engaged in the business of earning money through employment, then accessibility could be advantaged in a number of ways. For many reasons, though, this is unlikely to happen.

5.7.1.4 Status of Being an Individual with a Disability

In Subsection 5.7.1, proposals for creating some tax benefits specifically for people with disabilities were mentioned. Similar proposals could be made more narrowly, in connection with the costs of medical instrumentation only. But serious concerns are warranted that such an approach to identifying individuals with disabilities for tax benefits would have counterproductive and potentially very harmful effects.

As pointed out earlier and stressed again here, under any formulation that conditions the availability of tax benefit on the status of the taxpayer as an individual with a disability, there is always a risk that changing definitions of disability will create confusion and uncertainty. Anyone who has followed the series of court decisions interpreting the ADA will appreciate how this is so [16]. One of the themes running through these decisions has been the effort by courts to narrow the definition of disability, with the result that fewer and fewer people meet the legal test. If the availability of tax benefits is tied to an individual's status as a person with a disability, then rulings eliminating people from protection under civil rights laws will also have the effect of limiting the availability of disability-related tax benefits.

If the tax law were to use disability status as any sort of trigger or jurisdictional basis for the availability of any tax benefits, the definition of disability would inevitably become the focal issue in most cases. It is far better for the nature of the equipment and the circumstances of its use to determine the applicability of any tax benefits that may exist. If our goal is to increase the use and availability of accessible instrumentation, our approach must concentrate upon the equipment itself.

5.7.1.5 Flexible Spending Accounts

Our discussion would not be complete without mentioning one of the most important sources of funding for medical expenses not covered by insurance. This is the flexible spending account (FSA) offered by many employers as part of their fringe benefits program.

5.7.1.5.1 Current Law

Under the FSA, employees are allowed to set aside money each year to pay for noncovered medical costs with pretax dollars. Because the amounts set aside by the employees are excluded from their taxable income, the net effect is the same as if they had been able to claim a deduction for the expense. In fact, the value is often greater, among other reasons, because none of the complexities associated with itemizing need be confronted.

As it relates to AMI, the FSA presents two questions: Can funds be used to meet any incremental costs associated with accessibility, and is there any way that accessibility can be preferred over inaccessible items within the framework of the plans?

With respect to the first question, the law is ambiguous. To the degree that AMI or any other expense would qualify for the medical deduction if paid for out of pocket, fringe benefit plans have no legal basis for restricting coverage more narrowly than the IRS does. But at the same time the law grants plan administrators considerable discretion in what goods and services they will cover. This means that situations will arise in which plans refuse to reimburse, albeit out of one's own funds, for AMI.

5.7.1.5.2 *Potential Solution*

In many cases where such refusals occur, the reason may be lack of awareness on the part of plan administrators as to what accessibility means or as to its deductibility. Under those circumstances, it should often be possible, by explaining the facts fully to the plan administrator, to get the decision reversed. In some cases, this reversal may require amendment of the plan, and the difficulty of that may often be overestimated or overstated.

This leads us to the second question. Accessibility could be encouraged under the FSA format by requiring that where plans cover given items or services, they must cover accessible versions, where available. Failure to do so should be considered as putting the plan out of compliance with not only the IRC but with the other major laws governing fringe benefit plans.

5.7.1.6 Summary of Tax Provisions for Individuals

Viewed from the standpoint of the existing range of tax benefits available to individuals, little meaningful opportunity exists to build upon current law in ways that could materially increase demand or reduce costs for AMI. But this does not mean that consumers cannot be actively involved in the process. Even if the tax law as presently constituted can do little to help them directly, consumer behavior and demand remain key to the tax decisions that will influence the behavior of other target groups. Recommendations made in connection with the other target groups should result in significant cost reductions and availability enhancements. These developments should empower consumers in new and important ways.

5.7.2 Private Sector Health Care Providers

The private health care provider component of the health care system consists of physicians and other health care practitioners, certain hospitals, pharmacies, and many nursing homes, to name the most prominent examples. These health care providers purchase medical instrumentation for use in their work, typically at their facilities, on behalf of patients. They also directly distribute, prescribe, or recommend instrumentation of many kinds for home use.

As care providers, private sector medical facilities need to be concerned with the ability of their staffs to operate the equipment required to be used in the course of their work. They are also concerned with the ability of their patients to follow through on treatment programs, testing, and monitoring that may be indicated.

A number of existing business-related tax law provisions seem applicable to enhancing the use of AMI by these health care providers. Some of them are specific to entities that serve patients or customers (as these do), whereas others would be generally applicable in all for-profit settings.

5.7.2.1 Depreciation

5.7.2.1.1 *Current Law*

When businesses buy capital equipment (items expected to have a useful life exceeding 1 year) they generally deduct its cost over a period of years, rather than all in the year of purchase. The logic of this is that because the item will be used over a number of years, the tax deduction attributable to it should also be spread over a number of years, so that it is deducted as used. Generous provisions have been added to the law allowing many businesses to nevertheless deduct substantial amounts of their capital costs in the year the equipment is purchased [17]. When such costs are deducted or written off in the year incurred, it is called expensing.

Virtually anything that a for-profit business buys for use in conducting its activities is tax deductible. Accessibility considerations may change the amount of these costs, but they do not ordinarily alter the allocation of costs between depreciating and expensing. It is conceivable, however, that additional costs attributable to accessibility could bring otherwise expensable costs above the allowable dollar limit. Simple strategies exist for preventing this from happening.

5.7.2.1.2 *Potential Solution*

All limits on expensing should be waived for purchases by health care providers of equipment that meets accessibility standards. Although this would do nothing for AMI that is not capital equipment, which would have been expensed in any case, it will help with the big-ticket items such as imaging equipment, examination suites, and the like.

5.7.2.2 Disabled Access Credit

5.7.2.2.1 *Current Law*

As discussed earlier, small businesses that incur eligible access expenditures in order to meet their obligations under the ADA are allowed a significant tax credit [1]. Interestingly, most of the cases interpreting this provision have involved health care facilities' purchases of equipment for the purpose of better accommodating their patients with disabilities. Taken together, these cases reflect a narrow interpretation of the provision on the part of the IRS. A detailed analysis of the decisions is beyond the scope of our present inquiry; it is enough to note that the IRS has essentially taken the view that unless the equipment was obtained to avoid outright violation of the ADA, the DAC will not be allowed. Despite this unfortunate interpretation of the law, the DAC still represents an important tool for subsidizing the cost and encouraging the use of AMI.

5.7.2.2.2 *Potential Solution*

A number of steps are urgently required here. First, all instrumentation that complies with accessibility standards should automatically be made eligible for the credit. Second, the current \$5,000 limit on the size of the annual credit (50% of the first \$10,000 in eligible expenditures) should be eliminated, so that all expenditures for items that are accessible qualify for it.

Some will argue that application of the credit to all accessibility expenditures, whether or not required by the ADA or incurred in order to comply with the ADA, would create an undue risk of abuse. Their argument goes that without the baseline of the ADA, firms could pass off any number of unrelated expenditures as intended to accommodate customers or employees with disabilities.

The existence of accessibility guidelines would ensure that whatever is claimed under the credit will, in fact, be accessible. Moreover, it is a change in the credit that we are proposing, one that expands its focus from the ADA in particular to accessibility in general. What should be covered by the credit, without limit, are expenditures for AMI. There are many other expenditures made for the purpose of enhancing accessibility, but these are beyond the scope of the reforms being recommended here.

An additional issue relates to the size of businesses and medical facilities covered by the DAC. Existing upper limits on size of qualifying businesses (namely, fewer than 30 full-time employees or preceding year gross receipts under \$1 million) should be waived when it comes to AMI expenses. But there is another limit that also must be eliminated.

Many medical facilities have fewer than 15 full-time employees, and hence are not subject to the employment-related provisions of Title I of the ADA. Although not made clear in published rulings, IRS appears to take the position that such firms cannot claim the DAC in connection with expenditures incurred to accommodate their employees. Once again, the logic seems to be that as discrimination against these employees could not violate the ADA, the DAC does not apply.

This view is extremely short-sighted, both in light of the purpose of the DAC and because many small employers are covered by state employment antidiscrimination laws that may apply to firms with fewer than 15 workers. Why the benefits of the DAC should be denied them, especially when they are acting to comply with the law of their states, is hard to understand.

All size-based restrictions should be dropped, so that expenditures for the purchase, lease, or other use of AMI on behalf of employees (permanent or temporary, salaried or contractual) will be eligible for the credit.

5.7.2.3 Barrier Removal Deduction

5.7.2.3.1 Current Law

As described earlier, the architectural and transportation barrier (ATB) removal deduction is available to businesses of any size. One may ask why we need a deduction for these barrier removal costs. After all, aren't the ordinary and necessary expenses of operating a business deductible anyway? The answer is that yes, barrier removal expenses are deductible, but as they typically involve alterations to facilities, they will frequently be capital expenses. That means they would normally be deductible over a period of years. What the barrier removal deduction does is allow up to $15,000 in such expenses per year to be expensed. This acceleration in the rate at which they are written off constitutes a tax benefit.

As a guidelines-driven provision, the barrier removal deduction is conducive to application in other guidelines-based assessments. But its application to AMI is not possible now, because the barrier removal deduction is usable only with a narrow range of expenses.

5.7.2.3.2 Potential Solution

Realistically, as the proportion of public buildings and facilities built or renovated since enactment of the ADA increases, the role of the ATB has steadily declined. Inaccessibility certainly remains a barrier, but not limited to architectural or physical barriers only. Barriers to programmatic access and to the receipt of equal health care services, whether or not amounting to violation of law, are worthy of and much in need of being addressed by the ATB. As such, strong arguments exist for extending the deduction in ways that would contribute to the willingness and ability of health care providers to utilize AMI.

Once more, the principal area for this extension would be on behalf of firms that do not qualify for the DAC and that incur expenses for what would otherwise be capital equipment that would not qualify for any existing tax benefit.

5.7.3 Medical Instrumentation Manufacturers and Designers

5.7.3.1 Research and Development Credit

5.7.3.1.1 Current Law

One provision of the tax law that has been of benefit to many businesses is the research or research and development (R&D) credit [18]. Originally scheduled to expire on December 31, 2004, this credit has been extended for two years, through December 31, 2006. In essence, it converts certain expenses of R&D from capital expenses or ordinary deductions into a tax credit. Thus, the law is not creating any new tax benefits but it is accelerating the speed at which the benefit can be realized, because a tax credit comes off the bottom-line tax bill whereas a deduction simply reduces the income on which tax is paid.

5.7.3.1.2 Potential Solution

With a few minor modifications (which will be proposed with supporting statutory language in a subsequent technical paper), the R&D credit lends itself very well to developmental and basic research efforts on behalf of accessibility in the medical instrumentation area. Provisions should be included that will encourage and assure the participation of people with disabilities at the earliest possible stages of product conceptualization and development. To achieve this goal, provisions will be recommended to include interview or focus group research and other consumer outreach activities in the types of expenses eligible for the credit. In addition, the law should be clarified to recognize that accessibility is a permissible objective and to authorize application of accessibility standards to the evaluation of claims for the credit.

5.7.3.2 Work Opportunity Tax Credit

5.7.3.2.1 Current Law

The work opportunity credit (WOC) provides employers with a tax credit of up to $2400 for the hiring of members of designated target groups who face barriers to employment. People with disabilities are not explicitly included among the target groups, but two of those groups are, as a practical matter, composed almost entirely of people with disabilities. Those are supplemental security income (SSI) recipients and persons referred by state vocational rehabilitation (VR) agencies. By using the logic of the credit, it may prove possible to harness this provision of the tax law in the service of accessibility.

5.7.3.2.2 Potential Solution

In addition to using the credit for the hiring of people who need help finding jobs, it makes sense to use it to help businesses defray the costs of hiring personnel with special expertise in disability and accessibility, whose time will be dedicated to improving accessibility of the firm's products.

5.7.4 Nonprofit Medical Facilities

Public and nonprofit institutions play a key role in the delivery of facility-based health care and in the provision of medical instrumentation for home use. Any comprehensive strategy for making medical instrumentation accessible must include these institutions. But if it is a tax-based approach we are pursuing, how can we influence or assist entities that pay no income taxes?

Except for unrelated business income tax and except for the earnings of for-profit subsidiaries, it is certainly true that tax-exempt organizations do not pay income taxes. But that does not mean their activities and role are not heavily influenced by the taxes that others do or do not pay. And being income tax-exempt also does not mean these entities are relieved of the obligation to pay federal excise or state sales taxes, to name just a few of the nonincome taxes that tax-exempts still pay.

5.7.4.1 Income Taxes Paid by Others

5.7.4.1.1 Current Law

Even though nonprofits pay no income taxes, the income tax law largely accounts for their existence. This is so because a major source of financial support for the nonprofit sector, including medical research and treatment, is tax-deductible contributions made by individuals, bequests, and businesses. If you have a voluntary or other not-for-profit hospital in your area that added a new wing recently, the odds are good that the wing will bear some person's name. Odds are also good that without the tax deductibility to the donor of the contribution, the new wing would have been far more difficult to fund. It is in this light that tax cuts are a double-edged sword for much of the nonprofit community. Concerns are especially great over proposals for permanent elimination of the estate tax, with many fearing that bequests to charity will be significantly reduced once the tax benefit is lost.

5.7.4.1.2 Potential Solution

Within the framework of existing law, methods exist for enriching or increasing the value to the donors of certain kinds of charitable contributions. At various times deductions for certain kinds of technology donated by businesses, as well as contributions for the benefit of particular groups such as the ill, the needy, and children, have been favored with proportionally more deductibility than other gifts command. We will not go into the details here of the mechanisms used to achieve these goals. What is important to point out, however, is that if consensus emerged around the utility of encouraging charitable contributions on behalf of AMI, precedents exist for the technical and procedural means of doing this. If, for example, it were decided that universally-designed inventory equipment should command a deduction equal to its market price when contributed to medical facilities by its producers, this would make the value of such contributions far greater to the donor, because with ordinary contributions the value of the deduction is only the items' production cost, typically far lower than its fair market value or retail price.

5.7.4.2 Sales Taxes

5.7.4.2.1 Current Law

As this reference to other taxes suggests, a number of taxes do bear directly on the work of nonprofit institutions. Among these, state and local sales taxes are the most pervasive. Although some states provide sales tax exemption for certain medically related items purchased by consumers or by nonprofits, and some states grant broad sales tax exemptions to nonprofit purchasers, there is no general pattern that would ease the burden on accessibility by providing any general or nation-wide tax relief in this area.

5.7.4.2.2 Potential Solution

Options exist for cutting sales taxes in ways that create cost advantages for nonprofit end users (or, for that matter, even for individual or for-profit end users) who opt for accessible over inaccessible instrumentation. For example, over many years federal law barred states from charging sales tax on food purchased with food stamps. Why couldn't the imposition of sales taxes on purchases and sales of accessible medical instrumentation be similarly curtailed?

Some states already exempt medical devices, appliances, or supplies of various kinds from their sales tax, so for them, extending the exemptions should not be a great leap. As for possible federal involvement, if use of federal authority to exempt accessible items from state sales taxes seems heavy handed, it need only be remembered that comparable federal authority already restricts many state taxing activities, including the ability of states to tax most sales made over the Internet.

5.7.5 Health Insurance Carriers

5.7.5.1 Current Law

Every industry has manufacturers, retailers, and customers. One characteristic that makes the health care system unique and that most distinguishes it from any other sector of the economy is the role of third-party payers in the process. When I or my company buy a computer from a retailer, we pay for it ourselves, and the retailer pays the manufacturer. When we buy a house, we get a loan from a lender to pay for it. But when we buy medical services or devices, it is our hope, and generally our expectation, that somebody else — our employer or an insurance company or Medicare or Medicaid — will pay for it. Of course, we or someone has paid insurance premiums, but the normal expectation is that most of us who incur major costs will get back far more than we put in.

Under such a system, it becomes clear that what insurers want substantially determines what patients get and what modalities practitioners use. To understand this one need only ask this question: What would be the effect on the amount of time your doctor spends with you during an office visit if insurers dramatically raised their rate of reimbursement for consultations and advice but lowered it for ordering tests and carrying out procedures?

Insurance companies probably play more of a role in determining the nature and content of our health care than any other institution in society. Researchers may publish articles about what treatments work and what does not; doctors may prefer one drug over another; patients may want the treatment or medicine that did their friend so much good; legislatures may enact mandates or disclosure and appeals procedures. But insurers, who retain enormous legal discretion over what they pay for and when, play the largest role in determining the content, timing, and amount of the health care services we receive.

It follows from this that anything that changes insurance practices will have a powerful effect on our experience as patients. Our challenge, then, is finding ways to use the tax system to encourage insurers (including self-insured employers, fee-for-service where it still exists, and the numerous forms of managed care) to prefer accessible instrumentation, to use their market power to make it more available and cheaper, and to pay for it when it is available.

Insurance companies and insurance plans vary so much that it is difficult to generalize. Tax-based approaches that would be appropriate with one type of health insurance are not likely to work well with another. For instance, employers can already deduct from their income virtually all the costs incurred in providing health coverage to their employees. It is not clear what additional tax subsidization may be available within the fringe benefit context to encourage them to embrace AMI.

Of course, negative tax treatment could be used. The various tax advantages currently accorded to employer-sponsored medical care could be curtailed if the sponsors do not show evidence of having sought or used accessible versions of medical instrumentation wherever available. But even this, unlikely as it is to gain any political support, would have little or no effect on nonprofit employers, unless one were to take the extremely harsh and counterproductive step of revoking all the tax benefits attaching to their fringe benefit plans.

5.7.5.2 Potential Solutions

The insurance industry, meaning the companies that are in the insurance business (which still includes a variety of companies, depending on whether they sell coverage or simply administer coverage purchased by others, whether they provide coverage under contract with federal or state government or operate in the worker compensation system, whether they are primary or secondary carriers, whether they administer or provide disability as well as health coverage, and depending on a host of other factors), is governed by some unique tax laws. Generally, these laws already favor the industry to a high degree. The federal tax law may not be the most effective tool for influencing the insurance industry to adopt pro-AMI practices. But there may be some techniques available under state tax law that warrant further study.

In recent years, states have begun considering new taxation of HMOs and hospitals as one means of helping to meet the growing cost burdens of Medicaid. As a general matter, the federal statute called the Employment Retirement and Income Security Act (ERISA) bars state regulation, including taxation, of insurance providers or of activities conducted under ERISA's auspices. But recent court decisions interpreting ERISA have begun to give states a little more scope in levying excise, franchise, or other taxes. If states' costs for providing health care to the poor continue to rise, and if the trend of these court decisions continues, increased use of such taxes is foreseeable. That in turn may provide an opening for tax benefits for hospitals and private insurers who utilize, procure, disseminate, and otherwise add to the accessible component of medical instrumentation and health care.

If one lives in a state that has adopted any such taxes or is contemplating them, it might prove interesting to suggest that the tax should be reduced in some way that rewards the use of accessible technology and instrumentation. A subsequent technical paper will provide draft language for doing this under one typical state statute.

5.8 CONCLUSION

Technology has reached a point where greater accessibility in a wide variety of medical instrumentation is possible. Changes in the way medical services are delivered, evolving notions of consumer control and patient responsibility, increased use of home-based treatments and monitoring, and other factors also argue in favor of doing everything possible to increase the ability of patients, caregivers, and medical professionals and staff to fully and effectively use all the technologies, instrumentation, and devices at their disposal.

Many resources must be developed and mobilized for sustained and enduring progress in this area. As in all other areas of society, the tax law represents an important variable in determining the actions and decisions of individuals and institutions. Combined with other laws and strategies, the tax law can contribute to the accessibility of the medical system in many ways. This chapter has introduced some of the major areas in which the tax law can play this role most effectively. In no discussion of public policy can we afford to overlook or underestimate the importance of these opportunities.

ACKNOWLEDGMENT

This work is supported by a consulting contract with the RERC-AMI, funded by NIDRR, U.S. Department of Education Grant #H133E020729. All opinions expressed are those of the author.

REFERENCES

1. U.S. Department of Health and Human Services, Press Release, U.S. Surgeon General Issues First Call to Action on Disability (July 26, 2005, available at http://www.hhs.gov/news/press/2005pres/20050726.html).
2. U.S. Department of Education, Office of Special Education and Rehabilitative Services (July 19, 2002). Federal Register: National Institute on Disability and Rehabilitation Research — Rehabilitation Engineering Research Centers (RERC) Program; Notice Inviting Applications for Fiscal Year 2002, 16(118): 41768.
3. U.S. Access Board, ADA and ABA Accessibility Guidelines for Buildings and Facilities. July 23, 2004, amended August 5, 2005. Available at http://www.access-board.gov/ add-aba/final.htm.
4. Government Accounting Office, Business Tax Incentives: Incentives to Employ Workers with Disabilities Receive Limited Use and Have an Uncertain Impact. GAO-03-039, December 2002.
5. Sec. 508 of the Federal Rehabilitation Act, codified at 29 USC Sec. 794d.
6. Worldwide Web Consortium (W3C) Web Accessibility Guidelines (available at www.w3.org).
7. Internal Revenue Code, Title 26, Subtitle A, Chapter 1, Subchapter B, Part VI, Section 190. Expenditures to remove architectural and transportation barriers to the handicapped and elderly.
8. Internal Revenue Code, Title 26, Subtitle A, Chapter 1, Subchapter A, Part IV, Subpart D, Section 44. Expenditures to provide access to disabled individuals.
9. The DAC cases.
10. Story, MF (1998). Assessing usability: the principles of universal design. *Assistive Technology*, Vol. 10.1, pp. 4–12.
11. Rehabilitation Act, Section 508 (29 U.S.C. 794d), as amended by the Workforce Investment Act of 1998 (P.L. 105-220), August 7, 1998.
12. Miller, J.C., Imaging and Obese Patients. Radiology Rounds: A Newsletter for Referring Physicians, Massachusetts General Hospital, Department of Radiology. 3(7): 1–4, July 2005.
13. Graetz, M. & Shapiro, I (2005). Death By a Thousand Cuts: The Fight Over Taxing Inherited Wealth. Princeton: Princeton University Press.
14. Medicare Prescription Drug, Improvement, and Modernization Act of 2003. Public Law 108–173, December 8, 2003.
15. Internal Revenue Code, Title 26, Subtitle A, Chapter 1, Subchapter B, Part I, Section 67. Two Percent Floor on Miscellaneous Itemized Deductions.
16. National Council on Disability. Righting the ADA. December 1, 2004. Available at http://www.ncd.gov/newsroom/publications/2004/righting-ada.htm.
17. Internal Revenue Code, Title 26, Subtitle A, Chapter 1, Subchapter B, Part VI, Section 179. Election to expense certain deprecible business assets.
18. Working Families Tax Relief Act of 2004. P. L. 108–311, October 4, 2004.
19. Compare: Hubbard V. Commisioner of Internal Revenue, Tax Court Memo 2003–245, No. 1764-02, 2003. Tax Court Memo Lexis 243 (August 14, 2003), with Fan V. Commissioner of Internal Revenue, 117 T.C. 32, 2001 Tax Court Memo Lexis 34, 117 T.C. No. 3 (July 24, 2001).

Part II

Tools for Usability and Accessibility Analysis

6 Applying the Principles of Universal Design to Medical Devices

Molly Follette Story

CONTENTS

ABSTRACT

This chapter presents a brief history of the creation of the Principles of Universal Design and lists the principles and their associated guidelines. The chapter discusses relevance of the Principles of Universal Design to the field of health care and describes examples of devices that comply with the Principles. Finally, the chapter discusses the wide range of potential applications and users of medical instrumentation that should be taken into consideration during the design process, the importance of testing medical devices with as broad a diversity of potential users as practical, and the critical aspect of supportive procurement, implementation, and use policies.

6.1 INTRODUCTION

In the 1970s, Ronald L. Mace coined the term *universal design* to describe the process of designing all products and environments to be usable by people of all ages and abilities, to the greatest extent possible [1]. The universal design concept originates in the civil rights movement of the 1950s and

1960s, and its goal is to integrate people with disabilities into the social fabric of the U.S. to maximize participation in the widest variety of activities of daily living in a natural and holistic way.

Universal design can improve device accessibility for people with disabilities and, at the same time, improve usability for most users. This benefit has particular importance for health care because in most cases, all patients use the same medical devices. For example, no company would ever produce an "assistive" MRI machine, that is, one that is accessible to and used only with people who have disabilities. Universal design is also important for medical devices because the accessibility and usability of this equipment can affect the quality of health care provided.

6.1.1 Terms and Definitions

A number of terms have been used to describe the concept of accessibility and usability for the broadest spectrum of potential users. (Some of these terms are included in the glossary at the back of this book.) Two other terms popular in the U.S. are transgenerational design and inclusive design. The term *transgenerational design* was coined by James J. Pirkl in the late 1980s [2,3] to emphasize the multiage applicability of the design approach. The term *inclusive design* originated in England [4]. The Web site of Inclusive Design, developed by a consortium headed by the Royal Society for the encouragement of Arts (RSA) says the approach "… aims to include the needs of people who are currently excluded or marginalised (sic) by mainstream design practices and links directly to the concept of an inclusive society" [5]. The term has been adopted by some groups in the U.S. as well (e.g., Center for Inclusive Design and Environmental Access at the State University of New York at Buffalo).

Terms popular in other countries include design for all and *kyoyo-hin*. *Design for all* is the term used most widely in Europe. The European Commission uses the following definition: "Design for all means creating products, services and systems to cater for the widest possible range of user abilities and circumstances for use" [6]. Although the term *universal design* is widely accepted in Japan, "kyoho-hin," which means "shared design," is sometimes used to connote designs that are used concurrently by people with and without disabilities. The Kyoyo-Hin Foundation Web site states that "Kyoyo-hin and kyoyo services are designed to be used by as many people as possible, including the elderly and those with disabilities" [7].

Universal design differs from assistive technology and accessible design. Assistive technologies are typically designed for people with a specific type of disability without regard for any other disability. Some examples of assistive technologies are eyeglasses for people with visual disabilities, hearing aids for people who are hard of hearing, and wheelchairs for people with mobility impairments. Note, however, that any of these devices may be difficult to use for people who also have limited manual dexterity. Accessible design generally refers to environments, and a limited number of products, that comply with legislation that requires it, such as the Americans with Disabilities Act (ADA) [8], Section 508 of the Rehabilitation Act [9], or Section 255 of the Telecommunications Act [10]. The language of these laws usually requires that designs be "accessible to and usable by people with disabilities" and also "where readily achievable." These are antidiscrimination laws with specific, limited applicability to companies over a certain size or receiving federal funding. Chapter 8 of this book provides a definition that focuses on maximizing accessibility for products not currently under legal mandate.

Unlike assistive technologies, universal design seeks to design concurrently to suit the needs of people of all ages, sizes, and shapes, and with a wide range of abilities and disabilities, and unlike some accessible design, accessible features are integrated into universal designs so that they look as if they belong there. Although these requirements make achievement of universal design difficult, it is still possible and well worth striving for.

6.2 HISTORY OF THE PRINCIPLES OF UNIVERSAL DESIGN

From 1994 to 1997, the Center for Universal Design conducted a research and demonstration project titled, "Studies to Further the Development of Universal Design," funded by the U.S. Department of Education's National Institute on Disability and Rehabilitation Research (NIDRR). One of the activities of the project was to develop a set of universal design guidelines.

In April 1995, the project team convened a meeting of ten experts on universal design at the offices of the Center for Universal Design at North Carolina State University in Raleigh, NC. The group comprised ten professionals active in the field of universal design from seven institutions across the U.S., and included architects, product designers, engineers, and environmental design researchers. This group spent 2 days together, amassing their substantial collective knowledge of universal design, listing all the maxims and guidelines and concepts they could articulate that described the concept. They explicitly agreed that rather than claiming to be experts on all aspects of good design, the group would develop universal design guidelines to address only issues of design usability for the widest diversity of individuals.

Project staff subsequently analyzed the results, grouped and merged the bits of data, added to and shaped them and, in collaboration with the other authors, developed a list they called the "Principles of Universal Design." The draft principles were mailed to a dozen colleague universal design researchers and practitioners around the country for their review and comment, and their suggestions were incorporated into the final document (see Table 6.1).

In December, 1995, The Center for Universal Design published version 1.1 and in April 1997, version 2.0 of the Principles of Universal Design [11]:

Principle 1. Equitable use
Principle 2. Flexibility in use
Principle 3. Simple and intuitive use
Principle 4. Perceptible information
Principle 5. Tolerance for error
Principle 6. Low physical effort
Principle 7. Size and space for approach and use

Each of these principles had a definition and was followed by a set of four or five guidelines that described the key elements that should be present in a design that adhered to the principle.

The purpose of the Principles of Universal Design and their associated guidelines was to articulate the concept of universal design in a comprehensive way. They reflected the authors' belief that the basic universal design principles applied to all design disciplines, including environments, products, and communications. The principles were intended to guide the design process, allow the systematic evaluation of designs, and assist in educating both designers and consumers about the characteristics of more usable design solutions for diverse populations.

TABLE 6.1
The Principles of Universal Design and Their Definitions [11]

Principle	Definition
1. Equitable use	The design is useful and marketable to people with diverse abilities
2. Flexibility in use	The design accommodates a wide range of individual preferences and abilities
3. Simple and intuitive use	Use of the design is easy to understand, regardless of the user's experience, knowledge, language skills, or current concentration level
4. Perceptible information	The design communicates necessary information effectively to the user, regardless of ambient conditions or the user's sensory abilities
5. Tolerance for error	The design minimizes hazards and the adverse consequences of accidental or unintended actions
6. Low physical effort	The design can be used efficiently and comfortably and with a minimum of fatigue
7. Size and space for approach and use	Appropriate size and space is provided for approach, reach, manipulation, and use regardless of user's body size, posture, or mobility

Since their publication, several groups have developed universal design checklists. Some are focused on environments, such as the Americans with Disabilities Act Checklist for Readily Achievable Barrier Removal by Adaptive Environments [12]. Others are more product oriented, such as the Universal Design Performance Measures for Products by the Center for Universal Design at North Carolina State University [13]. For more information, see Chapter 9.

6.3 APPLICATIONS OF THE PRINCIPLES OF UNIVERSAL DESIGN IN HEALTH CARE

As stated earlier, universal design has particular importance to the design of medical devices because of the extremely diverse populations of people who use these devices, and because the design of medical devices can substantially affect the safety and efficiency of experiences people have using the devices and the quality of health care provided.

6.3.1 Principle 1: Equitable Use

Definition: The design is useful and marketable to people with diverse abilities.

Guidelines associated with Principle 1 and examples in health care:

1a. Provide the same means of use for all users: identical whenever possible, equivalent when not.
- A weight scale with a large platform that is recessed into the floor saves floor space and everyone can use the same scale, whether they walk or use a wheelchair or scooter. The scale may also have audio output, which is particularly advantageous for people with visual impairments.

1b. Avoid segregating or stigmatizing any users.
- A building map can be used by most visitors if it is simultaneously simple and easy to understand, has high contrast for legibility, and is tactile (so people who are blind can feel it).

1c. Make provisions for privacy, security, and safety equally available to all users.
- A door that has viewing windows both high and low enable people who are standing or seated or are shorter than average to see what is happening on the other side.

1d. Make the design appealing to all users.
- Medical devices that are attractive as well as functional are more appealing to a larger number of potential users.

6.3.2 Principle 2: Flexibility in Use

Definition: The design accommodates a wide range of individual preferences and abilities.

Guidelines associated with Principle 2 and examples in health care:

2a. Provide choice in methods of use.
- An examination table that adjusts in height can be lowered so that it is easier for the patient to get onto and off of the table; it can also be raised so that it is easier for the health care provider to examine and treat the patient at a level that is most effective and comfortable for him or her and the specific procedure.
- A dental chair with adjustable angles at the hip and knee accommodates nonaverage body shapes and individual position preferences.

2b. Accommodate right- or left-handed access and use.
- Devices that are symmetrical about a vertical or longitudinal access may be used equally well by someone who is right- or left-handed. Some devices may have

components that can moved from one side to the other to make them easier to use for people with one side dominance or preference.

2c. Facilitate the user's accuracy and precision.
  - Color and shape coding can facilitate correct connections between medical device components (e.g., cables, cords, tubing).

2d. Provide adaptability to the user's pace.
  - Some users are novices and need more guidance and time, and other users are experts who want to be able to move through the process of using a device quickly and efficiently. Medical devices should accommodate the entire range of expertise.
  - Large medical facilities should provide places to sit and rest along major paths of travel.

6.3.3 Principle 3: Simple and Intuitive Use

Definition: Use of the design is easy to understand, regardless of the user's experience, knowledge, language skills, or current concentration level.

Guidelines associated with Principle 3 and examples in health care:

3a. Eliminate unnecessary complexity.
  - Medical devices should be as simple as possible without eliminating any needed functions.
  - Some less frequently used functions may be located behind a panel that would be opened only when needed.

3b. Be consistent with user expectations and intuition.
  - Using easily understood or generally accepted standards and systems for component arrangements, color codes, and icons can make devices easier and faster for users to learn and to operate.

3c. Accommodate a wide range of literacy and language skills.
  - Color coding and icons can communicate more effectively (and quickly) than text with people who have limited literacy or language skills, and reinforce the content of text for those reading it.

3d. Arrange information consistent with its importance.
  - Important and most frequently used components, such as buttons on a monitor, should be easy to recognize visually and easy to reach.

3e. Provide effective prompting and feedback during and after task completion.
  - A defibrillator designed for use in a public place such as an airport can guide nonexpert users, both visually and audibly, through the entire process of use, from setup through shutdown.

6.3.4 Principle 4: Perceptible Information

Definition: The design communicates necessary information effectively to the user, regardless of ambient conditions or the user's sensory abilities.

Guidelines associated with Principle 4 and examples in health care:

4a. Use different modes (pictorial, verbal, tactile) for redundant presentation of essential information.
  - Medical devices that have visual output can also have audible output, such as a talking thermometer, weight scale, or exercise bike.

4b. Maximize legibility of essential information.
  - The message being sent should stand out against the background information. For visual displays, this involves visual contrast; for sound output, this involves auditory contrast.

- Auditory output should have a volume control; visual displays may offer choices of font types and sizes and color combinations used.

4c. Differentiate elements in ways that can be described (i.e., make it easy to give instructions or directions).

- Instruction manuals are easier to write and telephone help is easier to give if the components of a medical device are sufficiently different from each other so as to facilitate verbal descriptions. This is particularly important for home health care devices.

4d. Provide compatibility with a variety of techniques or devices used by people with sensory limitations.

- Medical devices should be compatible with peripheral devices or specialized assistive equipment or techniques that may used, such as hearing aids, videotape captioning, headphones, dynamic Braille machines.
- During procedures such as x-ray or MRI scans, when the medical professional is typically out of the room, communication with patients could be improved with lights or a visual display that says, for example, "Don't breathe." This would be particularly helpful for patients with hearing disabilities or patients who speak a language the professional does not know but that could be programmed into the display.

6.3.5 Principle 5: Tolerance for Error

Definition: The design minimizes hazards and the adverse consequences of accidental or unintended actions.

Guidelines associated with Principle 5 and examples in health care:

5a. Arrange elements to minimize hazards and errors, with the most used elements, being most accessible and hazardous elements eliminated, isolated, or shielded.

- Hazardous elements such as sharp corners or high voltage should be eliminated from medical devices whenever possible; if not, they should be located away from areas with which the user typically has contact, and whenever possible they should be covered or shielded to reduce the chance that the user will encounter them.

5b. Provide warnings of hazards and errors.

- Color coding of hazardous elements can make them easier and faster to recognize.
- Requesting confirmation of irreversible or potentially critical operations can reduce the chance of inadvertent actions.

5c. Provide fail-safe features.

- Having devices revert to benign settings when the operator takes no action for a period of time or with automatic shut-off capability (such as a ground-fault interrupter) in case of a power surge, can reduce the level of hazard.

5d. Discourage unconscious action in tasks that require vigilance.

- Medical devices may require multiple steps in a specific and unusual sequence, or may require two simultaneous actions, in order to force the user to pay attention during critical tasks.
- Bar coding of medications can help reduce errors by enforcing that there is a match between medication and patient.

6.3.6 Principle 6: Low Physical Effort

Definition: The design can be used efficiently and comfortably and with a minimum of fatigue.

Guidelines associated with Principle 6 and examples in health care:

6a. Allow user to maintain a neutral body position.
  - Keyboards can be split in the middle and angled to align with the forearm to prevent sustained ulnar deviation.
  - Handles on carts should be vertical rather than horizontal to prevent sustained forearm pronation, and they should be long enough to allow people of varying height to grasp them at the location that is most comfortable for each individual.

6b. Use reasonable operating forces.
  - Doors that open automatically when someone approaches eliminate all operating force.
  - Buttons that activate by body heat require no force (but are unusable for people with upper limb prostheses or cold hands).

6c. Minimize repetitive actions.
  - Multichannel pipettes allow more than one test tube to be emptied or filled in a single operation.
  - Some devices may be controlled with voice commands.

6d. Minimize sustained physical effort.
  - Providing physical support, such as a backrest or armrests, during long procedures can improve comfort and reduce fatigue.
  - A chair that has a narrow back and no armrests may be sat on backwards and support the chest during sustained reaching tasks.

6.3.7 Principle 7: Size and Space for Approach and Use

Definition: Appropriate size and space is provided for approach, reach, manipulation, and use regardless of user's body size, posture, or mobility.

Guidelines associated with Principle 7 and examples in health care:

7a. Provide a clear line of sight to important elements for any seated or standing user.
  - Reception desks or nurses' stations should have at least one section that is at standard desk height to suit visitors who use wheelchairs or are shorter than average, as well as people seated behind the desk who need to communicate with them.

7b. Make reach to all components comfortable for any seated or standing user.
  - Medical devices (such as mammogram machines) can be height adjustable or they can be placed on stands that are adjustable in height, or more than one device can be mounted on a wall at different heights, to suit people of varying heights who stand or sit during use.

7c. Accommodate variations in hand and grip size.
  - Gripping surfaces can be tapered to allow users to select a section that suits the size of their own hands as well as their needs and preferences for the task.

7d. Provide adequate space for the use of assistive devices or personal assistance.
  - At least a portion of medical examination and treatment rooms and public rest rooms should be large enough to accommodate people who use wheelchairs or scooters, or who are accompanied by a personal attendant or caregiver or service animal.
  - Equipment that typically includes a chair, such as eye exam equipment, should enable the chair to be removed so that patients who use wheelchairs could remain in their own chairs during the procedure.

6.4 DISCUSSION

Since their publication, the Principles of Universal Design have been accepted by a diverse collection of entities worldwide; they have been translated into several other languages and used for a variety of applications in a range of design disciplines.

6.4.1 Potential Applications and Users

The Principles of Universal Design can be applied to many types of health care equipment. The Rehabilitation Engineering Research Center on Accessible Medical Instrumentation (RERC-AMI) learned through its national survey (see Chapter 2 of this book) that some of the most basic and widely used types of equipment are the ones causing the most difficulty and discomfort: examination tables and chairs, weight scales, and imaging equipment. Clearly, these types of equipment should be designed to accommodate the widest possible range of patients. They should also accommodate a wide range of potential health care providers, including people who acquire disabilities, sometimes from aging or being injured on the job, as well as people who enter the professions who already have disability.

To as great an extent as possible, all medical equipment should accommodate a wide range of patients and disabilities, including people with disabilities and elders. As more people live to older ages and survive injuries and diseases that used to be fatal, the prevalence of disability in the U.S. populations is growing and it becomes increasingly important for medical equipment to serve the needs of a diverse population.

In addition, patients are leaving the hospital sooner and medical equipment that was designed for use only by trained professionals in a medical facility is now being used in the home. A variety of people now use the equipment, and its design must take this into account. Equipment must be designed for use by medical personnel, by personal caregivers, family members and friends, and by the patients themselves. Consideration should be given to equipment set up and use, storage, cleaning, repair, and disposal, and the many and diverse types of people who may perform each of these tasks.

6.4.2 Medical Device Testing

When considering the acquisition of a new piece of medical equipment, it is important to test the device before purchase to ensure that a wide variety of potential users can use it safely and effectively. Ideally, this would include testing users of all ages and abilities/disabilities, ethnicities and experience level, job titles, and use locations. While this is not practical, other methods can be used, such as reviewing survey data to determine a representative cross-disability mix, or using the "persona" approach described in Chapter 18 of this book. Testing can be done in focus groups [14,15] or in structured usability testing sessions [16–18] and may yield information about potential problems that may arise in actual use. An example of a systematic approach that incorporates universal design concepts is the RERC on Accessible Medical Instrumentation's Mobile Usability Lab, described in Chapter 13 of this book.

Medical facilities may also choose to evaluate devices they already own to assess how well they are serving the needs of the personnel and patients who are currently using them (see Chapter 7 of this book). If encouraged to voice their opinions in a frank manner without potential negative consequences, staff and clients may identify aspects of devices that could be made easier or safer or more effective to use. They may also be aware of alternative devices that may better meet the needs of the facility.

Finally, medical device manufacturers would be advised to test new designs under development with a wide variety of potential device users. It is best that this testing occur early and often during the development process to make best and most efficient use of the information that user testing can provide.

6.4.3 Policy Considerations

A critical component of any effort to improve broad accessibility and usability of medical equipment is to build consideration of these issues into procurement policies. Medical facilities should require, when feasible, that any equipment purchased or acquired be accessible to and usable by the widest possible and practical spectrum of potential health care professionals and patients. Without this commitment and leadership from management, procurement of accessible medical instrumentation will be haphazard, at best.

Another critical component of improvement of accessibility and usability in medical equipment is implementation. After equipment has been acquired, it must be installed and utilized in ways that will maximize its accessibility and usability for as many potential users as possible. This includes consideration of space allowances surrounding equipment such as examination tables and chairs, lighting requirements for control panels, and acoustic conditions for devices that provide essential auditory information.

Finally, the use of accessible medical instrumentation should be accompanied by policies that respect the individual needs and preferences of all staff members and patients, including the need to take more time sometimes and strategies for communicating appropriately and effectively with people with sensory or cognitive disabilities.

6.5 CONCLUSIONS

Universal design can be helpful in maximizing accessibility for people with disabilities and usability for all potential users, but it must be applied within the appropriate use contexts to be most beneficial. Consideration should be given to all potential locations, applications, and users.

The goal of universal design is cross-disability accessibility that maximizes usability for the highest percentage of users, both health care providers and patients. This can often be a challenge, particularly for more complex devices, but the human factors and ergonomics field offers many strategies for optimizing usability, which, if appropriately applied, may optimize accessibility as well.

ACKNOWLEDGMENT

This work is supported by the RERC-AMI, funded by the NIDRR, U.S. Department of Education Grant #H133E020729. All opinions expressed are those of the author.

REFERENCES

1. Mace, R.L., Hardie, G.J., and Place, J.P., *Accessible Environments: Toward Universal Design*, Center for Accessible Housing: Raleigh, NC, 1991, p. 32.
2. Pirkl, J.J. and Babic, A.L., *Guidelines and Strategies for Developing Transgenerational Products: A Resource Manual for Industrial Design Professionals*, Acton, MA: Copley Publishing, 1988.
3. Pirkl, J.J., *Transgenerational Design: Products for an Aging Population*. New York: Van Nostrand Reinhold, 1994, p. 260.
4. Helen Hamlyn Research Centre, Inclusive Design Education Resource [Available from http://www.designcouncil.org.uk/inclusivedesignresource/].
5. RSA, Inclusive Design Overview [Available from http://www.inclusivedesign.org.uk/index.php?filters=f4].
6. Dissemination Activities Supporting Design for All, Welcome to the Design for All Website by DASDA! [Available from http://www.design-for-all.info/].
7. Kyoyo-Hin Foundation, The Kyoyo-Hin Foundation Website, 1999–2001 [Available from http://kyoyohin.org/eng/].
8. U.S. Department of Justice, Introduction to the Americans with Disabilities Act, 2002 [Available from http://www.usdoj.gov/crt/ada/adaintro.htm].
9. 1998 Amendment to Section 508 of the Rehabilitation Act: Section 508 of the Rehabilitation Act (29 U.S.C. 794d), as amended by the Workforce Investment Act of 1998 (P.L. 105-220), August 7, 1998. Available from http://www.section508.gov/index.cfm?FuseAction=Content&ID=14

10. Federal Communications Commission, Section 255: Telecommunications Access for People with Disabilities, 2005 [Available from http://www.fcc.gov/cgb/consumerfacts/section255.html].
11. The Center for Universal Design, Principles of Universal Design, v. 2.0, N.C. State University: Raleigh, NC, 1997.
12. Adaptive Environments Center, I., The Americans with Disabilities Act Checklist for Readily Achievable Barrier Removal, Boston, MA, 1995.
13. The Center for Universal Design, Evaluating the Universal Design Performance of Products, N.C. State University: Raleigh, NC, 2000.
14. Story, M.F., Focus groups with participants who have disabilities, in *International Conference on Human-Computer Interaction*, Las Vegas, NV, 2005.
15. Krueger, R.A., *Focus Groups: A Practical Guide for Applied Research*, 2nd ed., Thousand Oaks, CA: SAGE Publications, 1994, p. 255.
16. Coyne, K.P., Conducting simple usability tests with users with disabilities, in *International Conference on Human-Computer Interaction*, Las Vegas, NV, 2005.
17. Dumas, J.S. and Redish, J.C., *A Practical Guide to Usability Testing*, Portland, OR: Intellect, 1993, p. 404.
18. Rubin, J., *Handbook of Usability Testing*, New York: John Wiley & Sons, 1994, p. 330.

7 Using Ethnographic Research to Develop Inclusive Products

Stephen B. Wilcox

CONTENTS

ABSTRACT

This chapter discusses the application of ethnographic research to the development of home health care products. The general goal of ethnographic research is to develop a thorough and accurate understanding of the worldview of different kinds of people. Such research is valuable for the development of home health care products because the users of such products are particularly likely to be different from the people who develop them. Good ethnographic research involves more than simply adding real-world observation to interviews. It involves a conceptual framework and a methodology that typically take a multiyear apprenticeship to acquire. Good ethnographic research also generally requires a number of sophisticated tools, both for conducting the research and for reporting it.

7.1 INTRODUCTION

The focus of this chapter will be on product development, particularly the area of home health care products. This is one area where the inclusive design approach is not controversial. Here inclusivity means the opposite of exclusivity — to be inclusive is to be usable by a broad cross section of the population regardless of whatever disabilities they may have. The reason for using the term *inclusive design* instead of the more common term (in the U.S.) *universal design* is that it is more appropriate. Virtually no product is truly universal. Products are designed for particular classes of users: golfers or teenagers or people with diabetes. However, in its niche, any product can be inclusive by failing to exclude potential users on the basis of their specific abilities.

Inclusivity is not controversial for home health care products because the target customer is typically defined as a person with a given condition, a condition that itself or via its common comorbidities creates disabilities. Thus, the developer of products for people with diabetes recognizes that many of his or her users will have arthritis or visual problems; the developer of a home dialysis system has to take congestive heart failure into account, and so on.

The situation in home health care contrasts with that of ordinary consumer products, whose developers are not always sympathetic to the issue of inclusivity, but that is, perhaps, a separate topic.

The aim of this chapter is to discuss how ethnographic research can be used as a powerful tool to develop better home health care products. The chapter starts by describing ethnographic research. Next, it describes how ethnographic research applies to the development of home health care products. Finally, it provides suggestions for how ethnographic research results can be presented effectively in the context of home health care product development.

7.2 ETHNOGRAPHIC RESEARCH

When this author started doing ethnographic research in the early 1990s, it was considered rather radical. At that time, it was generally accepted that there were two basic methods for developing an understanding of customer needs — qualitative research (i.e., focus groups) and quantitative research (i.e., surveys). These research methods came from psychology and sociology and, no doubt, replaced earlier methods that were much less effective.

The general notion was to begin with relatively informal group discussions (focus groups) to generate ideas, then to validate these ideas with relatively large sample-size surveys to predict whether or not the generated ideas would be accepted by the target population of customers. Such research certainly has its place. However, it only goes so far; it suffers the central limitation that it relies exclusively upon what people say. Unfortunately, one thing that psychologists have learned over the years is that what people say is often a poor predictor of what they will actually do. This is true because much of what is important to people and much of what they do is not fully conscious. Who can accurately describe, for example, where the left hand is as the right foot is planted while walking? Ironically, the more experience one has with something, the more the awareness of it tends to fade. The novice pianist concentrates on where his or her fingers are while playing a given passage. The skilled pianist is more likely, while playing, to be thinking about where he or she is going to have dinner that evening. Also, people tailor what they say to what they think you want to hear or what will put them in a better light or what they would like to be true. In other words, people's answers to questions are influenced by any number of things besides, or in addition to, the actual facts. And, when answering questions about the past, people have to rely upon memory, which is notoriously fallible.

Ethnographic research overcomes these limitations by supplementing such interview-based methods with direct observation. The general idea is that, rather than just talking to people directly or indirectly via questionnaires, time is spent with them in their "natural environment" [1–5]. This allows one to see what people actually do and to ask questions while the behavior of interest is actually taking place. What makes it ethnographic, however, is not just that it take place outside of a room with a one-way mirror. What makes it ethnographic is a conceptual framework and a methodology that comes from cultural anthropology — a conceptual framework and a methodology designed to allow one to see things from the other person's point of view.

7.2.1 Conceptual Framework

Ethnographic research was originally developed by cultural anthropologists (here "cultural anthropologist" and "ethnographer" will be used interchangeably) who wanted to understand other cultures, typically other cultures that were dramatically different from their own. They quickly recognized that the categorical structures derived from their own cultures did not equip them to understand fundamentally different cultures [6]. Indeed, they found that their own categorical structures got in the way. For example, it does not get you very far to go looking for mothers-in-law, or village heads, or occupations, if the culture of interest does not recognize these categories. Anthropologists acknowledge that they needed to develop a more general conceptual framework, one that could apply across cultures, instead of simply trying to "shoehorn" the facts of other cultures into the conceptual framework of their own culture.

Of course, as with any intellectual discipline, there are schools of thought about what this metaframework should be. The key, though, is that doing ethnographic research requires some form of more general conceptual framework in order to make sense of what one observes. Without this, the observer simply sees the new culture in terms of his or her old culture, which defeats the whole purpose of seeing it from the other person's point of view. Thus, the ethnographer talks (and thinks) in terms of broad concepts that apply across cultures — concepts such as norms, values, rules, and social hierarchies.

Thus, ethnographic research does not just involve observing and asking questions. It involves observing and asking questions with pairs of eyes and ears informed by a conceptual framework that makes it possible to find patterns that cannot be found otherwise. In other words, the ethnographer comes looking for the facts in the context of an insight-producing conceptual framework.

7.2.2 Methodology

As mentioned earlier, the other important aspect of ethnographic research is its methodology. Ethnographic methodology includes both an observational component and an interview component.

7.2.2.1 Ethnographic Observation

Not only do ethnographic observations rely upon a sophisticated conceptual framework, they are conducted in particular ways. They involve observation that:

- Takes place over periods of time
- Is conducted in a systematic manner
- Is carefully documented

Historically, ethnographic research involved spending months or years in another culture. Of course, in product development, such time spans are impossible. However, ethnographic research tends to involve more time at a given location than is spent in more traditional forms of product-related research. The ethnographer may, for example, spend a day or two at a given site, much of it spent simply staying out of the way and watching what unfolds. This is where one sees, for example, those lower-frequency glitches that people may not think of when discussing their experiences later.

Also, ethnographic research is systematic. It involves creating a careful research protocol that specifies what will be observed and how it will be observed. It is also typical to study the phenomenon of interest (for example, the underlying clinical issues for medical products) via the relevant technical literature beforehand, so that the researcher can understand more of what he or she sees.

Finally, ethnographic research must be carefully documented. For one thing, videotaping is invaluable because it is hard to see everything as it happens, and video can communicate the facts to others in ways that verbal descriptions cannot. It is also important to take careful notes. Some ideas for communicating ethnographic findings are presented in Subsection 7.3.3 of this chapter.

7.2.2.2 Ethnographic Interviews

Ethnographic interviewing differs from market research-related interviews in a number of ways. First of all, the ethnographer tries to fit questions in where they seem appropriate rather than asking them in a set order. The goal is to encourage the person to start talking, usually in the context of action. Thus, questions tend to be open ended, and ethnographers tend to tolerate a lot of discussion that a conventional interviewer might be tempted to cut short. Sometimes, allowing people to tell seemingly irrelevant stories will eventually lead to important information that would not have come to the surface otherwise.

One key goal of ethnography is to spend enough time with people to develop real rapport and to get beyond the "party line" that often characterizes initial answers to questions. In an ethnographic interview, a topic may come up initially, then be raised again when the person begins to perform a task that is relevant to that topic, then yet again toward the end of the day after the person has had a few hours to think about it. This sort of cyclical discussion, which can yield uniquely rich information, is hard to achieve without spending a significant amount of time with a given interviewee. Likewise, the ethnographer keeps his or her ears open for the time, for instance, while sharing a meal, when the interviewee leans forward and offers to explain the real situation.

In sum, ethnographic research is designed to produce a deeper and more accurate understanding (than one starts with) of what people do and how they see things, and it applies special observational and interview methods to achieve this understanding. In Section 7.3, these methods will be applied to the design of home health care products. First, however, the issue of validity needs to be addressed.

7.2.2.3 Validity

A fair question to ask at this point is how validity is achieved with ethnographic research. With survey research, for example, or clinical trials for new products, there are procedures, largely statistical, for determining the likelihood that research findings accurately predict the real-world situation they are designed to predict. Ethnographic research is a type of science, but one that has a different basis from the psychology- and sociology-based research that is more typical.

The key to conducting valid ethnographic research is to engage in cyclical hypothesis testing during the course of the research. As an ethnographer proceeds, he or she develops hypotheses, tests these hypotheses, and revises his or her hypotheses on an ongoing basis. Hypotheses (regarding, for example, what the social structure is, who communicates with whom about what, how decisions are made, what the unstated rules are, etc.) are tested by acting in certain ways and saying certain things, then observing the responses to these actions and comments or questions. By the end of a research project, the ethnographer should be able to provide convincing evidence for his or her conclusions, derived from this hypothesis testing.

In summary, ethnographic research does have a scientific basis and can yield valid results in the hands of a trained ethnographer.

7.3 THE APPLICATION OF ETHNOGRAPHIC RESEARCH TO THE DEVELOPMENT OF INCLUSIVE PRODUCTS

7.3.1 The Purpose of Ethnographic Research *vis-a-vis* Designing Home Health Care Products

The core concept for applying ethnographic research to home health care product development is that the users of such products have fundamentally different worldviews and ways of acting in comparison to the people who are developing products. Everything else aside, one reason that product users are always different from product developers (even if they are demographically similar) is they have a different focus. Users focus less on the product, and their focus is different. Ironically, the more sophisticated a product developer becomes, the harder it is for him or her to see things from the user's point of view. For the developers of a product, the design of a given product is tied up with such things as operating systems, manufacturing methods, product lines, distribution channels, niche markets, and so on. The development team constantly thinks and talks about the products that they have responsibility for.

In contrast, the typical home health care product is, for the user, simply a tool with a few functions that he or she sometimes uses.

The situation is much more complicated when target the product user lives with conditions such as those caused by diabetes or heart failure. Patients with chronic diseases have many experiences that inform their worldview. Of course, they experience various disabilities and use home health care products that are relevant to them, causing various alterations of their lives. They also develop relationships with caretakers and medical professionals, have to regularly go to medical facilities for diagnosis and treatment, join patient groups, read about their diseases, etc. All of these experiences are different from those of the people who develop medical products.

This is where ethnographic research comes in. Good ethnographic research can help the product developer to understand the basic facts — how people use products, where they store them, and so on. But perhaps more importantly, good ethnographic research can allow the product developer to see things from the user's point of view [5]. It provides a pathway out of the egocentrism that is one of the primary barriers to developing products that fit the needs of their users. Such egocentrism is particularly problematical for designing inclusive products because the gap between the developer and the user can be especially wide.

7.3.2 Conducting Ethnographic Research with Disabled Users

As should be clear by now, the general idea is to treat the target users of home health care products as members of a culture that is different from one's own and to use ethnographic methods to close the gap — to develop an understanding of this alternative culture, in the same way that a cultural anthropologist might study the Trobriand Islanders or members of a royal family. This means, among other things, to approach the problem of understanding with an open mind, to avoid assuming that the user of a home health care device will share behavior, knowledge, or attitudes with oneself. Of course, there will inevitably be overlap between the worldview of the product user and the product developer. But this overlap, where it exists, has to be verified, not simply assumed.

Ethnographic research, then, in this context, means spending time with the potential users of a home health care device. In practice, this usually means spending time with people in their homes (perhaps, even over the course of the night, if the product is used at night), in their workplaces, and anywhere else where they might use the relevant products — while shopping, visiting friends, engaging in recreational activities, etc.

The first step is usually to carefully construct a set of screening criteria to make sure that the participants are appropriate. Then they have to be recruited. Two sources for finding people are relevant clinical facilities and organizations for people with particular diseases or disabilities. The other alternative is to hire the same sort of professional recruiters who are used for market research and, of course, give them the appropriate screening criteria. In the meantime, as discussed earlier, it is crucial to create formal research protocols and to do some homework regarding technical issues. This includes information on the relevant disabilities so as to sensitize the researcher to issues that will emerge from the research.

In addition to the aforementioned methods for conducting ethnographic research, it is also worth noting that good equipment is crucial. Video has to have sufficiently high resolution to capture what needs to be seen, and specialized tripods or booms may be needed to get the right camera angles. Often, multichannel video systems are necessary to obtain an adequate perspective on what takes place. Infrared video is a useful tool for recording what takes place in dark environments. For recording long procedures, time-lapse video is a useful tool. It also may be helpful to have measurement devices for capturing key environmental characteristics, such as light levels, or even to take physiological measurements (e.g., heart rate) from participants. In general, it is prudent to carefully consider what needs to be captured and what equipment is needed to capture this before starting an ethnographic research project.

The final topic to be addressed is how ethnographic research can be reported in a way that is useful and effective.

7.3.3 Reporting Ethnographic Findings

Ethnographic research tends to be more complex and generally "messier" than traditional market research. This can make it challenging to report the results so that they make sense to product developers and that they serve effectively to support decision making. The following ideas come from many years of trying to make ethnographic research results as effective as possible for the development of home health care products. Some more novel approaches have been omitted because various reporting methods are increasingly seen by clients as part of their intellectual property.

7.3.3.1 Summarizing Procedures

One basic fact about the people who develop products is that they are disinclined to spend long hours pouring over reports. Also, products are developed by multidisciplinary teams, so decisions tend to be made in meetings. It follows that if information is to be used effectively, it really helps to put it into a form that does not require its users to spend large amounts of time reading reports and that can be easily used in a meeting.

Examples of reporting methods that meet these goals include:

- Procedure maps that present characteristics of procedures, such as timing and who does what when, in an abstract form, akin to a Gantt chart
- Scenarios that show how procedures are performed step-by-step in a cartoon- or storyboard-like fashion

7.3.3.2 Summarizing Environmental Conditions

A useful way to summarize the use environment is to show it as a hypothetical plan (overhead) view that shows how equipment is typically arranged. Such plan views can also include patterns of movement or even patterns of communication between different types of people.

7.3.3.3 Summarizing Users

One way of summarizing users is to create hypothetical individuals who represent classes of users. These personas can incorporate a wide variety of ethnographic findings about user opinions, attitudes, and habits.

7.3.3.4 Summarizing Usability Recommendations

A potential problem is that recommendations may have a powerful effect on design efforts right after the research was reported, but less of an effect over time, as a project proceeds through cycles of testing and revision. This is because the development team may or may not go back regularly to study research reports. One antidote for this phenomenon is to include the most important recommendations on a short summary document that can be easily kept on a desk or put up on the wall.

7.3.3.5 Using Video

If there is one thing that has proven to be true over the years, it is that video will be used to the extent that it is accessible and efficient. A box full of video tapes is not accessible. It helps to start by digitizing the video (or collecting digital video in the first place). Once it is digitized, the video can be structured into a searchable database, or relevant clips can be embedded, by category, into digital reports. Video is made efficient for use by careful editing that removes the inevitable 50% that is just not relevant.

Accessible and efficient video is an invaluable tool [7]. The aforementioned summary documents can provide information, but there is no substitute, especially for those who have not been in the field, to becoming immersed in the user's world indirectly via video. Such immersion can provide a deeper understanding of key issues than is achievable through more traditional reporting methods.

7.4 CONCLUSION

Developer egocentrism is always a problem in product development, but it is particularly a problem when developing products for users with disabilities, as is the case with most home health care products. Ethnographic research can reduce this egocentrism and, in general, can provide a body of information that other methods cannot — information that is deep, thorough, and accurate.

However, ethnographic research involves a lot more than simply going into the environment of use and taking notes. Doing it well requires a good conceptual framework, good methods that are supported by good equipment, and good tools for reporting the information.

Without these physical and conceptual tools, there is a risk that research will not be effectively used. A bigger risk is that the research will be effectively used but not be accurate, because the researchers have not applied methods that adequately address the validity of their work. This point is important because, as ethnographic research becomes more common, it seems that just about everyone is claiming to do it, regardless of whether or not they actually have any relevant training or even know what it is. Ethnographic research is at risk for becoming a synonym for any research that is conducted in the field instead of the lab or office — which it is not.

REFERENCES

1. Reese, W., Ethnography for business: optimizing the impact of industrial design, *DMI Review*, 15(2), 2004.
2. Wilcox, S., Applying universal design to medical devices, *Medical Device and Diagnostic Industry*, January 2003, p. 114.
3. Wilcox, S. and Reese, W., Ethnographic methods for new product development, *Medical Device and Diagnostic Industry*, September 2001, p. 68.
4. Wilcox, S., Ethnography as a product development tool, *Appliance Manufacturer*, July 2001, p. 58.
5. Wilcox, S., Designing out ego, designing in customer preferences, *Appliance Manufacturer*, March 2001, p. 68.
6. Wilcox, S., Why anthropology: a tool for design research, *Innovation: The Journal of the Industrial Designers Society of America*, 15, 10–11, 1996.
7. Wiklund, M. and Wilcox, S., *Designing Usability into Medical Products*, New York: Taylor and Francis, 2005.

8 Educating Engineers in Universal and Accessible Design

Robert E. Erlandson, John D. Enderle, and Jack M. Winters

CONTENTS

ABSTRACT

This chapter addresses the need for educating engineers in universal and accessible design by providing approaches for meeting this challenge. After introducing the problem, multiple definitions for universal and accessible design are provided, which show clear distinctions, and also synergies, between the two. This is followed by a review of considerations for medical devices and an overview of the educational challenges. A number of approaches for integrating educational material on universal and accessible design into the engineering curriculum are then reported. This includes the development of core educational materials, student design projects, and adding universal and accessible design content into other engineering courses.

8.1 INTRODUCTION

Dentist chairs and examination tables are just two examples of medical devices that serve a broad spectrum of people. Small people, tall people, overweight and obese people, people with physical or cognitive impairments — all need access to these and a host of other medical devices. Not only do people need access to such devices, the devices must be safe. Safe means one thing if you are physically fit and another thing if you have a balance disorder. Safety, accessibility, and usability for a spectrum of users are all essential considerations in the design of medical devices. In other words, the design of these devices should be based on the principles of universal or accessible design. They are not.

The problem is that engineering and related design professions do not systematically and consistently cover universal and accessible design principles, strategies, and methods in their curricula. As part of ABET requirements, economic, health, and safety considerations are covered in senior design projects, and students are typically required to include an analysis of these factors in their overall design approach. Usability is considered, but again most typically in relation to a relatively small population of users, and moreover as a concept rather than a process.

This chapter, written by three engineering educators with over 50 years of collective experience with design education, suggests approaches for mainstreaming universal and accessible design into engineering curriculums. Here, a basic description of universal and accessible design is provided in relation to medical devices and equipment. The chapter also provides strategies for and examples of the integration of universal and accessible design material into engineering education.

8.2 UNIVERSAL AND ACCESSIBLE DESIGN: DEFINITIONS

Both universal and accessible designs have inspired multiple definitions. A useful definition of universal design for this chapter is that provided by a Council of Europe resolution proposing the introduction of universal design principles into the curricula of all occupations working on the built environment, Resolution ResAP(2001)1 [1]. The aim of the resolution is to guarantee utilization of universal design so as "to ensure equal chances of participation in economic, social, cultural, leisure and recreational activities. Everyone of whatever age, size, and ability must be able to access, use and understand any part of the environment as independently and as equal to others as possible" [1].

Toward that end the Council of Europe, Committee of Ministers, provides the following definition of universal design.

> Universal design is a strategy, which aims to make the design and composition of different environments and products accessible and understandable to as well as usable by everyone, to the greatest extent in the most independent and natural manner possible, without the need for adaptation or specialized design solutions. [1]

This definition includes the term *accessible*. A problem with this definition for the U.S. is that accessible design has assumed a legal context for its meaning. Accessible design derives its legal meaning from laws such as the Americans with Disabilities Act of 1990 (ADA) [2], Section 255 of the Telecommunications Act of 1996 [3], and Section 508 of the Rehabilitation Act as amended in 1998 [4]. The latter includes procurement of electronic and information technologies (E&IT) by federal agencies. The Access Board provides technical assistance to the federal government regarding implementation of these laws and has published accessibility guidelines that provide specific design guidelines as related to each of the three laws mentioned [5]. These laws also mention that products need to be compatible with assistive technology devices used by people with disabilities or able to be modified so as to be rendered accessible. The following definition of accessible design emphasizes its legal roots [6].

> Accessible design is the design of entities that satisfy specific legal mandates, guidelines, or code requirements with the intent of providing accessibility to the entities for individuals with disabilities.

This definition of accessible design focuses on the legal implications of the term. The definition is an expansion of the 1991 Center for Accessible Housing's definition [7], which referred only to "code requirements." As the legal environment has evolved, the definition must reflect these changes.

Emerging and practicing engineers need to know and understand the legal mandates that will apply to their professional design activities. Emerging and practicing engineers need to know where to go to get specific design requirements and guidelines. It is the responsibility of engineering faculty to provide such knowledge to our emerging engineers. It is incumbent upon professional organizations to educate practicing engineers through professional development activities. It is the responsibility of practicing engineers to seek out knowledge. For these reasons it makes sense to define accessible design more narrowly from a legal perspective. The laws and Access Board guidelines provide a neat, readymade packaging of the required materials.

However, there is a limitation with this definition, especially as related to products. The legal standards and codes do not span the full array of products simply because the existing laws do not span this range. For instance, the Access Board's accessibility guidelines cover only three areas — architecture (e.g., ADA accessibility guidelines), transportation (ADA accessibility for transportation vehicles), and communication as related to electronic and information technologies (E&IT). The last of these, which focuses on devices, was developed in direct response to the aforementioned Section 255 and Section 508. The latter includes procurement of E&IT within federal agencies.

What about the two classes of medical products mentioned at the beginning of this chapter, dental chairs and exam tables? The Rehabilitation Engineering Research Center on Accessible Medical Instrumentation (RERC-AMI) has conducted a national survey and focus groups involving medical patients with disabilities that have documented that there are considerable access barriers for these products (see Chapter 2 of this book). Unfortunately, none of the top four categories identified in the survey as having the most significant access barriers (exam tables, imaging equipment, exercise and rehab equipment, weight scales) appear to be addressed under existing accessibility guidelines. Thus we see that there are gaps in applying the definition of accessible design when it is considered solely from a legal perspective as the existing guidelines are piecemeal and not yet complete.

For this reason, the RERC-AMI project on developing accessibility metrics for medical products does not use the accessibility guidelines in an explicit way. However, it is interesting that for the MED-AUDIT scoring instrument described in Chapter 22 of this book, about one-quarter of the roughly 600 possible questions related to design feature considerations are motivated by accessibility guidelines. Furthermore, there are degrees of accessibility for products. For instance, in accessibility studies using the RERC-AMI's Mobile Usability Lab (Chapter 13 of this book), the rater-observed access barriers are scored as "difficult or impossible." This reflects the reality that often an individual has access to only some of the capabilities of a product, or gaining access may pose greater risk because of a potentially unsafe activity. Thus an alternative definition for accessible design is maximizing accessibility. This is also noted in the Access Board's guidelines for federal procurement of E&IT: "If products that meet some, but not all, relevant provisions are commercially available, the agency must procure the product that best meets the standards."

These two alternative definitions fit well within the engineering design framework. Indeed, engineers tend to be trained to meet both design specifications and constraints (the legally mandated requirements), and to optimize a system based on maximizing or minimizing a performance criterion (e.g., maximizing accessibility). Even Section 508 recognizes this, and after providing a collection of accessible design specifications it then includes Subpart C — Functional Performance Criteria. Subpart C represents a shift in legal language that in essence encourages a multimedia approach to design by initiating most functional performance criteria with

"At least one mode of operation and information retrieval that does not require ..."

where each criterion continues by identifying one or more sensory or motor modalities [4]. In practice, a heuristic satisfaction approach is often used, i.e., finding design solutions that satisfy a collection of design criteria.

The generalized classic engineering optimization problem includes both constraint equations (e.g., design criteria that must be satisfied) and performance criteria (that are to be extremized, often by balancing relative importance of competing subcriteria):

$$\begin{aligned}&\text{maximize} \quad J_p = \sum_{i=1}^{n} w_i J_i(x,u); \\ &\text{subject to} \quad \Psi_k(x,u) \geq C_k; \quad k = 1, n_k \\ &\qquad\qquad\quad \Phi_l(x,u) = C_l; \quad l = 1, n_l\end{aligned} \tag{8.1}$$

where J_p is the overall performance criterion (degree of accessibility) to be extremized (here maximized); J_i is the ith performance subcriterion (which itself may have been an integrated function of time), w_i is the ith weight (giving relative importance of each type of subcriterion), Ψ_k is the kth inequality equation that must be greater or equal to the kth required accessible design feature C_k, Φ_l is the lth equality equation that specifies the lth required accessible design feature C_l, and x is the state vector and u is the input vector (both of which may be functions of time).

This is commonly called the *constrained optimization problem.* As provided in Equation 8.1, the accessible design features C_k are specifications that must first be satisfied to a "good enough" threshold level; the inequality suggests that there could be room for the feature to be improved over and above the specification, but in this formulation this does not matter. In some cases, there may be an exact specification that can be met only one way; these are accessible design specifications C_l. These features C_k and C_l are similar to the provision requirements of Section 508 and are necessary for conformance. In contrast, the set of performance criteria J_i bear similarity to recommended practices that augment or exceed the provision requirement but continue to enhance accessibility. To summarize, on the left of Equation 8.1 is an optimality performance criterion (or cost function) approach, whereas on the right is a design specification (or standards/guideline) approach; in engineering optimization, both can exist under the same umbrella, with the constraints on the right first needing to be met if there is a legal mandate.

An alternative to Equation 8.1 is often used in engineering optimization in which the equality constraints (and sometimes even inequality constraints) are nonlinearly mapped into the performance (or cost) function in which there is very high (but noninfinite) penalty for those not being satisfied:

$$\begin{aligned}J_p = \sum_{i=1}^{n} w_i J_i(x,u) \quad - \quad &\sum_{k=1}^{n_k} w_k [F_k(\Psi_k(x,u)) - C_k] \quad - \\ &\sum_{l-1}^{n_l} w_l [\Phi_l(x,u) - C_l]\end{aligned} \tag{8.2}$$

Note that if the J_p function does not exist, we default to the legal definition of accessible design. While the details do not matter, in this case the equality constraint weighted error terms w_k are often called Lagrange multipliers, whereas the asymmetry for the inequality constraints is trickier but can be handled by a clever approach called the Kuhn–Tucker conditions (hence the functional F_k) that give "slack" on one side but not the other. This formulation takes on a revised meaning in that overall accessibility is:

- Negative if accessible design criteria are not met (i.e., if not accessible)
- Roughly zero if minimally required accessible design criteria are met but nothing more
- Positive if, in addition to meeting minimal requirements, there are accessible features that further enhance accessibility

Also, different design features can be given different weights and thus relative importance. Notice that if the constraint equations are absorbed into J_p calculation in a manner suggested earlier, the legal definition can be viewed as a subset of the more general optimization problem.

The accessible design mandates, regulations, and guidelines specified in the laws and Access Board publications are in essence universal design strategies and methods. For example, Paragraph § 1194.25 (f) of Section 508 of the Rehabilitation Act Amendments of 1998 states that, "When products deliver voice output in a public area, incremental volume control shall be provided with output amplification up to a level of at least 65 dB. Where the ambient noise level of the environment is above 45 dB, a volume gain of at least 20 dB above the ambient level shall be user selectable. A function shall be provided to automatically reset the volume to the default level after every use." This exemplifies an accessible design requirement that calls for universal design.

A generalization of this design requirement is an example of a universal design strategy: Provide the ability for a person to increase or decrease the signal strength so as to increase the signal-to-noise ratio [6,8]. For example, one can control the sound volume on a car's radio to compensate for traffic and road noise. One can adjust the brightness on a TV screen to compensate for room illumination. One can adjust the vibration strength on a pager or cell phone. In all of these examples, the user could increase the desired signal strength so as to overcome ambient or background conditions. Such design approaches can increase product accessibility, usability, and understandability, and as such exemplify universal design, but in the context presented previously, they are not mandated by law and as such might not be called accessible design [6].

Accessible design need not be universal design. A fundamental universal design principle is equity. Universally designed entities should, if at all possible, provide the same means of use for all users. The products and processes should avoid segregating or stigmatizing any users, making the design appealing to all users [9]. Accessible design, as specified in the laws and Access Board guidelines, does not concern itself with equity [6]. A ramp may be legally required to ensure wheelchair access, but nothing is mandated or required about the aesthetic quality or stigmatizing effect. Accessible design, if defined as maximizing accessibility, also differs from universal design in such ways. A more sophisticated interface with multimodal options may maximize access for the largest possible number of users, but can make the interface more complex and thus lower the ease of use. At a basic level, accessibility operates on an "access" scale (from *not difficult to access* through degrees of difficulty to *impossible to access*, with the defined user group including everyone with a specific type of disability). Universal design has several roots, including usability, which tends to operate on a "use" scale (from *easy* to *hard to use* by a collective user group that includes as many people as possible).

8.3 LAWS AND REGULATIONS FOR MEDICAL EQUIPMENT

The design and operational features of medical equipment fall under the auspices of the FDA, at least as related to their mandated regulatory mission of product safety and efficacy. As with ISO certification, the FDA guidelines tend to focus on design and manufacturing processes. Specifically, the FDA's requirements for Good Manufacturing Practices (GMP) require manufacturers to establish and maintain plans for design and development activities, to ensure that design requirements relating to a particular device are appropriate, and to address how intended use of the device includes the needs of users and patients. Tied to this is the FDA's participation in the process of integrating of human factors concepts into the product design process through the ANSI/AAMI HE74:2001 (human factors design process for medical devices) standard and the emerging ANSI/AAMI HE75 standard (see also Chapter 15 and Chapter 16 of this book). These guidelines describe a recommended human factors engineering process for fulfilling user interface design requirements in the development of medical devices and systems, including hardware, software, and documentation.

More recently, the FDA's Human Factors Branch has emphasized the goal of minimizing use-related hazards so as to assure that intended users are able to use medical devices safely and effectively throughout the product life cycle (see Chapter 17 of this book). In a list of important characteristics of user populations, the authors mention a number of characteristics of physical, sensory, and cognitive abilities, and emphasize the importance of consideration of the abilities and limitations of the user. Thus there is an implicit, if not explicit, acknowledgement of the importance of considering user abilities in device design and evaluation. However, at a basic level, the FDA is not mandated to consider the right of access to a device, but rather that those who actually use a device can do so safely and effectively.

This does not imply that there may not be requirements that certain medical devices are accessible. The 1998 amendments to Section 508 of the Rehabilitation Act of 1973 mandates the accessibility of all E&IT purchased by federal agencies. The Department of Veterans Affairs manages the largest health care network in the country, and thus procures a tremendous volume of medical technology. Medical equipment is not explicitly covered under this law, but some medical equipment may be considered as E&IT such that dual-classified equipment may be subject Section 508 accessibility guidelines. At present, this does not appear to be an avenue that is being pursued, but it does represent an intriguing possibility.

8.4 EDUCATIONAL ENVIRONMENT

Universal and accessible design concepts, methods, and strategies are not typically taught in engineering programs. The basic reason is that there is no perceived need, on the part of academicians, for the inclusion of this material into an already overloaded curriculum. As reported in "The Movement of Accessible Design Principles into Mainstream Engineering: Now and Then" [10], practicing engineers in industries affected by the accessibility laws are well aware of the need for knowledge of the laws, the Access Board, and its published guidelines. Likewise, academicians in certain disciplines, for example, civil engineers and architects, are very aware of the ADA accessibility requirements and the Access Board's *ADA Accessibility Guidelines for Buildings and Facilities (ADAAG)* [11]. The ADA has been around since 1990 and its influence has found its way into textbooks in the affected disciplines. However, many academicians are still not aware of the legal requirements for accessibility of telecommunications products and services, and electronic and information technology, which also apply to online teaching. This is a serious knowledge gap.

The driving forces for including universal design into engineering programs are not as obvious, but nonetheless, significant. Global competition and markets present the most compelling reasons for introducing universal design principles and strategies into our educational programs [6,12]. Toyota Corporation [13] and OXO International, Ltd. [14] are just two examples of international corporations dedicated to the use of the universal design approach in its products and services.

Global educational pressures are also at work. Kennig and Ryhl, in the publication, *Teaching Universal Design: Global Examples of Projects and Models for Teaching in Universal Design at Schools of Design and Architecture* [15], describe the spectrum of international educational models and examples currently being practiced in the global educational community. The Council of Europe Resolution [ResAP(2001)] mentioned earlier is but one example of the mounting international pressures [1].

From a consumer products perspective, a global market presents a variety of design challenges. Language is an obvious challenge, but so is the anthropometric and ethnographic diversity seen in the peoples of this world (see also Chapter 7 of this book). The following is a quote from the Toyota Universal Design Web site: "Tall, short, male, female, plump, slim, young, mature, elderly — we're all so different in so many ways. This showroom offers you an opportunity to notice for yourself the importance of universal design, a design approach that strives to accommodate the differences in the ways individuals use a product" [13]. The fact that universal design can address the needs of a diversity of people, including people with disabilities, is a huge benefit.

8.5 STRATEGIES FOR INTEGRATING UNIVERSAL AND ACCESSIBLE DESIGN MATERIAL INTO ENGINEERING PROGRAMS

Figure 8.1 provides an overview of the various instructional strategies being used by the authors. These range from broad program-based philosophies such as the action research model, to the utilization of federal grant initiatives designed to achieve specific project goals and objectives, to the creative integration of universal and accessible design methods and concepts into a variety of classes.

The discussion will move from the big picture to the classroom and describe how federal grant programs are utilized to achieve the goal of integrating universal and accessible design material into engineering programs.

8.5.1 Action Research as an Integration Tool

The Enabling Technologies Laboratory (ETL) at Wayne State University has a unique approach, based on an action research model, to the integration of universal and accessible design concepts and methods into its curriculum. According to Stringer, action research "is a systematic and rigorous inquiry or investigation that enables people to understand the nature of problematic events or phenomena by including in the inquiry process those whose lives are affected by the problem under study, and seeking to implement some change or development that is tested by its ability to enhance the lives of the people with whom it is engaged" [16]. Action research methods orchestrate the actions and activities of the participants in order to solve problems, develop new methods, and create educational materials that directly impact the participants' lives. ETL has developed an action research model that naturally allows the integration of education, research, and community service.

The ETL's operational procedures and interactions with the community exemplify universal design strategies and methods. Action research methodology is closely linked to *kaizen* or continuous improvement methodologies, which in turn exemplify universal design principles [17,18]. Stringer's model of observation, reflection, and action is basically the same as the plan-do-check-action (PDCA) cycle that is fundamental to the kaizen or continuous improvement methodologies so familiar to business and industry [19,20]. Kaizen language and methods are more familiar to the business and education communities than action research; thus, by promoting and utilizing kaizen methodologies, strategies, and language when working with its community partners, ETL exemplifies, by default, universal design philosophies and approaches.

Design classes have provided a natural opportunity to educate engineering students about universal and accessible design principles, methods, and strategies as they pertain to the needs of people with disabilities and the broader community. Concurrently, ETL staff and participating students have been able to educate the community as to the practical benefits of products and services designed using universal and accessible design concepts. The following provides an example of how this has worked.

As part of ETL's initial plan to develop meaningful student design classes, ETL entered into a consortium with eight intermediate school districts in southeast Michigan (collectively known as Region IV). The consortium provided 6 years (1993 to 1999) of funding to support the design, prototyping, and sale of devices to special education teachers and vocational classrooms and

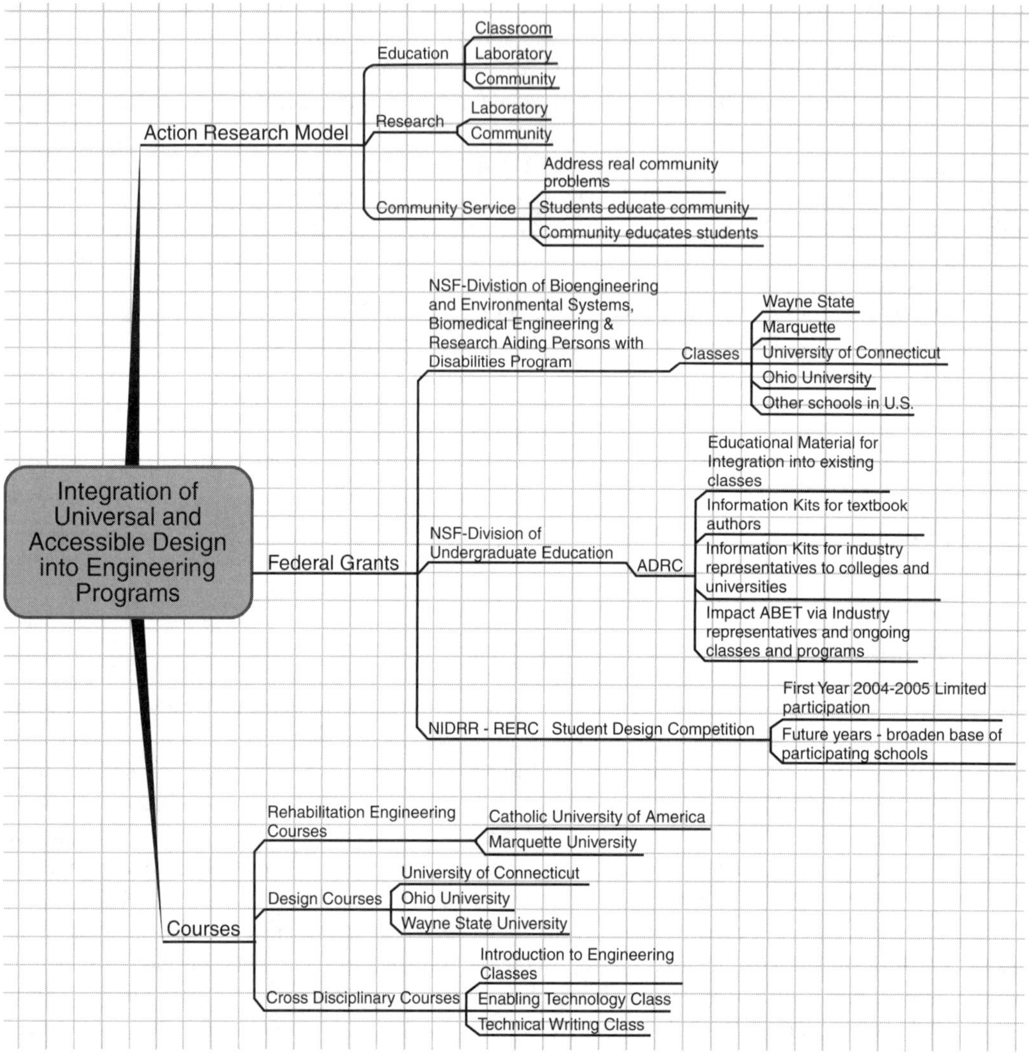

FIGURE 8.1 Overview of the current programs and projects utilized by the authors.

activities throughout the region. Teacher and student needs assessment generated project ideas and interdisciplinary teams of engineering students, under the guidance of co-author Erlandson, designed and built prototype devices. Based on user feedback, two to three products a year were selected by consortium representatives to be reengineered into more robust and durable products for sale throughout the region and beyond, if appropriate. The consortium provided financial support for a full-time engineer and part-time student help to effect the redesigns and prepare the products for distribution [21]. (Special care was taken to set up an appropriate account to manage these limited sales so as not to jeopardize the university's nonprofit standing.)

ETL also utilizes professional development initiatives as a way to promote universal and accessible design to practicing professionals. Project Enable, a cooperative venture among ETL, the General Motors Knowledge Center, and participating United Auto Workers (UAW) members, was created to promote and advance the utilization of kaizen techniques (process improvement) in special education and vocational classrooms [22]. Erlandson, in collaboration with staff from General Motor's Quality Network group, both salaried and hourly (UAW) personnel, conducted 3 to 6 workshops each year over a 10-year period, reaching over 2000 special education and vocational educators, individuals with disabilities and their caregivers, and, of course, Wayne State University engineering students. As noted, the kaizen techniques are essentially universal design principles by another name [18].

Another spin-off of Project Enable is the Agile Systems (Creform) Workshops and seminars. The workshops were originally held at the General Motors Knowledge Center, Productivity Laboratory, in Warren, MI. When that lab was closed, the workshops moved to Creform's Wixom, MI, facility. Funding for the workshops come from a grant from General Motors and support from Creform. Participants at these workshops (general and special education teachers, occupational, physical, and speech therapists, parents, vocational guidance personnel, and engineering students) are taught the principles of universal and accessible design and how to embody these principles in the design of their specific devices. Over the past 10 years, about 400 to 500 participants have designed and built over 200 different devices. The devices range from customized, adjustable workstations, to augmentative communication device holders, to sensory stimulation frames and tents [23]. What makes these workshops and devices so unique is that the participants are not engineers or technicians, nor do they have any special technical training, and yet they are able to bring their designs to the workshop at 8:30 a.m. and leave by 4:00 p.m. with a completed device.

ETL has a research focus on universal and accessible design. The student design projects are an integral part of ETL's R&D mission and community service. The student projects move theory to practice in a real context. The student projects, the client's utilization of the project devices and systems, the clients' reactions, and the observed process improvements are all components within a broader action research model [16] which seeks to include the clients as part of the research and development effort.

The ultimate and real test of the action research model is that the associated changes or projects truly enhance the lives of the people with whom it is engaged. ETL has had a significant impact on the community partners with which it has worked. Over 100 different products and devices have been delivered and utilized by schools, sheltered workshops, and small businesses. ETL has sold a limited number of these devices and requests for product information is received regularly [24]. Thousands of people from working professionals to students have directly participated in ETL sponsored and run professional development workshops and seminars.

ETL and its community partners have received a variety of state [25,26] and national awards for their programs — those that have clearly and directly responded to community needs. The programs are based on and derived from universal and accessible design concepts and methods.

How a specific academic institution would implement and operationalize such a model will vary greatly, depending on faculty interests, the resources, and needs of the academic institution and community partners [27,28]. The other key element is funding. The following section provides examples of federal grant programs that are currently being used by the authors for the execution of their respective initiatives.

8.5.2 Use of Federal Programs in Addressing the Integration of Universal and Accessible Design into Engineering Programs

The three federal programs described in the following text are programs that the authors have utilized to achieve their respective goals, but there are many more federal and private foundation programs that could be utilized.

8.5.2.1 The National Science Foundation's Research to Aid Persons with Disabilities Program: Support for Designs for Individuals with Disabilities

In 1988, the National Science Foundation (NSF) began a program to provide funds for student engineers at universities throughout the U.S. to construct custom-designed devices and software for disabled individuals. Through the Bioengineering and Research to Aid the Disabled (BRAD) program of the Emerging Engineering Technologies Division, NSF* competitively awarded funds to 16 universities for supplies, equipment, and fabrication costs for the design projects. Funding for this program has continued each year with the goal to enhance educational opportunities for students and improve the quality of life for persons with disabilities. Approximately 15 universities have been involved with this program on a yearly basis, with thousands of projects completed. Students and university faculty provided, through their normal senior design class, engineering time to design and build the device or software.

The purpose of the NSF program is threefold. The first purpose is to provide an opportunity for practical and creative problem solving in addressing a well-defined problem to students for meeting the required design component of their study. In many cases, development of devices and software for an individual may lead to applications for others with similar disabilities. Students are also exposed to a body of applied information on current technology in the area of rehabilitation design. The second purpose is to motivate students, graduate engineers, and other health care professionals to work more actively in rehabilitation, toward the creation of a larger technology and knowledge base, to effectively address the needs of people with disabilities. The third purpose is to provide universities an opportunity for a unique service to the local community. The students participating in this program have been singularly rewarded through their activity with persons with disabilities and have experienced a sense of purpose and pride in their accomplishment.

One student or a team of students designs each project for a disabled individual or a group of disabled individuals with a similar need. Local school districts and hospitals have participated in the effort by referring interested individuals to the program. A positive outcome of this involvement is that persons with disabilities receive devices that provide significant improvement in quality of life and independence at no cost to the recipients. The students are provided an opportunity for practical and real creative problem solving in addressing a well-defined problem; the person with disability receives the product of that process. There is no financial cost incurred by the recipients participating in the program and, upon completion, the finished project becomes the property of the individual for whom it was designed. Some of the projects are custom modifications of existing devices; modifications that would be prohibitively expensive to the person with disabilities were it not for the student engineer and this NSF program. Other projects are unique one-of-a-kind devices wholly designed and constructed by the student for the disabled individual. Project selection is highly variable depending on the university, and the local disability support services.

Each year, the NSF publishes a book describing each of the successfully completed projects. For over 10 years, this book has been edited by coauthor Enderle [29,30]. Each year, this annual review is mailed free of charge to the program participants, all U.S. bioengineering and biomedical engineering academic programs, federal and state agencies involved with persons with disabilities, and other interested individuals and organizations. The overall goal for this publication is that it serves as a catalyst and a source of information for future design projects to aid people with disabilities. An indirect goal of the publication is to motivate other biomedical engineering programs to work more actively in rehabilitation design and provide service to their local communities.

All three of the coauthors of this chapter have, at one time, coordinated grants in this program and, indeed, this activity helped set the stage for many of our subsequent activities. Collectively, we have supervised well over 500 senior design projects involving over a 1000 students that were either directly funded by this program or involved other rehabilitation-related design projects.

* In January of 1994, the Directorate for Engineering (ENG) was restructured. This program is now in the Division of Bioengineering and Environmental Systems, Biomedical Engineering and Research Aiding Persons with Disabilities Program.

8.5.2.2 National Science Foundation's Division of Undergraduate Education Programs

NSF's Division of Undergraduate Education Programs administers a variety of programs to promote and improve science, mathematics, and engineering education. With funding from one such program [31] the ETL has created the Accessible Design Resource Center (ADRC), which has a collection of material suitable for integration into existing courses [32]. Topic modules, notes, PowerPoint material, resource material, homework, and project ideas are available and can be freely downloaded and integrated into existing classes. The universal and accessible design material developed for the ADRC is being regularly used in Wayne State University's College of Engineering introduction to engineering class, as well as senior design classes. The ADRC material has been further organized and collected into a book dealing with universal and accessible design that is pending publication [6].

In order to encourage the inclusion of universal and accessible design materials in textbooks, author information kits for textbook authors were developed and distributed to textbook publishing houses. The author information kit is posted on the ADRC Web site and can be freely downloaded.

Industry must communicate to the academic community the importance of including universal and accessible design material in engineering programs. The Accreditation Board for Engineering and Technology (ABET) strongly encourages the creation of industry advisory boards for engineering programs and every college of engineering, and every engineering department has such an industry advisory board. In order to facilitate the communication process between industry representatives and the academic community, including ABET accreditation requirements, an industry representative information kit has been developed and distributed to companies involved in telecommunications, electronic and information technology, Web design, construction, and architecture. The industry representative information kit is also posted on the ADRC Web site and can be freely downloaded.

8.5.2.3 NIDRR: RERC- AMI's Annual Student Design Competition on Universal Design for Accessible Medical Instrumentation

The National Institute on Disability and Rehabilitation Research (NIDRR) administers the Rehabilitation Engineering Research Center (RERC) program. This program provides grant support for broad-based initiatives. One such initiative is the annual student design competition, sponsored by the RERC-AMI for the past 2 years based on input from a national survey and follow-up focus groups, and interaction with participating universities. The goal of this initiative, which is implemented through a subcontract to the University of Connecticut and coordinated by coauthor Enderle, is to raise awareness of and support training on accessible medical instrumentation. Student teams accepted into the competition received reimbursements up to $2000 for each project. The first year was a test of concept with a small number of projects funded (see http://www.rerc-ami.org/ami/projects/d/2/2/year1).

During 2004 to 2005, the second year of the competition, three design challenges were presented in the following areas — accessible weight scale, accessible syringe dosing, and an accessible ergometer. These projects were to be designed for a fictitious group of clients with a variety of disabilities, including (in various combinations) paralysis, fragility and weakness, multiple sclerosis, diabetes, poor eyesight and blindness, limited limb function due to stroke, Parkinson's disease, and hearing impairment.

For this competition, each team was required to create a Web site that was used to evaluate the design and help select the winners of the competition. At a minimum, each Web site contained a final report, detailed photos, and a digital video clip of the project in action. The final report also fully described the project, including detailed drawings and photographs, full engineering analysis of the optimal design and at least one alternative design, consideration of universal and accessible design principles and how the design addresses the needs of the hypothetical clients, all expenses incurred to build the prototype, and a projected cost to produce a manufactured product. For full credit, the project was tested with representative intended users, with their feedback used to improve the project. The use of appropriate terminology was stressed when communicating with and describing people with disabilities and assistive technologies (see http://www.lsi.ku.edu/lsi/internal/guidelines.html), and a brief resource on universal and accessible design terminology and principles was made available (http://www.rerc-ami.org/ami/projects/d/2/udg/). The Web sites were requested to and for the most part followed Web accessibility guidelines (http://www.w3.org/WAI/).

In August 2004, an announcement was sent to BME programs in the U.S. and other programs in which we were aware of faculty with rehabilitation interests. Nineteen teams from sixteen universities submitted entries into the competition by end of the spring 2005 semester. The projects were evaluated by 11 judges from government, industry and academia. At least four judges evaluated each entry. Six teams received awards in the competition for first, second, and third places. The results were posted on the RERC Web site (see http://www.rerc-ami.org/ami/projects/d/2/2/year2/reports/).

For the 2005 to 2006 academic year, three challenges have been presented — blood glucose monitor, accessible medication dispensing device, and a patient positioning aid, based on input from the RERC-AMI national survey and focus groups. As in the first year, these projects were designed for a fictitious group of clients with a variety of disabilities. As of the end of May 2006, 22 of the 24 accepted projects had been received.

8.6 EXAMPLES OF INTEGRATION OF UNIVERSAL AND ACCESSIBLE DESIGN MATERIAL INTO ENGINEERING PROGRAMS

The most obvious strategy for integrating universal and accessible design into engineering curricula is to create a class dedicated to them. Such a strategy is most likely to succeed within disciplines that are directly impacted by laws mandating accessibility. However, even in such cases, there is little likelihood that this will occur. More realistic is that existing classes will start to incorporate universal and accessible design topics into their syllabi. Curricula in architecture, civil engineering, rehabilitation engineering, occupational therapy, law, and a few other disciplines incorporate accessible design as related to ADA mandates. Increasingly, computer science and computer engineering classes are including sections on Web accessibility, Section 508 requirements, and the broader notions of universal accessibility advocated by the World Wide Web Consortium's (W3C's) Web Accessibility Initiative (WAI).

Another mechanism of change, while more long term, is to change ABET's professional component and program outcomes criteria for accrediting engineering programs to include universal and accessible design. This action must go through the Engineering Accreditation Commission before ABET can act on it.

Three examples are presented of the integration of universal and accessible design content into courses: (1) rehabilitation engineering courses, (2) engineering design courses, and (3) cross-disciplinary courses.

8.6.1 Integration of Accessible/Universal Design Content into Rehabilitation Engineering Courses

Rehabilitation engineering courses provide a natural entry point for universal and accessible design content. Coauthor Winters has taught courses in this area at the senior graduate level for most of the past 15 years. This section shares some of these experiences, which interestingly also provides a historical perspective of how conceptual frameworks related to universal and accessible design have evolved.

The first of these courses, a survey course taught from 1991 to 1998 at The Catholic University of America, included at least one guest lecture each year on universal design; details on this course are published elsewhere [33]. For several years this lecture was given by James Mueller, author of Chapter 18 of this book; each year there was also a presentation in this area by a senior rehabilitation engineer from the National Rehabilitation Hospital. Based on course evaluations, these were very popular lectures. During that time, the focus of the lectures was much more on the built environment, including everything from door knobs to fixtures. There was also a strong focus on the design of containers for products that can be difficult for older adults as well as persons with disabilities to use, such as the types of products that end up stored in a refrigerator or kitchen cabinet. This included medications. Many of these universal design challenges involved manual operation, such as twisting off a lid; others involved labeling (e.g., challenges of small fonts). A beauty of many of these applications was that many wonderful examples of biomechanical principles could be woven into the course. This was especially true for applications in which the proposed design modifications involved changing the mechanical advantage of a required task so that less strength or dexterity was required. During most of these years, students were given a homework project in which they proposed their own novel universal design for a household product. The assignment required that they employ a rather classic design analysis protocol — recognition of need, professional quality drawings, a simple bench engineering (as appropriate), and a heuristic usability analysis. In some years, a class period was allocated to having students present their design to the class; 5 min was usually sufficient. In such cases, they often fabricated a physical form of their proposed universal design as part of their demonstration. On several occasions, there was serious consideration of whether some of the ideas might have been patented, but this option was never pursued.

During the last 4 years, when coauthor Winters taught similar courses at Marquette University, the concept of universal design has been extended to a much broader suite of devices. Specifically, the conceptual framework is now routinely applied to E&IT products. In an indirect way, this probably reflects Sections 255 and 508 of the laws mentioned in Section 8.2, but it also reflects changes in society. Current society is much more dependent on the Internet and telecommunications technologies, and in the process, barriers to universal design in these areas have become more apparent. Additionally, many of the types of universal design solutions that were being suggested in the 1990s have now been implemented — door levers rather than knobs are now common within the built environment, and there have been improvements in the packaging of containers, especially those containing fluids.

In the present course taught by coauthor Winters, universal design and accessible design are covered in distinct ways. Universal design is covered as a topic, whereas accessible design is covered within the conceptual framework of universal access, similar to the way it is presented in Chapter 25 of this book. This approach in part reflects the author's interest and experience in telerehabilitation [34]. Interestingly, the term *universal access* is probably even more challenging than accessible design in that it also has legal implications, in this case, related to a telecommunications industry that is regulated by the Federal Communications Commission (FCC). For instance, it addresses rights related to receiving and supplying services to rural communities for any lawful purpose in a nondiscriminatory manner. Within the context of this rehabilitation course, universal access involves extending the classic consideration of accessibility of a product to include the access barriers of distance and cost ([34]; Chapter 25 of this book). Thus, it includes an additional dimension that is beyond the scope of the present discussion, except perhaps for certain electrical or rehabilitation engineers. In terms of material, laws that relate to accessible design, such as the ADA and Sections 255 and 508, are covered. Guidelines associated with these laws, such as those maintained by the Access Board as noted previously, are viewed as both design specifications and as a collection of hints for developing appropriate design strategies.

Human sensorimotor performance is also covered, and human factors and usability concepts are covered within the context of human performance assessment. Accessibility is treated as having a continuum within a "difficulty" domain, with the extreme being "impossible." Within the context of universal access, accessibility is recognized at both the level of the individual and of the collective community of all persons. Typically there has been a homework assignment that uses the RERC-AMI's Mobile Usability Lab (see Chapter 13 of this book) as a tool to evaluate human performance. Students perform goal-directed tasks associated with using products or services while experiencing varied abilities (e.g., wearing a glove, blind-folded, wearing ear-muffs, having a weight strapped to their wrist). As part of the assignment, they perform a simple video-based task analysis, and have their peers fill out questionnaires that they designed. Their write-up includes identification of access difficulties and barriers within their results section and a discussion section that often brings up accessible design concepts.

8.6.2 Integration of Accessible/Universal Design Content into Design Courses

8.6.2.1 University of Connecticut and Ohio University

In the University of Connecticut's (UConn's) biomedical engineering (BME) program, the senior design course provides an opportunity for practical and creative problem solving. Particular focus in the design experience is placed on the creation of a commercial product. Many of the projects built by UConn students are created as an outreach program to benefit persons with disabilities that reside in an economically deprived Appalachian region of southeast Ohio. The goal is to have students from one of the most prosperous states in the U.S. building projects that make a difference for people in one of the poorest states. This experience is comprehensive, reflecting all aspects of the engineering design process and industry practice. Students use the Web to document and report progress on their project. (The senior design home page is located at http://www.bme.uconn.edu.) BME senior design consists of two required courses, BME Design I and II. Design I is a three-credit-hour course in which students are introduced to a variety of subjects. These include working on teams, design process, planning and scheduling (timelines), technical report writing, proposal writing, oral presentations, ethics in design, safety, liability, impact of economic constraints, environmental considerations, FDA, patents, manufacturing, and marketing. Design II, a three-credit-hour course following Design I, requires students to implement their design by completing a working model of the final product. Prototype testing of the paper design typically requires modification to meet specifications.

Ohio University (OU) is well suited to serve as a partner with the UConn senior design project experiences, not only because the two faculty members (coauthor Enderle and Brooke Hallowell) working on the project have complementary areas of expertise, but also because of the university's facilities and clinical affiliations. The College of Health and Human Services houses six health-related professional schools. In addition to its own on-campus communication disorders and physical therapy clinics, the college has 22 active off-campus clinical contracts serving persons of all ages with a wide variety of disabilities, such that contacts with persons with disabilities in the surrounding Appalachian region are numerous. OU also houses its own College of Medicine, with active clinical components in geriatric, family, and specialty medicine, providing additional possible sources for the identification of specific needs of individuals in the region. Once the projects are completed at UConn, they are sent to OU for delivery to the clients.

To facilitate working with sponsors, a Web-based approach is used for reporting progress on projects. The students provide a weekly report on their home pages. The report structure includes project identity, work completed during the past week, current work within the last day, future work, status review, and at least one graphic inserted into the report.

The global marketplace is one in which engineering and professional teams are working on projects simultaneously at distant sites. It is vitally important that students be exposed to working in local teams and global teams at distant sites before working in industry. Part of this experience has included video conferencing, telephone, e-mail, and the use of the Web in communicating project progress between the sponsor, the student team, and the faculty. For the most part this has worked well. At first, the use of video conferencing was thought to be the best way to communicate, but the difficulty of arranging video conferencing and cost of video conferencing has limited it usefulness. E-mail and the Web have been the most successful methods of communication, along with the telephone.

8.6.2.2 Wayne State University's Enabling Technologies Laboratory (ETL)

ETL student design activities are key elements in its action research model. The student design projects implement accessible and universal design concepts into products and services. The ETL has been awarded two NSF student design project grants described in Subsection 8.5.2.2 [35,36]. These grants built on the Region IV and Project Enable support and allowed an expansion of activities beyond the Region IV partners. The ETL continued its "client-oriented" approach to student design and has continued to sell devices as the need arises.

Some examples of the devices that have been designed and delivered to clients include an automated page turner [37], a switch-operated ribbon-cutting device [38], and a paper dispensing and counting system [39]. Devices that originated as student design projects and have been redesigned for limited sale include a Poka-Yoke (error-proofing) controller [40,41], which is used to control talking scales and counting and sorting conveyor belt operations [42], an inexpensive turntable [43], and an inexpensive electronic counter [44].

In addition to devices, the ETL projects included a number of multiyear process analyses and redesigns. A number of ETL student design teams worked with the Josephine Brighton Skills Center over a 3-year period to analyze, redesign, and implement major changes to their vocational, special education operations. Industrial engineering student teams analyzed and developed redesigns for the commercial baking, commercial cleaning, and commercial kitchen classrooms [45]. These process redesigns resulted in a diverse collection of device and product-based student design projects. A similar long-term, multi-semester, multi-team, interdisciplinary team approach has been taken with other schools and organizations [22,46–49].

8.6.3 Integration of Accessible/Universal Design Content into Other Courses

8.6.3.1 Introduction to Engineering Courses

Introducing universal and accessible design concepts, methods, and examples into introductory engineering courses is an effective way to reach students from all engineering disciplines. Not only does this approach reach a broad array of students, it also serves to educate and raise the awareness of engineering faculty.

At Wayne State University the Introduction to Engineering course is required for all lower division engineering students. Faculty from different departments rotate through as coordinators, and faculty from different departments act as quest lecturers. Co-author Erlandson volunteered to teach a section on universal and accessible design. He used this opportunity to test the educational material being developed for the ADRC. Universal and accessible design modules are now part of the course topics.

8.6.3.2 Cross- Disciplinary Courses

In addition to the engineering-based design classes, ETL offers Enabling Technology, a 6000-level class, meaning both undergraduate seniors and masters-level graduate students can take the class. The class is cross-listed between electrical and computer engineering and occupational therapy. The class is cotaught by coauthor Erlandson (engineering) and Case (occupational therapy). Having both professors in the classroom and engaged in discussions is a key ingredient of the class. The class is an elective in engineering and occupational therapy, but is required for undergraduate Special Education majors and people in the Developmental Disabilities Program. The class has been offered for about 10 years and has continued to attract a diverse body of students. Universal and accessible design principles, methods, and strategies are an integral part of this class. Students are required to form interdisciplinary teams and conduct a community-based class project.

8.6.3.3 Other Undergraduate Courses

The ADRC has material on universal and accessible design that can be integrated into a variety of undergraduate courses, for example, technical writing, social sciences, political science, and ethics. There is no shortage of technical material related to universal and accessible design; in addition, a wealth of ethical, social, and political issues also exist. As practitioners of universal and accessible design, we are in a unique position to influence and provide material to our liberal arts colleagues.

8.7 CONCLUSIONS

Different but complementary pressures are at work to mainstream universal and accessible design. A variety of federal laws and associated regulations and guidelines drive the need for engineers to know about accessible design. Global manufacturing and marketing, changing demographics, and a variety of international educational initiatives drive the need for engineers to know about universal design.

The design of medical devices and equipment falls in the realm of universal design with the objective of maximizing accessibility if feasible. Figure 8.2 illustrates that both aspects of accessible design, conforming to legal requirements and constraints, and maximizing accessibility, share common features with universal design. Yet both aspects of accessible design and universal design also have features unique to themselves. At present, the design of medical devices has no legal requirements for accessibility. However, as Equation (8.1) and Equation (8.2) emphasize, the design of medical devices and equipment must typically satisfy a collection of possibly conflicting safety- and health-related constraints and performance criteria.

Practicing engineers and emerging engineers in our institutions of higher learning must become aware of these universal and accessible design concepts if they are to design systems and devices that can successfully compete in today's global economy. Generally speaking, engineering schools in the U.S. have not integrated the concepts and methods of universal and accessible design into their engineering programs. There are pockets of exception and a small sample of these exceptions have been presented and discussed. The programs, courses, and project initiatives discussed in this chapter will hopefully spark ideas and motivate others to more actively promote the integration of universal and accessible design into engineering programs.

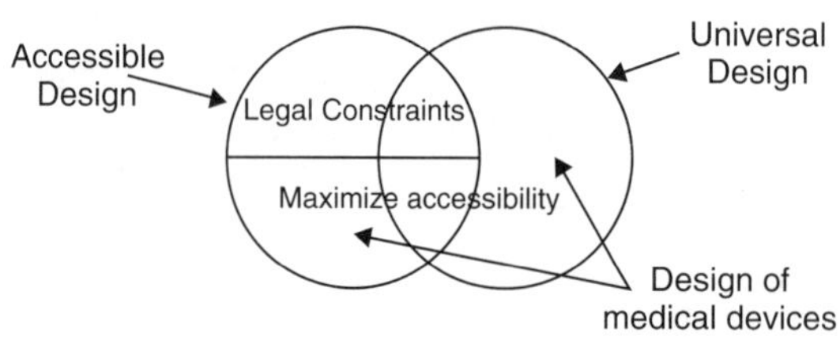

FIGURE 8.2 A Venn diagram illustrating the relationship among aspects of accessible design and universal design.

REFERENCES

1. Council of Europe Committee of Ministers, Resolution [ResAP(2001)1] on the introduction of the principles of universal design into the curricula of all occupations working on the built environment, 15 February 2001. Available from: http://www. logos-net.net/ilo/159_base/instr/coe_adj.htm#sl2
2. U.S. Access Board, Americans with Disabilities Act Accessibility Requirements, Washington, D.C., http://www.access-board.gov/bfdg/adares.htm, 1999.
3. U.S. Access Board, Telecommunications Act Accessibility Guidelines: Final Rule, Washington, D.C., Federal Register, 36 CFR Part 1193, 1998.
4. U.S. Access Board, Electronic and Information Technology Accessibility Standards, Vol., http://www. access-board.gov/sec508/nprm.htm. Washington, D.C.: 36 CFR Part 1194, Docket No, 2000-01, RIN 3014-AA25, 2000.
5. U.S. Access Board, Access Board Home Page, http://www.access-board.gov/, 2001.
6. Erlandson, R.F., *Universal and Accessible Design for Products, Services, and Processes*. Boca Raton, FL: CRC Press, in press.
7. Center for Accessible Housing, Definitions: Accessible, Adaptable, and Universal Design (Fact Sheet), North Carolina State University, Raleigh, NC, 1991.
8. Erlandson, R.F., Universal and Accessible Design Principles, Accessible Design Resource Center (ADRC), Wayne State University, MI, 2003.
9. Connell, B.R., Jones, M., Mace, R., Mueller, J., Mullick, A., Ostroff, E., Sanford, J., Steinfeld, E., Story, M., and Vanderheiden, G., Principles of Universal Design, North Carolina State University, The Center for Universal Design, 1997.
10. Erlandson, R.F. and Babbitt, B.C., The movement of accessible design principles into mainstream engineering: now and then, in *Emerging and Accessible Telecommunication and Information Technologies*, Winters, R.J., Simpson, R.C., and Vanderheiden, G.C., Eds., Arlington, VA, RESNA Press, 2002, pp. 1–18.
11. U.S. Access Board, ADA Accessibility Guidelines for Buildings and Facilities (ADAAG), 2002.
12. Erlandson, R.F., Universal Design/Accessible Design/Adaptable Design Introductory Module, http:// www.etl-lab.eng.wayne.edu/adrc/, 2003.
13. Toyota Corporation, Toyota Universal Design Showcase, http://www.megaweb.gr.jp/Uds/English/, 2004.
14. OXO International, What We're About, http://www.oxo.com/oxo/about_what.htm, 2006.
15. Kennig, B. and Ryhl, C., Teaching Universal Design: Global Examples of Projects and Models for Teaching in Universal Design at Schools of Design and Architecture, AAOutils, ANLH, Brussels, 2002.
16. Stringer, E.T., *Action Research*, 2nd ed., Thousand Oaks, CA, Sage, 1999.
17. Erlandson, R.F., Universal Design for Learning: Curriculum, Technology, and Accessibility, in *ED-MEDIA 2002 World Conference on Educational Multimedia, Hypermedia and Telecommunication*, June 26–29, 2002, Denver, CO: 2002.
18. Erlandson, R.F., Accessible Design and Employment of People with Disabilities, in *The Sourcebook of Rehabilitation and Mental Health Practice*, Moxlley, D., Ed., New York: Plenum, 2003, pp. 235–252. chap. 19.
19. Imai, M., *Kaizen*, 1st ed., New York, McGraw-Hill, 1986.
20. Imai, M., *Gemba Kaizen*, New York, McGraw-Hill, 1997.
21. Enabling Technologies Lab, Enabling Technologies Laboratory: Home Page, Wayne State University, MI, 2000.
22. Erlandson, R.F., Greenwood, L., Perrin, M., and Zapinski, R., *Kaizen and Kids*. Dearborn, MI, 1997.
23. Enabling Technologies Lab, Agile Devices and Creform Applications, Wayne State University, MI, 2004.
24. Enabling Technologies Lab, ETL Products and Applications, Wayne State University, MI, 2003.
25. Michigan Association for School Boards, Education Excellence Award 1997: Bovenschen School Award for work with ETL (WSU) and GM, MI, 1997.
26. Michigan Campus Compact, Erlandson-Michigan Campus Compact 2000 Faculty/Staff Community Service-Learning Award, Michigan Campus Compact, 2000.
27. American School Board, Magna winners 2000: Macomb Intermediate School District, *American School Board Journal*, 2000.

28. Engineering Society of Detroit, Ms. Linda Ray, Hardy Elementary School, South Lyon, MI, A 2004 da Vinci Awards™ Winner, 2005.
29. Enderle, J.D., An Overview on the National Science Foundation Program on Science Design Projects to Aid Persons with Disabilities, *International Journal on Engineering Education*, Vol. 15, No. 4, 288–297, 1999.
30. Enderle, J.D. and Hallowell, B., Eds., *National Science Foundation 2003 Engineering Senior Design Projects to Aid Persons with Disabilities, Creative Learning Press*, Mansfield Center, CT, 405 pp. (Available for viewing at: http://nsf-pad.bme.uconn.edu)
31. National Science Foundation, Accessible Design Curriculum and Educational Materials, grant DUE-0088807. 2/1/2001-7/31/2006.
32. Erlandson, R., ADRC-Home Page, http://www.etl-lab.eng.wayne.edu/adrc/, 2005.
33. Winters, J.M., Rehabilitation Engineering Training for the Future: Influence of Trends in Academics, Technology, and Health Care, *Assistive Technology*, Vol. 7, 95–110, 1995.
34. Winters, J.M., TeleRehabilitation Research: Emerging Opportunities, *Annual Reviews of Biomedical Engineering*, Vol. 4, 287–320, 2002.
35. National Science Foundation, Enabling Technologies Laboratory: Student Design Projects, 2002–2007, BES-0204099.
36. National Science Foundation, Enabling Technologies Laboratory: Student Design Projects, 1997–2002, BSE-9707720.
37. Abdul-Mujeeb, N., Antaran, M., Kivac, M., Rauf, S., and Slack, G., Automated page-turner, in *National Science Foundation Engineering Senior Design Projects to Aid Persons with Disabilities*, Enderle, J.D. and Hallowell, B., Eds., Mansfield Center, CT, Creative Learning Press, 1999, pp. 292, 293.
38. Brolh, H., Chuong, M., Barlow, W., and Sant, D., Switch operated ribbon cutter, in *National Science Foundation Engineering Senior Design Projects to Aid Persons with Disabilities*, Enderle, J.D. and Hallowell, B., Eds., Mansfield Center, CT, Creative Learning Press, 1999, pp. 302, 303.
39. Sant, D. and Gummadi, V., Parts dispensing and counting system, in *National Science Foundation Engineering Senior Design Projects to Aid Persons with Disabilities,* Enderle, J.D. and Hallowell, B., Eds., Mansfield Center, CT, Creative Learning Press, 1999.
40. Enabling Technologies Lab, PokaYoke Controller, 2000. Available at http://eng.wayne.edu/legacy/etl/Products/PokaYoke.html.
41. Erlandson, R.F. and Sant, D., Poka-yoke process controller designed for individuals with cognitive impairments, *Assistive Technology*, Vol. 10, 102–112, 1998.
42. Erlandson, R.F., Noblet, M.J., and Phelps, J.A., Impact of poka-yoke device on job performance of individuals with cognitive impairments, *IEEE Transactions on Rehabilitation Engineering*, Vol. 6, 269–276, 1998.
43. Enabling Technologies Lab, *ETL Indexing Turntable*: http://ece.eng.wayne.edu/etl/ Products/Indexing Turntable.html, 2000.
44. Enabling Technologies Lab, *ETL Counter Controller*: http://ece.eng.wayne.edu/etl/ Products/Counter-Controller.html, 2000.
45. Enabling Technologies Lab, The Jo Brighton Skills Center, http://ece.eng.wayne.edu/etl/design/jobrighton.html, 2000.
46. Hudson-Biggens, E., Flis, E., and Fayvusovich, V., Redesign of Kennedy center vocational classroom, in *National Science Foundation Engineering Senior Design Projects to Aid Persons with Disabilities*, Enderle, J.D. and Hallowell, B., Eds., Mansfield Center, CT: Creative Learning Press, 2000, pp. 277–278.
47. Champion, T. and Ricaurte, C., HVAC disassembly process and workstation design, in *National Science Foundation Engineering Senior Design Projects to Aid Persons with Disabilities*, Enderle, J.D. and Hallowell, B., Eds., Mansfield Center, CT: Creative Learning Press, 2001, pp. 310–311.
48. Erlandson, R.F., Kierstein, I., and McElhone, D., Assembly Techniques to Sheltered Workshops and Community Worksites: Working Smarter not Harder, presented at *Council on Exceptional Children — Annual State Conference*, Grand Rapids, MI, 1998.
49. Powell, K., Hardin, S., and Erlandson, R.F., Stop The Juggling Act: Structure for Success, presented at Closing the Gap, St. Paul, MN, 1998.

9 Assistive Technology Devices and Universal Design Assessments: Theoretical Relationships and Implications on Measurement

Roger O. Smith, Kathy Longenecker Rust, and Stephanie Siegler

CONTENTS

ABSTRACT

This chapter proposes a relationship between assistive technology (AT) and universal design (UD), describing the efforts of practitioners and researchers to measure both, and recommending approaches suited to the understudied needs in medical instrumentation. Both the use of assistive technology devices (ATDs) and the application of UD strategies provide concurrent interventions/preinterventions that can improve functional outcomes of people with disabilities. Specifically, the IMPACT^2 model and A3 Model are discussed, and both of these models address a person's interaction with the environment. Commonly used items, such as the telephone, were originally developed to assist a specific population with a disability and are now accepted universally by society. Developers have struggled to make AT and medical instrumentation universally designed, due to the limited number of assessments currently available on UD. Two strategies are listed to support the incorporation of UD and medical instrumentation. The first strategy is to use traditional methods of functional assessment. A second strategy involves developing an assessment that will specifically measure the level of UD for medical instruments.

9.1 INTRODUCTION

Minkel defines assistive technology (AT) outcome as "the cumulative result of the application of a measured bundle of technology resources, services, and devices, on the functional needs of the individual, consistent with the mutually decided goals of the consumer, family and AT provider, bounded by available resources" [1]. Indeed, this complex definition addresses several issues inherent in measuring AT outcomes. One issue related to measuring AT outcomes is to understand its relationship to universal design (UD). How does AT impact the use of other technological devices such as medical instruments? Does understanding AT outcomes measurement help understand measures issues related to individualized and universal environments? This chapter addresses this question by hypothesizing a relationship between AT and UD, describing the efforts of practitioners and researchers to measure both and recommending approaches suited to the understudied needs in medical instrumentation.

9.2 THEORETICAL MODELS THAT DEPICT THE RELATIONSHIPS OF AT AND UD

The use of assitive technology devices (ATDs) and the application of UD strategies provide concurrent interventions/preinterventions that can improve functional outcomes of people with disabilities. Two models developed at the University of Wisconsin–Milwaukee describe this relationship, the IMPACT^2 model and the A3 model. Both of these models portray the generic relationships and concurrent use of AT and UD. Although each can be discussed at much greater length, they are summarized here to help explain this theoretical relationship. Following the introduction of these models, we explore the implications for the design of medical instrumentation.

9.2.1 THE IMPACT^2 MODEL

IMPACT^2 (see Figure 9.1) stands for the integrated multi-intervention paradigm for assessment and application of concurrent treatments model described by Smith [2] and based on the earlier models of Smith [3] and Christiansen [4]. IMPACT^2 illustrates the theoretical relationship of key intervention approaches used to optimize function of people with disabilities. Several assumptions underlie this model.

- The model projects that the level of a person's functional performance is the result of interactions among the person, the task, and the environment. It follows, therefore, that interventions are created for the individual and their unique situation. In regard to services, the person is conceptualized as being in the center, with varied systems that need to integrate as they all revolve around the individual. The individual's personal goals form the basis of intervention. Individualized needs and objectives dominate.
- AT is only one of multiple interventions available to improve functional performance. When functional performance is not at a satisfactory level, there are several intervention approaches used in the attempt to bring the degree of participation to the satisfactory level, including the use of ATDs and services. The six intervention approaches depicted in this model are described as common intervention approaches used for and by people with disabilities. They include (1) reduce the impairment, (2) compensate for the impairment, (3) use ATDs and services, (4) redesign the activity, (5) redesign the environment, and (6)

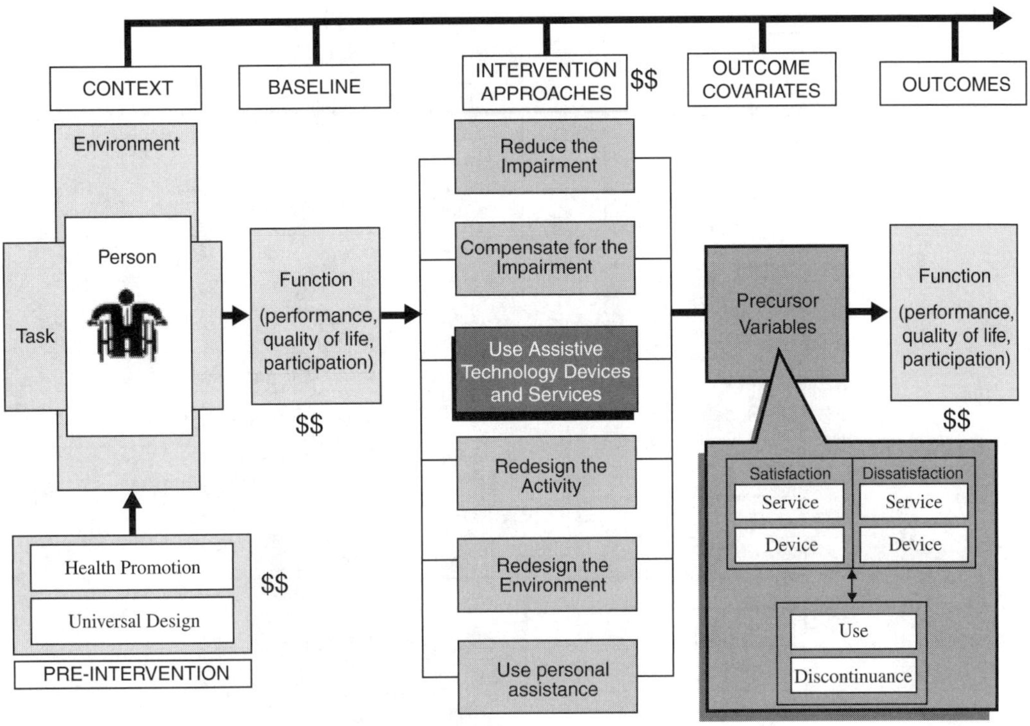

FIGURE 9.1 The IMPACT² model.

use personal assistance. Redesigning the environment, in this context, represents specific accommodation measures. Figure 9.2 shows examples of the ATD interventions created specifically to meet a specific accommodation need related to medical instrumentation.

- If we do not document the intervention carefully, then we will not know what causes any particular outcome. It is not unique to this model to mandate the documentation of the specific moderating variables of AT service delivery. In this model, however, it is not only the AT service intervention that must be documented. To understand AT outcomes we must account for concurrent interventions. As noted earlier, it is not unusual for several interventions to be occurring at the same time. The individual with an acute spinal cord injury is engaged in a rehabilitation program with goals of improving strength, endurance, and balance while at the same time learning to use AT to compensate for functional limitations. The individual recovering from total hip arthroplasty uses adaptive equipment during a prescribed period while healing occurs. Children use AT in conjunction with their educational activities. Hospice workers, to reduce the burden of personal assistant care, provide adaptive equipment. The need to document these other intervention approaches, in addition to the specific AT services delivered, is crucial.
- The natural environment is the context in which AT outcomes must be assessed if we are to garner true outcomes. All too frequently, AT outcomes are measured in the clinical or laboratory context. However, AT consumers must use their devices outside of these settings, for example in their home environments that can vary in their ability to support the disabled individual to use their assistive devices to optimize their capabilities.
- Although the model presented appears linear, moving from the person with current limited function to enhanced function, there resides an implicit iterative loop. As the function changes, so does the person and the relationship with the environment and the task. AT outcomes must be studied in this context, both to isolate the effects of AT from all the approaches that might be serving as covariate influences on the enhanced outcome

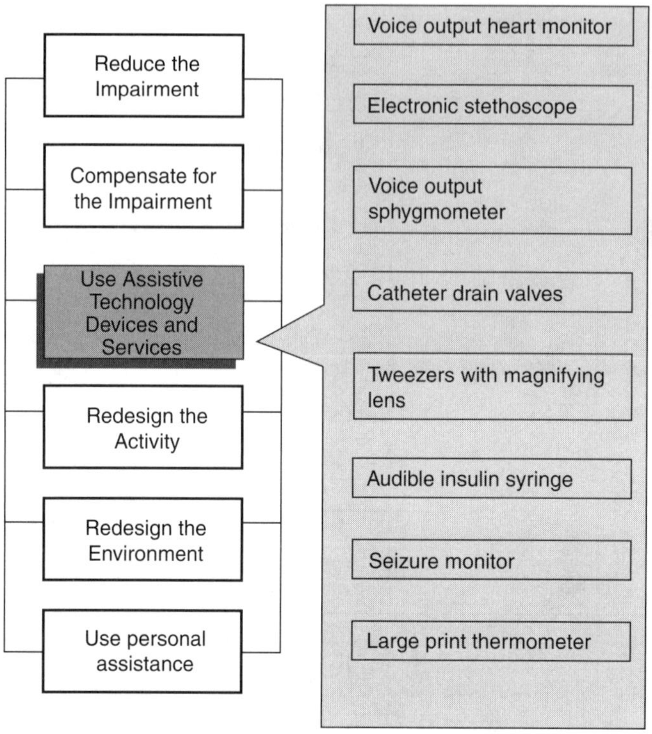

FIGURE 9.2 Personal/consumer medical AT devices.

function and the interactions and relationships of AT and other approaches related to the enhanced outcome (or lack thereof). It is clear that this will lead to the interdisciplinary and integrated application of AT and UD strategies.

- Interventions can be effected and even the need for them can be reduced through the use of preinterventions. The IMPACT^2 model specifically includes the application of preinterventions. Both health promotion and UD are considered essential components in this model of significant contribution. The sequencing of the model components clarifies that the earlier components set the stage for functional problems and even define the need for interventions that are delivered later in sequence.

9.2.2 The A3 Model

The advocacy, accommodation, and accessibility model, or A3 model (see Figure 9.3), was initially developed as an instructional tool to clarify different methods or approaches to creating accessibility for people with disabilities. The term *accessibility*, describing the third phase of the model, is used in the context of UD [5]. Its purpose is to describe accessibility beyond the common standard of individual accommodation. The first, or advocacy, phase describes the anticipation of needs of persons with disability to access their environment. In the second, accommodation, phase the primary focus is to meet the needs of the disabled person through individualized accommodation. For example, common architectural accommodation includes the installation of grab rails or the addition of ramps in the home after the need is identified for the person. Other examples of ATDs to provide accommodation include the use of a long stick to push an elevator button for the person with limited reach and Braille signage for blind individuals. These examples demonstrate how access to the typically constructed environment is enhanced by individualized ATDs.

The accessibility phase demonstrates that as the UD of the environment increases, there is less need for individualized accommodation. If a curb-cut already exists, all people, whether in

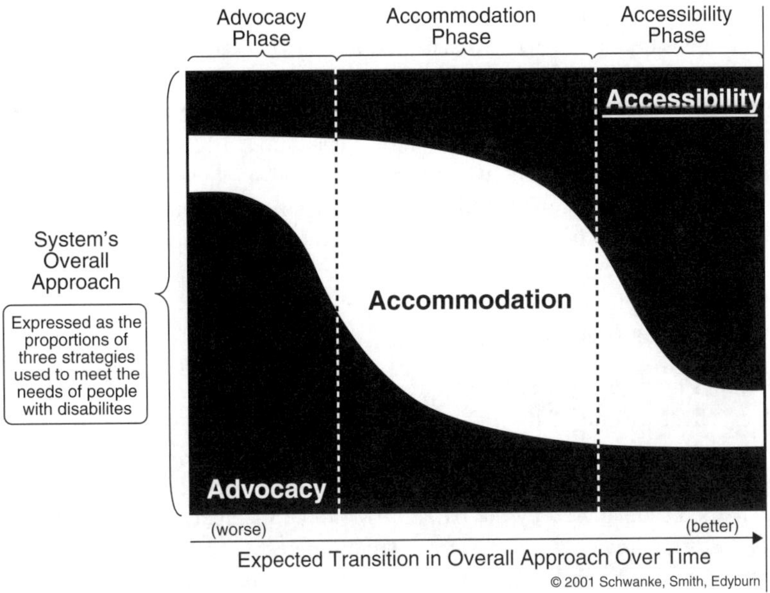

FIGURE 9.3 The A3 model.

wheelchairs or not, can use the sloped access to a sidewalk and a special ramp is not needed. If "alt-text" verbally describes visual items within a computer operating system, a special reader is not required. If a professor automatically faces the class when lecturing, the deaf student who lip-reads does not need to obtain special lecture notes as an individual accommodation.

9.3 IMPLICATIONS FOR MEDICAL EQUIPMENT DESIGN

9.3.1 Mutual Interdependence of AT and UD

AT and UD can work together, the former as an intervention and the latter as a preintervention. Both affect the functional performance of people with disabilities. This includes enabling their participation and use of medical environments and instrumentation, known to be problematic for persons with disabilities [6–8]. These models explain that functional performance cannot be considered separate from the environment and the proportions of the overall relationship between the accommodation strategies of ATDs with the accessibility afforded by UDs, which is directed toward an environment, tool, or technology. These relationships imply a very interesting phenomenon. If UD is successfully embedded in a total technology environment, people with disabilities would require less AT. Conversely, a certain logic can be applied resulting in the statement that for people with disabilities, "The more we identify AT needs, the greater the mandate for UD solutions."

9.3.2 AT Solutions Can Lead the Way to UD Strategies

AT solutions for functional problems for some people frequently lead to more universally designed solutions that benefit much larger numbers of people. For example, the telephone was created by Alexander Graham Bell as he searched for a hearing device for people with hearing impairment. We know that sidewalk curb cuts were created for people who use wheelchairs. Closed caption decoders on television sets were legally mandated for people who are deaf. Motion analysis systems were designed to assess gait of individuals with disabilities, such as children with cerebral palsy. The Bowden cables that enable a cyclist's hands to control braking on most bikes were designed for upper extremity prostheses fabricated for veterans of World War II. Lever door handles were created as alternatives to round door knobs for people with limited dexterity. All of these technologies are now incorporated into mainstream life and are accepted by the general public as universal technologies from which many people benefit. Widespread use of telephones, convenience of curb cuts, public television viewing with captions available, and opening doors with an elbow while carrying packages have all demonstrated the successful application of AT solutions becoming UD solutions.

Consequently, this relationship between the design and application of assistive technologies and the UD approach suggests consideration of how specific AT solutions and interventions may contribute to improved approaches to accessibility of medical instruments for people with disabilities (and measures of their success).

9.3.3 AT as a Type of Medical Equipment

The Rehabilitation Engineering Research Center on Accessible Medical Instrumentation (RERC-AMI) delineates ATDs as one of its four subcategories of medical equipment. Specifically, the subset of assistive technologies that the U.S. Food and Drug Administration (FDA) classifies as medical equipment or that federal programs (e.g., Medicare) reimburse as medical equipment, such as wheelchairs, is considered by the RERC-AMI to be medical equipment. While the RERC-AMI takes the position that certain assistive technologies could benefit from UD principles (e.g., see Chapter 6 of this book), in fact, most devices have not been designed with this approach and for many it would make no sense for them to be. Often ATDs have been designed for specific types of impairment or disability.

Interestingly, designing ATDs so they include a UD strategy becomes an enormous and somewhat special challenge. Ironically, many ATDs represent the poorest universally designed medical instrumentation examples because by their very nature, their design is rooted in the concept of accommodation for a specific and focused type of impairment or disability or personal preference.

Of the 20,000 plus ATDs that are available on the market, each, almost by definition, has been created to solve a very focused problem specific to an impairment area. As a result, the devices inadvertently neglect the needs of individuals with other types of disabilities and impairments including those associated with aging. For example, this paradox is seen in many devices that have been developed for people who are blind where the solution has been to create audio output of information. The audio-only display of information excludes individuals who depend on visual information because they have hearing impairments. Similarly, augmentative communications systems designed for people who have a speech impairment often assume average or well above-average cognitive abilities. Indeed, some assistive technologies fit better within the framework of personalized interface design, which is an alternative strategy of interest to the RERC-AMI where an interface is personalized to the abilities and preferences of a specific user (e.g., see Chapter 25, Chapter 27, and Chapter 28 of this book).

The consideration of a large part of ATDs as a subclass of medical instrumentation logically suggests that there is a great need for more UD specific to ATD design. There is also a need for better conceptualizing the personalized interface designs of the future. Thus solutions in the ATD design area may inform strategies to employ for medical instrumentation design. In the same way that animal or simulation models move science forward, a case can be made that ATDs can serve as an important research platform for discovering improvements in UD and engineering overall, a topic that could be of value in engineering education (see Chapter 8 of this book). In this manner, as breakthroughs in AT-UD are forwarded, solutions to some of the most difficult problems for accessible medical instrumentation may be developed.

As an example, a large proportion of ATDs are orphan technologies with very low production volumes each year and manufactured by very small companies. Consequently, whereas product accessibility is desirable, it is often economically impractical to invest too much R&D resource into the accessibility component of the initial device design. If we can solve this for small AT manufacturers, we create a realistic process for other larger product developers and manufacturers.

9.4 AT ASSESSMENTS AND THEIR CONTRIBUTION TO MEASURING THE NEEDS AND OUTCOMES OF UD OF MEDICAL INSTRUMENTATION

As one part of its comprehensive needs assessment, the ATOMS Project (Assistive Technology Outcomes Measurement System) at the R_2D_2 Center, University of Wisconsin–Milwaukee, conducted a two-phase comprehensive search for instruments used in AT interventions. The purpose was to identify whether existing instruments are used primarily for assessment or whether they may be used for outcomes measurement [9]. The review of more than 50 instruments, those both commercially available and those that have not progressed to commercial development but have been discussed or used in published research, resulted in a broad classification scheme that represents the intents of the instruments [10].* Each was categorized by purpose, technology categories, formats, and populations for which they were designed. Purposes included screening, referral, comprehensive assessment, matching person and technology, acquisition, implementation, follow up, impact, and outcome. For example, the Efficiency of Assistive Technology and Services (EATS) [11] serves the needs of AT referral, follow-up and impact while the Seated Postural Control Measure (SPCM) [12] accommodates individual screening and technology acquisition needs. Some instruments are applicable to all ages of consumers, whereas others are age specific. Similarly, the disability population may be specific to the instrument (e.g., cognitive, sensory) or generic. A final category explains the type of AT that the instrument was developed for. Examples include augmentative and alternative communication, computer access, electronic aids of daily living, organizers, mobility, reading supports, seating and positioning, vision access, writing supports, or activities of daily living (ADL).

The School Funtional Assessment (SFA) [13] includes medical devices in their ATD Checklist as a part of the overall assessment. Additionally, the SFA protocol allows ATDs, including medical devices, to be used during scoring of performance. However, though, the SFA is very progressive in its conceptual inclusion of ATDs and medical instrumentation, it does not isolate ATD need or outcome. Furthermore, the SFA leaves the ATD Checklist optional. Therapists and educators do not need to use the checklist as a required step while using the SFA. Consequently, the SFA, though demonstrating promise and leadership in the assessment field as an ATD and medical instrumentation needs assessment, was not developed with this as a primary purpose and falls short as a medical instrumentation or ATD needs or outcomes assessment.

So, what might an AT assessment focusing on medical instrumentation look like? Does it require a functional assessment strategy? The purpose of this type of assessment would be to identify needs for independent use of medical equipment on a more general and functional outcome level. This approach would focus on medical equipment-related tasks as opposed to device features or device application. Additionally, it would also depend on a high level of expertise on the part of the assessor in the same manner that functional assessments do in the general rehabilitation area. Another possibility to consider would be to use a consumer selection purchase assessment strategy. No other assessments have that orientation although some of the AT device assessments do ground themselves in selecting the appropriate device from a consumer standpoint. The potential approaches to the development of an instrument for medical instrumentation are varied and require study. Such an instrument must describe the match, or lack, among the person's functional ability, features of the AT device, and the AT services that are needed.

The mandate for such an endeavor is that the use of tools to measure medical instrumentation and AT in the area of medical instrumentation would highlight and measure the need for UD because of the previously delineated relationship between accommodation and UD. Again, as UD increases, the need for specialized accommodations decreases.

* Database resource: ID-AT-Assessments (Informational Database of Assistive Technology Assessments). http://www3.uwm.edu/CHS/r2d2/atoms/idata/

9.5 UD ASSESSMENTS

Currently, established instruments that examine and quantitatively measure UD are scarce. We lack guidelines for measuring UD. Holmes-Siedle states, "most access audits are launched with only a vague idea of what they are intended to achieve, high expectations of what they will achieve, and a lack of perception of the management procedures involved in implementing the changes that are required" [14]. Many checklists have not been published and also do not have reliability or validity established for their criteria. Of the 13 instruments identified in a search for UD, accessibility, and usability indices (see Table 9.1), 4 of these assess UD.

TABLE 9.1
Categorization of ID- AT Assessments

Assistive Technology Areas Covered in Tool
AAC
Assistive listing
Computer access
Electronic aids of daily living
Organizers
Mobility
Reading supports
Seating and positioning
Vision access
Writing supports
ADL
Disability Population Tool
Behavior
Cognitive
Hearing
Physical
Speech
Vision
Age/Program Population Tool
Birth - 5
Elementary
Middle and high school
Vocational
College
Business
Adult home
Continuum of Assessment Measurements
Screening
Referral
Comprehensive assessment
Matching person and technology
Acquisition
Implementation
Follow up
Impact
Outcome

The Universal Design Audit Checklist was developed at the University of New York at Buffalo. The instrument uses a trichotomous objective scale and is broken down into sections consisting of site issues, building issues, environmental systems, communication systems, and program spaces [15].

The Universal Design Checklist was developed at Kansas State University [16]. It is a list of items adapted from several residential facility checklists. North Carolina State University (NCSU) provides a listing of UD features in housing available to consumers in the document *Universal Design in Housing* [17]. A detailed definition of UD is provided, but the housing features are not presented in checklist or audit format. NCSU has also created "The Universal Design Performance Measures for Products," a checklist that is scored on a Likert scale of "strongly agree" to "strongly disagree" with the additional option of "not applicable." Because of its scoring methodology, it does not determine the overall accessibility of a product. However, it recognizes that UD is not a purely architectural construct and that manufactured products need to be evaluated as well [18].

As observed from the review of AT assessments, no UD assessment is currently available that focuses on the unique or detailed needs in measuring the UD characteristics of medical instruments. In this regard, the RERC-AMI's Mobile Usability Lab (see Chapter 13 and Chapter 14 of this book) appears to be a novel attempt at integrating UD principles into assessment of the usability and accessibility of specific medical instrumentation, used both for the early planning stage prior to use by research participants with disabilities, and as part of the postactivity questionnaire that is administered to participants.

9.6 ACCESSIBLE MEDICAL INSTRUMENTATION UD MEASUREMENT STRATEGIES

Given what is currently available for measuring UD and AT needs or outcomes, we suggest two strategies to measure the degree of need for UD with medical instrumentation. The first is an indirect measure as implied earlier in this discussion. The second is a direct measure of accessibility.

The first strategy would apply traditional methods of functional assessment to measure the need for UD. The strategy is based on measuring the functional problems that people encounter with medical instruments using a traditional rehabilitation style functional assessment strategy — the higher the functional deficit, the greater the need for UD. In a sense, the development of a structured rating scale observing specific aspects of an individual's ability to participate in medical instrumentation procedures would provide a proxy to the need for a UD. This approach is analogous to the structure of the widely used and accepted functional independence measure (FIM) that conceptualizes a difference between the types of assistance needed to perform tasks [19]. The FIM delineates the differences of independent performance, independent performance with devices, and performance requiring personal assistance.

The second strategy is to create an assessment specifically to serve the purpose of directly measuring the level of UD for medical instruments. This prompted the RERC-AMI to work on developing the MED-AUDIT (medical equipment device accessibility and UD information tool). This strategy focuses on the device and not overall functional performance. This is somewhat similar to the approach taken by the NCSU Universal Design Performance Measures for Products, but is much more detailed and medical device specific. It pays attention to the client, the practitioner, and a self-administered perspective. However, the challenge revolves around creating an objective and reliable rating system. This work is described in more detail in other RERC-AMI reports [20–21] and is also the primary focus of Chapter 22 of this book.

9.7 CONCLUSION

Examining the issues surrounding measuring the need and outcomes of AT and UD interventions related to medical instrumentation reveal a multifaceted problem. Hopefully, there also seems to

TABLE 9.2
Universal Design/Accessibility Checklists

Instrument	Authors	Source
	Universal Design	
Universal Design Audit Checklist — State University of New York at Buffalo	The Center for Inclusive Design and Environmental Access (2003)	www.nyc.gov/html/ddc/pdf/udny/17checklist.pdf
Universal Design Checklist — Kansas State University	Department of Apparels, Textiles, and Universal Design	www.ksu.edu/humec/atid/UDF/udchecklist.htm
Universal Design in Housing — North Carolina State University	The Center for Universal Design (revised 2003)	http://www.design.ncsu.edu/cud/pdf_files/UDinHousing.pdf
Universal Design Performance Measures for Products—North Carolina State University (2000)	The Center for Universal Design (2000)	http://www.design.ncsu.edu/cud/events_news/UD_Performance.html
	Accessibility	
ADA Checklist for Hotels and Motels	American Foundation for the Blind (2005)	www.afb.org/section.asp?SectionID=3&TopicID=136&DocumentID=531&Mode=Print
Checklist for Universal Access — Oak Park Universal Access Program for Places of Public Accommodation	Adaptive Environments Center, Inc. and Barrier Free Environments (1992)	http://academics.triton.edu/faculty/fheitzman/Checklist.html
Checklist for Existing Facilities — ADA Checklist for Readily Achievable Barrier Removal	Adaptive Environments Center, Inc. and Barrier Free Environments (1995)	www.usdoj.gov/crt/ada/racheck.pdf
UFAS Accessibility Checklist	U.S. Architectural and Transportation Barriers Compliance Board (1990)	http://www.access-board.gov/ufas/UFASchecklist.txt
Handicap Accessibility Self-Evaluation Checklist	WI Department of Commerce	http://commerce.wi.gov/CDdocs/CD-bcf-cdbg-pf-SelfEvalChcklst_000.pdf
Minimum Requirements Summary Sheets and ADAAG	ADAAG (last amended 2002)	http://www.access-board.gov/adaag/html/adaag.htm
ADA Standards for Accessible Design — Code of Federal Regulations	Department of Justice (revised 1994)	http://www.usdoj.gov/crt/ada/adastd94.pdf
McClain and Todd Food Store Accessibility Survey	McClain and Todd (1999)	Food Store Accessibility. *AJOT*,44(6), 487–491
Environmental function independence measure (Enviro-FIM).	Danford and Steinfeld (2001)	Center for Inclusive Design and Environmental Access, University at Buffalo

be a growing set of ideas that could light the way for better measures in the future. Additionally, the inherent interaction between the AT intervention and UD preintervention provides us with new ways to consider how we measure the needs and outcomes of each.

We also need to point out that this chapter neglects an important factor in measurement of AT and UD. This chapter discusses only the objective measurement of AT and UD, but certainly, we acknowledge the subjective component of universally designed environments and products. Although UD aims to accommodate everyone, it is not perfect for everyone as individual differences are not just about performance (see Chapter 18 of this book). Costs, perceived cost, and perceived aesthetics influence response, acceptance and, very importantly in our capitalistic society, marketability. Steinfeld writes "most successful universal design often expresses the usability features of the product or environment as strong aesthetics qualities and are successful precisely because they are beautiful as well as useful" [22]. This subjective response of the user should also be considered when considering UD and measuring the need and success of UD. Such an observation ties to the ethnographic research methodology for inclusive design advocated by Wilcox (Chapter 7).

This chapter reflects on strategies of measuring UD, particularly in relation to the measurement of AT outcome. AT and functional assessments may provide an additional contribution to the measurement of UD for medical instruments. Additionally, developing knowledge about needs and outcomes measurement systems for people with disabilities may excite and generates new ideas and strategies for specifically measuring the UD of medical instruments.

ACKNOWLEDGMENT

This chapter has been supported in part by the National Institute on Disability and Rehabilitation Research (NIDRR), grant numbers H133A010403 and H133E020729. The opinions contained in this chapter are those of the authors and do not necessarily reflect those of NIDRR and the U.S. Department of Education.

REFERENCES

1. Minkel, J.L., Assistive technology and outcome measurement: where do we begin?, *Technology and Disability,* 5, 285, 1996.
2. Smith, R.O., The Impact² Model: Integrated Multi–Intervention Paradigm for Assessment and Application of Concurrent Treatments, retrieved September 28, 2005 from http://www.uwm.edu/CHS/r2d2/archive/impact2model.html, 2005.
3. Smith, R.O., Technological approaches to performance enhancement, in *Occupational Therapy: Overcoming Human Performance Deficits*, Baum, C. and Christiansen, C., Eds., Slack Publishers, Thorofare, NJ, 1991, p. 747.
4. Christiansen, C., Occupational therapy: Intervention for life performance, in *Occupational Therapy: Overcoming Human Performance Deficits*, Christiansen, C. and Baum, C., Eds., Slack Publishers, Thorofare, NJ, 1991.
5. Schwanke, T.D., Smith, R.O., and Edyburn, D.L., A3 model diagram developed as accessibility and universal design instructional tool, in *RESNA 2001 Annual Conference Proceedings*, RESNA Press, Arlington, VA, 2001.
6. Mace, R.L., Removing Barriers to Health Care: A Guide for Health Professionals, The Center for Universal Design, North Carolina State University, retrieved January 11, 2005 from http://www.fpg.unc.edu/%7Encodh/RB-HealthCare.pdf, 1998.
7. Veltman, A. et al., Perceptions of primary healthcare services among people with physical disabilities, Part I: Access issues, *Medgenmed [Computer File]: Medscape General Medicine,* 3, 2001, 18.
8. Wilcox, S.B., Applying the Principles of Universal Design to Medical Devices, retrieved October 11, 2004 from http://www.devicelink.com/mddi/archive/03/01/contents.html, 2003.

9. Rust, K.L. et al., Technical report — Assistive Technology Instrument Update and Review (Version 1.0), retrieved September 28, 2005 from http://www.uwm.edu/CHS/ r2d2/atoms/archive/technicalreports/fieldscans/tr-fs-ati.html, 2005.
10. ATOMS Project, ID-AT-Assessments (Informational Database of Assistive Technology Assessments), retrieved September 28, 2005 from http://www3.uwm.edu/CHS/r2d2/ atoms/idata/, 2005.
11. Hellbom, G., and Persson, J. EATS: Efficiency of Assistive Technology and Services, available at www.siva.it/research/eats/info1_ing.htm, 1998.
12. Gagnon, B., Seated Postural Control Measure for Adults, CIRRIS, Quebec, 2002.
13. Coster, W. et al., School Function Assessment, The Psychological Corporation/ Therapy Skill Builders, San Antonio, TX, 1998.
14. Holmes-Siedle, J., Barrier-free design, *A Manual for Building Designers and Managers*, Butterworth-Heinemann, Oxford, 1996.
15. Kansas State University, Department of Apparel, Textiles, and Interior Design, Universal Design Checklist, retrieved June 8, 2005 from http://www.ksu.edu/humec/atid/ UDF/ud_checklist.htm, 2005.
16. Kansas State University, Department of Apparel, Textiles, and Interior Design, Universal Design Checklist, retrieved June 8, 2005 from http://www.ksu.edu/humec/atid/ UDF/ud_checklist.htm, 2005.
17. North Carolina State University, The Center for Universal Design, Universal Design in Housing, retrieved June 8, 2005 from http://www.design.ncsu.edu/cud/pdf_files/ UDinHousing.doc, n.d.
18. Story, M.F. and Mueller, J.L., *Universal Design Performance measurements for Products: A Tool for Assessing Universal Usability*, Winters, J.M. et al., Ed., RESNA Press, Arlington, VA, 2002, chap. 2.
19. State University of New York at Buffalo, Guide for the Uniform Data Set for medical rehabilitation (Adult FIM), Version 5.1., State University of New York at Buffalo, 1997.
20. RERC-AMI, MED-AUDIT Expert User System (EUS) Taxonomy, retrieved from http://www.uwm.edu/ CHS/r2d2/rerc-ami/archive/eustaxonomy.html, 2005.
21. RERC-AMI, MED-AUDIT Black Box System (BBS) Taxonomy, retrieved from http://www.uwm.edu/ ctts/r2d2/rerc-ami/archive/bbstaxonomy.html, 2005.
22. Steinfeld, E., Center for Inclusive Design and Environment Access, State University of New York at Buffalo, The concept of universal design, retrieved June 5, 2005 from http://idea.ap.buffalo.edu/ publications/The%20concept%20of%20Universal%20Design.htm, 1994.

10 Tools for Sensor-Based Performance Assessment and Hands-Free Control

Gerald E. Miller

CONTENTS

ABSTRACT

This chapter provides a review of tools and approaches for sensing and using signals from speech, eye movements, head movements, and upper limb movements to operate devices. The focus is on the functional performance characteristics of these movements, which in turn sets limits as to their possible use as signals for controlling devices. It is seen that each of the motor modes of speech, eye and head movements, and arm-based signals have the possible strengths and weakness, and examples of their use are presented.

10.1 INTRODUCTION

Activity limitations of individuals with disabilities that limit their ability to control everyday devices in the home and workplace have been well recognized. The Americans with Disabilities Act has provided much needed guidance in the modification of facilities-based access for individuals with motor-related disabilities, but has not been able to easily coordinate devices and systems which such individuals can readily access to assist in the functions of their daily lives. Activities associated with various National Institute on Disability and Rehabilitation Research (NIDRR)-based programs and centers, as well as several rehabilitation engineering programs have provided more focused assistance in such assistive technologies. Of considerable importance are those types of assistive technologies that can be developed and utilized as hands-free or limited-mobility controllers. Such controllers could be used, for instance, as universal remote consoles for target medical devices such as described in Chapter 27 and Chapter 28 of this book. The sensor technologies that have been developed in this category include eye tracking, head tracking, speech recognition, and various signals associated with arm movements (the latter utilizing approaches based on limited motor function or range of motion). Several of these technologies are described in the following text.

10.2 SPEECH RECOGNITION TECHNOLOGIES

Speech is an excellent and natural hands-free method of communication with the outside world, which can also be utilized to control various devices and systems with the aid of appropriate technology. The use of a computer or dedicated microprocessor to recognize human speech has become more prevalent, particularly for individuals without speech distortions. A computer-based speech recognition system is based upon an utterance — a vocalization (speaking) of a word or words that represent a single meaning to the computer. Utterances can be a single word, a few words, a sentence, or even multiple sentences.

Speech recognition can be designed to be either speaker independent or speaker dependent. The speaker-independent systems are usually smaller-vocabulary systems or systems with embedded tree-based vocabularies, with each branch having limited vocabularies. In addition, a speaker-independent system should consist of words that are phonetically different, as there are already differences in speaker pitch, loudness, and tone that must be accounted for. An example of a speaker-independent system is an airline automated reservation system, which is based upon simple answers such as numbers between 0 and 100 as well as "yes" and "no." Many embedded speech recognition systems are also speaker independent as they are based on a limited vocabulary. One example would be a design to control a motorized wheelchair, in which the controlling words would consist of "left," "right," "stop," "go," and "back."

The constraints on using such a technology by individuals with disabilities are far more important than for speaker-dependent systems such as airline reservations. If the airline system does not understand your spoken words, you are routed to a human operator. This cannot be the case for control of a wheelchair or other hands-free environment for people with disabilities. In addition, there are issues with ambient noise, other speakers nearby, and stress-related changes in speech — all of which can degrade the ability of a dedicated speech recognition system to accurately serve as a reliable agent for accessibility. A more robust system is the speaker-dependent system that allows for speaker variability and a broader vocabulary. Most commercially available speech recognition systems are speaker dependent and include such popular software packages as IBM Via Voice and Dragon Systems Naturally Speaking, among others. For use in quiet environments, with the system pretrained for the speaker's voice, word accuracies of 95% are quite possible for such applications as word processing and control of standard computer functions. Unfortunately, the word recognition degrades significantly if ambient noise, voice changes with stress, or multiple speakers exist nearby. In addition, such issues as continuous vs. discrete speech are important, as many commercially available systems have difficulties with adequate pauses between utterances.

Because speech requires a relatively low bandwidth, most medium- to high-quality 16-bit sound cards will be adequate for the host computer, with sound "enabled" in the kernel, and with the correct drivers installed. Sound cards with the cleanest analog-to-digital conversions are recommended, but most often the clarity of the digital sample is more dependent on the microphone quality and even more dependent on environmental noise.

Electrical noise from monitors, computer slots, hard-drives, etc., is usually negligible compared to ambient noise from the computer fans, squeaking chairs, or heavy breathing. The microphones that come free with a speech recognition system tend to be worth their price. The two most popular types of microphones for professional use are the dynamic type and the condenser (sometimes called an electret) type. The primary difference — as far as sound cards are concerned — is that condenser microphones require a source of DC power to operate. Dynamic microphones do not require any external power. Automated speech recognition (ASR) applications can be heavily dependent on processing speed. This is because a large amount of digital filtering and signal processing can take place in ASR. As with just about any CPU intensive software, the faster the better, and the more memory the better. Although it is possible to handle some ASR with 100 MHz and 16 M RAM, for fast processing (of large vocabularies, complex recognition schemes, or high sample rates), most software packages list minimum requirements for the computer, which are commonly 400 MHz and 128 M RAM.

Vocalization of human speech occurs in the trachea. Examples of the basic speech units, called phonemes, are shown in Figure 10.1a. A speech waveform in the time domain (amplitude in decibels vs. time) is shown in Figure 10.1b, but commercially available speech recognition systems employ a frequency domain based description (Figure 10.1c), as the time domain waveforms look similar for many words.

Research has been conducted that addresses modified speech recognition systems for individuals with disabilities. Systems employed by individuals with altered speech (such as people with cerebral palsy and advanced Parkinson's disease) have been described by Prasad and Miller [1] that utilize combined neural networks and hidden Markov models for advanced speech recognition for people with speech impairments as well as motor impairments. This method extends earlier work [2–4]. More global speech recognition issues also have been addressed [5,6], and issues related to the impact of ambient noise on speech recognition also have been described [7–11].

Speech recognition has long been a mainstay as a means of controlling devices by individuals with disabilities. Miller et al. [12] described a simple system to control wheelchairs through speech. Speech is an excellent mechanism for hands-free control of devices either as a stand-alone system or in conjunction with other technologies, such as eye-tracking, head-tracking, or motor-controlled/EMG systems. Research is continuing by mainstream software manufacturers, such as Microsoft, into the design of robust, context-sensitive speech recognition systems to control computer functions. In addition, there is considerable ongoing research into the design of more robust voice controllers for individuals with a broad spectrum of disabilities.

10.3 EYE-TRACKING TECHNOLOGIES

The measurement of eye movement is also a commonly utilized technique by individuals with limited motor function to serve as a hands-free controller actuator in the home and work environment. Eye movement, as was the case with voice, is based upon a complex interaction of numerous anatomical components and physiologic subsystems. The motivation for such binocular movement of the eyes is that the fovial region of the retina, where there is highest clarity is only for a region with under 2° of arc. As with speech recognition, eye movement is described by components and waveforms that can be complex. Eye movements are often conjugate (or versional) eye movements, in which the eyes move in the same direction with equal amplitude, thus shifting the direction of gaze. A specialized vergence system (described in the following text) controls disjunctive eye movements, in which the eyes move in opposite directions but with equal amplitude, thus changing the depth of focus. There are a number of distinct types of eye movements that are generated by different parts of the brain, but converge to the same ocular muscles to move the eye.

Saccadic eye movements (or saccades) are rapid conjugate movements by which fixation is voluntarily changed from one point to another [13]. The characteristics of saccades include:

- High initial acceleration and deceleration, up to $40{,}000°/sec^2$
- Peak velocity may be as high as 400 to 600°/sec, with the value increasing with amplitude
- Duration is also dependent on amplitude and varies between 30 and 120 msec
- Normal size of saccades during searching ranges between 1° and 40°
- Approximately 85% of all saccades are less than 15° (except when in high gravity)
- Probability of a saccade increases with target displacement
- Head movement in conjunction with the saccade occurs when target motion is greater than about 30°
- Response latency is between 100 and 300 msec, and is amplitude dependent

(a)

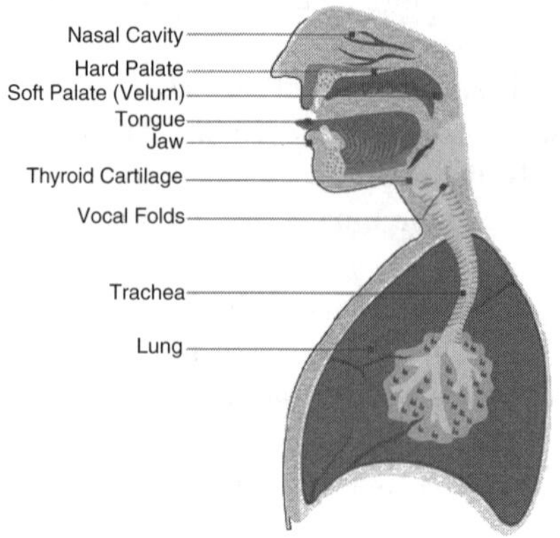

PHONEME	EXAMPLE	PHONEME	EXAMPLE	PHONEME	EXAMPLE
/iʸ/	beat	/s/	see	/w/	wet
/ɪ/	bit	/š/	she	/r/	red
/eʸ/	bait	/f/	fee	/l/	let
/ɛ/	bet	/θ/	thief	/y/	yet
/æ/	bat	/z/	z	/m/	meet
/ɑ/	Bob	/ž/	Gigi	/n/	neat
/ɔ/	bought	/v/	v	/ŋ/	sing
/ʌ/	but	/ð/	thee	/č/	church
/oʷ/	boat	/p/	pea	/ǰ/	judge
/ʊ/	book	/t/	tea	/h/	heat
/uʷ/	boot	/k/	key		
/ɝ/	Burt	/b/	bee		
/ɑʸ/	bite	/d/	Dee		
/ɔʸ/	Boyd	/g/	geese		
/ɑʷ/	bout				
/ə/	about				

(b)

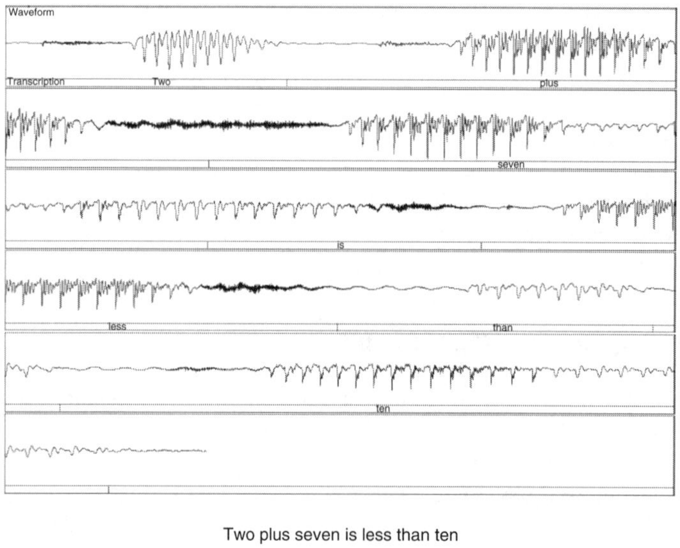

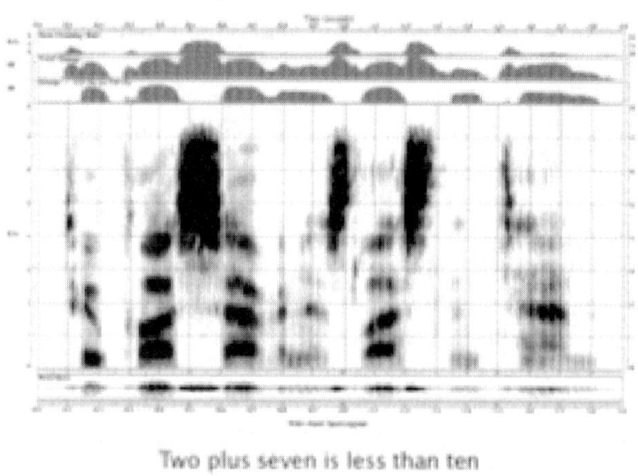

FIGURE 10.1 (a) Example of vocalization of human speech, with the basic speech units called phonemes. (b) Example of a speech waveform in the time domain, amplitude in decibels. (c) Example of speech waveform in frequency domain.

- Threshold for visual detection increases considerably prior to and during the saccade, thus helping prevent the perception of a "spinning" world during these fast movements
- Predictive operator minimizes phase lag during time- and space-predictable tracking patterns

Pursuit eye movements are conjugate movements that are used to track slowly (1 to roughly 30°/sec) moving targets in order to stabilize an image of the moving target on the retina. The characteristics of smooth pursuit are as follows:

- Not under voluntary control and thus for most individuals require some form of moving visual field or target
- Pursuit gain is limited and may be influenced by characteristics of the target
- Latency of the pursuit system is less than the saccadic system (approximately 130 msec)
- Increases in target velocity beyond the capabilities of the smooth pursuit system lead to additional contributions from the saccadic system so as to minimize retinal slip
- Predictor operator minimizes phase lag during tracking

Compensatory eye movements are also smooth movements, but they compensate for active or passive motion of the head or trunk. The purpose of these movements, also called the vestibulo-ocular reflex (VOR), is to stabilize the retinal image of fixed objects during head motion. Compensatory movements are attributable to stimulation of the semicircular canals due to head turning and stimulation of proprioceptors located in the neck, with a documented "3-neuron arc" for some of the signal, thus enabling a latency for this eye movement system that is very small relative to other types of eye movements (e.g., 20 msec).

Vergence eye movements are disjunctive movements in response to changes in target depth. Vergence can either involve convergence or divergence of the eyes. The characteristics of vergence are as follows:

- Can also be elicited by changes in accommodation as well as binocular disparity
- Dynamics are much slower than those of the pursuit system
- Maximum velocity is about 10°/sec for a 15° eye movement

Miniature (or fixation) eye movements are those smaller than 1° in amplitude and serve to make minor corrections to the fixation point. Some subcategories of miniature eye movements are as follows:

- Drift — Slow random movement of the eye away from the target at velocities approaching several arc minutes per second.
- Microsaccades — Small rapid eye movements with amplitudes of several arc minutes up to 1° separated by as little as 30 msec. Dynamic properties are similar to those of larger amplitude saccades in terms of peak velocity and accelerations.
- Tremor — High frequency tremor (30 to 150 Hz) of the eyes during normal fixation. Peak amplitudes are on the order of 30 arc seconds at 70 Hz.

Eye movements can be measured by a variety of techniques. Electrooculography (EOG) involves measurement of the electrical potential between surface electrodes placed around the eye. The eye is an electrical dipole that is more positive at the front than at the back (this results in the so-called corneal-fundal potential [CFP]). Therefore, as the eye moves, the electrical potential between the surface electrodes changes, with the following features:

- Cornea is positively charged with respect to the retina due most likely to the higher metabolic rate of the retina
- The 1 mV (CFP) difference between the cornea and retina can be treated as a rotating dipole

- Theoretically, the change in voltage is related to the sine of the eye position angle
- Recorded signals range from approximately 15 to 200 mV
- Eye movements up to ±70° with sensitivity about 4 mV per degree
- Accuracy is 0.5° to 2°

Possible artifacts include the following:

- EMG, EKG interference
- Changes in baseline CFP (e.g., due to diurnal, hormonal, adaptation factors)
- Changes in electrode potential
- Cross coupling
- AC or DC coupling
- Frequency response limited to less than 130 Hz

The use of direct contact lens systems (search coils) as an eye tracking method involves measuring the movement of a coil, attached to the eye, relative to an external magnetic field, with the following features:

- Highly accurate, on the order of several arc seconds
- Lenses subject to slip
- Require topographical anesthetic
- Cannot be used for extended periods
- Analog output

The most commonly employed techniques for eye tracking now involve photoelectric, boundary reflection, and pupil/corneal reflection approaches.

The photoelectric technique involve measuring changes in the amount of infrared light reflected from the surface of the eye as it moves relative to the light source, with the following features:

- Differential measurement of reflected light between the iris and scleral boundaries
- Linearity limited to approximately 15°
- With stabilized head, accuracy to better than 0.1°
- Vertical measurement is often indirect
- Must compensate for cross-talk
- Analog output

Boundary reflection (Purkinje image) techniques involve monitoring the relative positions of the reflections of a light source from various boundary surfaces within the eye. For instance, in the most simple corneal-reflection implementation, eye position is measured by determining the angle between the reflected light and a line normal to the cornea. The corneal reflection moves in the direction of eye movement. The reflex moves roughly half as much as the eye. It has the following features:

- Limited to approximately 15°
- Range can be increased with linearization or by adding additional corneal reflections
- Highly sensitive to translation

Pupil/corneal reflection techniques represent an improvement of the corneal reflection techniques whereby eye position is estimated by taking the scaled differences between the pupil center and the location of the corneal reflection, with the following features:

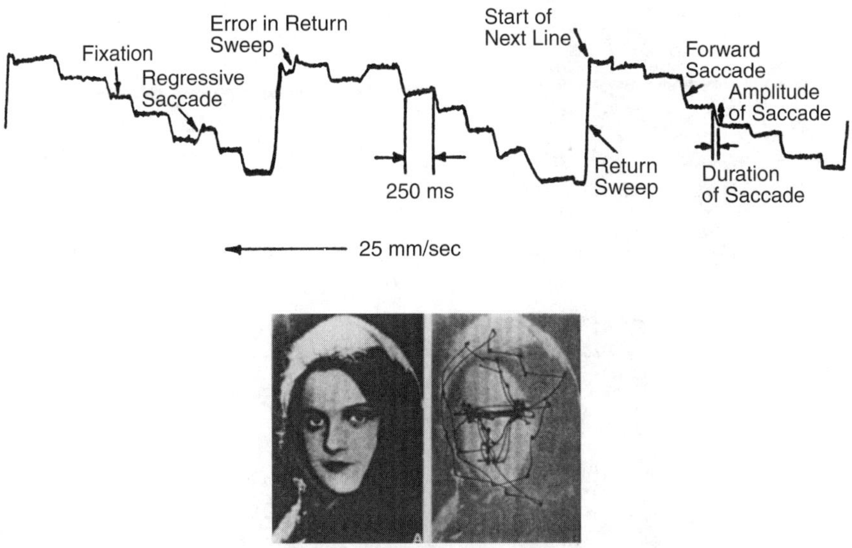

FIGURE 10.2 (a) Example of a typical eye movement waveform as a function of time, here for reading. Note the small target jumps representing rightward saccadic eye movements across the page, and the larger saccadic movements to begin reading the next line. (b) Example of a typical eye scan path made while looking at an image. Notice that most of the focus is on key features of higher informational content, such as the eyes and nose.

- Less sensitive to translation
- Bright pupil methods
- Dark pupil methods

A typical eye movement waveform (during reading) is shown in Figure 10.2a, with eye movements during a typical visual scan shown in Figure 10.2b.

The pupil corneal reflection technique is shown in Figure 10.3a, with an integrated system that also employs a head-mounted scene camera (to monitor head motion) shown in Figure 10.3b.

Research into the use of eye tracking and head tracking by individuals with disabilities and for use by clinicians and researchers as a clinical tool to evaluate the level of disability has been conducted for many years (e.g., [13–21]). Numerous studies regarding the development of technologies for eye tracking have been conducted [22–26].

Eye tracking and head motion measurement have become primary mechanisms of analyzing impaired motor function in Parkinson's patients and for individuals with multiple sclerosis or cerebral palsy. It is a very useful tool for hands-free control of assistive technology and as a means of providing accessibility for individuals with disabilities. As was the case with speech recognition, there are issues still to be addressed, such as tremors affecting eye motion and head movement technologies and the effect of unfocused gaze by the user.

Nonetheless, the use of both eye tracking and head tracking, either as a stand-alone technology or in combination with speech recognition, offers considerable promise as a means of augmenting assistive technology or standard technology for individuals with disabilities.

10.4 HEAD-TRACKING TECHNOLOGIES

The use of head tracking is a natural extension of eye tracking and is often a required element in proper eye-tracking approaches, as the movement of the head changes the position of the eye gaze.

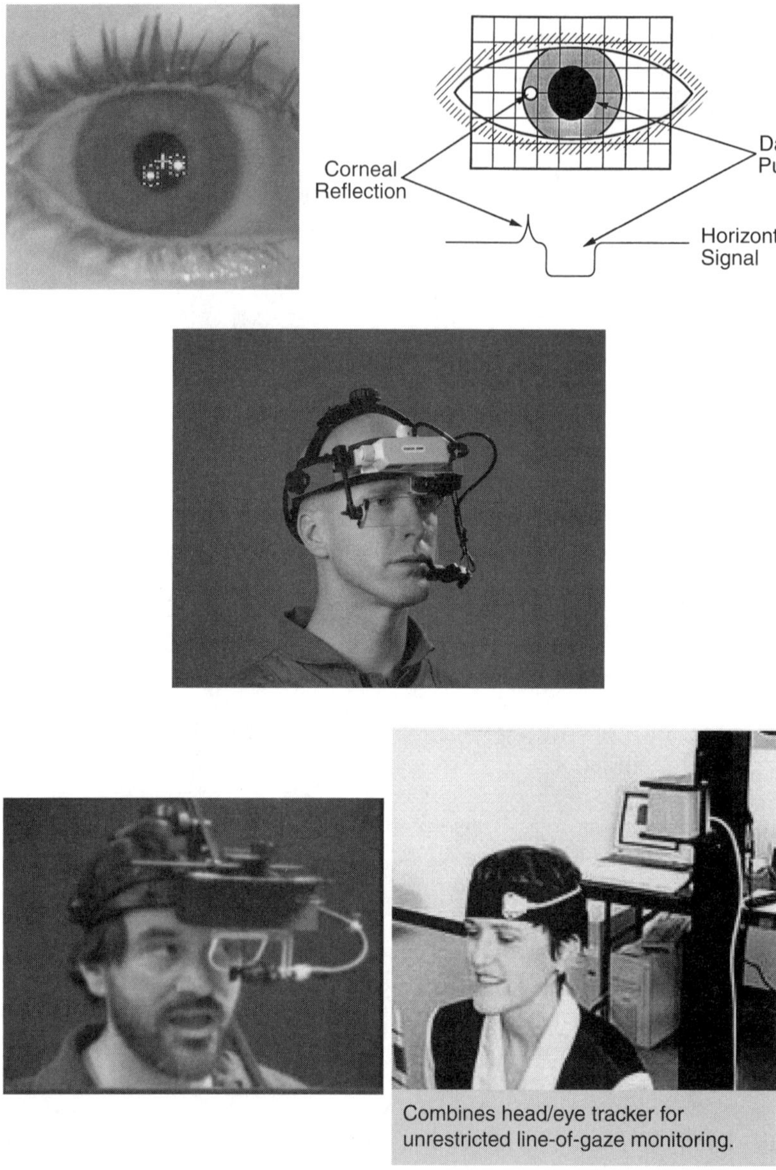

FIGURE 10.3 Examples of eye- and head-tracking systems. (a) A pupil corneal reflection technique. (b) Various integrated eye and head system that employ a head-mounted scene camera. Photos courtesy of Ascersion Technology Corporation. [27]

In fact, the determination of gaze is a combination of head tracking and eye tracking in a coordinated system [28].

Most head-tracking technologies consist of head mounted, forward projecting, miniature cameras such as that shown in Figure 10.3b. Several examples are shown in Figure 10.4. Applied Science Laboratories (ASL) is a leading manufacturer of eye-tracking and head-tracking technologies. The specifications of their combined eye tracker/head tracker (models 501 and 504) are shown in Figure 10.4.

The head tracker provides a two-dimensional (2-D) frame of reference for the eye tracker, such that the true gaze point in 2-D is determined by the addition of eye-tracking data in reference to the head position.

(a) **Features and Benefits**

Factory integrated head/eye tracking	• Easy to use and highly accurate.
6 degrees-of-freedom head tracking	• Unrestriced eye tracking. • No operator intervention.
Remote pan/tilt	• Operator never has to manually aim pan/tilt module • Correct for error by changing head position.
Automatic reacquisition	• Data unaffected by sudden head movements or subject looking away.

(b) **Specifications**

ASL Models 501 & 504	
CONTROL UNIT	
Dimensions (HxWxD):	3" x 9.75" x 10.25"
Weight:	4.25 lbs
Power:	100-240 VAC; 25 watts
Display:	9" B/W Monitors for eye and scene cameras
HEAD MOUNTED OPTICS (501) / Remote Optics (504)	
Sampling and Output Rates:	50 Hz or 60 Hz 120 Hz amd 240 Hz (optional)
Measurement Principle:	Pupil-corneal Reflection
System Accuracy:	0.5 degree visual angle
Resolution:	501: 0.1 degree visual angle 504: 0.25 degree visual angle
Head Movement:	501: Unlimited 504: 1 sq. foot
Visual Range:	50 degrees horizontally, 40 degrees vertically
Weight:	501: 8.5 oz. (includes headband, optics module monocle and scene camera 504: 2.5 lbs

FIGURE 10.4 3(a) Features and benefits and (b) specifications of the Applied Science Laboratories (ASL) combined eye tracker/head trackers (models 501 and 504) [27].

10.5 ARM/MOTION SENSOR TECHNOLOGIES

Movement analysis for control of external devices is accomplished by a variety of techniques. One commonly employed technique is the use of the electromyogram (EMG) to determine the underlying electrical excitation of muscles and soft tissue resulting from voluntary movement. By analyzing the muscle activity of nearby muscles, one can then remotely control rehabilitation devices, including assistive technology and prosthetic limbs.

Measurement of the EMG can employ surface mounted sensors or subsurface (needle) electrodes. The advantage of needle electrodes is that surface mounted sensors may be susceptible to motion artifacts. However, surface electrodes involve more preparation and are, of course, invasive. For this reason, most rehabilitation systems employ surface electrodes. The EMG frequency range for surface electrodes normally falls within 20 to 200 Hz, making it relatively easy to filter out other physiological signals or extraneous noise. Unfortunately, as 60 Hz electrical noise falls within

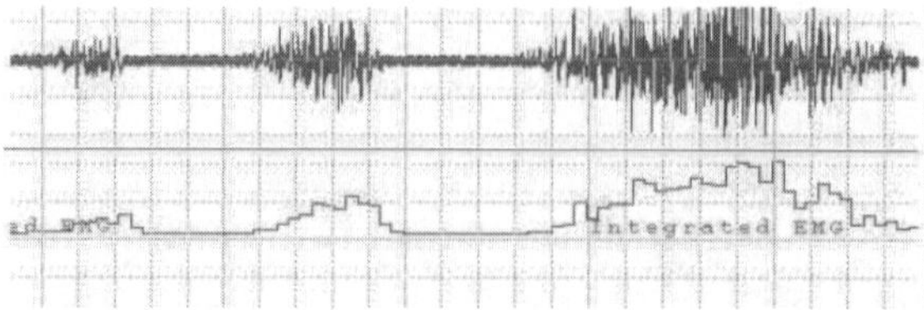

FIGURE 10.5 Example of raw and integrated EMG collected during a hand-tracking movement task.

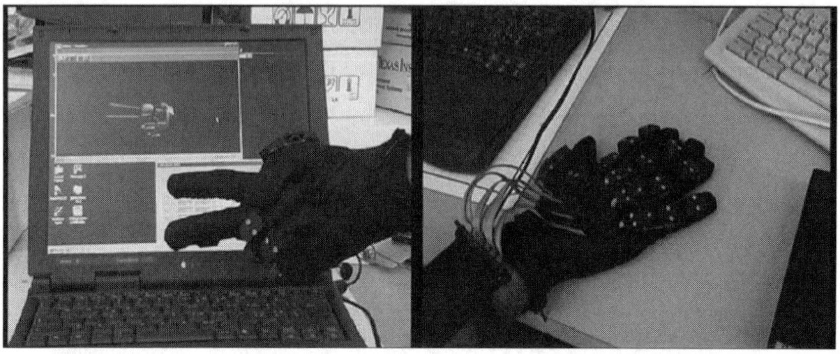

FIGURE 10.6 Images of specialized gloves that utilize piezoelectric sensors that measure the strain of each finger joint.

this band, it is necessary to filter such noise out of the signal in order to properly control devices, many of which are electrical in nature.

A typical EMG waveform generated by surface electrodes is shown in Figure 10.5 indicating bursts of activity as muscles move. In this example these signals are processed by creating an envelope around the waveform (after removing spurious signals/noise via filtering) and then creating a spike train, which would serve as a controlling input to a device. This can be done by controlling a servomotor or similar technology to operate an assistive device. The envelope approach using a modified spike train is shown, which is based on integration of the EMG signal. An example of the strategy is EMG-control upper extremity prostheses.

A variety of sensors have been explored for measuring movements and using these for device control. Shoulder shrugs often have been used as control signals for upper extremity prostheses. Hand motion/movement can also be analyzed by specialized gloves, for instance as shown in Figure 10.6. Such gloves utilize piezoelectric sensors, which measure the strain of each finger joint as an indirect measure of joint motion [29]. The challenge of using such sensor-based signals for device operation is that often performance is low because the required capability is very different from normal functional use of the body component.

10.6 SUMMARY

There are several modalities used to analyze human performance in order to control devices and assistive technology for individuals with disabilities. The hands-free technologies of speech recognition and eye tracking/head tracking offer advantages in the control of systems that require a geometric basis, such as opening and closing specific devices based upon their location. These systems also remove the constraint of limited motor function by people in a rehabilitation setting. However, the use of EMG and other motion-based approaches are more suited for control of prosthetic systems or in the direct control of devices that are remote to the end user, in which the motion of the device directly mirrors the movement of the user.

The proper utilization of any or all of these approaches is determined after analyzing the capabilities of the user. Some users have severely distorted speech, such that speech recognition unfortunately may be inappropriate until there are further improvements in the technology. This is often true for individuals with cerebral palsy caused by traumatic brain injury. Other individuals may have spastic motion where motion-based systems are not appropriate. Luckily, there are a sufficient number of different approaches and system that one or more may likely be available to the end user. In addition, continuing advances in technology, particularly in the area of miniaturization, are ongoing, which bodes well for the future of assistive technology and interfaces that enhance accessibility.

REFERENCES

1. Prasad, P.D. and Miller, G.E., Effect of high-frequency spectral components in computer recognition of dysarthric speech based on a Mel-cepstral stochastic model, *J. Rehabil. Res. Dev.*, Vol. 42, No. 3, 363–372, 2005.
2. Noyes, J.M. and Frankish, C.R., Speech recognition technology for individuals with disabilities, *Augmentative Alternative Commun.*, Vol. 8, 297–303, 1992.
3. Sy, B.K. and Horowitz, D.M., A statistical causal model for the assessment of dysarthric speech and the utility of computer-based speech recognition, *IEEE Trans. BME*, Vol. 40, No. 12, 1282–1298, 1993.
4. Jayaram, G. and Abdelhameid, K., Experiments in dysarthric speech recognition using artificial neural networks, *J. Rehabil. Res. Dev.*, Vol. 32, 162–169, 1995.
5. Mak, B., Tam, Y.C., and Li, Q., Discriminative auditory-based features for robust speech recognition, *IEEE Trans. Speech Audio Process.*, Vol. 12, No. 1, 27–36, 2004.
6. Rabiner, L.R., A tutorial on hidden Markov models and selected applications of speech recognition, *Proc. IEEE*, Vol. 77, No. 2, 257–286, 1989.
7. Dendino, M., Bakamidis, S., and Carayannis, G., Speech enhancement from noise: a regenerative approach, *Speech Commun.*, Vol. 10, 45–57, 1991.
8. Etter, B.D. and Miller, G.E., Voice controls for manufacturing environments, *Manuf. Rev., ASME*, Vol. 2, No. 4, 242–249, 1989.
9. Juang, B.H., Speech recognition in adverse environments, *Computer Speech and Language*, Vol. 5, 275–294, 1991.
10. Le Bouquin, R., Enhancement of noisy speech signals: application to mobile radio communications, *Speech Commun.*, Vol. 18, 3–19, 1996.
11. Bitzer, J., Simmer, K.U., and Kammeyer, K., Multi-microphone noise reduction techniques as front-end devices for speech recognition, *Speech Commun.*, Vol. 34, 3–12, 2001.
12. Miller, G.E., Brown, T.E., and Randolph, W.R., Voice controller for wheelchairs, *Med. Biol. Eng. Comput.*, Vol. 23, 597–600, 1985.
13. Cook, G. and Stark, L.W., The human eye-movement mechanism. Experiments, modeling and model testing, *Arch. Ophthalmol.*, 79(4): 428–436, 1968 April.
14. Bahill, A.T., Clark, M., and Stark, L., The main sequence, a tool for studying human eye movements, *Math. Biosci.*, 24, 191–204, 1975.
15. Ciuffreda, K.J., Kenyon, R.V., and Stark, L., Saccadic intrusions contributing to reading disability: a case report, *Am. J. Optom. Physiol. Opt.*, Vol. 60, No. 3, 242–249, 1983.
16. Alpini, D., Milanese, C., and Berardi, C., Value of otoneurological tests in the staging of multiple sclerosis, *Ital. J. Neurol. Sci.*, Suppl. 6, 103–108, 1987, June.
17. Shapira, Y.A., Jones, M.H., and Sherman, S.P., Abnormal eye movements in hyperkinetic children with learning disability, *Neuropadiatrie*, Vol. 11, No. 1, 36–44, 1980.
18. Berryhill, M., Kveraga, K., and Hughes, H.C., Effects of directional uncertainty on visually-guided joystick pointing, *Percept. Motor Skills*, Vol. 100, No. 1, 267–274, 2005.
19. Ketelaer, P., Interaction between eye and hand movements in multiple sclerosis patients with intention tremor, *Movement Disord.*, Vol. 20, No. 6, 705–713, 2005.
20. Muir, L.J. and Richardson, I.E., Perception of sign language and its application to visual communications for deaf people, *J. Deaf Stud. Deaf Educ.*, Vol. 10, No. 4, 390–401, 2005.

21. Baheux, K., Yoshizama, M., Tanaka, A., Seki, K., and Handa, Y., Diagnosis and rehabilitation of hemispatial neglect patients with virtual reality technology, *Technol. Health Care*, Vol. 13, No. 4, 245–260, 2005.
22. Wetzel, P.A., Geri, G.A., and Pierce, B.J., An integrated system for measuring static and dynamic accommodation with a canon Autoref R-1 refractometer, *Ophthalmic Physiol. Opt.*, Vol. 16, No. 6, 520–527, 1996.
23. Orban de Xivry, J.J., Bennett, S.J., Lefevre, P.P., and Barnes, G.R., Evidence for synergy between saccades and smooth pursuit during transient target disappearance, *J. Neurophysiol.*, 95(1): 418–427, 2006 Jan.
24. Zeevi, Y.Y., Wetzel, P.A., and Geri, G.A., Preferences and asymmetries in saccadic responses to delayed bihemifield stimuli, *Vision Res.*, Vol. 28, No. 10, 1145–1155, 1988.
25. Erkelens, C.J., Coordination of smooth pursuit and saccades, *Vision Res.*, 46(1–2): 163–170, 2006 Jan.
26. Traisk, F., Bolzani, R., and Ygge, J., A comparison between the magnetic scleral search coil and infrared reflection methods for saccadic eye movement analysis, *Graefes Arch Clin Exp Ophthalmol.*, 243(8): 791–797, 2005 Aug.
27 Acension Technology Corporation. Products: Eye Tracken, 2005. Retrived from www.ascension-tech.com/products/eyetracker.php.
28. Zangemeister, W.H. and Stark, L.W., Active head movements and eye-head coordination, *Ann. N.Y. Acad. Sci*, Vol. 374, 540–559, 1981.
29. Dipietro, L., Sabatini, A., and Dario, P., Evaluation of an instrumented glove for hand-movement acquisition, *J. Rehabil. Res. Dev.*, Vol. 40, No. 2, 179–190, 2003.

11 Ergonomic Evaluation and Design of Handheld Medical Devices

David M. Rempel, Thomas J. Armstrong, and Ira Janowitz

CONTENTS

Ergonomic principles can play an important role in the evaluation and design of handheld medical devices. Traditionally, the process involves identifying gaps between worker capacities and the requirements of the task and tool, with the ultimate goals of preventing pain and disability (primary and secondary prevention), and improving productivity. However, the approach can also be applied to the use of medical tools by people with disabilities in order to improve function (tertiary prevention). For example, the principles can be applied to evaluating equipment used by patients with disabilities, healthcare practitioners with disabilities, or healthcare practitioners who are treating or assisting patients with disabilities.

Examples of hand-manipulated medical devices that may be difficult to use by health care providers or patients with disabilities are listed in Table 11.1. The patient list comes from a recent

TABLE 11.1
Medical Devices That May Be Difficult to Manipulate Depending on the Task Demands

Medical Providers	Patients
Ultrasound	Wheelchairs
Syringes	Syringes
Pipettors	Thermometers
Endoscopes	Blood pressure cuffs
Minimally invasive surgical tools	Bandages
Tubes/catheters/valves	Tubes/catheters/valves
Humidifiers	Inhalers/nebulizers
	Pill splitters and dispensers
	Blood glucose monitors
	Insulin pumps and pens

survey of people with disabilities (see Chapter 2 of this book) [1]. The use of syringes can be problematic for patients, depending on their disability, and for nurses, depending on their task. For patients, the process of drawing up medications for self-injections (e.g., insulin) is sometimes difficult due to unsteady hands, poor grip strength, or arthritis. For patients with visual impairments, the numbers on the syringe may be difficult to read. For nurses who perform occasional injections, the use of a syringe is not problematic. However, when the task requires repeated injections, for example, while administering flu shots, then the repetitive pinching involved in uncapping vials and drawing the medication into the syringe may cause hand fatigue and hand disorders.

11.1 ERGONOMIC ANALYSIS METHODS

Ergonomic analysis entails measurement of factors that affect the demands as people interact with equipment to achieve one or more goals. The elements of the interaction between humans and machines (the human–machine system) includes objectives, machine components, human components, and interactions between the human, machine, and an environment, which collectively provide a framework for understanding what people do and why. To achieve the system goals, humans must interact with equipment or other humans to gather and process information about the state of the system. They then interact with the system by issuing control inputs to maintain or alter the state of the system. This input may entail pressing keys on a keyboard, operating a machine or tool, moving an object from one location to another, or giving a verbal command. The gathering and processing of information and the resulting actions place physical and mental demands on the user.

Task demands can be identified from the system objectives and physical properties of the machine components. For example, a system goal in a medical laboratory might be to transfer 50 μl of reagent to a vial containing a blood sample, using a pipette. The interactions can first be described as a sequence of steps or task elements:

1. Get pipette from rack.
2. Apply pipette tip.
3. Get reagent.
4. Dispense reagent into vial.
5. Eject pipette tip.
6. Place pipette in rack.

Each element involves one or more machine components (i.e., the rack, the pipette, the tip, the vial, and the container for discarding the used pipette tip). Each of these machine components has physical qualities that affect the task demand. For example, the locations of the pipette rack, the reagent, the vial, and the container for used tips in relation to the worker affect how far the worker has to reach, and so does the worker's posture. Coincidentally, the locations of work objects also affect the workers' postures and their ability to see and gather necessary information. The locations and weights of work objects, such as the pipette, further affect loads on the workers' joints and their ability to exert the required forces. The capacity of the human to achieve the system objectives may also be affected by environmental conditions such as space, lighting, or temperature.

In some cases where the task is performed occasionally, the task demand can be compared directly with corresponding human capacity. For example, the force required to eject a pipette tip (approximately 30 N of thumb flexion force) can be compared with first percentile strength capability of a given individual or population to make sure that the individual or 99% of the population in question can perform that task. If the task is performed many times per day, it may be necessary to consider other factors, such as frequency and duration of use, hand or wrist posture, and the demands of other hand-intensive tasks. Tools for assessing these other factors will be described later in this chapter, but first we will describe the human–machine system as it relates to understanding how people interact with equipment to achieve a given task objective.

11.1.1 Human–Machine System

The starting point for all ergonomic analyses should include a description of the human–machine system, with the following information:

1. Goals
2. Machines and tools
3. Human–machine interactions
4. Environment
5. Humans

11.1.1.1 Goals

The goals include why the system exists and what the user, customer, employer, investor, or other concerned party wishes to derive from the system. For example, the objective for a system of measuring a patient's blood pressure might be: "Measure blood pressure with an error less than ±5 mm Hg 90% of the time." This is the goal of the clinician treating the patient and of the patient wishing to receive health care. Additionally, there are professional and societal goals that pertain to the well-being of the patient and the caregiver, and to the integrity of the health care system.

Objectives can often be divided into a set of subobjectives. For example, the objective of measuring blood pressure might be divided into: (1) select a suitable location for attaching cuff, (2) attach cuff, (3) attach and position stethoscope, and (4) measure blood pressure.

11.1.1.2 Machines and Tools

The machines and tools description includes the machines, tools, parts, materials, input and output devices, controls, displays, etc. Machine components may be divided into subcomponents; e.g., subcomponents of a computer might include the monitor, keyboard, mouse, and case. Details about machine components that affect task demands should be included (e.g., location, weight, and visual displays). A system for measuring blood pressure should include the blood pressure cuff, the stethoscope, the patient, patient chart, and device for recording the results. Details about the blood pressure cuff (e.g., cuff size and fastener, pressure display [analog, digital, and audio], bulb size, and force requirements) affect demands on users and should be reported. Also, information about the patient's size that affects which size cuff to use should be reported.

11.1.1.3 Human–Machine Interactions

Human–machine interactions include the gathering of information about the system components, processing that information, and actions that affect the state of the system. It is often convenient to divide the interactions into groups that correspond to a given objective or subobjectives. Each objective is associated with a set of actions, which collectively are called a "task." For example, the subobjective "select a suitable location for attaching cuff" entails visual inspection of the patients and perhaps asking them to roll up their sleeves or remove clothing. If the patient is unconscious, the caregiver may have to position the limbs and expose the patient's arm. The basic interactions can be described as a list of steps or elements. For example, to achieve the goal of "measure blood pressure," the caregiver must perform the steps shown in Table 11.2a. Individual steps sometimes can be decomposed into smaller steps, as shown in Table 11.2b. The steps required to achieve a given objective are sometimes called "work elements" or just "elements." The smallest division of an element that corresponds to movements of the body or actions of the mind is called a "movement." The process of decomposing tasks into successively smaller steps is referred to as "hierarchical task analysis" [2].

TABLE 11.2a
The Human–Machine Interactions for Measuring Blood Pressure are Listed as a Sequence of Steps or Elements

A.	Attach cuff	
	1.	Identify a suitable site for measuring blood pressure
	2.	Position cuff on patient
	3.	Secure cuff
B.	Put on and arrange stethoscope	
	4.	Place stethoscope in ears
	5.	Place stethoscope over artery
C.	Measure blood pressure	
	6.	Inflate cuff
	7.	Deflate cuff
	8.	Determine systolic and diastolic blood pressure

TABLE 11.2b
The Work Elements Required to Inflate and Deflate the Cuff to Determine Blood Pressure (Steps C6 and C7 of Table 11.2a) can be Divided into Subelements that Correspond to Discrete Movements

a.	Reach for bulb	
b.	Grasp bulb	
c.	Apply pressure to bulb	Repeated × 10
d.	Release grip	
e.	Reach for valve	
f.	Grasp valve	
g.	Move valve while watching pressure gauge to set bleed rate	
h.	Listen for systolic pressure sounds	
i.	Identify systolic pressure	
j.	Listen for diastolic pressure sounds	
k.	Identify diastolic pressure	

TABLE 11.3
Work Elements Affected by Environmental Factors

1. Detect sounds that indicate systolic and diastolic pressures	→ Noise
2. Observe pressure	→ Lighting, vibration

The process is continued until the value of additional information exceeds the cost of obtaining it. The sequence of elements or movements used to achieve a system goal is called a "method."

11.1.1.4 Environment

The environment includes information that might affect people's ability to accomplish each of the actions, e.g., lighting, noise, vibration, temperature, and chemicals. For example, blood pressure may be measured in a quiet and well-lit examining room that is much hotter or colder and where the air temperature is 20°C, or it may be measured in a flying helicopter that is much hotter or cooler and where high background noise and vibration make it hard to detect the systolic and diastolic pressures. Environmental conditions that affect the human-machine interactions can be identified by examining the list in Table 11.2. An example is shown in Table 11.3.

11.1.1.5 Humans

The human components include people who are responsible for achieving the system goals. In the case of the system for measuring blood pressure, the human might be a physician, nurse, medical technologist, an emergency medical technician, a layperson caregiver, or the patient. Information about the humans should relate to their capacities to meet the task demands and achieve the system goals. The list of interactions can be used to identify the qualities of the humans that are related to their capacities for completing the systems goals. Table 11.4 shows how hand size, dexterity, strength, hearing, vision, writing, and speaking correspond to the human–machine interactions required to "measure blood pressure."

11.1.2 Task Analysis Methods

Ergonomic analysis draws on a number of generic task analysis tools and methods. These methods generally involve observations and interviews. Observations may include observing people doing the task or physical measurements of the equipment and site where the task is performed. Observations also may include the use of instrumentation for recording forces, postures, or muscle activity of people as they perform a task. Interviews may include informal discussions with individuals, formal individual or group interviews, or questionnaires.

TABLE 11.4
The Human–Machine Interactions and the Related Human Qualities with Reference to their Capacities to Perform the Job

1.	Grasp inflation bulb	→ Vision, hand size, dexterity, strength
2.	Squeeze bulb to inflate cuff	→ Hand size, dexterity, strength
3.	Grasp release value	→ Vision, hand size, dexterity, strength
4.	Adjusting release valve	→ Hand size, dexterity, strength
5.	Detect sounds that indicate systolic and diastolic pressures	→ Hearing
6.	Observe pressure	→ Vision
7.	Remember pressures	→ Memory
8.	Recording pressures	→ Vision, writing or speaking

11.1.2.1 Observational Methods

Observational methods include direct observations, video analysis, instrumentation, and time-and-motion study. Observational analyses may be time-based or event-based. Time-based implies that the job is observed continuously or at discrete intervals, and selected system attributes are recorded. Event-based implies that the state of the system is examined only when certain events occur. In many instances we are interested in only one task or instrument used by a worker. For example, we might be interested only in the use of a control for adjusting a patient's bed position. To study this event, we might wait for it to occur and then record the information of interest, or we might ask the caregiver and the patient to demonstrate this task while we observe.

11.1.2.2 Direct Observations

Direct observations entail observing and recording human–machine interactions as they occur. Observations may be continuous or they may be spaced at fixed or random intervals. Continuous observations are best suited for highly structured jobs in which the human–machine interactions follow the same pattern over time. Random or equally spaced observations can be spread over longer periods of time and are suited for jobs with low structure in which the human–machine interactions are highly variable. Observation methods based on periodic observations are referred to as work sampling [3]. The overall aim of continuous and periodic observations is to determine the sequence and frequency of the human–machine interactions and the corresponding machine and human qualities as described above.

Even in highly structured jobs, the sequence of elements or methods may vary from one occurrence and one person to another. These variations should be explored to the extent possible by observing or interviewing multiple people. The analyst may record the prescribed or most common method in detail. Brief descriptions and explanations for some of the variations also should be included.

11.1.2.3 Video Recordings

Video recordings are commonly used in task analysis. Permission should be obtained from all subjects and, potentially, the facility management. The camera should be positioned to capture a full view of all human–machine interactions. Additional close-up views can then be recorded of the body parts of interest, e.g., the hands entering data on a keyboard. Usually, multiple complete repetitions of the human–machine system under normal conditions are recorded. It is often desirable to record irregular or difficult cases as they provide insight into barriers to the system objectives that merit further study. By their nature, irregular work elements may occur infrequently, and the analyst may have to rely on interview techniques to gather information about them.

Most video can now be converted or directly recorded in digital format for easier review. The video may be evaluated frame-by-frame to identify human–machine interactions. QuickTime® from Apple is well suited for both time-based and event-based analysis. The video segment can be reviewed one frame at a time, or it can be advanced to specific events of interest. QuickTime® also enables the user to capture individual frames for inclusion in reports. Specialized software (e.g., see Chapter 12 of this book) can be purchased that permits frame-by-frame observations of the job and recording of ergonomic attributes [4].

11.1.2.4 Verbal Protocols

Individual interviews are widely used to gather information from users, supervisors, and customers about the human–machine system. Interviews should be systematic and unbiased. Some key points from McCormick [5] for conducting interviews include: (1) explain the purpose of the interview to the interviewee, (2) list all topics to be included in the interview, (3) be careful not to ask leading questions, (4) periodically summarize what the interviewee has said, (5) steer the interview to keep the interviewee focused, (6) preserve the interviewee's confidentiality, and (7) use appropriate recording devices.

Because *group interviews* include multiple people, it may be possible to obtain a more reliable result in less time than with individual interviews; however, care must be exercised to avoid a biased sample. Some people in a group may be inclined to go along with the group rather than voice their own opinions. A high degree of interviewer skill is required to draw out opinions of all members. At the conclusion of a given question, the interviewer may want to summarize the question and assess the degree of group agreement. The term "focus groups" refers to group interviews that are often designed to gather information from users of a given product or procedure. They are also used to gather information from potential customers about a new product so that the manufacturer can "test the water" before committing to production. The results of a focus group may be affected by the experience of the participants. Experienced users are often able to share specific examples of problems, but they are sometimes biased to traditions and stereotypes. Inexperienced or potential users may provide more useful feedback about a new procedure or tool than experienced users in some cases.

Questionnaires can be used to standardize the questions and fixed response sets. Questionnaire results can be tabulated and analyzed statistically more readily than interview data. However, questions are sometimes interpreted differently by the respondent than the person who designed the questionnaire, and respondents may interpret the questions differently based on their background and experience. A good questionnaire requires considerable time to design and test.

Critical incidence method technique is an interview method for collecting information about past "incidents" that could adversely affect the performance or safety of the system. Experienced users are asked to recount person errors or mistakes that they have made or directly observed someone else make that could have adversely affected the operation of the human–machine system. Incidents are then grouped into similar categories, and recommendations are developed for each category to prevent future occurrences. Confidentiality is important for a critical incidence survey to work.

Fitts and Jones [6,7] conducted a classic study of pilot errors associated with controls and displays in aircraft. In their first study, pilots were asked to describe in detail an error in operation of a cockpit control that they themselves had made or they had directly observed someone else make. Four hundred and sixty errors were tabulated and classified into six major categories:

1. *Substitution errors:* confusing one control with another
2. *Adjustment errors:* moving a switch to the wrong position, or following the wrong sequence in operating two or more controls
3. *Forgetting errors:* failing to set or adjust a control at the proper time
4. *Reversal errors:* moving a control in a direction opposite to the required direction
5. *Unintentional activation:* inadvertently operating a control without noticing it
6. *Unable to reach a control:* loss of control when reaching for a control or the inability to reach a control at all

These methods are readily adaptable to errors made by caregivers (or patients) using medical instrumentation.

11.1.3 Special Ergonomic Analysis Methods for Upper Extremity Musculoskeletal Disorders

Many jobs entail repeated exertions, often in combination with forceful exertions and extreme postures. These factors have been shown to be associated with elevated risk of upper extremity work-related musculoskeletal disorders (WMSDs), such as carpal tunnel syndrome, hand–wrist tendonitis, and nonspecific forearm pain [8,9]. These disorders are a serious cause of work disability and workers' compensation in health care providers. Some of the common tools that are used for assessment of WMSD risk factors include Rapid Upper Limb Assessment (RULA) [10], Strain Index [11], Liberty Mutual (Snook) psychophysical tables [12,13], and American Conference of Governmental Industrial Hygienists® Threshold Limit Value (ACGIH TLV) for Hand Activity Level (HAL) [14] (see Table 11.5). These tools are best suited for highly structured jobs in which the same sequence of human–machine interactions is repeated throughout the work shift. In these cases, the analyst can estimate the factors listed in Table 11.5.

All of the tools shown in Table 11.5 include a metric for repetition. RULA, Strain Index, and ACGIH HAL consider the frequency of hand exertions, while Snook considers the frequency of wrist motions. Strain Index and ACGIH HAL consider duty cycle — the percent of time the hand is actually exerting force. RULA, Strain Index, and ACGIH HAL consider the speed of hand motions as a factor of repetition. All of the scales consider force. RULA and Snook specify actual forces, while Strain Index categorizes forces as light, somewhat hard, hard, etc. ACGIH specifies force as a fraction of maximum where 0 is no force and 10 is the greatest imaginable force. For posture, RULA specifies specific ranges of joint angles. Strain index specifies ordinal values: very good, good, fair, etc. Neither ACGIH HAL nor Snook mention specific joint angles. None of the tools consider contact stress, low temperature, or vibration. All of these tools are intended for repetitive work similar to that found in manufacturing plants or on assembly lines. Each of the factors can be estimated by observing the task as is performed. Time-based force and posture plots as described by Armstrong et al. [15,16] can be particularly helpful; however, the time required to construct a plot for long cycle jobs such as performing a surgical operation or bathing a patient may be excessive for practical purposes.

Many jobs involving medical instrumentation are relatively unstructured. That is, the tasks and human–machine interactions may vary from one minute, one hour, or one day to the next. Although persons performing these jobs may be at elevated risk of WMSDs, identification and control of the causes can be difficult. First, the evaluation tools listed in Table 11.5 may not be appropriate. These tools were developed primarily for analyzing highly structured, very repetitive jobs. A case can be made for applying these tools if the job entails repetitive use of the hands, even if what the hands are doing changes from one exertion to the next. In some cases, the job can be divided into tasks that correspond to different goals or subgoals of the human–machine system. Each task can be analyzed separately and combined as a time-weighted average [17]. In cases where the tasks themselves vary from occurrence to occurrence, a work sampling method approach in which the job is observed at fixed or random intervals over the course of one or more work shifts may prove fruitful [18]. Application of the tools shown in Table 11.5 and similar tools to jobs with low structure or jobs with multiple tasks that vary from patient to patient presents several problems. In most work situations, it will be found that health care providers utilize many medical devices in addition to handling materials and patients. This makes it difficult to determine the contribution of one medical device to hand fatigue or aggravating a WMSD. In these cases, it is necessary to systematically evaluate all of the activities and consider the relative duration and intensity of use. The tools in Table 11.5 may be helpful for this purpose. Finally, the stresses associated with the use of a medical device on the user can vary greatly from one job or setting to another, so the context in which it is used should be well documented as described above.

11.2 APPROACH TO THE DESIGN OF HAND- MANIPULATED MEDICAL DEVICES

The process of designing a device must consider the purpose of the device in light of the associated performance, comfort, and aesthetics. These factors are, in turn, informed by the capabilities of the intended users. If the device is a new design, then the process might consider the designs of earlier

TABLE 11.5
Tools for Assessing Job Demands as they Relate to Risk of WMSDs

	Body Parts	Exertion Frequency	Duty Cycle	Dynamics	Work Duration	Force	Contact Stress	Posture	Low Temperature	Vibration	Specified Limits
RULA [10]	Upper limb and torso	Yes Exertion frequency and duration categories	No	Static/dynamic	No	Loads <2 kg, 2–10Kg, >10Kg	No	Wrist, elbow, shoulder, neck, trunk variable categories	No	No	Yes
Strain Index [11]	Hand, wrist, forearm	Efforts/minute <4, 4–8, 9–14, 15–19, >19	<10, 10–29, 30–59, 60–79, >80%	Very slow, slow, fair, fast, very fast	<1, 1–2, 2–4, 4–8, >8 h/d	Light, somewhat hard, hard, very hard, near max	No	Hand/wrist 5 categories	No	Hand, wrist, forearm	No
TLV® for Hand Activity Level (HAL) [14]	Upper limb	Included in HAL rating and HAL calculation	Ratings: Hands idle — difficulty keeping up; calculations: <20%, 20–40%, 40–60%, 60–80%, >80%	Rating only	Applies to 4 or more hours monotask hand work per day	None to maximum, continuous scale	Defers to expert judgment	Defers to expert judgment	Defers to expert judgment	Separate guideline	Yes
Psychophysical tables [12,13]	Wrist flexions or extensions per minute	Wrist motions per unit time	No	No	No	Finger force	No	No	No	No	Yes

TABLE 11.6
Example of Prioritized List of Barriers to Use of a Blood Pressure Cuff

1. Force required to squeeze bulb
2. Visibility of pressure gauge
3. Audibility of blood flow sounds
4. Force required to detach blood pressure cuff
5. Manipulation required to position cuff on patient's arm
6. Manipulation required to roll up sleeve on patient's arm

devices that have a similar function. If the design involves a modification to a current design, then the design process can be informed by the ergonomic analysis. In this case, the design should address the high priority risk factors or barriers first. For example, the list of Table 11.6 is a possible prioritized list of barriers to use of a blood pressure cuff. Items 1, 2, and 3 on the list should be addressed first in the design process.

11.2.1 Display of Information: Perception and Cognition

Location and design of displays are guided by the importance of the information, the ease of seeing and interpreting the display, and the expected reaction of the user to information on the display (e.g., perception, cognition, and action). The ability to perceive the information is based on the character size, character stroke width, contrast or brightness of characters, color, glare, and the ambient environment (e.g., background lighting or noise and vibration). There are guidelines for computer workstation design that can be used in the design of information on displays [19–21]. For example, the ratio of the character height to distance from eyes should be greater than 0.007 for critical information but can be not lesser than 0.0025 for routine information. A display may be augmented by audible or tactile information, which could help individuals with sensory impairments get access to information that would otherwise be inaccessible.

Cognition has to do with how persons interpret the information they receive. The goal is for the user to take correct actions and to avoid dangerous misinterpretations and wrong actions. Mental overload can occur if there are distractions by nonimportant information, such as too many buttons on the device or too much information displayed. Overload can also occur if the displayed information is too complex or the expected actions are too complex for the capabilities, training, or experience of the users. For medical devices that are intended to be used by individuals with cognitive disabilities, there can be many potential challenges, and more guidance for designers and analysts is needed, as developed in Chapter 15 of this book.

11.2.2 Manipulation of Device

The user interacts with a medical device by pushing or pulling switches, connecting cables or tubes, or performing some other hand manipulation. In considering where to place switches, the designer must consider the location of the corresponding display, the importance of the action, the risk of accidentally activating the switch, the posture of the hand when using the device, and the location of the device when it is set down. Switches should provide clear feedback that an intended action has taken place. This can be tactile or audible (e.g., microswitch) or visible (change display), or as preferable to improve accessibility, all of these. The feedback should be rapid, so the user is not left wondering whether or not the device is working. If the device is processing information, it should alert the users not to take an action until the process is completed (e.g., moving bar, clock with moving second hand).

The forces used to activate switches or to insert and connect cables and tubes and turn valves should consider the strength of the weakest intended users. For occasional use, the switch force can be 20% of strength. For repeated use, approximately a maximum of 5% of strength should be used [22]. On the other hand, if the switch must be protected from accidental activation, it should have a lock-out mode or be covered.

The size and weight of the device should consider the population of users [23]. Anthropometry tables can be consulted to design for the hand sizes of the smallest intended users. Frequently, the 5th to 25th % female dimensions will be used when considering distances involving reach or stretching of the hand. On the other hand, the 75th to 95th % male dimensions will be used for considering distances between switches, so that the switches are not too close together. Of course, from the perspective of accessibility, such an approach implies that some of the population may not have optimal access to the intended use of the device.

11.2.3 Holding a Device: Reducing Static Loads

If the device is handheld, usually the nondominant hand will support the device while the dominant hand manipulates it, or the device may be used with just one hand. If it is held for longer periods of time, the hand may become fatigued. The shape of the device should allow easy support by the hand without an awkward grip or posture. Devices can be designed with finger recesses, hooks, or curves that allow them to rest on the side of the hand or fingers in order to reduce sustained grip force. When possible, the device should be designed so that it can be used without holding it for long periods. For example, it could be designed for easy use after it has been set on a surface or attached to a fixture. If it must be held for long periods, the attributes of the contact points of the device on the hand should be considered to reduce uncomfortable stress points. An alternative is to rethink the design of the interface from a more fundamental level (e.g., see Chapter 21 of this book).

11.2.4 Prototype Development and Testing

Usually the design process contains several rounds of building and evaluating prototypes. The first round involves building nonfunctional wood or foam models. The weight of the model should be the same as and distributed as it would be in the finished product (e.g., consider battery placement, cable attachment points, etc.). These can then be evaluated by people of different sizes and capabilities [24]. Usually there are several designs, and users are asked to evaluate the usability of different features. This is useful to evaluate the size, button location, display location, balance of device in hand, etc. The second round will involve prototypes that are not robust but are nearly fully functional. Here it is critical for users to perform the complete task, perhaps several times. They should provide feedback on usability, comfort, and aesthetics. This feedback can be provided using a questionnaire after or as running dialogue of the "good" and "bad" elements while they are using the device.

The subjects selected to test the devices should match, as closely as possible, the ultimate users in terms of age, gender, anthropometry, education level, and medical status. Within these broad ranges it may be useful to also include subjects who are at the extremes of a category (e.g., hand size, strength, and visual acuity).

11.2.5 Case Study: Laboratory Pipettes

The pipette is one of the most commonly used hand tools in the hospital laboratory (Figure 11.1). The pipette is used to transfer precise volumes of liquid between containers, and improper use may lead to incorrect test results and mistakes in treatment. While occasional pipette use does not pose a problem for people without hand disabilities, repeated use of the pipette for more than 60 min has been associated with hand ailments. The primary risk stems from the sustained grip on the pipette handle and the high thumb forces required to depress the plunger or eject pipette tips.

In a study of pipetting by Asundi et al. [25], the peak thumb forces for depressing the plunger were between 23 and 35 N, which was 23 to 34% of the mean thumb strength (101 N). For

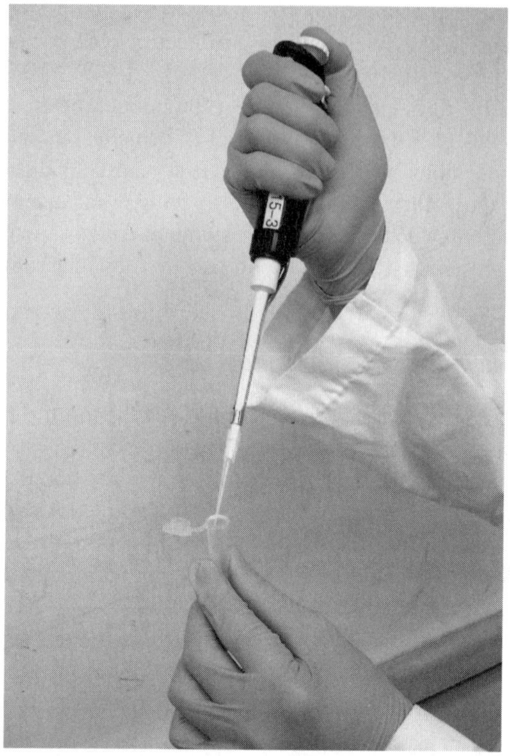

FIGURE 11.1 A conventional pipette which requires 23 to 35 N of thumb force to operate. A gloved right hand is grasping the pipette with the thumb over a button on the top of the pipette and the tip of the pipette is in a small vial being held by the left hand. (Used with permission from D. Rempel.)

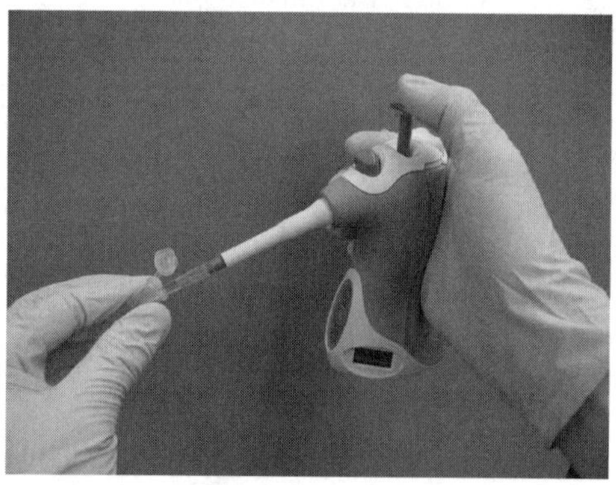

FIGURE 11.2 An electric pipette design that requires less thumb and grip force to operate and moves the tip to a location that requires less shoulder elevation. The pipette held by the right hand is a different shape from the conventional pipette. The pipette tip is closer to the knuckles so that the right and left hand are closer together while pipetting and therefore the right arm does not have to be elevated as high as with a conventional pipette. (Used with permission from D. Rempel.)

occasional use, these forces are reasonable for the stronger half of the population. But the forces will be too high for people with weaker thumb flexion strength. Workers with hand or arm weakness or disorders may have difficulty manipulating the pipette or may rapidly develop hand or shoulder fatigue. However, for repeated use, the forces are well beyond the endurance limits of even the stronger half of the population [22].

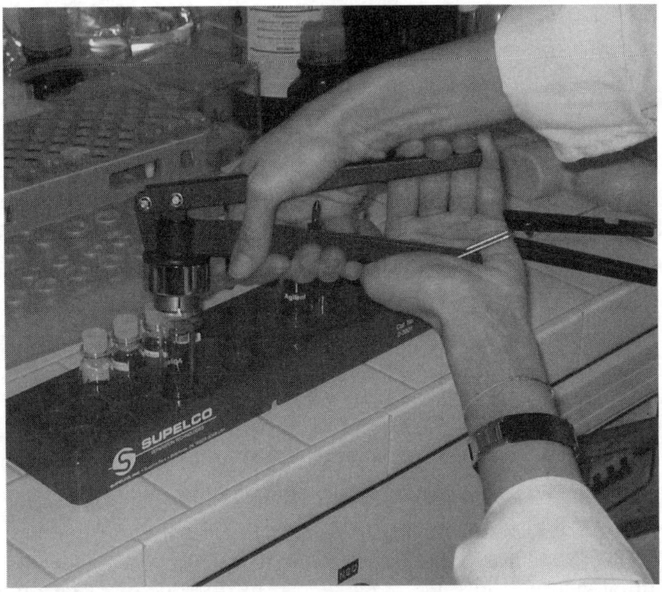

FIGURE 11.3 Traditional crimping tool for capping medication vials requires high grip strength and good motor control. Two hands are grasped tightly around a pair of handles that look like the handles of large pliers. The other end of the tool is holding a glass vial, about 1 in. high, and the tool is sealing a metal cap onto the top of the vial. (Used with permission from T. Armstrong.)

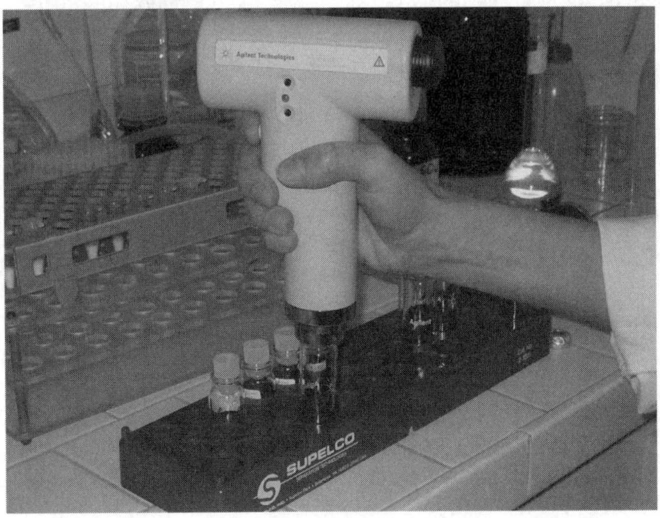

FIGURE 11.4 Electric crimper requires less grip force to cap medication vials. A tool about the size of small soup can is held with one hand. The tool has buttons. The tool is held on top of a glass vial and is sealing a metal cap onto the vial. (Used with permission from T. Armstrong.)

There are modified pipette designs that reduce these risk factors. For example, the electric pipette shown in Figure 11.2 has small motors for drawing up fluid. In addition, the pipette has a modified tip design that requires less force to load or eject. Both changes reduce thumb forces. This design also includes a hook that allows the device to be suspended on the top of the hand, thereby reducing the grip force. Finally, the pipette tip is closer to the hand. This will reduce shoulder flexion and make the tip easier to see and manipulate. Another modification (not shown) is to suspend the pipette on a fixture to hold and stabilize it.

11.2.6 Case Study: Capping Medication Vials

Medication preparation may involve the sealing of solutions in small vials (Figure 11.3). These solutions are later drawn out of the vial with a syringe and needle. The sealing of the vials is typically done by a crimping tool that requires high grip force and good dexterity to perform (Figure 11.3). A modification is to use an electric tool which crimps the aluminum shield over the vial using a motor. This device requires much less force to use although it still requires the user to hold the device over the vial (Figure 11.4). For those with poor motor control, this tool could be suspended using a balancing system to reduce forearm and shoulder load.

11.3 FUTURE DIRECTIONS

The systematic approach of matching the demands of a handheld medical device to the capabilities of the user can benefit from methods developed in the ergonomics literature. One of the keys to using ergonomics approaches for enhancing the accessibility of medical devices is to expand the consideration of the intended users so as to include individuals with a greater diversity of abilities, for instance, using the types of methods suggested by Mueller (Chapter 18).

Although the ergonomics methods presented here have primarily focused on biomechanical loads such as force, repetition, and postures, the methods can incorporate other factors such as cognitive and visual capabilities. The ergonomic tools listed in Table 11.5 are undergoing constant rethinking and revision, based on new information on the contributions of the risk factors to fatigue and disorders. For example, the contribution of peak pinch force to risk is likely to be higher than is reflected in these tools. Thus, the improving ergonomics framework has great potential as a methodology for making medical devices more accessible and usable for persons who could benefit from their use.

REFERENCES

1. Winters, J.W.M., Story, M.F., Barnekow, K., Kailes, J.I., Premo, B., Schwier, E., and Winters, J.M., Accessibility of medical instrumentation: A national healthcare consumer survey, in *Proc RESNA 2005 Annual Conference*, Atlanta, GA. 2005.
2. Shepherd, A., *Hierarchical Task Analysis*, New York, Taylor and Francis, 2001.
3. Barnes, R.M., *Motion and Time Study: Design and Measurement of Work*, John Wiley & Sons, New York, 1980, p. 407.
4. Yen, T.Y. and Radwin, R.G., A comparison between analysis time and inter-analyst reliability using spectral analysis of kinematic data and posture classification, *Appl Ergonomics*, 33(1), 85–93, 2002.
5. McCormick, E., Task analysis, in *Handbook of Industrial Engineering*, John Wiley & Sons, New York, 1982, pp. 2.4.4–2.4.6.
6. Fitts, P. and Jones, R., Analysis of Factors Contributing to 460 "Pilot-Error" Experiences in Operating Aircraft Controls, Memorandum Reported TSEAA-694-12, Aero Medical Laboratory, Air Material Command, WPAFB, Dayton, OH, July 1947.
7. Fitts, P. and Jones, R., Psychological Aspects of Instrument Display. I: Analysis of 270 "Pilot-Error" Experiences in Reading and Interpreting Aircraft Instruments, Memorandum Report TSEAA-694-12, Aero Medical Laboratory, Air Material Command, Wright-Patterson Air Force Base, Dayton, OH, Human factors in the design and use of control systems, Sinaiko, H.W., Dover Publications, 1947, pp. 359–395.
8. Rempel D., Harrison R..J., Barnhart, S., Work-related cumulative trauma disorders of the upper extremity, *J Am Med Assoc*, 267(6), 838–842, 1992.
9. National Research Council and Institute of Medicine, Musculoskeletal Disorders and the Workplace, National Academy Press, Washington, D.C., 2001.
10. McAtamney, L. and Corlett, E., RULA: a survey method for the investigation of work-related upper limb disorders, *Appl. Ergonomics* 24(2), 91–99, 1993.

11. Moore, J. S. and Garg, A. The Strain Index: a proposed method to analyze jobs for risk of distal upper extremity disorders. *Am Ind Hyg Assoc J*, 56(5), 443–458, 1995.
12. Snook, S.H., Vaillancourt, D.R., Ciriello, V.M., and Webster, B.S., Maximum acceptable forces for repetitive ulnar deviation of the wrist, *Am Ind Hyg Assoc J*, Vol. 58, 509–517, 1997.
13. Snook, S.H., Ciriello, V.M., and Webster, B.S., Maximum Acceptable Forces for Repetitive Wrist Extension with a Pinch Grip, *Int J Ind Ergonomics*, 24, 579–590, 1999.
14. ACGIH, Documentation of the TLVs and BEI with Other Worldwide Occupational Exposure Values, Cincinnati, OH, 2005.
15. Armstrong, T.J., Foulke, J.A., Joseph, B.S., and Goldstein, S.A., Investigation of cumulative trauma disorders in a poultry processing plant. *Am Ind Hyg Assoc J* 43(2), 103–16, 1982.
16. Armstrong, T.J., Keyserling, W.M., Grieshaber, D.C., Ebersol, M., and Lo, E., Time based job analysis for control of work related musculoskeletal disorders, in *Proc 15th Triennial Cong. Int Ergonomics Assoc*, Seoul, Korea, 2003.
17. Latko, W.A., Armstrong, T.J., Franzblau, A., Ulin, S.S., Werner, R.A., and Albers, J.W., Cross-sectional study of the relationship between repetitive work and the prevalence of upper limb musculoskeletal disorders. *Am J Ind Med*, 36(2), 248–259, 1999.
18. Homan, M. and Armstrong, T., Evaluation of three methodologies for assessing work activity during computer use, *Am Ind Hyg Assoc J*, 64(1), 48–55, 2003.
19. ANSI/HFS Standard No. 100-1988, American National Standard for Human Factors Engineering of Visual Display Workstations, Human Factors and Ergonomics Society, Santa Monica, CA, 1988.
20. ISO 9241, Ergonomic Requirements for Office Work with Visual Display Terminals (VDTs), ANSI, New York, 1992.
21. Department of Defense Design Criteria Standard — Human Engineering, MIL-STD-1472E, Department of the Navy, Philadelphia, PA, October 1996.
22. Bjorksten, M. and Jonsson, B., Endurance limit of force in long-term intermittent static contractions. *Scand J Work Environ Health*, 3(1), 23–27, 1977.
23. Pheasant, S., *Bodyspace: Anthropometry, Ergonomics, and the Design of Work*, 2nd ed., Taylor & Francis, London, 1996.
24. McClelland, I. and Suri, J., Involving people in design, in *Evaluation of Human Work*, Wilson, J. and Corlett, E.N. Eds., Taylor and Francis, New York, 2005, pp. 281–333.
25. Asundi, K., Bach, J., and Rempel, D., Thumb force and muscle load are influenced by pipetting tasks and pipette design, *Hum Factors*, 47, 67–77, 2005.

12 Usability Testing by Multimedia Video Task Analysis

Thomas Y. Yen and Robert G. Radwin

CONTENTS

ABSTRACT

An iterative cycle of usability testing is often employed to evaluate a product for its strengths and weaknesses. Video offers objective, quantitative, temporal, and motion-based information that would be very difficult and tedious to obtain through direct observation. Multimedia Video Task Analysis (MVTA™) is a software tool for analyzing observational data from video recordings that are both qualitative and quantitative, facilitates the analysis, and offers features that would be difficult to accomplish without a computer. MVTA offers flexibility in maintaining observational records and cataloging events from video recordings that can easily accommodate intentional and unexpected changes in the analyses. The software can extend the observational task analysis by providing time-based and posture-based data used to identify difficulties and barriers related to medical device accessibility. The richness of the qualitative and quantitative data adds a great deal of information to the iterative design process, which can help developers produce better and more usable products, and obtain a better understanding of the user and environments in which they are used.

12.1 INTRODUCTION

Usability testing involves the collection of empirical data by observing end users of a product while performing representative tasks. An iterative cycle of testing is often used to evaluate a product for its strengths and weaknesses, applying redesign strategies to reduce the weaknesses, and then reevaluating it until the weaknesses are eliminated as much as practicable.

Video recordings provide off-line and detailed review of the user's actions that may not be possible in real time. Usability data generally involves qualitative information (e.g., was the user able to complete a task, what were the steps needed to complete a task, or which steps did the user have the most difficulty with and why?). Video offers objective, quantitative, temporal, and motion-based information that would be very difficult and tedious to obtain through direct observation. Quantitative data includes objective performance measures such as the time to complete a task or the number of errors made.

Multimedia Video Task Analysis (MVTA™) is a software tool for analyzing observational data from video recordings that are both qualitative and quantitative. This chapter is not intended to be a user's guide or tutorial to the MVTA™ software. The methods presented here can be accomplished using alternative means but MVTA™ is one tool that facilitates the analysis and offers features that would be difficult to accomplish without a computer. See also Chapter 11 for a review of approaches that relate to ergonomic analysis.

12.2 MULTIMEDIA VIDEO TASK ANALYSIS

12.2.1 General Description

The MVTA™ system, developed at the University of Wisconsin–Madison, contains software for observational time-based activity and event analysis and synchronized analog data sampling. It helps reduce or eliminate tedious activities associated with manual timing and video analysis. An optional module allows the capture of video and sensor-based analog data that can be displayed simultaneously in synchronization with the video, allowing interactive exploration of relationships between the data and video recordings.

The software user interface facilitates information entry, data management, time analysis, and reporting. The computer keeps track of the time codes in video recordings that enable the program to link each occurrence of observed activities with the time it occurred. This makes it possible to locate previously identified events by having the computer find it in the video recording.

Arbitrary events are discerned by interactively identifying terminal break points in the video record. Break points are characteristic occurrences that define the start and end of an event. The video record may be reviewed at any speed and in any sequence (real time, slow motion, fast motion, or frame-by-frame in either forward or reverse direction). Analysts can review any event as long as desired, by stop-action or replaying it in a continuous loop. The software produces time study reports and computes the frequency of occurrence for each event. One of the unique features of this software is its ability to classify interactions among events. This feature enables the analyst to identify the occurrence of simultaneous events, and the computer can tabulate the frequency and duration of each incident.

Basic angle and distance estimation tools are also provided. By clicking on a frame of the recorded images, distance and angle estimations can be made. This application may be used for quantifying included angles between adjacent body segments or for estimating distances relative to an object of known size or other standard.

12.2.2 Current Areas of Use

The MVTA software system was designed to be flexible and adaptable to many different applications and types of analyses [1]. Some of the analyses that the MVTA system can be used for include:

- Activity sampling
- Checklists
- Behavior observation
- Detailed job analysis
- Elemental analysis
- Event analysis
- Left-hand and right-hand analysis
- Micromotion analysis
- Posture analysis
- RULA or OWAS
- Task analysis
- Time and motion study
- Usability testing
- Work sampling

Typical fields of application include:

- Industrial engineering
- Biomechanics and kinesiology
- Work physiology
- Ergonomics
- Psychology
- Zoology
- Human factors engineering
- Training
- Sleep labs
- Sports and athletics
- Rehabilitation
- Human–computer interaction

This chapter will focus on just one type of application, usability testing of medical devices, which is the primary focus of this book. The human subjects data reported here was obtained from the Rehabilitation Engineering Research Center on Accessible Medical Instrumentation (RERC-AMI), which has used MVTA at Marquette University for a number of studies (see also Chapter 13).

12.3 USABILITY TESTING

Built into an iterative product development cycle is the ability for usability testing to detect design flaws and deficiencies. It is important that the focus is on the understanding of the product. This can be accomplished through four types of tests: (1) exploratory, (2) assessment, (3) verification, and (4) comparison tests, as described by Rubin [2].

12.3.1 Exploratory Test

The exploratory test is conducted early in the development cycle. The main objective of this test is to explore or examine the effectiveness of the preliminary design. The assumptions about the user are also verified (e.g., does the user perceive the design as intended?). It is at this stage that the foundation design is set, and all future design decisions are based. Wrong assumptions must be corrected before continuing. A great deal of interaction between the tester and the user occur at this stage to establish the effectiveness of the preliminary design concepts through the use of prototypes [2].

12.3.2 Assessment Test

The assessment test is the most typical of usability tests due to its simplicity. The assessment test is used to expand the findings of the exploratory test by evaluating performance of the lower level operations and aspects of the product. Beyond testing the intuitiveness of the product, how well the user performs the specified tasks is also assessed, such as developed in Chapter 14. The use of an actual working prototype is needed. The researcher's interaction with the user is reduced, and more quantitative data is collected [2].

12.3.3 Verification Test

The verification test, conducted later in the development cycle, is intended to verify the product's usability by comparing the current product to some predetermined usability standard or benchmark. These benchmarks can be either performance standards from previous tests, company or historical standards, or a competing standard. The verification test can also be used to ensure that all the components of the product work together especially when the components were developed in relative isolation from each other. This test ultimately must make sure that no flaws exist in the product, and necessary corrections are made before the product gets into the user's hands. Mostly quantitative data is collected [2].

12.3.4 Comparison Test

The comparison test can be used at any stage of development, especially when a comparison is needed between two or more alternative designs. The test helps the researcher to better understand the strengths and weaknesses of the different designs. Performance data and preference data are collected for each of the alternative designs. A comparison test using objective, quantitative data allows the identification of the best design components from each of the alternative designs, especially when no single design produced the best outcome on the whole. Why one component preformed better than another must be understood. The best components from all the alternative designs can be combined to produce a new composite design [2].

12.4 USING MVTA™

An MVTA screen containing both the Task Analysis and Data Analysis windows is shown in Figure 12.1, which illustrates the analysis of a medical weight scale. The Data Analysis module provides the interactive link between analog sensor data and the video recordings, such as wrist flexion and extension, measured using an electrogoniometer. Although a great amount of data can be collected using sensors, which are especially useful for ergonomics analyses, the additional time and cost of equipment and its setup may not be necessary or practical in most cases. This chapter will deal mainly with the observational task analysis.

12.4.1 Records and Events

12.4.1.1 Representation of Time Information

Timelines are used for visualizing activities and events as a series of occurrences in order to understand temporal aspects of the events. An ordered sequence of related events can be organized by using a left-to-right timeline.

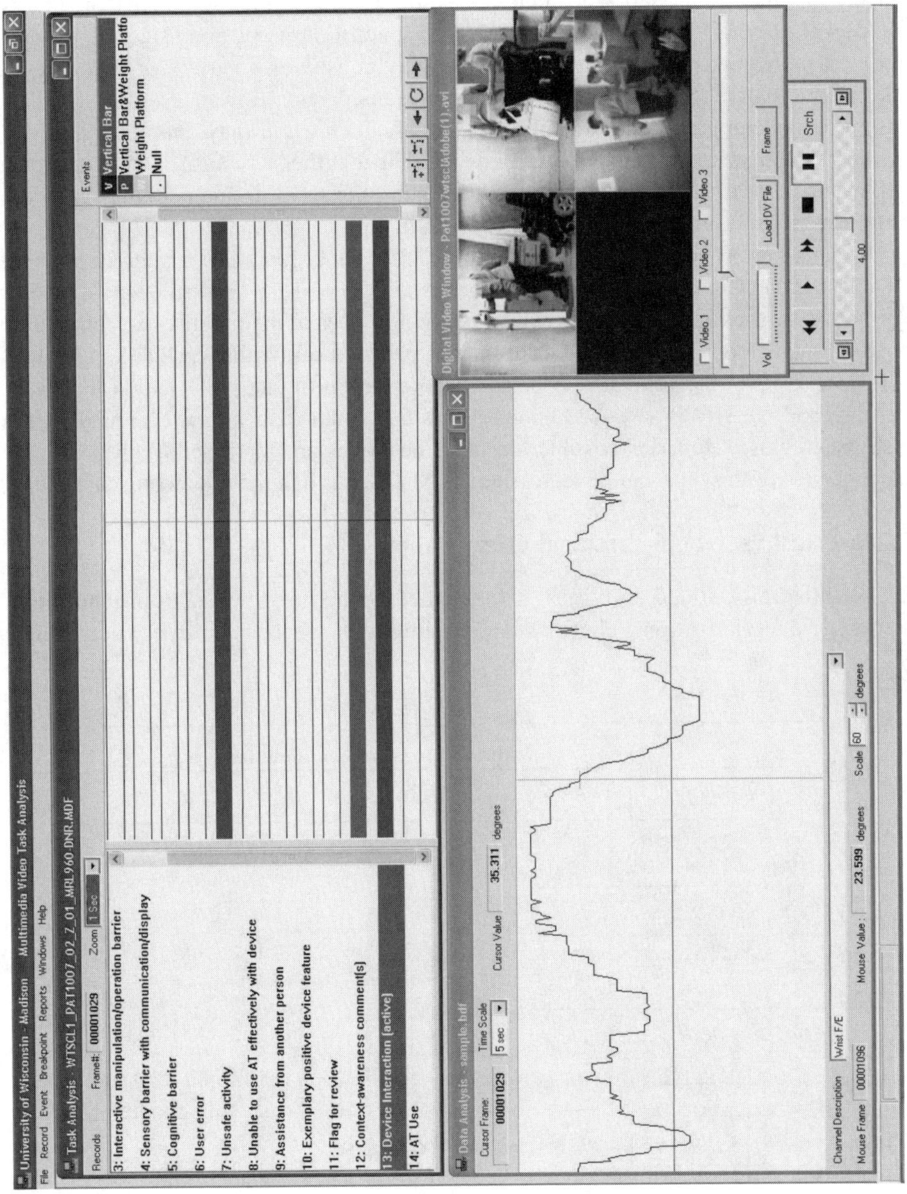

FIGURE 12.1 MVTA software showing the main Task Analysis (observational) and Data Analysis (analog sensor–wrist flexion and extension) windows for the analysis of a weight scale. (Data file courtesy of Melissa Lemke of the RERC-AMI and Marquette University.)

12.4.1.2 Representation of Activities in Time

Activities may be described using a hierarchical framework as shown in Figure 12.2 (e.g., activities in a work shift). Such an organization provides a useful method for systematically documenting an activity using various levels of detail. The level of detail needed depends on the specific activity under study.

The top level of the hierarchy is the job in the example shown in Figure 12.2. A job delineates work performed by an individual and represents a specific work assignment, usually on a daily basis. The next level of detail breaks down the job into specific tasks or activities. A job may consist of one task performed throughout a shift, or it may consist of a variety of tasks. Tasks include all productive work activities in addition to scheduled rest allowances such as lunch breaks. Repetitive tasks can be reduced further into cycles. Each cycle may contain a series of elements. Elements represent sequential units of work that together constitute one cycle of a task. The bottom and most detailed description of work activities reduces each element to micro movements and exertions such as a reach, a move, or a grasp.

The hierarchical framework for usability studies (Figure 12.3) can be represented from the top level as the product to be evaluated (e.g., an ECG monitor). The next level of detail breaks down the product into the different tasks or activities that the user must perform to operate the product (e.g., turning on or off the device, adjusting monitor brightness, or displaying patient data). Within each task, a series of elements is identified (e.g., for the task "display patient data" the elements are press *data* key, press #2 key, turn input dial, and press *enter* key). Additional levels below the element, such as fundamental operations (like reach, grasp, etc.), are possible but often not necessary for usability analysis. Any hierarchical arrangement of this type can be represented in MVTA through the use records and events.

12.4.1.3 Hierarchical vs. Nonhierarchical Organization

Structured tasks with well-defined activities, as described in the previous section, lend themselves to hierarchical organization. There are also situations where no direct hierarchical

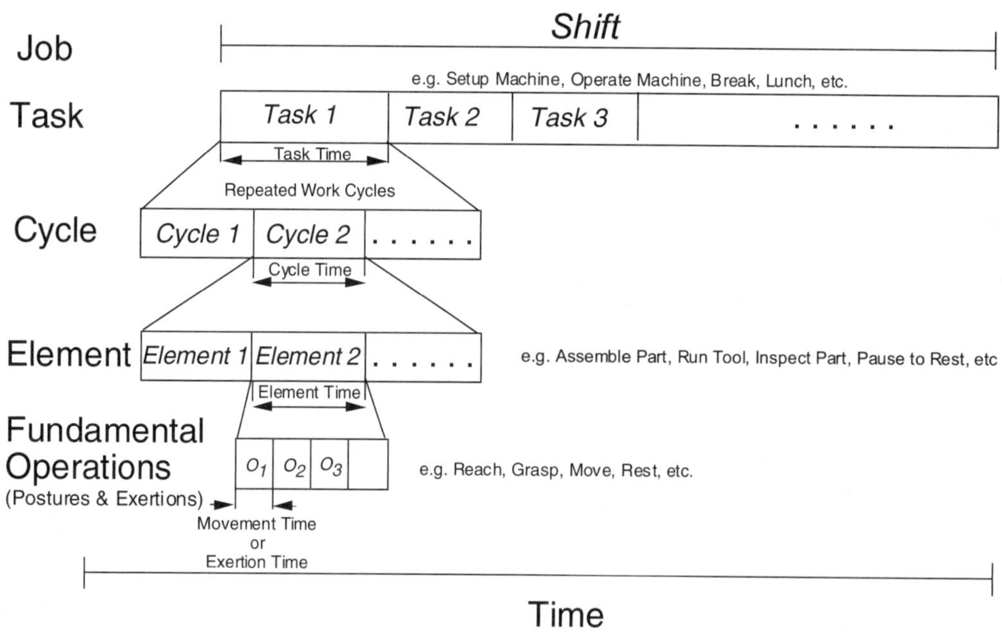

FIGURE 12.2 Example of hierarchical relationship between work elements, work cycles, tasks, and jobs.

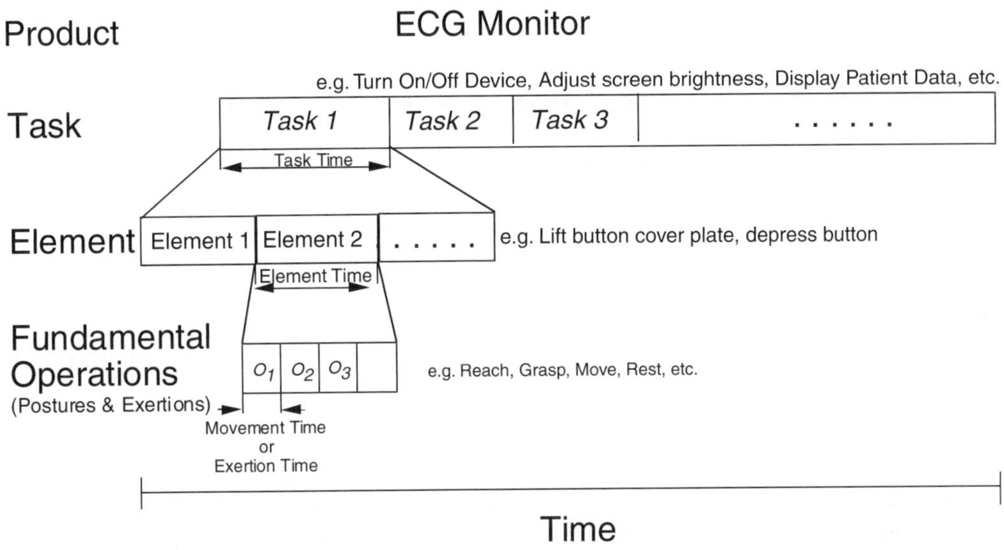

FIGURE 12.3 Example of hierarchical relationship for the analysis of an ECG monitor.

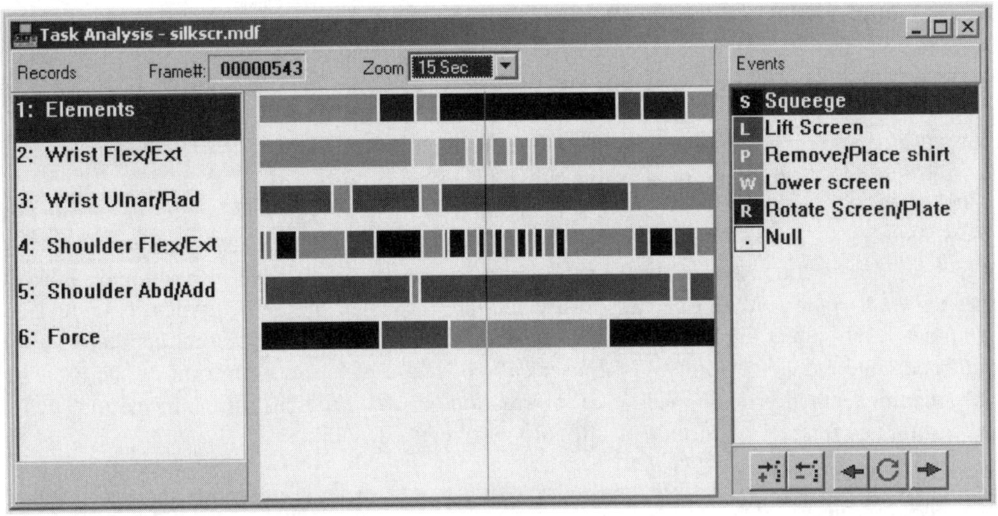

FIGURE 12.4 Task Analysis window highlighting the key controls and displays for a silkscreening task.

relationship exists between the record elements, but they can be grouped together in the same record list because they have the same nonhierarchical relationship. Two examples of nonhierarchical relationships are the right- and left-hand analysis, and the multiple operators (teamwork) analysis.

- *Right and left hand:* The individual activities of the right and left hands have no hierarchical relationship but have a clear relationship to how the activity is performed.
- *Multiple individuals and groups:* Members of a group may be represented as individual records. Activities of each group member are recorded as individual events, where each member represents a separate record.

12.4.2 Task Analysis

An example of the task analysis window is shown in Figure 12.4. The *Record List Window* displays the different records associated with the analysis file. Each record is represented by a timeline in the *Timeline Window.* The *Frame Number* identifies the current video frame and timeline location of the *Time Cursor. Timeline Zoom* sets the time range displayed by the timeline window. The *Event List Window* shows the events associated with the currently selected record. Each event can have a different color to represent the different event segments in the timeline window. The *Event Speed Button* allows quick access to the assignment, editing, and deletion of event break points.

The graphical timeline representation interface permits quick navigation between the records and events. Additions, deletions, or modifications of the records and events are permitted at any time during the analysis.

12.4.2.1 Record and Event Setup

Usability testing typically starts by doing a task analysis. The individual activities and elements needed to operate the product are systematically identified. The activities and their corresponding elements are represented in MVTA in the Records List and Events List, respectively. For example, the following activities shown in Figure 12.5 might be specified as records: (1) turn on or off the patient monitor, (2) adjust screen brightness, and (3) display patient data. The elements for each corresponding record can be: record 1 (lift cover plate; depress button), record 2 (press *screen control* button; press #1 key; turn input selection dial for desired brightness; press *enter* key), record 3 (press *data* button; press #2 key; turn input selection dial until patient name highlighted; press *enter* key). Figure 12.5 shows that record 3, “display patient data,” is selected and its corresponding events. If at anytime during the analysis, additional activities are identified, a new record or event can be inserted without losing or affecting previous entries.

The usability analysis of a patient’s interaction with a weight scale and the surrounding environment are shown in Figure 12.6. The study goes beyond a task analysis (Figure 12.6c) by not just looking at the tasks involved in the operation of the product but also studying how the user’s personal equipment and barriers to use that are presented by the equipment (Figure 12.6a and Figure 12.6b) affect use of the product. The events in Figure 12.6b represent qualitative levels of difficulty and reduced stability of the user caused by use of barriers confronting the user. Not only does this method provide qualitative information but also provides time information such as the duration and interval of periods of difficulty and reduced stability.

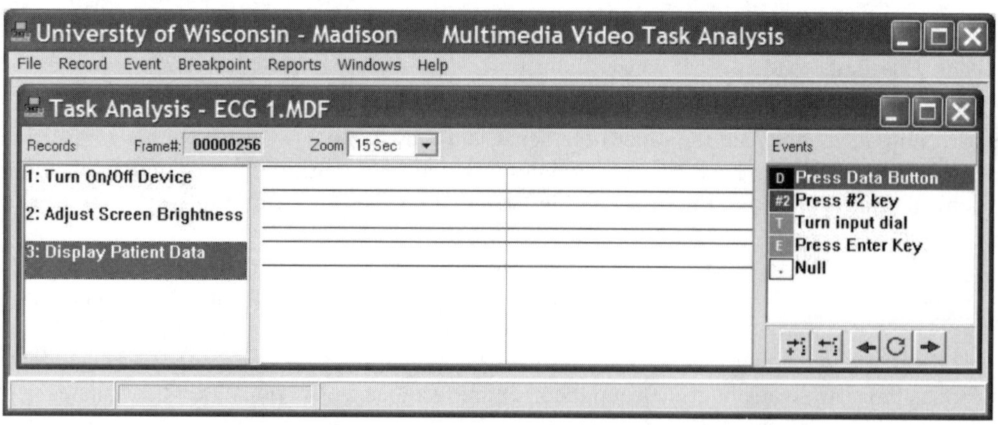

FIGURE 12.5 Records and Events list for a task analysis for an ECG collection task.

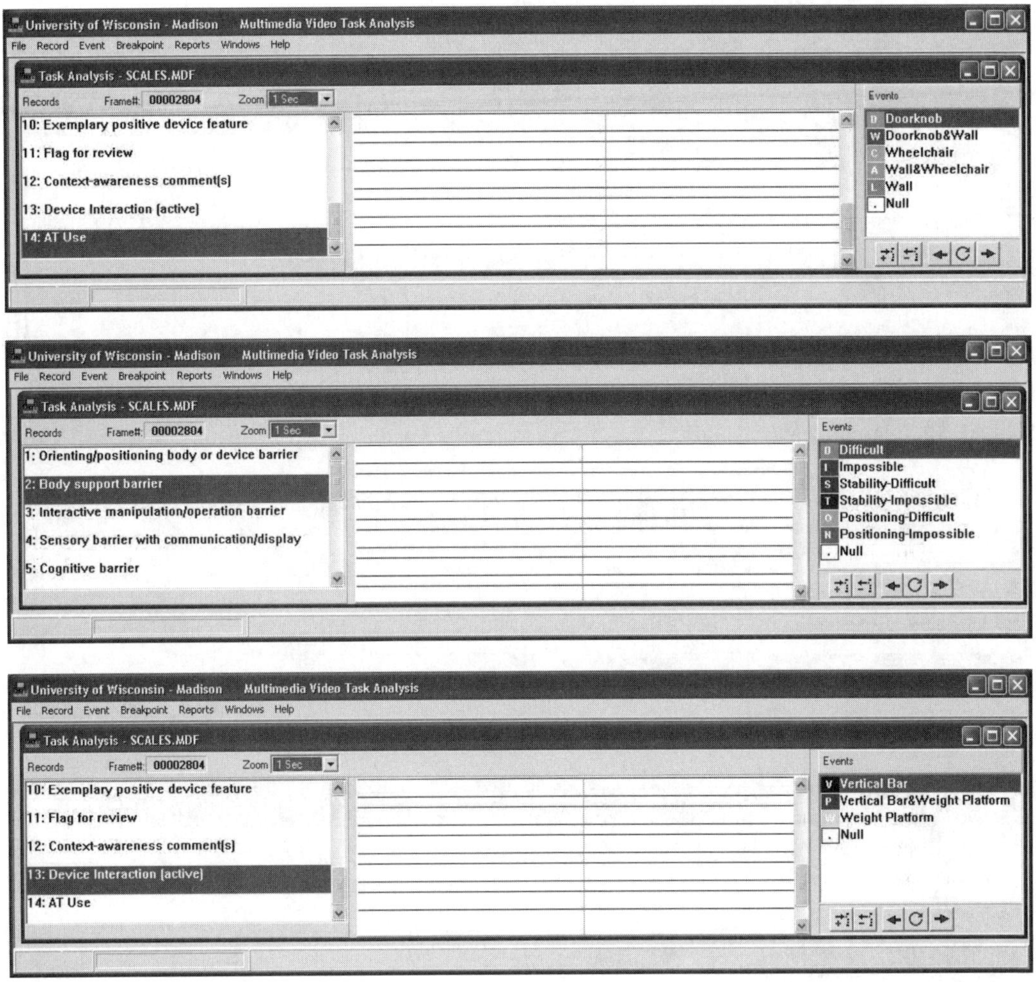

FIGURE 12.6 Task Analysis windows for studying a patient's use of a weight scale, emphasizing records categories used by the RERC-AMI as a core set for an integrated accessibility and task analysis. (a) AT (assistive technology) use, (b) Body Support Barrier, (c) Device Interaction (active). (Records courtesy of Melissa Lemke, RERC-AMI.)

12.4.2.2 Event Break Point Editing

The MVTA™ program contains features for event break point assignment and editing. An overview will be presented to provide a better understanding of the break point editing process used by MVTA™.

- *Inserting new event break points:* Event labels are created in the event list window. Each event list element can have a unique alphanumeric key associated with it. The corresponding key is pressed to mark the beginning of the event at the desired video frame. The timeline window is updated with the new break point. The break point can be edited at any time. Break points inserted in the timeline, after the "D," "2," and "T" keys were pressed, are shown in Figure 12.7.
- *Deleting and changing event break points:* Two commonly occurring assignment errors are: (1) inserting a break point at the wrong video frame, and (2) marking the desired video frame using the wrong event break point. Break points marked at the incorrect video

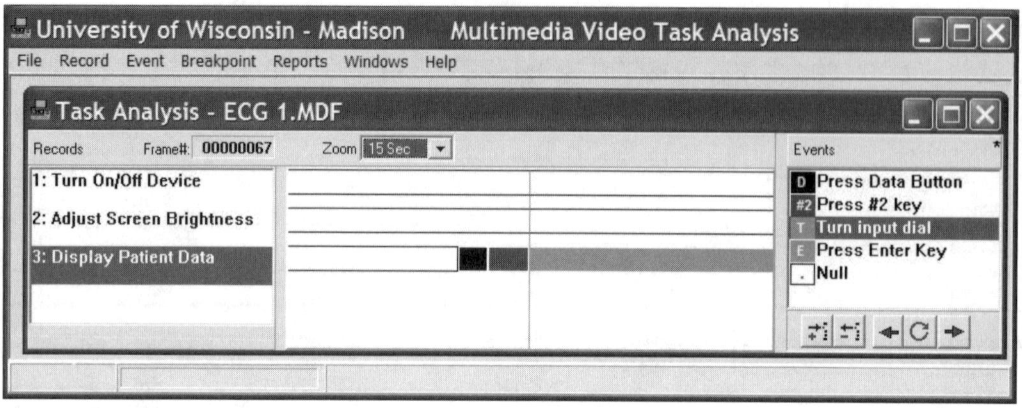

FIGURE 12.7 Inserting break points.

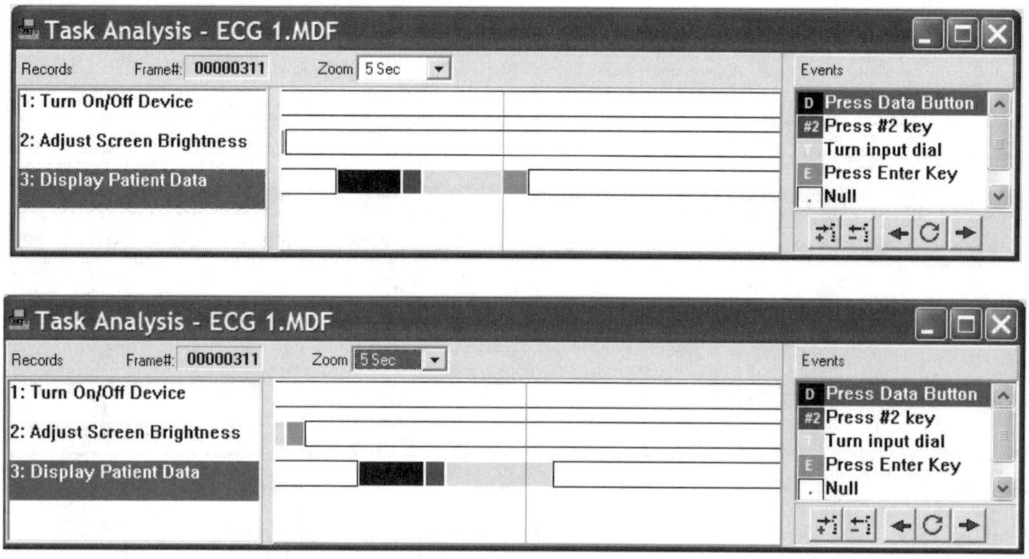

FIGURE 12.8 Deleting break points.

frame are corrected by moving the timeline cursor to any video frame in the event, deleting the event, then moving the timeline cursor to the correct video frame location and inserting a new event break point. A break point marked using an incorrect event label can be corrected by moving the timeline cursor into any video frame in the event, selecting the correct event from the event list window, and changing the event. The currently selected event label replaces the incorrect event label for the event break point. (see Figure 12.8.)

- *Undefined events:* There are situations when the analyst may be unable to determine which event is occurring until continuing to review activities later in the video record. Marking break points in this situation would require constantly shuttling the video to a video frame where the event can be determined, and then shuttling back to the beginning of the event. The "undefined" event feature can help solve this problem. At the video frame when the event begins, the analyst inserts an "undefined" event to mark the time by pressing the Escape key. After the video frame is advanced and the event is identified, the analyst marks the appropriate event by selecting the correct event label. The undefined event is then replaced by the actual event. This feature saves a great deal of time.

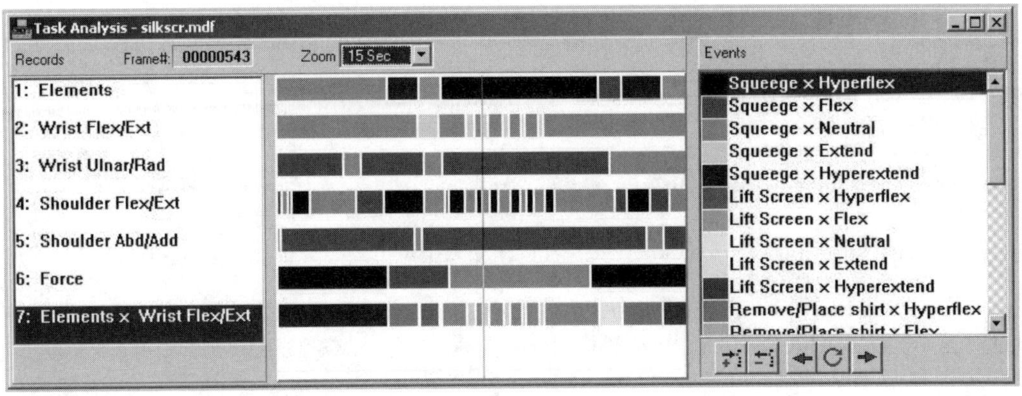

FIGURE 12.9 Interaction record for a silkscreening task.

- *Null event:* A "null" event is a special predefined event that is excluded from the analyses. Often this is because a portion of the recording is not stored. All new analyses begin with all record list elements initialized as null events. Null events are ignored by MVTA™ when generating reports and analyses. Null events should be used for segments of video that have discontinuities in time (such as when the recording was paused) or to break up unrelated analyses in the record timeline. Duration and frequency intervals are never calculated across null events.
- *Record interaction:* A very useful feature of the MVTA™ program is record interactions. Interactions reveal the relationship between two activities at the record level. MVTA™ allows two independently observed events to be combined to produce a new event that represents the coincidence of the two. For example, one may be interested in determining the intersection between events in record 1 and record 2 in order to determine the duration and frequency of the simultaneous occurrence of each combination of events. If record 1 contains five events and record 2 contains three events, the analyst would have to keep track of fifteen (3 × 5) different combinations. In Figure 12.9 the interaction between the Elements record and the Wrist Flex/Ext record was created and displayed at the bottom of the records list. Note the interactions visible in the event list.

12.4.2.3 Annotation

Supplemental information associated with an event can be entered and displayed in the annotation window (See Figure 12.10). This information may be any alphanumeric string desired. Only a single annotation can be associated with an individual event, up to 255 characters. With the timeline cursor located at an element of the desired record, pause or stop the video. Click in the edit box for the text bar to appear, and type the desired annotation. If previous annotations were assigned and the annotation window is displayed, the annotation message will appear in the edit box as the timeline cursor moves while the video advances.

12.5 TIME- BASED USABILITY DATA WITH MULTIMEDIA VIDEO TASK ANALYSIS

After a task analysis has been completed, the exploratory and assessment stages of usability testing begin. Some of the basic quantitative timing data is collected. In some cases, the verification stage is completed with respect to the subjective and qualitative data on the user and product interaction (e.g., were the tasks completed and what difficulties were encountered?). The verification stage

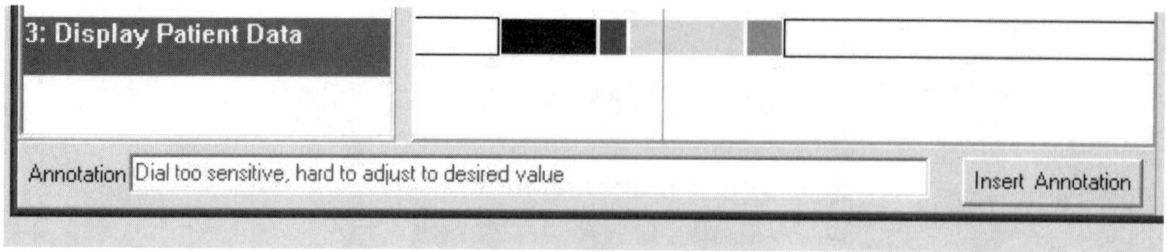

FIGURE 12.10 Annotation window for an ECG collection task.

can be extended by extracting time-based data from the task analysis. By using the timing information associated with the recordings used in the task analysis, data such as the time needed to complete tasks and the frequency of task failure can be collected.

MVTA reports time data in two ways: (1) time study and (2) frequency analysis. Time study computes the time for individual events, whereas frequency analysis computes the interval of occurrence or repetition rate of all events such as the frequency of failure or the need to repeat a particular element too many times.

If multiple replications are recorded, a statistical analysis is provided including the mean, standard deviation, the number of data points, along with confidence intervals, percent error, sample size needed for a given percent error, total cumulative event time, and percent of total cycle values. The upper and lower 95% confidence interval values are provided. The percent error (%error) is the ratio of the 95% confidence interval to the average event time as a percentage. The sample size required (N (5% Err)) value provides an estimate of how many data samples are needed for a percent error of 5%. Percent error levels of 1, 5, 10, and 20 are selectable.

The time-based data can be used in the comparison stages of the testing as changes are made to the product during the iterative design process. The designers can use this data to compare competing product designs. The quantitative data can also show how subsequent reiteration in design may not substantially improve the product, when a barrier to further improvement has been reached or a design approach is yielding negative outcomes.

12.6 POSTURE- BASED USABILITY DATA WITH MULTIMEDIA VIDEO TASK ANALYSIS

MVTA can provide basic estimations of distance and angle. An object of known dimensions must be identified in the frame of the recording, and after some simple calibration procedures, distances and angles can be determined. By clicking on two points in the image frame to define a line segment, the distance can be computed. By clicking on three points to define two line segments, the angle between the line segments can be computed. Parameters such as reach distances and elbow or shoulder angles can influence the time to complete a task by affecting the physical requirement to do the task. The accuracy of the angle or distance estimation is dependent on the view of the video to the object. An orthogonal view of the object is essential for accurate estimations.

12.7 CONCLUSIONS

Usability testing is a very important part of the design and evaluation of a product. MVTA offers flexibility in maintaining observational records and cataloging events from video recordings that can easily accommodate intentional and unexpected changes in the analyses. Observational task analysis provides data that are subjective and qualitative. The MVTA software can extend observational task analysis by providing time-based and posture-based data that are objective and quantitative. As shown here, it has also been used to identify difficulties and barriers related to medical device accessibility (see also Chapter 13 and Chapter 14). The statistical reports of the quantitative data can provide additional validity to the results. MVTA provides the additional benefit of offering a detailed, frame-by-frame analysis. The richness of the qualitative and quantitative data provided by MVTA adds a great deal of information to the iterative design process, which can help developers produce better and more usable products, and obtain a better understanding of the user and environments in which products are used.

REFERENCES

1. Wisconsin Alumni Research Foundation, *MVTA User's Manual*. Quebec: NexGen Ecgonomics, 1997–2006.
2. Rubin, J., *Handbook of Usability Testing: How to Plan, Design, and Conduct Effective Tests*, John Wiley & Sons, New York, 1994, chap. 2.
3. Yen, T.Y. and Radwin, R.G., A video-based system for acquiring biomechanical data synchronized with arbitrary events and activities, *IEEE Trans. Biomed. Eng.*, 42(9), 944–948, 1995.

13 The Mobile Usability Lab Tool for Accessibility Analysis of Medical Devices: Design Strategy and Use Experiences

Jack M. Winters, David M. Rempel, Molly Follette Story, Melissa R. Lemke, Alan Barr, Sean Campbell, and R. Sarma Danturthi

CONTENTS

ABSTRACT

This chapter describes the Mobile Usability Lab (MU-Lab), a structured tool for performing systematic analysis of the accessibility of a targeted medical product or class of products. MU-Lab helps guide a research team through the assessment process. The system consists of Web-based Protocol Manager (PM) software, plus hardware that can be transported within a customized suitcase. The process starts with preliminary steps such as an initial heuristic analysis guided by universal design principles, plus the important step of determining an appropriate population of users with disabilities and documenting their abilities. This is followed by video-based usability data collection sessions that also include a structured postactivity analysis questionnaire. Data analysis includes a special focus on task analysis of events related to accessibility barriers.

13.1 INTRODUCTION

The Rehabilitation Engineering Research Center on Accessible Medical Instrumentation (RERC-AMI), to fulfill its mission, has needed to develop and then use an effective tool for cross-disability evaluation of how medical products are used. A key objective has been to understand access barriers that limit effective use of a medical device. For instance, needs assessment research by the RERC-AMI may identify a given medical product or class of products where there is a high-priority need to better understand problematic or exemplary features associated with product use. A usability analysis is then performed that systematically documents use strategies, difficulties, and access barriers. Data collection involves recruiting a sample of volunteers with a diversity of abilities, including individuals who represent subpopulations with known functional limitations. It also requires, for ecological validity, that the tool be mobile in order to enable data collection in the field, whether the site is within, for example, a hospital, home, or clinic. Often the on-site researcher is alone and must multitask under time pressures, having to both interact with the subjects and collect sensor-based and observational data. Thus a key practical consideration is that the system be easy to use in the field and indeed serve as an "enabler" for the researcher. Finally, it must support data analysis by a team of experts that, at least for some analyses, may be located at different sites (e.g., Wisconsin and California).

The obvious first step toward addressing these needs is to build on past knowledge and work, specifically in the interrelated fields of usability engineering, human factors engineering, and ergonomics. After all, these relatively mature fields have developed a rich variety of approaches and tools [1–3; see also many chapters in Parts 2 and 3 of this book]. Other resources include the Principles of Universal Design [4], accessibility guidelines for certain types of products [5,6], and a rich variety of approaches for human performance analysis tools. But based on the aims identified in the previous paragraph, none of these existing approaches have been found to completely satisfy the identified need.

In developing an approach, one important observation is that the use of most medical technologies is procedural and goal-directed. The focus of the device use evaluation can be on activities and tasks that are performed when using devices that have clearly identifiable performance goals. Thus, a task analysis of product use is viable, albeit challenging, as humans will often adapt their strategy based on their abilities. Often each activity can be broken into a sequence of subtasks (e.g., stages related to positioning, mobility, reaching, manipulation, and communication). Each of these subtasks can be broken down further, and many such classification schemes exist (see Chapter 11 and Chapter 9).

Building on these considerations, a process evolved to create a novel approach that, as appropriate, extracted useful ideas and approaches from a number of fields. The result of a collaborative effort of over 2 years is a new technology called the Mobile Usability Lab, or MU-Lab. This mobile system is specifically designed to study the accessibility and usability of targeted medical devices for individuals with diverse functional impairments and disabilities.

This chapter shares some of the internal decision-making behind its design (especially in contrast to conventional human factors and usability approaches) and describes how this system integrates a comprehensive Web-based evaluation procedure with data collection hardware and software, and a structured data analysis methodology. Finally, it describes experiences using the MU-Lab technology for a number of completed and ongoing pilot studies involving human subjects with disabilities.

13.2 BACKGROUND

A key challenge was to determine which of the many alternative approaches and methods to include in the MU-Lab. This section provides the motivation behind the selection of the components of this tool and may serve as a resource for groups interested in integrating considerations of accessibility or universal usability into a usability analysis activity.

13.2.1 Insights from Usability Analysis

Usability refers to the extent to which a product can be used by specified users to achieve specified goals in an effective and efficient manner, to the satisfaction of these users. In our case, the specified users included individuals with a diversity of abilities. Indeed, often individuals were recruited with disabilities that were known, based on our national surveys and focus groups, to have experienced difficulties with or lack of access to the device [7; Chapter 2 of this book]. The specified goals relate to roles played by a device to support and enable access by an individual to medical procedures and services. And finally, satisfaction includes both an indication of whether the procedure associated with device use was successful (e.g., collecting useful medical information) and opinions of the users (e.g., patient or health care provider).

Usability testing encompasses a number of evaluation methods that range from those typically used early in the design process that do not require a usability lab (e.g., cognitive walkthrough of the goals of and steps involved in using the interface and heuristic evaluation of whether a user interface follows established usability principles), to operational evaluations and human performance testing. Universal usability has a focus on designing products so that they are usable by the widest range of people operating in the widest range of situations as is commercially practical [8].

13.2.2 Insights from Universal Design

Universal design aims to design products (and environments) to be usable by people with a wide range of abilities, to the greatest extent possible, without the need for adaptation or specialized design [4; Chapter 6 of this book]. Universal design overlaps substantially with (and is sometimes considered a synonym for) the concepts of "design for all" (a term popular in Europe) and "inclusive design" [9,10; Chapter 7 and Chapter 8 of this book]. Seven consensus principles were developed that articulate universal design [see Chapter 6], and they are quite relevant to design and analysis of medical devices [4]: equitable use; flexibility in use, simple and intuitive use, perceptible information, tolerance for error, low physical effort, and size and space for approach and use.

Of note is that there is overlap between these and the usability approach called "heuristic evaluation." There is also overlap with accessibility (covered in subsequent pages), and indeed the Council of Europe's consensus definition of Universal Design includes the phrase: "*... products accessible and understandable to as well as usable by everyone ...* ."[11] But there are distinctions, as will be seen below. Device-oriented, more pragmatic performance measures have been developed [12], and evaluation method development is ongoing [13]; Chapter 18 and Chapter 9 of this book].)

13.2.3 Insights from Accessible Design

Accessibility addresses access to the intended use of a product (or service) by all for whom there is benefit, including any person with disability. There are degrees of this ability to access, both at the level of the individual (e.g., device use may be difficult or impossible; inaccessible device components or features may be optional or essential) and at the level of the population (e.g., more difficult or impossible for certain groups of users, integration of design features known to benefit people with similar functional capabilities). One important distinction between universal design and accessible design is that the former strives to satisfy the needs of all users concurrently, as far as practicable, whereas the latter may add features specifically intended to accommodate the access needs of some groups of users who would otherwise lack access by providing approaches that might not be accessible (or even of interest) to other users (see Chapter 8 and Chapter 25).

We suggest that the MU-Lab tool provides a cross-disability *accessibility evaluation* rather than a universal usability evaluation in that our focus is on performing a usability analysis primarily for the parts of an activity (or task sequence) where access is difficult or impossible for any user. In other words, we prioritize the task analysis based on identification of difficult or impossible access barriers. We further consider the importance of the subtask or design feature associated with the access barrier. From this perspective, universal usability is a subset of the accessibility domain because it considers the needs of *all users,* with accessibility considering the role of assistive technologies in helping provide access, and also access through device options or multimodal interfaces.

Note that at times, making an interface more fully accessible for some people may lower the degree of usability for others. For instance, an interface may become more complex when multimodal options are added or as the number of options grow, but these may be the very features that make it accessible to groups of people with certain functional limitations. Thus while we call our technology the MU-Lab, the desired form of the usability analysis actually needs to be based on accessibility analysis considerations. A task analysis should be performed that targets understanding the nature and extent of barriers to use of the device. Thus the nature of this tool differs in some key ways from those used in conventional usability analysis.

For this project we avoid the use of the term "accessible design." *Accessible design* includes two classes of definitions:

1. It is a legal term that mandates for accessible products in certain categories where standards and guidelines exist, such as Access Board [5] guidelines, which were developed to help implement certain laws including the Americans with Disabilities Act of 1990 (ADA, [14]) and Section 508 of the Rehabilitation Act of 1973 as amended in 1998 [Rehab Act, [15]].
2. It describes the more general design methodology of maximizing accessibility and minimizing barriers that prevent individuals from using a product and participating in activities associated with it. Degrees of accessibility have been proposed to be captured by the words "difficult" [6] and "handicap" [16], each capable of describing a continuum while also having natural qualifiers (e.g., somewhat difficult and partially handicapped).

There are two basic design strategies for enhancing access:

1. Direct access — Modify a product to significantly improve its accessibility as related to the intended use of the product.
2. Assistive access — Make product interfaces compatible with add-on assistive technologies to provide the user with full access, or support other reasonable accommodations.

Legislation such as Section 508 of the Rehab Act allows either strategy [6]. Unfortunately, the legal definition of accessible design is not particularly beneficial to the aims of the RERC-AMI because, as far as we have been able to ascertain based on review of existing laws and discussions with federal experts, most medical instrumentation is currently not considered to fall under the scope of the guidelines. In contrast, regulations for implementing the ADA include a broad set of building design specifications called the "Americans with Disabilities Act Standards for Accessible Design" that hold facilities providing health care to an even higher standard than other businesses. Also, Section 504 of the Rehab Act requires that any program or service receiving federal financial assistance, either directly or indirectly, be accessible to everyone. This includes some health care facilities. Thus in terms of the universal ability to access, the laws are considerably stronger for health care facilities than for health care devices.

13.2.4 Insights from Human Factors, Ergonomics and FDA

The fields of human factors and ergonomics offer additional analysis tools and approaches from which the MU-Lab technology could potentially benefit. Often defined as the "science of work," human factors or ergonomics removes barriers to safe human performance, productivity, and quality by fitting products, tasks, and environments to people. Notice that this definition mentions barriers, but the barriers relate to safety and productivity rather than accessibility. Often human factors is considered to have more of a base in cognitive performance while ergonomics has more of a base in biomechanics ([2]; see also Chapter 11 of this book). Both matter. Notice also that, by definition, human factors and ergonomics professionals are concerned primarily with the safety and productivity of the worker, in this case the health care provider, and less so with the product, in our case, the patient.

There are two key points to make. First, the human factors or ergonomics field has a longer history than the aforementioned fields. For this reason, many more approaches and tools exist, some with roots in biomechanics and others originating in psychology. The second key point is that one strong proponent of the use of human factors methodology is the U.S. Food and Drug Administration (FDA) and its Center for Devices and Radiological Health (CDRH), which has the responsibility for regulating medical devices (including "durable medical equipment"). Product "safety" (for health care provider and patient) and "efficacy" (for the patient) are the key criteria for the FDA, and the CDRH has developed a strong interest in encouraging the use of human factors principles and processes in the design of medical products [17–19]. The FDA's Human Factors Branch has produced documents and supported standards activities that emphasize a systems perspective to help companies minimize user risks and maximize error tolerance (see also Chapter 17). One example is the current ANSI/AAMI/ISO HE74 standard (Human factors design process for medical devices) [20], and even more importantly, the emerging HE75 standard that is discussed in Chapter 15 and Chapter 16. Both involved active FDA participation. These FDA efforts are not surprising, given that medical error is said to be the eighth leading cause of death in the U.S., [21] and that many medical products initially approved for use by health professionals in controlled settings have migrated to home use. Often these products are used by persons with functional limitations, and indeed there is reason to believe that there is synergy between accessibility and safety. The FDA also attributes a significant proportion of injuries to what it classifies as use errors. Therefore, the MU-Lab technology should address safety as part of its analysis, including identification of both unsafe activities and use errors.

Risk management frequently mentions the importance of understanding user abilities and limitations, often in the context of identifying "use scenarios." Kaye and Crowley [18] provide a useful distinction:

- Analytic approaches — Heuristics that involve systematic decomposition and analysis of device use (e.g., use scenarios and descriptions, descriptive functional and task analysis, heuristic analysis, and expert review).
- Empirical approaches — Use studies that involve evaluation of data from actual or simulated use of the device by a representative sample of test participants (e.g., walk-throughs and full usability testing).

Taken in the context of the aims for the MU-Lab technology, the analytical component of MU-Lab should be structured into the early part of the analysis, whereas the empirical component should be the heart of MU-Lab system.

13.2.5 Practical Considerations and Key Specifications

Prior work in the relevant fields described in sections 13.2.1–13.2.4 provided a foundation for the design of the MU-Lab system, summarized as follows:

1. From practical considerations related to RERC, the MU-Lab needs contextual field evaluations that meet certain criteria:
   - For high ecological validity, feasible evaluations should be done at a representative health care or home site.
   - The system should be mobile and modular, with wireless components used when feasible.
   - All hardware must fit within a rugged suitcase that meets airline requirements for carry-on luggage.
   - The system should enable the field researcher to effectively multitask, and include instructional documents.

2. From practical considerations related to the logistics of a multisite RERC team:
   - A password-protected Web site should be used as the primary mode for protocol planning, data collection and storage, and data analysis.
   - The cost of the MU-Lab technology must not be prohibitive, and must integrate commercial products whenever possible.
   - The technology will be developed and evaluated by the multisite team, communicating through e-mail and videoconferencing sessions.

3. From considerations and insights of usability analysis, we recognize that
   - Usability involves specified users who may have disability.
   - Specified goals normally relate to the role that the device plays in the context of goal-directed procedures.
   - One important approach is to solicit measures of user satisfaction.
   - Usability analysis is best done in stages, and use of multiple methods that extract information from different sources (e.g., experts, audio–video, and users) is often advantageous.

4. From considerations and insights of universal design:
   - Take advantage of project team member Molly Story's long history of leadership in universal design to heuristically integrate these concepts into the device evaluation protocol.
   - Apply the Principles of Universal Design at an early stage of the evaluation process to identify what difficulties users may have.

5. From considerations and insights of accessible design:
   - Carefully identify the intended use of the device.
   - Craft the analysis in terms of identifying barriers to use, and classify these barriers as "difficult" and "impossible."
   - Identify device features that affect accessibility, and study task procedures that may require use of these features, at least for some potential users.
   - Identify device features and access barrier events related to the use of assistive technologies (assistive access).
   - Consider involving test subjects who have a diversity of affected disabilities.

6. From considerations and insights related to human factors, ergonomics, and the FDA:
   - Take advantage of the experience of project team members at the University of California Ergonomics Lab, led by David Rempel, and at Marquette University, particularly

Jack Winters's experience in neuromechanical performance assessment, to refine task analysis breakdown categories.

- Take advantage of existing ergonomics software packages for event-based task analysis.
- In addition to an accessibility-oriented task analysis, include identification of use error, unsafe activities, and exemplary positive features within the analysis.
- Build on the foundation provided by existing FDA documents [17–19] that support and guide the inclusion of a human factors process in the design of medical instrumentation.

13.3 METHODS

The MU-Lab system development process attempted to synthesize the diversity of requirements and specifications, identified in Section 13.2.

13.3.1 General Framework

The MU-Lab system includes:

1. A Web-based Protocol Manager (PM) that helps guide the multisite research team and on-site experimenters through all the stages involved in performing accessibility and usability analyses, including preactivity preparation and postactivity data evaluation tools and procedures.
2. A portable usability lab consisting of a collection of hardware and software that can be transported within a suitcase for on-site task analysis.
3. A task analysis procedure that is event-based and focuses primarily on identification and analysis of access barriers and also documents unsafe activities and use errors.

Although it is possible to use the first two of these technologies separately, the package is designed as an integrated system.

The PM is an integral part of MU-Lab when it is used as a comprehensive accessibility analysis tool:

- It helps manage a multipart research study involving many devices because it is organized hierarchically with the IRB approval code for a study at the highest level.
- It helps coordinate, implement, and document data and filenames associated with a study, as it structures and guides data collection and documentation.
- It provides a structured way to screen potential subjects and to determine if any accommodations are needed for their participation.
- It provides structured methods to conduct universal design analyses of medical instrumentation and user pre- and postactivity scoring instruments that complement the task-based analysis tools.
- It supports integrated analysis of a single device or classes of devices with a "parent–child" structure that facilitates grouping and comparison of similar devices within the same class for a population of users.
- It supports multisite data sharing for approved members of the team, with an additional password protection beyond the initial user login that supports sharing of large files by uploading and downloading mechanisms among the researcher team.

The PM, developed by the team over the course of more than a year of meetings, guides the research team through various procedures that constitute the device evaluation process, including: formation of a research problem statement, understanding all aspects of instrument usage, universal design analyses, prescreening and tracking of subjects (both health care patients and practitioners), activity performance observations during data collection, postactivity interviews of subjects, post-activity data analysis and documentation, and data tracking for each targeted medical device. The PM also includes tools to summarize the preactivity and postactivity questionnaire data, which are selectable by either instrument name or anonymous patient and provider codes. It is implemented in ASP.NET, C#, and XML in the Microsoft Video Studio.NET environment.

The PM has several choices for site navigation and data saving, including a "save and lock" mechanism to protect data from being accidentally overwritten once a form has been completed. It can be implemented on a single computer with the help of Internet Information Server on the computer's localhost Web site, in a standalone mode (where the data is stored on the computer's hard drive) or online whenever an Internet connection is available (where the data is stored directly to the network database).

13.3.2 Preactivity Preparation Protocol

13.3.2.1 Use of the Protocol Manager

The team recognized early on that efficient collection of the most relevant and useful data would benefit substantially from diligent and thorough preparatory work to describe the problem and plan usability testing in the field. Before collecting any data in the field with the MU-Lab, the research team takes advantage of the PM to develop and organize the details surrounding a particular research study.

The advance preparation portion of the PM is discussed within this section, which contains all of the PM sections that are completed prior to bringing in subjects to collect data. These forms include:

1. Section I: Problem statement page — This PM form is used to identify the specific device class (parent) and device model (child) of the medical instrumentation under investigation, as well as to describe the key access problems or concerns to be investigated.
2. Section II — Planning and preparation for usability testing.
   - Section IIA: Instrumentation usage page — This PM form documents practical aspects of the medical devices under investigation (e.g., medical facilities to be used for field testing, the manufacturer's intended and expected uses of the device (class), estimates of the intended and actual conditions of use at the test facilities, and the range of potential device users).
   - Section IIB: Universal design analysis of device (patient and provider perspectives) pages — These PM sections are motivated by the Principles of Universal Design [6, 9, Chapter 6], and are used to collect data on:
     - Sensory usability (e.g., ease of use for a patient or provider who is hard of hearing, deaf, or blind)
     - Cognitive usability (e.g., ease of understanding of how to use a device)
     - Physical usability (e.g., ease of use for a person who is very tall or short, has large or small hands, or can use only one hand)
     - Assistive technology accommodation (e.g., ease of use for a person using a cane, crutches, walker, or manual or powered wheelchair)
     - Error tolerance (e.g., device safety from damage, user safety from injury, and device tolerance of mistakes)
     - Equitable use (e.g., whether every user finds at least one way to use the device without stigma)

     Note that this approach bears some similarity to the usability approach of heuristic evaluation, which is also usually employed at an early stage of the process.
   - Section IIC: General requirements for test subject performance page — This PM form is used to document desired types of test participants (e.g., quantity, ability

characteristics, and experience level), pilot testing needs, tasks and number of repetitions to be conducted, and data collection tools needed for the data collection sessions. It supports a team-based, interactive (either synchronous or asynchronous) approach to developing the field testing protocol.

3. Section III: Prescreening subject interview pages (patient and provider) — These PM forms are used to document interview responses from potential subjects and include sections on:
   - Demographic data (e.g., gender, race, and education)
   - Disabilities (e.g., vision, hearing, and paralysis)
   - Functional difficulties (e.g., reaching, grasping, and tremor)
   - Previous experience with this type of device
   - Provider experience level, treating patients with specific conditions (e.g., vision impairment, hearing impairment, or arthritis), if relevant
   - Assistive technology use (e.g., cane, walker, or wheelchair)

All of the above data are entered directly into the PM, using the software version on either the Web (www.rerc-ami.org/D1Two/UserLogin.aspx) or the local computer. The user must first have a username and password, which are allocated and managed by the RERC-AMI. If an Internet connection is available, the PM can be accessed directly on the Internet, in which case the subject data collected during the research session can be stored directly on the remote server. Otherwise, the information is stored locally and the MU-Lab computer acts as the server until the data is uploaded to the network database.

13.3.2.2 Preparation of Hardware

The following steps were adopted:

- Preparation for multimedia data acquisition: Figure 13.1 displays a hardware schematic of the core MU-Lab technologies that are available for a usability analysis involving a targeted medical device or class of devices. The first step is to gather the appropriate technologies prior to travel to the field site. For some studies or locations alternative cameras, camera stands, or specialized sensors may be needed. The MU-Lab supports a variety of audio and video components, so the researcher can optimize the system for a particular device and research setting.
- Suitcase and components: All the MU-Lab hardware components fit within a standard carry-on suitcase (approximately 9" × 14" × 22"), as shown in Figure 13.2. The laptop computer is carried in a separate case that can be stored in the larger suitcase, if desired. The suitcase is protected with hard plastic shielding and contains a customized foam insert to secure the hardware components during travel. All of the hardware has specific locations within the suitcase that are labeled and several pockets within the case are used to house the cables and remote controls. Laminated copies of the informational documents included in electronic format in the PM (i.e., Quick Start, System Diagram, and Pocket Inventory) are also included as hard copies in the suitcase.
- Color quad processor: Because data collection software (i.e., Synchronized Video Data Acquisition — SVDA) currently supports only one video input for data collection, a color quad processor is used to compile up to four video streams into one output (to the laptop computer). Several display modes are available with the quad processor, depending on the number of cameras in use and different research requirements, including modes to view a single video feed, two video feeds via picture-in-picture (PIP), or up to four video feeds with a quadrant display. Either the remote control or the buttons on the front of the quad processor can be used to switch between the different modes, and more settings can be used to display the time, date and separate channel names.

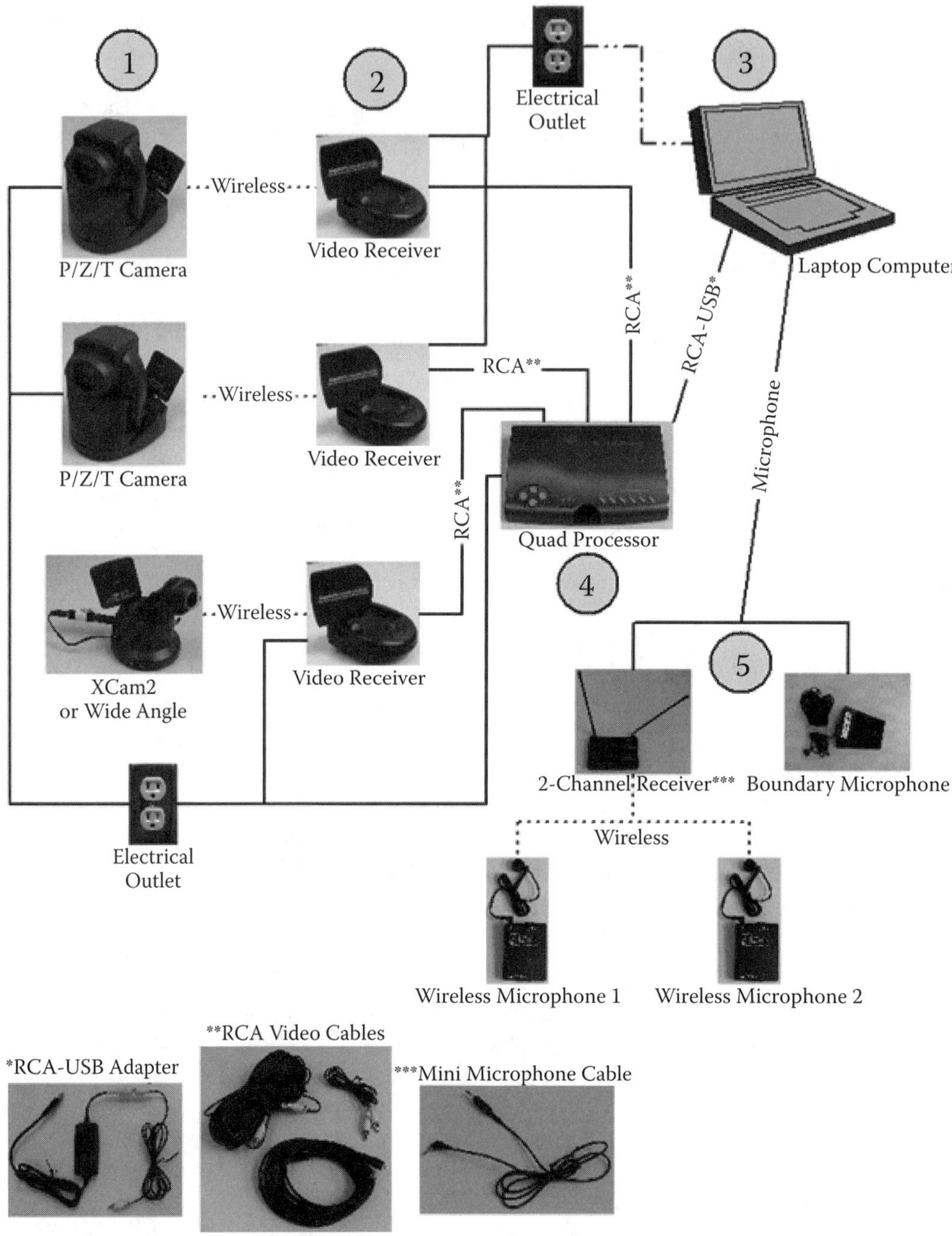

FIGURE 13.1 Schematic of the hardware technologies of the MU-Lab.

- Cameras: Several remote-controlled wireless video cameras were evaluated prior to selecting the models for inclusion in the MU-Lab, and it was desired to maximize signal quality while minimizing size and weight. Three different models were selected for inclusion in the MU-Lab, including higher-cost digital video cameras that can be automatically panned, tilted, and zoomed (Vanguard), and lower-cost digital video cameras that have 60° (XCam2) and 120° (WideEye) fields of view.

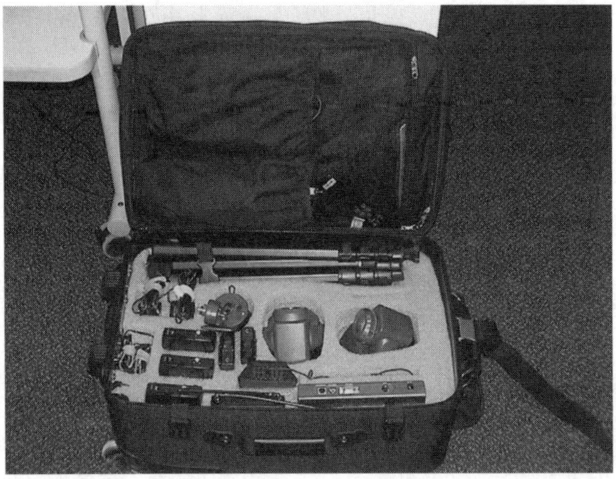

FIGURE 13.2 Photograph of the MU-Lab hardware components stored within the roll-aboard suitcase.

- Wireless video receivers: If multiple wireless video cameras are used for testing, a separate video receiver must be used for each camera. Each camera and receiver pair is tuned to the same unique channel (A, B, C, or D). Camera and receiver pairs can transmit signals up to 100 ft, although the highest quality signal is obtained when the receiver is placed near the corresponding camera.
- Microphone system: A discrete two-channel wireless microphone transmitter–receiver system and a boundary microphone are included in the MU-Lab to enable audio collection, if desired. The wireless (169–172 MHz transmission) microphones may be clipped directly onto a subject or a researcher, which is helpful in noisier environments. The protocol includes a process for checking for the amount of interference within the research environment before collecting data. A boundary microphone is available to enable audio collection inside a room without having to attach the microphone transmitter to subjects. The omnidirectional microphone can pick up audio in the hemisphere above and in front of the mesh area, but not below or behind it, and the protocol includes a process for checking the quality of the audio signal.
- Camera stands: Several camera stands can be included in the MU-Lab, and all of them have the necessary fittings for attachment to the stands. The carrying case has space for up to three camera stands (or they can be carried separately). The height ranges for the current camera stands are 7.5 in., 12.7 to 47.7 in., and 6 to 64.1 in. A ceiling amount is also available.

13.3.3 On- Site Usability Testing

This section describes the technical data collection process that occurs during usability testing with human subjects. Normally two components of usability testing data are collected from subjects: data collected with the PM, if used (e.g., subject questionnaires and recording of observations), and data collected using Synchronized Video Data Acquisition (SVDA) software (e.g., audio, video, and possibly sensor data files).

13.3.3.1 Use of the Protocol Manager for Preparation for Data Acquisition

The PM supports collection of field data only to guide the process and document activities. The PM software is available on a password-protected site on the Internet whenever there is web access at the field facility, and this is the preferred method for PM data collection since the subject interview data collected during the research session is stored directly online. Otherwise, if the information is stored locally, the MU-Lab computer acts as the server until the data is uploaded to the remote server. Data is automatically stored within a folder structure (as XML files), which are readily available for further review in the field. Normally the field researcher will run both the PM and SVDA software (see Section 13.3.3.2) simultaneously on the same laptop computer.

Assuming the PM was used during the advance preparation phase (see Subsection 13.3.2.1), all of the collected data is available to the field researcher to help implement the sequence of tasks in the testing protocol. The PM can be used to record on-site observations and document file names, and then after data collection, to collect postactivity interview data.

13.3.3.2 Using SVDA to Collect Data

Synchronized Video Data Acquisition (SVDA, NexGen Ergonomics) software, developed by the authors of Chapter 12 (Yen and Radwin), is used to simultaneously collect video, audio, and sensor data. It supports a wide range of compression algorithms. Several other software tools are available for subsequent data reduction and analysis.

Steps required to use SVDA in the field are outlined in the MU-Lab manual, available to the on-site research both in hard copy stored within the suitcase and electronically on the laptop. The MU-Lab User's Manual also provides a suite of troubleshooting capabilities.

13.3.3.3 Use of the Protocol Manager to Administer Postactivity Questionnaire

After a subject conducts the specified sequence of tasks to use a medical device, the researcher has the option of using the PM to conduct a structured interview. The postactivity questionnaire complements video-based data collection of subject performance by systematically assessing the subject's opinion of the accessibility and usability of the devices.

The postactivity questionnaire covers the following areas: sensory usability, cognitive usability, physical usability, error tolerance, safety and comfort, and AT accommodation. Open-ended comments are also recorded at the end of each area. Many of the questions within the postactivity questionnaire are similar to the preliminary universal design analysis (in Section IIB of the PM; see Subsection 13.3.2), with an emphasis here placed on the subjects' impressions of their experiences during the testing session and their satisfaction with the device.

While the core set of questions are designed to apply to any type of medical instrumentation, the researcher can also add up to eight customized instrumentation-specific questions. This ability to add questions directly to the Web-based PM postactivity questionnaire is an important feature that has been used for every IRB-approved study conducted to date.

13.3.4 Postactivity Evaluation Tools and Procedures

13.3.4.1 Accessibility- Centered Task Analysis

The team evaluated a range of commercial products for video-based data analysis. One viable approach is to use video editing cards (i.e., Canopus DVStorm2 and Matrox RT.X100) that use Adobe Premiere for enhanced video editing capabilities. However, after evaluating many approaches, it became apparent that an event-oriented ergonomics package adapted for barrier-oriented accessibility analysis, was most suited to our needs.

Multimedia Video Task Analysis (MVTA, NexGen Ergonomics, developed at the University of Wisconsin–Madison) is used for data and task analysis procedures, specifically interactive time and motion analyses of video recorded activities by researchers (Chapter 12). In general, MVTA is used to identify events with terminal break points during a timed activity for usability analyses. Multiple video and sensor data streams are synchronized so they can all be viewed on the same timeline during video playback, and video files may be viewed at any speed (i.e., real time, slow motion, fast motion or frame by frame) in both forward and reverse directions. Optionally, an event may be replayed in a continuous loop or an arbitrary event or point in time may be displayed. MVTA can also be used to produce conventional time study reports or to study the frequency of occurrence of any particular event, which may be helpful in usability analyses but has not been used with the MU-Lab thus far.

A standard protocol and template were created for conducting medical device usability analyses with MU-Lab and MVTA. The default set of MVTA records for all usability analyses, based on an evolutionary internal development process, consists of the following:

1. *Orienting and positioning body or device barrier* — Consider: dynamic support needs, such as at setup or beginning and end of device use, e.g., transferring, body balance or stability, physical obstruction, movement requirements, reaching, strength requirements, etc.
2. *Body support barrier* — Consider: static support needs for body or extremities without which there is loss of stability or fatigue, e.g., seat, back, leg, arm, and head support.
3. *Physical interaction, manipulation, and operation of controls barrier* — Consider: physical interactions with controls (e.g., switches and levers), reaching, handling, strength, dexterity, motor control, physical obstructions to hands (or other appropriate body part), etc., during use.
4. *Sensory barrier with communication or display* — Consider: device exceeds sensory capabilities for vision, hearing, touch, etc. (e.g., sightlines, letter size, sound volume, ambient noise, and tactile features).
5. *Cognitive barrier* — Consider: misunderstanding device, misinterpreting visual cues, memory demands, cuing, and language (often difficult to interpret).
6. *Use error* — Consider: misuse from manufacturer's intended manner of use.
7. *Unsafe activity* — Consider: activity that may put subject or other person at risk of injury. Note that this is a very important record and special attention should be paid to accurate identification and classification.
8. *Environmental barrier with device* — Consider: architectural elements, auxiliary furniture, or equipment other than device.
9. *Unable to use assistive technology effectively with device* — Consider: device impedes effective use of assistive technologies.
10. *Assistance from another person required with device* — Consider: must directly affect subject's normal, intended, and expected use of device; may be physical (does not include device use tasks normally performed by someone else) or verbal (does not including subject prompting needed for task performance).
11. *Exemplary positive device features* — Consider: device features that enable or facilitate use (does not include environmental features).
12. *Flag for review* — Consider: need for further review or discussion.
13. *Context-awareness comments.*

Notice that records 1 to 5 classify accessibility barriers. For each of these, three possible events may be marked:

- Impossible — a critical barrier that makes intended device use impossible for this person.
- Difficult — a substantial barrier that makes device use difficult but still possible.
- Mildly difficult — a very minor barrier to device use or inconvenience (use of this category is optional).

Of note is that this approach diverges from the conventional "task analysis" that is common in usability engineering and human factors and ergonomics. Rather, the focus here is on accessibility barriers, scored using the "impossible" and "difficult" terminology that is common for accessibility guidelines such as the Web Accessibility Initiative Guidelines, Priority Levels 1–3 ([22]; see chapter 23). This is an important point, and perhaps more than any other helps us distinguish between usability analysis (where the focus is on task performance) and accessibility analysis (where the focus is on identifying and then trying to understand barriers). In essence, the focus of accessibility analysis, as developed here, is on using barrier analysis as a form of "triage" for targeted (and detailed) analysis of strategic subtasks.

Notice also that records 6 and 7 identify use error and unsafe activity, events of interest to the FDA that are clearly worth documenting. Of particular interest to the RERC-AMI and others is a better understanding of when these events correlate with accessibility barriers.

Finally, records 8, 9, and 10 identify barriers or support provided by other objects and people that may be in the vicinity and affect use of the device. The project team decided that no barrier should be marked if subjects use an assistive technology (e.g., glasses, prosthesis, or wheelchair), and they are successful in using the device.

Importantly, custom MVTA records and events can also be added for more specific data analyses. This is an important feature, one that was used, for instance, for the study reported in Chapter 14. Examples of custom records include:

- Active device interaction (consider: device features that the subject actively engages for use).
- Shoulders or arms supporting body weight.*
- Contact pressure on hands or arms.

Examples of custom events include:

- Wrist range of motion — Moderate and Extreme**
- Reaching AND grasping — Moderate and Extreme***

13.3.4.2 Integrated Analysis of Subject Populations and Devices

A hierarchical "parent–child" structure with summary reporting capabilities of the PM enable a researcher to easily compare data from different subjects for any given device or class of devices. The researcher can generate reports for a group of subjects who use the same device, for one subject who uses a class of multiple devices, and for the comparative rating and ranking survey for several devices within the same class. For instance, if a researcher collects data for a group of individuals, who use several different examination tables, pre- and postactivity survey data can be summarized (1) for several subjects and one examination table, (2) for a group of subjects and several examination tables, (3) and for a subject's rating and ranking comparison of the examination tables. These summary tools within the PM automate much of the data reduction process, so the data is presented in an organized, tabulated manner with the total number of respondents for a given response summed.

13.4 RESULTS AND DISCUSSION

Two sets of the core components of the MU-Lab technology were first successfully transported in suitcases and demonstrated at an RERC-AMI Advisory Council meeting in February 2004 in Oakland, CA. At this stage the PM software was still being refined, and an aim was to solicit input from the project's advisors.

---

* Custom records can be added as custom events if they can be categorized within a default record. For example, "Shoulders or arms supporting body weight" could become an event under the "Body support barrier" record.

** We can always assume a custom window-event is an instance of the default window-event. So if custom events are used in place of the default events, the default information still exists, as well as more detailed information for those who are interested.

*** "AND" events can be used when there is more than one barrier (event) occurring simultaneously.

The first human subjects studies started in the summer of 2004. To date, MU-Lab has been used or is in use for eight IRB-approved human subjects studies. Of note is that several of these studies were designed specifically to evaluate MU-Lab as part of the development process [23] and were performed by graduate students from Marquette University as part of their master's projects. For these projects, a wide range of medical devices were purposely selected to be evaluated by samples of subjects with diverse abilities. Part of one of these is highlighted in Chapter 14. In all, these evaluations involved five to twelve subjects using one to three sample products for each of the following types of devices:

- Exam table, hospital beds, and weight scales
- Dental chairs, dental monitor, and portable (dental) x-ray
- Cycle ergometers, heart rate monitors, blood pressure monitors, and pulse oxymeter

These evaluations served multiple purposes. First, because these studies were performed by members of the team developing MU-Lab (and coauthors on this chapter), feedback from these experiences has been used to considerably refine the MU-Lab technology, especially as related to the PM. For instance, two versions of the PM were developed, versions 1.0 and 1.1, with the latter including a refined reporting structure and more capabilities for comparative data analysis. Second, these studies helped establish a secure database of examples of accessibility barriers for a range of device–disability conditions. The database has been critical to a reliability study of the barrier data analysis protocol used within MVTA, in which a collection of members of the California–Wisconsin team have independently scored videotape segments in MVTA using the core categories of records from Subsection 13.3.4.1. This internal study, which is especially focused on examining reliability of identifying "impossible" and "difficult" events, is nearing completion. Third, these studies have refined instructional materials such as the MU-Lab manual [24].

The other studies that have used MU-Lab are varied in nature. One study targeted videoconferencing technologies where the participants on either side of goal-directed tele-encounters had differing disabilities and was performed at the Telerehabilitation and Performance Assessment Lab at Marquette University. Several studies have targeted analysis of innovative technologies designed for use in stroke neurorehabilitation, including one study at the Veterans Affairs Medical Center in Milwaukee. Two recently approved studies relate to use of MU-Lab for projects associated with the RERC-AMI's Development Program D3 — Emerging and Accessible Health care Technologies (see http://www.rerc-ami.org/ami/projects/d/3). Both relate to usability evaluation of innovative interface technologies.

Several human subjects studies related to Research Program R2 — Usability Analysis (see http://www.rerc-ami.org/ami/projects/r/2), such as examination tables, imaging equipment, home monitors, and infusion devices are in preparation. Recently started is a study related to Development Program D2 — Design Projects (see http://www.rerc-ami.org/ami/projects/d/2) that will evaluate, for a diversity of users, an exercise ergometer. This will include an integrated collection of potentially exemplary accessibility features that are largely based on the work of student design teams from around the country. Their work targeted lower-cost accessible ergometers in the RERC-AMI national design competition (see also Chapter 8). The titles and principal investigator for all of the RERC-AMI sponsored human subjects studies that use MU-Lab are posted at http://www.rerc-ami. org/ami/projects/human/, a site that is updated as new projects are approved.

Notably, a side benefit of MU-Lab use is that it serves as a natural training tool for learning about accessibility analysis, usability analysis, universal design, and human factors and ergonomics. MU-Lab provides a structured process for integrated accessibility and usability evaluation. This is not a self-evident process, and indeed MU-Lab is the consequence of an evolutionary process that, upon reflection, differs from what any member of this team could have conceptualized two years ago. This is, in many ways, its added value. It is both a procedural tool for protocol development and implementation, and an educational tool.

Finally, MU-Lab complements the MED-AUDIT tool that is being developed for Research Program R3 — Accessible Metrics (see Chapter 22). The key distinction is that for MED-AUDIT there are no human subjects. Recent insights gained from the expert survey compared MU-Lab and MED-AUDIT approaches that are reported in Chapter 14. Based on these insights, it is becoming clear that these two alternative approaches are, in fact, quite complementary as we strive to establish excellence in performing systematic accessibility analysis of medical instrumentation.

13.5 FUTURE DIRECTIONS

The integrated collection of technologies called MU-Lab that is described in this chapter will continue to be a critical vehicle in the RERC-AMI's quest to better understand barriers to accessible medical instrumentation and to identify strategies for removing such barriers. From the initiation of this project in 2003, the aim of this tool has been to serve other RERC-AMI activities, in particular projects within Research Program R2 (for detailed usability analysis of specific, targeted problematic and potentially exemplary medical products), Development Programs D2 and D3 (for evaluation of accessibility and usability of innovative medical technologies), and Research Program R3 (as a complementary approach to the MED-AUDIT accessibility metric described in Chapter 22). Because a MED-AUDIT accessibility analysis requires less investment of time and resources than a comprehensive MU-Lab human subjects study, it makes sense that MED-AUDIT eventually be integrated into the preactivity component of the PM, where it can be used as a sort of accessibility triage filter that helps identify strategic types of users who may be predicted to have use barriers as well as suggest task procedures that should be part of the testing protocol for the device.

Use of MU-Lab is gradually becoming habitual for staff members of the RERC-AMI. This is important. A considerable advantage of such habitual use is that it influences how we approach research and design evaluation activities. Based on planned use, the main improvements will relate to refining the PM so that it better supports advanced statistical analysis. This is a challenge because unlike for conventional studies with highly controlled subpopulations, we proactively desire subjects with disabilities and indeed comorbidities because our national consumer survey has found this to be the norm (Chapter 2). Thus we are looking into advanced methods for statistically correlating assessment scales made at the preactivity stage (e.g., impairment and independence) with postactivity metrics related to performance and identification of barriers. We will also continue ongoing activities related to assessing and improving reliability.

Against the advice of several members of the RERC-AMI Advisory Council, we have chosen not to patent or sell this technology. Information on and about this technology is freely disseminated, and RERC-AMI staff is available to provide technical assistance to teams that may want to implement the hardware at their site or use aspects of the software. The core PM web software, written in C# and hosted on a password-protected site, is only available by way of first building a collaborative relationship with the RERC-AMI at some level. The main criteria for collaboration with an entity outside of the RERC-AMI is that they have interest in accessibility and usability analysis, and that they agree to provide periodic feedback on their experiences with MU-Lab. This in turn may help improve MU-Lab, which is our intent.

We would like nothing better than to have the MU-Lab technology used by dozens of groups interested in usability or ergonomic or accessibility analysis; because of the nature of the package, such users will likely find that they end up employing an integrated accessibility–usability approach to conduct their research, which benefits all.

ACKNOWLEDGMENT

This work is supported by the RERC-AMI, funded by the National Institute on Disability and Rehabilitation Research, U.S. Department of Education Grant #H133E020729. All opinions expressed are those of the authors.

REFERENCES

1. Sanders, M.S. and McCormick, E.J., *Human Factors in Engineering Design*, McGraw-Hill, New York, 1993.
2. Nielsen, J., *Usability Engineering*, AP Professional, Boston, MA, 1993.
3. Cook, A.M. and Hussey, S.M., *Assistive Technologies: Principles and Practice*, St. Louis, Mosby, 1995.
4. The Center for Universal Design, The Principles of Universal Design, NC State University, Raleigh, 1997, retrieved from http://design.ncsu.edu/cud/univ__design/ princ_overview.htm.
5. U.S. Access Board, A Federal Agency Committed to Accessible Design, 2005, retrieved from http://www.access-board.gov.
6. Section 508 federal site, 2005, retrieved from http://www.section508.gov.
7. Winters, J.M.W., Story, M.F., Barnekow, K., Premo, B., Kailes, J.I., Schwier, E., Rempel, D., and Winters, J.M., Problems with Medical Instrumentation Experienced by Patients with Disabilities, *Proc. Human Factors and Ergonomics Society 48th Annual Meeting*, Santa Monica, CA, 2004.
8. Vanderheiden, G. Fundamental Principles and Priority Setting for Universal Usability, 2000, retrieved from http://trace.wisc.edu/docs/fundamental_princ_and_priority_ acmcuu2000/.
9. Preiser, W.F.E. and Ostroff, E., Eds., *Universal Design Handbook*, McGraw-Hill, New York, 2002.
10. European Institute for Design and Disability, retrieved from http://www.design-for-all.org/, 2005.
11. D4.1 Report on update of Design for All and Design for All related higher education and research policies in EU member countries and U.S., IST-2001-38786 IDCnet, 2004, available at http://www.idcnet.info/html/IDCnet_D4.1.html.
12. The Center for Universal Design, Evaluating the Universal Design Performance of Products (Universal Design Performance Measures for Products), 2000, Raleigh: NC State University.
13. Story M.F. and Mueller J.L., Universal design performance measures for products: a tool for assessing universal usability, in *Emerging and Accessible Telecommunications, Information and Health Technologies*, Winters, J.M., Robinson, C., Simpson, R., Vanderheiden, G., Eds., RESNA Press, Arlington, VA, 2002, pp. 19–28, chap. 2.
14. U.S. Access Board, ADA and ABA Accessibility Guidelines for Buildings and Facilities. July 23, 2004, amended August 5, 2005. Available at http://www.access-board.gov/ada-aba/final.htm
15. Rehabilitation Act, Section 508 (29 U.S.C. 794d), as amended by the Workforce Investment Act of 1998 (P.L. 105-220), August 7, 1998.
16. World Health Organization, International Classification of Functioning, Disability and Health, Geneva, 2001.
17. Sawyer, D., Do It By Design: An Introduction to Human factors in Medical Devices, FDA's Center for Devices and Radiologic Health, Rockville, MD: FDA CDRH. 1996, (see http://www.fda.gov/cdrh/humfac/doit.html.)
18. Kaye, R. and Crowley, J., Guidance for Industry and FDA Premarket and Design Control Reviewers — Medical Device Use-Safety: Incorporating Human Factors, 2000, retrieved from http://www.fda.gov/cdrh/humfac/1497.html.
19. Medical Device Use-Safety: Incorporating Human Factors Engineering into Risk Management, FDA Guidance Document, issued January 2000, see http://www.fda.gov/cdrh/humfac/1497.html.
20. ANSI/AAMI HE74:2001, Human Factors Design Process for Medical Devices, Arlington, VA: Association for the Advancement of Medical Instrumentation, 2001.
21. Kohn, L.T., Corrigan, J.M., Donaldson, M.S., Eds., *To Err is Human: Building a Safer Health System*, Washington: National Academy Press, 2000.

22. Web Content Accessibility Guidelines Working Group, Web Content Accessibility Guidelines, Version 1.0, May 1999, Available at http://www.w3.org/TR/WCAG10.
23. Lemke, M.R., Winters, J.M., Campbell, S., Danturthi, S., Story, M.F., Barr, A., and Rempel, D.M., Mobile Usability Lab: A Tool for Accessibility and Usability Testing of Medical Instrumentation, *Proc. IEEE Eng. Med. Biol.*, San Francisco, CA, 2004.
24. Lemke, M., Winters, J.M., Story, M.F., Campbell, S., Barr, A., Omiatek, E., Rempel, D., *User's Manual for Mobile Usability Lab (MU-Lab)*, Tech Report AMI-001, Rehabilitation Engineering Research Center on Accessible Medical Instrumentation, Milwaukee, Version 1.1, 2005, see http://www.rerc-ami.org/ami/tech/tr-ami-001_mu-lab.aspx.

14 Comparison of Accessibility Tools for Biomechanical Analysis of Medical Devices: What Experts Think

Melissa R. Lemke and Jack M. Winters

CONTENTS

ABSTRACT

Accessibility analysis tools can be used to better understand the nature and extent of access barriers related to medical devices so better designs can be implemented. Expert comparisons of the utility of three tools for determining biomechanical accessibility are discussed, including (1) Mobile Usability Lab (MU-Lab) Protocol Manager (PM) questionnaires, (2) interactive MU-Lab barrier analyses using Multimedia Video Task Analysis (MVTA) software, and (3) Medical Equipment Device-Accessibility and Universal Design Information Tool (MED-AUDIT) software algorithm for estimating accessibility. MVTA was most often rated the highest of all the tools. The strengths, weaknesses, advantages, and disadvantages were documented for each tool.

14.1 INTRODUCTION

As documented by the Rehabilitation Engineering Research Center on Accessible Medical Instrumentation (RERC-AMI) national surveys [1–2; Chapter 2 of this book], individuals with disabilities are often denied adequate health care services because of various equipment barriers. Thus, though the U.S. spends more per person on health care than any other country [1], a significant proportion of our population still lacks access to health care products and services because of potentially correctable design limitations. Tools of accessibility and usability analysis can be used to help better understand the nature and extent of access barriers (see Chapter 6 and Chapter 13 of this book) so that better medical device designs can be implemented.

Three tools are discussed within this chapter, and they represent alternate, yet perhaps complementary, approaches to assessing accessibility. Each tool is covered elsewhere in this book, so they need not be developed in detail here. For the study presented, experts were asked their opinions about the following tools, comparatively:

- MU-Lab PM prescreening and postactivity questionnaires (Chapter 13 of this book)
- Interactive MU-Lab device barrier analyses using MVTA software [2,3; Chapter 12 and Chapter 13 of this book)
- MED-AUDIT software algorithm for estimating accessibility (Chapter 22 of this book)

Each tool helps researchers assess accessibility and usability of medical devices (or classes of devices) through detailed analyses that consider users with a diversity of abilities within the contexts of product design and task performance. Unfortunately, assessing accessibility often is challenging because there are numerous degrees of accessibility. There are often cases in which individuals lack access because of barriers that can be clearly identified without a detailed task analysis, but other analyses are not so straightforward because a task is difficult or unsafe, instead of impossible. However, accessibility and usability challenges often are comparable for groups of individuals with similar functional impairments, in which case it may be possible to develop population-based accessibility metrics for different products, including medical devices.

Thus, many questions can be raised regarding how to quantify medical device accessibility, and the RERC-AMI has been striving to address these questions. For instance:

- Because task analysis is critical in any accessibility assessment, can methods from the fields of human factors and usability engineering be transferred to accessibility analysis?
- Is it beneficial to have human subjects participate in accessibility analyses, and if so, at what stages of the process?
- Given the diversity of abilities within the population of individuals with disabilities, how does one select a representative sample of participants?
- Should an analysis focus on the observations of accessibility experts, on opinions and comments from usability testing participants, or on video-based task analyses of person–device interactions?

This chapter reports opinions from a sample of accessibility and ergonomic analysis experts who participated as human subjects to help address some of the aforementioned questions. Specifically, experts were presented summary analyses from the three alternative accessibility and usability assessment methods for a variety of medical products. Analyzed data were presented to experts in reduced form for "patient" users with diverse self-reported impairments or health problems (e.g., back or spine condition, arthritis or rheumatism, chronic pain, paralysis, low vision). For each device, experts completed a short survey to document their opinions of the device and the utility of the tools with that device. Experts also completed a comprehensive survey after reviewing all the data to document their overall opinions of the tools.

Each tool represents a unique methodology, design, and data set, while also providing accessibility and usability information useful for dissemination (e.g., product standards, design guidelines). It is important to note that an emphasis was placed on biomechanical accessibility and patient positioning, and as presented in Chapter 2, several of the devices presented were found problematic for respondents in the 2004–2005 RERC-AMI national consumer survey (i.e., examination table, weight scales, examination chairs).

14.2 BACKGROUND

The MU-Lab and MED-AUDIT were designed by teams of individuals with expertise in areas such as human factors engineering, ergonomics, universal design, rehabilitation engineering, and biomechanics. The Principles of Universal Design [4], further discussed in Subsection 14.2.3, also were incorporated into the design of each tool (e.g., questions within the PM and MED-AUDIT, barrier template in MVTA). Although many different methods exist to evaluate and improve product design, few, if any, integrate accessibility considerations for individuals with motor, sensory, and cognitive disabilities, and especially for the vast diversity of medical devices currently available. Assessing medical device accessibility is a demanding task, to say the least, so it is important to understand some key components relevant to accessibility for individuals with disabilities, including: human movement and biomechanics, disability prevalence, accessibility and accessible design, universal design, human factors engineering and ergonomics, and current medical device design guidelines and standards.

14.2.1 Human Movement and Biomechanics

Understanding how humans integrate different processes to coordinate movement is important for designing effective systems for humans to interact with, and indeed many disciplines exist to research different components of human motion (e.g., normal and abnormal gait, reach patterns). However, describing the complex and intricate processes involved in human movement are beyond the scope of this chapter. Globally, the skeletal system provides the structure, the motor system provides the ability, the sensory system provides the feedback, and the neurological system provides the commands that allow the human body to move in space [5]. The motor system is organized hierarchically, and movements are obtained by activating systems of muscles that, through dynamic interactions with skeletal structures and the environment, change configurations of the body. Muscles have spring-like properties, and tension generated by muscles varies in proportion to length and velocity.

Movements of slow or moderate speed often are thought of as sequential transitions in posture, which are carried out through contracting different skeletal muscles according to voluntary commands integrated with continuous peripheral sensory information. It is often necessary to simultaneously control multiple muscles at the same joint or different joints to obtain or maintain particular body positions (e.g., elbow and shoulder extension, reaching while standing). Many degrees of freedom exist within human joints, typically more than required to specify endpoints (e.g., hand position and orientation). The brain and spinal cord often select from numerous alternative postural sequences to complete a given task. The brain and spinal cord organize numerous possible movement patterns into a connected hierarchy within the premotor cortex, sensorimotor cortex, brainstem, spinal cord, and other structures such as the cerebellum and peripheral nerves. Some autonomic reflexes (e.g., knee jerk, flexion withdrawal) are organized at the spinal cord level, while other complex motions are organized in higher brain centers [5,6]. Although described in very minimal detail here, coordinated movement often requires many physiological systems to be fully synchronized so that motor commands for maintaining or changing postures can be effectively selected, executed, and attuned.

Many biomechanical studies use sensors (e.g., EMGs, force plates, goniometers) and quasi-static analyses or inverse dynamic calculations to study motion and joint loading. Because body movement and loading is involved in every interaction between a person and medical device, the application of biomechanical methods to investigate medical device accessibility and usability is appropriate. Some applications of traditional biomechanical principles include static force analysis to determine joint loading and stability during tasks, dynamic motion analysis to investigate and quantify movement patterns and muscle interactions, and dynamic analysis of movement patterns and compensatory mechanisms to optimize rehabilitation and design.

Several criteria documents from the National Institute for Occupational Safety and Health (NIOSH) have been developed that are based primarily on biomechanical studies, including recommendations for manual lifting, pushing and pulling, and asymmetric load handling, to name a few. These documents were written to help prevent disease and hazardous conditions in the workplace, and recommendations often are conveyed as formal publications to organizations such as the Occupational Safety and Health Administration (OSHA) for use in mandated standards [7]. Many tasks investigated and outlined in NIOSH documents and other biomechanical studies seem appropriate to apply to improving medical device design, and these types of mandates show the importance of considering tasks when investigating accessibility.

14.2.2 Disability Prevalence

Today nearly one out of every five individuals in the U.S. has a documented disability [8], and the most common self-reported causes of disability among adults in 1999 are shown in Table 14.1 [9]. Thus, a significant proportion of the U.S. population would benefit from the use of accessible medical instrumentation. Many causes of disability affect body positioning and biomechanics, therefore it is presumed that many commonly used medical devices may be difficult or impossible to use for the nearly 20% of the U.S. population of individuals with disabilities. However, when normal movement mechanisms are disrupted and users have limitations, individuals should not be prevented from accessing necessary medical devices.

14.2.3 Accessibility and Accessible Design

Since the passage of several U.S. laws (e.g., Americans with Disabilities Act (ADA) in 1990), access for individuals with disabilities has been addressed more, especially related to employment, state and local government services, public accommodations, commercial facilities, and transportation. However, specific guidelines and requirements for medical devices have not yet been developed. Of relevance are the ADA Accessibility Guidelines for Buildings and Facilities (ADAAG), which are technical requirements for making buildings and facilities accessible to individuals with disabilities that are applied during the design, construction, and alteration of establishments covered by titles II and III of the ADA. These regulations are mandated to the extent required by federal agencies, including the Department of Justice and the Department of Transportation, and it seems some of these guidelines could be applied directly to medical device designs, such as: space allowance and reach ranges (ADAAG Section 4.2), ground and floor surfaces (4.5), ramps (4.8), stairs (4.9), handrails, grab bars, and tub and shower seats (4.26), controls and operation mechanisms (4.27), alarms (4.28), detectable warnings (4.29), and signage (4.30) [10].

TABLE 14.1
Self- Reported Causes of Disability among 41.2 Million Adults in the U.S. in 1999

Cause of Disability	Percentage
Arthritis or rheumatism	17.5
Back or spine problem	16.5
Other	15
Heart trouble/hardening of the arteries	7.8
Lung or respiratory problem	4.7
Deafness or hearing problem	4.4
Limb/extremity stiffness	4.2
Mental or emotional problem	3.7
Diabetes	3.4
Blindness or vision problems	3.3
Stroke	2.8
Broken bone/fracture	2.1
Mental retardation	2
Cancer	1.9
High blood pressure	1.7
Head or spinal cord injury	1.1
Learning disability	1
Alzheimer disease/senility/dementia	0.9
Kidney problems	0.8
Paralysis	0.8
Missing limbs	0.7
Stomach/digestive problems	0.7
Epilepsy	0.5
Alcohol or drug problem	0.5
Hernia or rupture	0.5
AIDS/AIDS-related condition	0.3
Cerebral palsy	0.3
Tumor/cyst/growth	0.3
Speech disorder	0.2
Thyroid problems	0.2

Section 508 of the Rehabilitation Act is another mandate for federal agencies and departments that may be important in accessible medical instrumentation. Section 508 specifies accessibility requirements for electronic and information technology, and this mandate is legally applied in many different sectors, but not including medical device design. However, much the same as with parts of ADAAG, it seems appropriate to apply several of these mandates to medical device design, such as: software applications and operating systems (Section 508, 1194.21), telecommunications products (1194.23), functional performance criteria (1194.31), and information, documentation, and support (1194.41) [11,12].

14.2.4 Universal Design

Although rehabilitation engineering was founded in part on the principle of augmenting products to better serve individuals with disabilities, universal design and universal access are becoming more commonplace. Assistive technologies, or products used to increase or improve the functional capabilities of individuals with disabilities, have long been used to make certain technologies accessible and usable for individuals with disabilities [13]. Yet some products that were originally designed for individuals with disabilities have even been discovered to be beneficial for everyone (e.g., larger knobs, automatic door openers, curb cuts, large visual displays). The Seven Principles of Universal Design, developed in 1997, further enhance this goal (see also Chapter 6). Also, a set of Universal Design Performance Measures for Products was subsequently created which are used to evaluate existing designs, guide the design process, and educate consumers and design students [14].

Universal design is often referred to as inclusive design (see Chapter 7), because universally designed products are intended to include satisfactory use by as many people as possible regardless of their abilities. Furthermore, the key to applying universal design is to aim to make products usable by all individuals, without stigmatizing the product as being designed for individuals with disabilities. So, in essence, universal design has two major parts — making products appear as normal and desirable as possible while trying to accommodate everyone, including individuals with disabilities [15]. For example, using a low-force control mechanism can allow an individual with low strength to perform a desired device function that could not otherwise be performed, while it also may benefit someone with a sprained wrist, or someone using their nondominant hand, and so on. Including individuals with disabilities during the design phases, consulting disability experts, and simulating functional impairments of users are good ways to apply universal design to improving medical device usability [15; Chapter 18 of this book].

In medical device design, universal design is especially important because many medical technologies need to accommodate a large group of diverse users, regardless of their abilities and preferences. Whereas it also may appear that medical professionals are less likely than the general population to suffer from a disability and more likely to have above-average abilities required to operate medical devices, it is well-known that many home-health care consumers have disabilities. Also, many caregivers are middle- or older-aged women who may have chronic diseases, have dexterity or mobility problems, or have visual or auditory difficulties [15], and it seems appropriate to assume that many individuals seeking health care services and using medical devices are not in peak performance condition. Essentially, many individuals seeking health care services may be classified as having temporary disabilities, thus integration of accessible and universal design principles in any medical device design is beneficial, and indeed necessary for many individuals with disabilities.

14.2.5 Human Factors Engineering and Ergonomics

Human factors engineering and ergonomics are fields that play critical roles in designing safe and effective devices, and in recent years increasing attention in these fields has been placed on optimizing medical device design. Both human factors engineering and ergonomics apply knowledge of human performance (e.g., capabilities and limitations) to the design of systems and equipment, while considering interactions between the user, environment, and product. These fields exist to optimize the efficiency, safety, effectiveness, and reliability of systems [16], and although many commonalities exist between these two fields, there are some distinctions that can be made: ergonomics focuses more on biomechanical interactions and performance; human factors engineering focuses more on cognitive usability and performance; and human factors engineering originated in the U.S., whereas ergonomics originated in Europe. Some well-established ergonomics methods include document reviews, exploratory studies, product analysis, and usability testing [17].

Many performance recommendations and guidelines have been developed and refined throughout the history of these fields, but applying such guidelines to populations of individuals with disabilities can be challenging. The vast continuum of human performance capabilities that must be considered is extremely complex, because some people are capable of performing highly technical and complex activities, yet others may have physical, perceptual, or cognitive limitations that prevent them from performing seemingly routine tasks [18]. However, users often can be grouped according to physical characteristics or limitations (e.g., range of motion, strength, vision), and established human factors methods allow product designers to address these limitations within the context of "interface points" between users and products. Interface points are the areas of a device that users control or maintain to facilitate desired outputs from the system (e.g., controls, displays, training, documentation) [16], and many interface points are directly relevant to accessibility for individuals with disabilities. Applying human factors and ergonomic principles to medical device design for individuals with disabilities also can impact this population more than a nondisabled population, because health care access plays a greater role in their overall quality of life [18].

People are capable of making mistakes, but effective design can help medical devices mitigate positive and negative user effects, especially related to use error. Safety has become an extremely important focus within the medical device industry, especially because the FDA pays close attention to the safety of medical devices made available on the market. Medical device safety can be improved by applying good human factors principles, and safety improvements often result from detailed risk analysis and reduction efforts, such as identifying possible failure modes and effects, eliminating hazards, and providing protections [19].

The use environment, user, and device are all important factors in ergonomic analyses related to developing safe and effective (or unsafe or ineffective) products. Most important to accessibility of medical devices for individuals with disabilities seem to be user abilities and limitations, use environment (e.g., light, noise), and the device operation requirements and procedures (including complexity and user interface characteristics). Furthermore, some important user characteristics include health and mental state (e.g., relaxed, stressed, tired, diseased), physical size and strength, sensory capabilities, coordination, cognitive ability and memory, knowledge, previous experience, motivation, and ability for adaptation to adverse circumstances [20].

Usability testing often is conducted to provide detailed analyses of product design and usage, and the FDA currently requires manufacturers to conduct usability testing to demonstrate that products are suitable for use. Therefore, medical device designers are seeking detailed information on acceptable human factors principles and practices. In 2001, following discussions between human factors professionals and medical device regulators, the following guidelines were developed to allow more intuitive, ergonomic, and smart device development [19]:

1. Guard critical controls
2. Confirm critical actions
3. Make critical information legible and readable
4. Simplify and ensure proper connections
5. Use tactile coding
6. Prevent the disabling of life-critical alarms
7. Present information in a usable form
8. Indicate and limit the number of modes
9. Do not permit settings to change automatically
10. Reduce the potential for negative transfer (e.g., arrow keys then arrow keys/enter)
11. Design in automatic checks

14.2.6 Current Medical Device Guidelines and Standards

Although design guidelines and suggestions are helpful for improving product designs for individuals with disabilities, federal mandates receive the most attention from manufacturers. In 2001, the American National Standards Institute (ANSI) and the Association for the Advancement of Medical Instrumentation (AAMI) released an ergonomics and human factors standard for medical device design — HE74. This important process-oriented standard describes design approaches and techniques, training programs, and learning tools to help manufacturers interpret and satisfy relevant national and international regulations to make devices safer, more effective, and easier to use [21]. A follow-up document, HE75, is currently under development and planned for release in 2006.

More recently, a working group has been established to create an international guideline for standards developers related to accessibility of products, services, and environments for older adults and individuals with disabilities (Chapter 15). This document is intended to supplement the ISO/IED Guide 71 with ergonomic methods, principles, and data for individuals with disabilities [22]. With the development and implementation of human factors standards such as these, medical device design will be better matched to the capabilities and limitations of real users, including individuals with disabilities.

However, because individuals with disabilities still lack access to numerous medical technologies, it seems obvious that federally mandated standards and guidelines need to exist so more medical devices are designed and implemented to better serve this population. Most importantly, if accessible medical devices exist yet are not mandated and used in clinical settings, our health care system is falling well below the mark for individuals with disabilities.

14.3 METHODS

Each accessibility analysis tool presented in this IRB-approved study (i.e., MU-Lab PM, MU-Lab analysis with MVTA, and MED-AUDIT) was used to collect, analyze, and summarize data for expert participants to review in this study. Representative reduced and summarized data from each tool were presented to five experts in the fields of accessibility, biomechanics, ergonomics, and design, in order to determine their opinions on the three tools. With each tool, the biomechanical accessibility of seven different medical devices also was investigated, including an examination table, two weight scales, two dental chairs, and two power-adjustable hospital beds. For the MVTA and PM tools, data were collected and reduced for 12 participants with various disabilities. For MED-AUDIT, several representative impairment types similar in nature to characteristics of the 12 participants with disabilities (i.e., low vision, lower body paralysis, overall body balance impairment) were used to generate accessibility scores.

14.3.1 Expert Research Packet

The 51-page research packet contained introductions, executive summaries of reduced data, and surveys for expert participants to document their opinions, insights, and suggestions for each tool. Numerous colleagues were involved in the iterative process used to refine the content included in this research packet, so the most meaningful and representative information was presented to expert participants for each tool.

The expert packet contained the following summary and data documents:

1. Introduction to purpose and methodology of MED-AUDIT, MVTA, and PM surveys
2. Summary data for the 12 participants with disabilities who used the 7 medical devices presented
3. Data sets for 7 different medical devices (i.e., examination table, hospital beds, dental chairs, weight scales), which included:
   - Summary of the medical device with 2 to 6 color pictures and usability testing protocol for each device
   - Summary data from each of the three accessibility tools (i.e., MED-AUDIT, MVTA, PM)
   - Targeted survey to complete for each medical device after reviewing each data set
4. Comprehensive survey to complete after reviewing all data presented

Data sets were presented in randomized order, except pairs of similar devices were presented sequentially, to eliminate any effects of presentation order on the opinions of the experts. Device introductions also described the uses, features, and task scenarios attempted by participants, and each device had text descriptions that pointed out targeted accessibility information for each device (i.e., dimensions, important features, weight limits).

Summary data for each tool (described in detail in Subsection 14.3.4, Subsection 14.3.5, and Subsection 14.3.6) were included to present key observations and findings about each of the seven different medical devices. Data from each tool were presented in randomized order. Each data set also contained a targeted survey to document expert opinions about ease of use and safety of each medical device, and effectiveness of each tool in providing insights into general biomechanical challenges or barriers and specific biomechanical accessibility features needed for each device.

A comprehensive survey also was completed by the expert participants after reviewing all the data sets to document their opinions on the following:

- Effectiveness of each tool in providing insights into challenges or barriers related to targeted biomechanical tasks
- Effectiveness of each tool in providing insights into specific barriers encountered related to assistive technology (AT) use
- Effectiveness of each tool in providing insights into specific biomechanical accessibility features that are needed on a device
- Utility for providing accessibility and usability data for targeted audiences, and the practical aspects of collecting and reducing data and effectively disseminating results
- Strengths and weaknesses of each of the three tools
- Advantages and disadvantages of each of the three tools

Forced response rating and ranking questions were included in the surveys, as well as open-ended questions about the devices and tools. For all surveys, an ordinal scale ranging from "not at all" (0) to "extremely" (5) was used to determine the degree of effectiveness, utility, strengths, weaknesses, advantages and disadvantages of each tool, and the safety and accessibility of each medical device. Survey results are described in detail in Section 14.4.

14.3.2 Expert Participants

Five experts in the fields of accessibility, biomechanics, design, human factors engineering and ergonomics, and usability analysis (i.e., in academia, engineering, and research) were participants in this study. Experts were mostly male (80%), and all were between the ages of 51 to 61, with an advanced degree (i.e., M.S. or Ph.D.). Three experts (60%) self-reported having impairments or disabilities that affect their daily lives. None of the experts reported previously working on any RERC-AMI related projects or tools, and they spent an average of 2 h and 40 min reviewing the packet and completing the surveys. It should be noted that experts were exposed to a lot of information in a limited amount of time.

14.3.3 Expert- Testing Protocol

The research packet was mailed to expert participants, with instructions asking them not to evaluate the quality of information presentation within the documents, but instead to focus on the content and ability of the tools to assess and portray biomechanical accessibility and usability of medical devices for patient subjects with disabilities. Specifically, experts were asked to focus on the subject tasks outlined in each device introduction, so an emphasis was placed on the ability of the tools to evaluate biomechanical accessibility of medical devices. Furthermore, because these experts are very busy people, they were asked not to spend more than 3 h on the entire study.

14.3.4 Collection and Reduction of MVTA Data

MVTA software (see also Chapter 12 of this book) was used to document specific time instances when biomechanical accessibility barriers occurred during attempted device uses. Participants with disabilities attempted seemingly routine tasks that would likely be part of a medical procedure

TABLE 14.2
Tasks Attempted by Human Subjects during Usability Testing Procedures

Device Class	Tasks Attempted
Examination table	Get onto table; sit on table; lie supine on table; lie prone on table; if female, use stirrups; get off table
Weight scale	Get onto scale; measure weight; obtain weight readout; get off scale
Power adjustable hospital bed (head and foot sections)	Get into bed; adjust bed to eat; adjust side safety rails; get out of bed
Dental chair	Get into dental chair; sit in dental chair; lie back in dental chair; get out of dental chair

involving each medical device, as outlined in Table 14.2. Each subject–device interaction was audio and video recorded with the MU-Lab, and interactive barrier analyses were later conducted using MVTA. Specific biomechanical barriers considered and observed during at least one subject's attempt to use the medical devices, in order of most prevalence, included transferring, safety, positioning/postural support, reaching, leg strength/weight bearing on lower extremities, manipulation, visual sensing (related to biomechanics), orienting into position, exertion, gross balance/postural control, auditory sensing (related to biomechanics), and tactile sensing (related to biomechanics).

MVTA breakpoint reports were generated for each biomechanical barrier subset, and the total number of occurrences and number of participants who experienced each barrier were presented for each device, as shown in Figure 14.1. Numerical data in the table were supported with representative comments (e.g., detailed descriptions of documented barriers, researcher observations, and proposed solutions). Furthermore, because video is such an integral part of the MVTA tool, tabulated data for each device also were supplemented with representative video snapshots in the form of MVTA screenshots, several sequential video screenshots with text descriptions, or a quadrant screenshot of the subject–device interaction (see Figure 14.2).

14.3.5 Collecting and Reducing Protocol Manager (PM) Data

Pre- and postactivity questionnaire data were collected from participants with disabilities as part of MU-Lab PM to document their opinions regarding the accessibility and usability of medical devices (see also Chapter 13 of this book). Preactivity questionnaire data were compiled into a one-page summary of the 12 participants, which included information such as gender, age, task difficulties (e.g., reaching, grasping, keeping your balance while sitting) and functional impairments (e.g., vision, hearing, paralysis). Targeted biomechanical data, from the postactivity interview, collected from participants with disabilities were presented, including the number of respondents for each response set for each device.

Average values were calculated for each PM question by assigning numerical values to the PM response set (i.e., 0 for "N/A," 1 for "Not at all," 2 for "A little," etc.) and then multiplying the number of respondents for each question by the corresponding response set value across all devices. Vertical arrows (see Figure 14.3) were used to help guide the expert to focus on answers that were outside the expected norm, upward for higher than expected and downward for lower.

Representative biomechanics-related comments from the free-response sections of the postactivity questionnaire also were included to supplement the forced-response data, because comments obtained during the free-response portions of the postactivity surveys proved to be a valuable part of the PM tool. Narrative comments were grouped according to common themes, and then the number of similar occurrences and total number of participants who made similar comments were indicated with each representative quotation.

MVTA Barrier Report Summary: Green Dental Chair

Category	Rating	# of Subj.	# of Occur.	Level	Representative Comments for Events Identified by Researcher
Orienting into position (dynamic)	Difficult	8	14	Difficult:	Threshold causes imbalance Patient cannot position wheelchair right next to dental chair seat due to threshold Patient expects device to be higher, bends way over to feel device and orient to device Patient keeps one or both feet on floor while seated to help with balance and orienting
Transferring	Difficult	11	21	Difficult:	Threshold causes balance difficulty-patient trips Patient cannot do side transfer so has to slide from end of device backwards to seat Patient has to lean way over for balance aid because there are no armrests Patient has difficulty getting out of device because of contouring
	Impossible	2	3	Impossible:	Patient cannot get out of device without provider assistance with leverage Patient cannot swing legs onto device
Positioning	Difficult	12	23	Difficult:	No where to rest arms while seated, no upper arm support while supine No armrests to help patient feel secure or balance upper body on chair Patient is not comfortable with headrest position Patient's lower body is not aligned in dental chair Patient has unsupported gap in lower back while sitting
	Impossible	5	11	Impossible:	Headrest is too far back for patient to reach it comfortably
Gross Body Balance	Difficult	5	9	Difficult:	There is nothing to support or stop patient's upper body during transfer (armrest) There are no armrests to assist patient with balance
	Impossible	1	1	Impossible:	No balance aid for patient when rolling to side to place transfer board under body
Reaching	Impossible	1	1	Impossible:	Patient attempts but is unable to adjust headrest
Manipulation	Impossible	1	1	Impossible:	Patient attempts but is unable to adjust headrest
Safety	Moderate	3	4	Moderate:	No balance aid (armrests), threshold causes imbalance and patient has nothing to grab Patient doesn't have upper body stability so doesn't feel safe when device is in motion Patient falls back into seat when getting on device
	Extreme	3	3	Extreme:	Patient almost falls off side of device while getting on-researcher has to stop descent Patient has nothing to stop body from going off side of device when transferring

FIGURE 14.1 Example of Multimedia Video Task Analysis software (MVTA) barrier analysis summary data presented to experts for each device. Figure includes data for "newer green dental chair."

14.3.6 Collecting and Reducing MED- AUDIT Data

A preliminary black box version of MED-AUDIT (see also Chapter 22), further referred to as *pre*MED-AUDIT, was used to generate accessibility estimates presented for the seven medical devices. A subset of the tool was used to generate the estimates, specifically 50 device tasks, 100 device features, and 3 user impairment types. Tasks and features were selected to be relevant for one or more of the devices used by participants with disabilities, and functional impairments were selected to some of those experienced by the usability testing participants (i.e., low vision, lower body paralysis, overall body balance impairment). The accessibility and usability "importance" matrices (described in Subsection 14.3.5.2) also used the aforementioned subsets of device tasks and features, as well as several representative user impairments. This subset was used to make the data set more manageable in this first-round use of *pre*MED-AUDIT and to narrow the scope of the tool to a biomechanical focus.

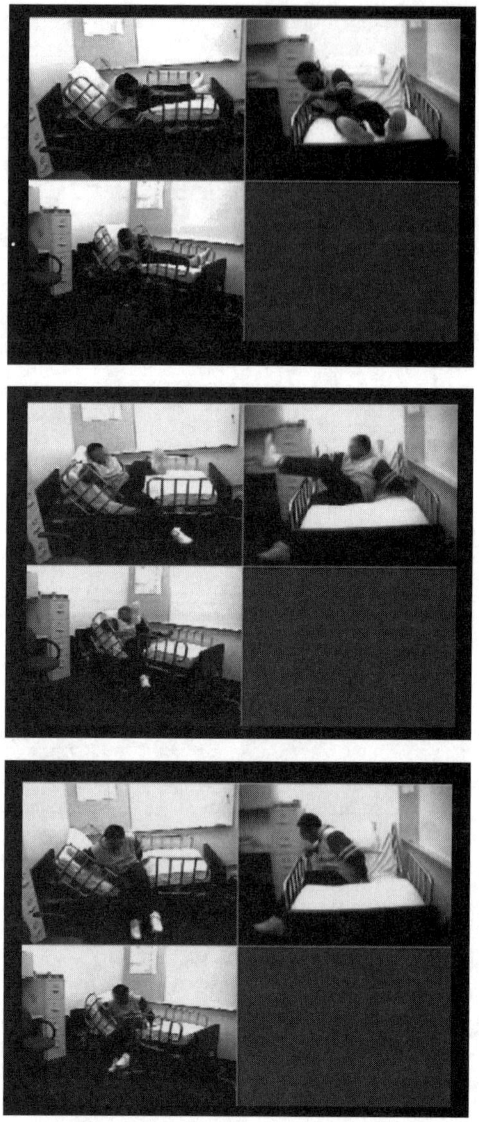

FIGURE 14.2 Examples of supplemental Multimedia Video Task Analysis (MVTA) software screen shots presented to experts: (a) MVTA analysis screenshot, (b) several sequential video screen shots with text descriptions describing subject actions: a subject who attempts but cannot find/operate side rail buttons; he then gets frustrated and climbs over the rails.

14.3.6.1 Rater Data

Assuming the role of a MED-AUDIT user, *pre*MED-AUDIT matrices were created for each device, which contained the following information:

Section I: Tasks required to use the medical device (x_{rt})

- Does the device require the user to do this task (e.g., sitting, standing, lying)?
- (2 = yes, 1 = somewhat, 0 = no or N/A)

Section II: Medical device accessibility feature availability (x_{rd})

- Does the device have this accessibility feature (e.g., head/neck positioners and supports, rails)?
- (2 = yes, 1 = somewhat, 0 = no or N/A)

PM Post-Activity Survey Data: Standing Weight Scale

↑ and ↓ indicate values >1 above and below the average number of responses across all devices (for relevant questions in top portion of table).

Question	Not at all	A little	Somewhat	Very	Extremely	N/A
How well could you see (or feel) the labels?	2	0	2	4	4	0
How important is this?	0	0	0	9	3	0
How well could you find all the buttons/knobs/levers?	1	0	1	8↑↑↑↑	2	0
How important is this?	0	0	0	9	2	1
Did the arrangement of the parts of the device make sense to you?	2	0	1	7↑↑	2↓	0
How important is this?	0	0	0	9	3	0
How well could you reach everything you needed to?	3↑	3↑	2	3	1↓	0
How important is this?	0	0	0	8	4	0
How well could you operate everything you needed to?	3↑	1	2	5↑	1	0
How important is this?	0	0	0	9	3	0
Was the arrangement of the parts of the device convenient for you?	5↑↑	0↓	1↓	1↓	4↑	1
How important is this?	0	0	0	9	3	0
Were the postures you used comfortable?	2	0	4	4	0↓↓	2
How important is this?	0	0	0	10	2	0
Was the amount of strength needed okay?	1	1	3	4	1↓	2
How important is this?	0	0	1	10	1	0
Was the amount of fatigue you had okay?	0	1	3	2	3	3
How important is this?	0	1	0	8	2	1
How easy was it to use the device without making any mistakes?	0	1	3	3↓	2	3
How important is this?	0	0	0	8	3	1
If you had made a mistake, how safe would you have been?	5	1	1	1↓	1	3
How important is this?	0	0	0	6	5	1
Did you feel safe?	2	0	3	2	2↓	3
How important is this?	0	0	0	7	2	3
How well could you use your assistive technology with the device?	3↑	1	1	4	1	2
How important is this?	0	0	0	5	5	2
How easy was it to maintain your balance while using the device?	3	2	2	1	0	4
How important is this?	0	0	0	6	3	3
How easy was it to obtain the readout of your weight?	3	0	3	2	0	4
How important is this?	0	0	1	6	2	3
How easy was it to get on the weight scale?	2	0	6	0	0	4
How important is this?	0	0	1	6	2	3
How easy was it to get off the weight scale?	2	0	2	4	0	4
How important is this?	0	0	0	7	2	3

Representative Comments from Subjects (P=# subjects who commented similarly, C= total # comments made)

Perceptible Information:

- It would be much easier to use if it was electronic or the numbers were larger. (2P-3C)
- It would be better if there was sound info. (1P-1C)
- I was able to read the scale easily. (1P-1C)

FIGURE 14.3 Compiled post-activity Protocol Manager (PM) questionnaire data and comments from 12 participants with disabilities. Arrows indicated how much above (i.e., up arrows) or below (i.e., down arrows) the average subject responses were for particular questions. For example, one up-arrow indicated the number of respondents for a particular question was at least one above the average across all devices and two down-arrows indicated the number of respondents was at least 2 below the average across all devices for that question. Figure includes data for "older standing weight scale."

14.3.6.2 Expert- Based "Importance" Matrices for Mapping across Domains

Besides the rater data collected directly from the MED-AUDIT user, two expert-knowledge matrices (accessibility and usability importance) were used to help weigh the importance of the rater data when determining estimated scores of accessibility. The following information is stored in the expert-created accessibility and usability importance matrices:

- Accessibility importance matrix: Relationship between user impairments and medical device features ($x_{e\text{-}id}$): How much does this device feature help a person with this impairment?
- (2 = substantially, 1 = partially, 0 = not at all)
- Usability importance matrix: Relationship between medical device features and required tasks ($x_{e\text{-}dt}$): How well does this feature accommodate this task?
- (2 = highly accommodates, 1 = partially accommodates, 0 = not at all accommodates)

$X_{e\text{-}id}$	Device Feature			
Impairment	Adequate approach	Adequate w/c turning space	Avoids mobility/transfer obstacles	Clear overhead
Low Vision	1	0	2	2
Lower Limb Paralysis	2	2	2	1
Overall Balance	1	1	2	1

$X_{e\text{-}dt}$	Required Task		
Device Feature	d. Understand display info	1). Locate device	2). Detect orientation
Adequate approach space	1	1	1
Adequate wheelchair turning space	1	1	1
Avoids mobility/transfer obstacles	1	1	1
Clear overhead	0	1	1

FIGURE 14.4 Example of subset of: (a). Accessibility Importance Matrix ($x_{e\text{-}id}$); (b). Usability Importance Matrix ($x_{e\text{-}dt}$)

These mapping matrices were generated using different scoring schemes, because the accessibility matrix was assumed to have more merit and value than the usability matrix because a feature required for accessibility is more important than a feature needed for usability. A <0, 2> scheme was used to create the accessibility matrix and <0, 1> for the usability matrix. Examples are provided in Figure 14.4.

14.3.6.3 preMED- AUDIT Scoring Algorithm

Equation 14.1 is the algorithm used with *pre*MED-AUDIT to generate the accessibility estimates presented to expert participants. In general, the estimates generated (i.e., on the interval of <0,1>) represent device accessibility scores through systematically considering tasks that are accessible or inaccessible to users with specific impairments, based on the presence or absence of important accessibility features.

$$y_i = \frac{\sum_{j=1}^{n_d}\left[\sum_{k=1}^{n_t}\left[w_{jk}(x_{rd}-1)\right]\right]}{2\left(\sum_{j=1}^{n_d}\left[\sum_{k=1}^{n_t} w_{jk}\right]\right)} + 0.5 \tag{14.1}$$

where:

y_i = estimate of device accessibility on the range of <0..1> for user with specific functional impairment

n_d = number of device features in complete taxonomy

n_t = number of device tasks in complete taxonomy

x_{rt} = rater matrix with <0,1,2> scores representing "task essentiality" vectors

x_{rd} = rater matrix with <0,1,2> scores representing "feature present" vectors

w_{jk} = $(x_{e\text{-}dt})$j $(x_{e\text{-}id})$k (x_{rt})k scaling vector with products of <0,1,2,4>

x_{rt} = rater matrix with <0,1> scores representing "task required" vectors
$x_{e\text{-}dt}$ = expert matrix with <0,1> scores representing "usability importance" vectors
$x_{e\text{-}id}$ = expert matrix with <0,1,2> scores representing "accessibility importance" vectors

Product relationships are summed in this algorithm, and four product terms (multiplied by a normalizing constant) are included: two generic expert entries multiplied together (i.e., impairment–device feature accessibility [$x_{e\text{–}id}$], multiplied by device feature–task usability [$x_{e\text{–}dt}$]), multiplied by the device-specific rater value for tasks required [x_{rt}], multiplied by the rater "feature present" entry minus one [x_{rd}–1]. This means an x_{rd} (device feature presence) of "2" affects the estimate positively, "1" becomes neutral, and "0" affects the estimate negatively. Also notice, a "0" for any of the w_{jk} terms (i.e., $x_{e\text{–}id}$, $x_{e\text{–}dt}$, x_{rt}) within the multiplication negates the entry as unimportant, while a really important entry has a scaling value of ±4 (2×2). Each score presented represents an impairment specific accessibility estimate on the interval <0,1>, which is scaled to 0% to 100% accessibility. Normally, "+" represented important and accessible terms, and "-" represented important and inaccessible terms.

14.3.6.4 Reduced preMED- AUDIT Data for Expert Research Packet

Generated accessibility estimates for three impairments (i.e., low vision, lower limb paralysis, and overall body balance) were provided to experts for each device, as well as an abbreviated list of essential tasks required to use the device (i.e., x_{rt} terms that received a rater score of "2") and accessibility features present (i.e., x_{rd} terms that received a rater score of "2") (see Figure 14.5). Data were selected in an attempt to display the best information in the time and space permitted, although it may have been more beneficial to present more detailed and descriptive information from the tool. Again, it should be noted that the MED-AUDIT tool was at the most preliminary development stage compared with the other tools, so this should be taken into account when reviewing the overall results.

14.4 RESULTS

Overall, experts most often rated MVTA the highest out of all the tools, although the PM surveys and MED-AUDIT also were rated highly for some aspects related to determining biomechanical accessibility. One expert in the fields of biomechanics, ergonomics, work physiology, musculoskeletal disorders, and job analysis and design also felt very strongly about using MED-AUDIT (with suggested modifications). It also is believed that the presentation method of MED-AUDIT should have been more in-depth and could have been more effective, because several experts noted difficulty with conceptualizing the tool. Because the MED-AUDIT is at an earlier development stage as compared to the MU-Lab, it is at a disadvantage and results may be lower as compared to the other tools. Nonetheless, the availability of input from experts was beneficial even at this early stage of development.

Figure 14.6 shows the average expert response across all devices for questions related to the effectiveness of the tool in providing insights into biomechanical challenges or barriers related to orienting into position, transferring, sensing, static positioning and postural support, reaching, manipulation, balance and postural control, exertion, safety, AT use, and biomechanical accessibility features needed on a medical device. On average, experts thought MVTA was the most effective tool for providing biomechanical accessibility insights, and it was the only tool to receive ratings of "extremely effective" (5) from one expert. MVTA was rated the highest for all questions except for exertion, safety, and AT usage, where the PM and MVTA were scored near equally. MED-AUDIT had the greatest diversity of opinions from expert participants overall, with ratings between "A little" (1) and "Very" (4). Also, average ratings for MVTA and the PM were generally lower for questions related to understanding AT usage and accessibility features needed on a device.

MED-AUDIT Estimated Accessibility Scores: Hospital Bed with Casters

Low Vision: 0.448 Lower Body Paralysis: 0.431 Overall Body Balance Imp.: 0.377

(0=0% and 1=100% accessibility for biomechanics subset of MED-AUDIT questions for given impairment type)

Essential Tasks Required to Use Device [2]

- Position during use:
  - Locate device
  - Detect orientation
  - Approach-ambulate to device:
    - Get into position
    - Leave position
  - Physical Interaction with device: Manipulate body-in use:
    - Sit:
      - Get into position
      - Maintain position
      - Leave position
    - Lay:
      - Get into position
      - Maintain position
      - Leave position
    - Roll to side lying:
      - Get into position
      - Leave position
    - Twist:
      - Get into position
      - Leave position
    - Bend/straighten trunk:
      - Get into position
      - Maintain position
      - Leave position
    - Bend/straighten upper limbs:
      - Get into position
      - Leave position
    - Bend/straighten lower limbs:
      - Get into position
      - Maintain position
      - Leave position
  - Ambulate away from device:
    - Get into position
    - Maintain ambulation
    - Leave position
- Operate device:
  - Manipulate controls:
    - Locate controls

Accessibility Features Present on Device [2][1]

- Environment:
  - Adequate wheelchair turning space
  - Avoids mobility/transfer obstacles
  - Clear overhead
- Overall device features:
  - Overall adjustability:
    - Adjustable height
  - Portability aids:
    - Locks
  - Finish material:
    - Smooth
- Overall labeling:
  - Meaningful, consistent, concise:
    - Consistent
  - Viewing characteristics:
    - Background contrast
  - Abbreviations, acronyms, graphics:
    - Number of pictorial symbols
  - Text and character design:
    - Simple character
    - Font type
- General control aspects:
  - Motor aspects:
    - Depth
- Component specific features:
  - Positioners and supports:
    - Head/neck positioners and supports:
      - Adjustable height
    - Leg/lower limb positioners/supports:
      - Adjustable position:
        - Adjustable angle
    - Full body positioners and supports:
      - Adjustable height:
        - Upper height
      - Width
    - Rails:
      - Load limit
    - Component control types:
      - Pushbutton controls:
        - Travel distance

FIGURE 14.5 Example of Medical Equipment Device – Accessibility and Universal Design Information Tool (MED-AUDIT) data presented to experts for each medical device. Figure includes data for "older hospital bed with casters."

Figure 14.7 shows the average expert rankings for the utility of each tool for items listed along the x-axis. On average, expert participants ranked MVTA first, the PM second, and MED-AUDIT third for utility of providing accessibility and usability data for product designers, consumers, safety analysts, public dissemination, and reliably documenting device accessibility for individuals with disabilities. Experts ranked, on average, MVTA first, MED-AUDIT second, and the PM third for utility in providing accessibility and usability data for students and academics and amount of setup required. The PM was ranked first, followed by MVTA, and then MED-AUDIT for the amount of training required to use the tools for data collection and analysis, ease of collecting qualitative data, and readiness for public dissemination. Experts ranked the PM first for amount of setup required to use the tool and ease of collecting quantitative data, whereas MED-AUDIT came in second and tied with MVTA for each of these questions, respectively.

Table 14.3 shows the strengths and weaknesses, advantages and disadvantages, and other comments listed by expert participants for each tool. One expert felt using all the tools together had an advantage because it, "give[s] the most complete picture from all perspectives-experts, users, etc., [it] yields the most data [and] helps ensure that nothing is missed." Another expert felt, "MED-AUDIT should be the starting point for all analyses. It provides a framework for

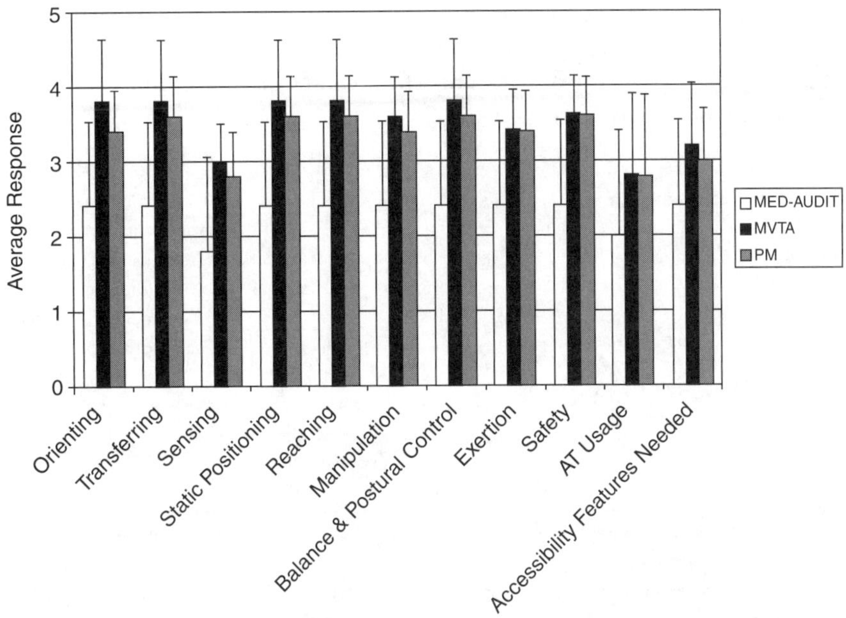

FIGURE 14.6 Average expert ratings and standard deviations for the effectiveness of each tool in providing insights into biomechanical challenges or barriers related to items along the x-axis. Response set included: N/A (0), Not at all (1), A little (2), Somewhat (3), Very (4), and Extremely (5).

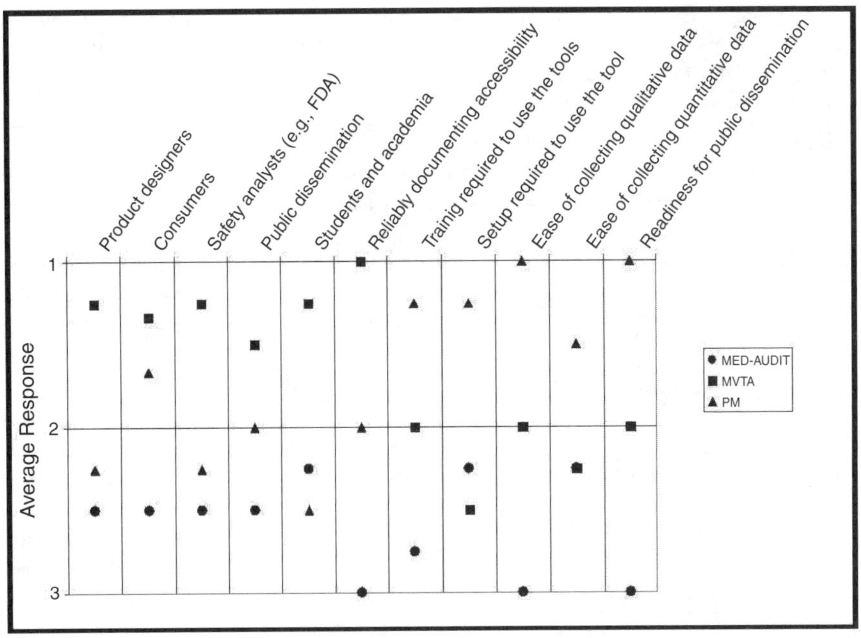

FIGURE 14.7 Average expert rankings for utility of each tool for providing accessibility and usability data related to items along the x-axis. Response set included rankings of 1–3, with 1 being the best.

linking problems to design parameters. The MVTA and PM survey help with user experience data. It should be the backbone of the task analysis." When asked about the disadvantage of using all the tools together, several experts commented on cost, time, and effort. An expert also commented, "Only time and money. Need method for determining when the cost of additional

TABLE 14.3
Strengths and Weaknesses, Advantages and Disadvantages, and Other Comments from Expert Participants for Each Tool

	MED- AUDIT	MVTA	PM
Strengths	• Good … at all levels-including conceptual level … group of users (not required). • Lists of tasks	• Very visual • Observational • Video clips provide useful information, observational analysis • Visual record immensely helpful, best source of information … on assistance required … real data on users who found tasks difficult or impossible	• Good survey tool requires representative study populations • Comment section • Useful information • Good perspectives on the user sense of the product
Weaknesses	• … include more quantitative information and standard methods • … relationship between task and accessibility • … [ineffective] for determining access and biomechanical data (qualitative and quantitative) • … general/nonspecific and too reliant on expert opinion … would miss a lot, unless the tool itself contains an incredible amount of knowledge about real user behavior	• Should be linked to standard method in MVTA • Video information can show bias and therefore affect results • … less quantitative	• Information based on a limited number of users could be misleading; each deficiency should be explained, lends itself to a focus group • … limited when trying to collect information beyond questions • … lack of specificity on reasons for certain problems, user importance data generally not that helpful
Advantages	• Provides framework for identification of gaps and hazards • Potential for systematically considering all aspects of a device if algorithms are complete	• Enables analyst to view task, helps identify problems not anticipated • Observational • Very rich data set, real-world illustration of problems, good sense of problem prevalence	• … [good] for obtaining feedback from broad range of users • User comments • Good, quick, and orderly evaluations, ability to compare across products on a number of key aspects, user friendly
Disadvantages	• Requires good conceptual understanding of task • Lacks sufficient detail • Results seem rather abstract …	• Can be misleading, still requires knowledge of what user is doing, need to look at multiple users • Time intensive	• May not provide information about cause of problem and how to fix, sensitive to user background, problems, and experiences • Importance data not useful, nonspecific as to cause of problems in some respects

information exceeds its value." Another commented the disadvantages were "Cost and effort required [and] potential for inconsistencies."

Most experts agreed that MVTA was a thorough enough tool to be used alone, whereas one expert also thought the PM was thorough enough. Experts claimed "MVTA with its video clips is a little bit better as a standalone product" and "MVTA-visual record is helpful, compelling, essential, gives problem prevalence, gives good 'log' of all problems, comments sufficient for user perspective, video also yields this, gives good sense of difficulties versus impossibilities in terms of user tasks."

Unfortunately, most of the experts felt uncomfortable scoring and commenting about MED-AUDIT, which is likely due to the early stage of development of this tool at the time of analysis, and especially the approach for extracting and summarizing information. Several experts commented on the representation of this tool, indicating they "... didn't get a good sense of what it was doing, based on the output presented for each case." Because the experts felt the *pre*MED-AUDIT summary and data presented were not adequate compared to the other tools, it is likely that the MED-AUDIT results were negatively affected. One expert suggested trying a "cross-impact matrix, something that explicitly shows the relationship" for the accessibility and usability importance matrices to "show how the accessibility features are explicitly tied to a task (diagram in survey)," which would likely have been more beneficial than some of the content presented for MED-AUDIT.

14.5 FUTURE DIRECTIONS

From the expert opinions presented in this study, it can be seen that each of the tools is useful and beneficial for one or more stages of assessing the accessibility of medical devices for individuals with disabilities. It also is apparent that using the tools together is probably the best solution, and each of the tools needs to be used to conduct further accessibility analyses so more improvements in the methodologies and outcomes produced can be made. Specific suggestions for each of the tools are discussed in the following text.

14.5.1 MED- AUDIT

Because MED-AUDIT is at the most preliminary developmental stage, so this tool seems likely to benefit the most from continued improvement. Specifically, the most pressing improvement for this tool is probably the development of reporting capabilities, such that the accessibility estimates generated can be explained further and devices "diagnosed." This capability likely would have improved the opinions of experts for MED-AUDIT, because the report is intended to explain the estimate(s) as well as the good or bad features that affected the accessibility estimate(s). Also, continued improvements within the task requirement and device feature taxonomies will be beneficial, as well as using the MED-AUDIT algorithm in future studies to determine its validity and reliability. Finally, it will be helpful to integrate insights gained from usability testing with the MU-Lab and PM into the MED-AUDIT matrices, in an effort to increase the robustness of MED-AUDIT, as the RERC-AMI learns more about medical device accessibility. Overall, MED-AUDIT seems to provide a thorough and systematic approach to initially assessing accessibility, and it offers individuals who do not necessarily have an expertise in accessibility the opportunity to evaluate product accessibility and usability for individuals with disabilities.

14.5.2 MVTA

Although MVTA may appear to be the best solution for assessing accessibility, there are some limitations to note. Most importantly, MVTA analyses are time consuming, because subjects with disabilities have to be recruited to participate in usability testing, audio and video data have to be collected and refined using the MU-Lab, interactive analyses have to be performed by one or more accessibility experts, and then MVTA reports have to be generated and analyzed. Therefore, although the data set generated with MVTA is rich and valuable, a substantial amount of time and effort goes into using this tool for accessibility analysis. Nevertheless, there are many benefits associated with conducting usability analyses with MVTA, including the ability to perform detailed frame-by-frame analyses (if desired) the benefit of directly observing real users using real medical devices in real environments, and the ability to create visual demonstrations from the data collected.

Overall, MVTA provides the best visually represented data out of all of the tools presented and is beneficial to the RERC-AMI and other groups seeking to investigate accessibility. Ultimately, using this tool to document specific barriers and develop logic may be complementary to MED-AUDIT.

14.5.3 PM Surveys

The PM is another valuable tool available to the RERC-AMI for conducting accessibility assessments, and data collected with this tool provide a good understanding of user opinions of devices used. Although this tool may seem an effective solution for assessing accessibility, it is also time consuming to use and relies on the collection of subject opinions that are gathered in a limited time immediately after they use a particular device. Subject opinions may depend on the circumstances surrounding the testing procedure. However, this tool provides researchers an excellent means of determining the ways subjects envision making products more accessible for them, which are based on real-world experiences with devices that are usually video and audio recorded for post hoc analysis. Furthermore, with some refinement efforts suggested by expert in this study, this tool provides the opportunity to efficiently obtain design improvement suggestions from individuals who know the most about their interactions with medical devices. Overall, the PM yields the best user opinion-based data of all of the tools presented.

ACKNOWLEDGMENT

This work is supported by the RERC-AMI, funded by the National Institute on Disability and Rehabilitation Research, U.S. Department of Education Grant #H133E020729. All opinions expressed are those of the authors.

REFERENCES

1. Grabois, E. and Young, M.E., Managed care experiences of persons with disabilities, *Journal of Rehabilitation*, 67(3), 13, 2001.
2. Lemke, M.R. and Winters, J.M., Experiences using the mobile usability lab to investigate medical device biomechanical barriers, in *Proceedings of RESNA*, Atlanta, GA, 2005.
3. Lemke, M.R., Winters, J.M., Story, M.F., Campbell, S., Barr, A.B., Omiatek, E., and Rempel, D., TR-AMI-001: User's manual for Mobile Usability Lab (MU-Lab), v.1.1, June 2005. RERC-AMI, Milwaukee, WI, (see http://www.rerc-ami.org/ami/tech/tr-ami-001-mu-lab.aspx).
4. The Center for Universal Design, The Principles of Universal Design, v.2.0., Raleigh, NC: North Carolina State University, 1997.
5. Popovic, D. and Sinkjaer, T., Mechanisms for natural control of movement (chap. 2), Pathology of sensory-motor systems and assessment of disability (chap. 3), *Control of Movement for the Physically Disabled*, 2000.
6. Winters, J.M. and Crago, P.E., *Biomechanics and Neural Control of Posture and Movement*, Springer-Verlag, New York, 2000.
7. National Institute for Occupational Safety and Health (NIOSH), Work Practices Guide for Manual Lifting, Washington, D.C., 1981.
8. U.S. Census Bureau, Economics and Statistics Administration, 2000.
9. CDC, Prevalence of disabilities and associated health conditions among adults — U.S., 1999, *Morbidity and Mortality Weekly Report,* 50, 120, 2001.
10. Americans with Disabilities Act (ADA) Accessibility Guidelines for Buildings and Facilities, U.S. Architectural and Transportation Barriers Compliance Board (Access Board), as amended through September 2002.

11. Baquis, D., Section 508 drives accessible technology, in *Emerging and Accessible Telecommunications, Information and Healthcare Technologies*, Winters J.M, Robinson C.J., Simpson, R.C., and Vanderheiden G.C., Eds., RESNA Press, VA, 2002, chap. 3.
12. Section 508 Standards, http://www.section508.gov
13. Cook, A.M. and Hussey, S.M., *Assistive Technologies: Principles and Practice*, Mosby-Year Book, Inc., St Louis, 1995.
14. Story, M.F. and Mueller, J.L., Universal design performance measures for products: a tool for assessing universal usability, in *Emerging and Accessible Telecommunications, Information and Healthcare Technologies*, Winters J.M, Robinson C.J., Simpson, R.C., and Vanderheiden G.C. Eds., RESNA Press, VA, 2002, chap. 3.
15. Wilcox, S.B., Applying universal design to medical devices, *Medical Device and Diagnostic Industry*, 2003.
16. Fries, R.C., *Reliable Design of Medical Devices*, Marcel Dekker, New York, 1997.
17. Sawyer, D., *Do It By Design: An Introduction to Human Factors in Medical Devices*, Office of Health and Industry Programs, Washington, D.C., 1996.
18. Kumar, S. and Berg Rice, V.J., Ergonomics for special populations: an introduction, in *Ergonomics in Health Care and Rehabilitation*, Berg Rice, V.J. Ed., Butterworth-Heinemann, MA, 1998, chap. 7.
19. Wiklund, M.E., Eleven Keys to Designing Error-Resistant Medical Devices, *Medical Device and Diagnostic Industry (MMDI)*, 2002.
20. Medical Device Use-Safety: Incorporating Human Factors Engineering into Risk Management, U.S. Department of Health and Human Services, FDA, CDRH, Division of Device User Programs and Systems Analysis, Office of Health and Industry Programs, Washington, D.C., 2000.
21. AAMI/ANSI, HE74-2001: Human Factors Design Processes for Medical Devices, 2001. Association for the Advancement of Medical Instrumentation (AAMI), Arlington, VA, 2001.
22. ISO/TC159. ISO Technical Committee 159 Working Group 2, Ergonomic Requirements for People with Special Needs, Geneva, publication pending.

Part III

Considerations in Design Guideline Development

15 Accessibility Standards and their Application to Medical Device Accessibility

Daryle Gardner-Bonneau

CONTENTS

ABSTRACT

Accessibility standardization efforts are accelerating, both nationally and internationally. One purpose of this chapter is to identify and describe some of the most relevant U.S. and international standards that could be applied or adapted for use in ensuring the accessibility of medical devices and medical instrumentation. A second purpose is to discuss other ergonomics standards-related work in the areas of home health care and medical instrumentation that have the potential to incorporate accessibility-related guidance. This chapter emphasizes the need for coordination and cooperation among the various affected stakeholders to ensure successful standardization.

15.1 INTRODUCTION

"What we have here is a failure to communicate," was said to Paul Newman's character in the film, *Cool Hand Luke*. This could just as easily be said with regard to the people involved in various aspects of the design of medical instrumentation. Many fields of endeavor are relevant to medical device design — medicine, biomedical engineering, human factors engineering, disabilities and rehabilitation, and aging. Each discipline has its own methods and approaches, and for too long the disciplines have existed independently of each other, in some cases deliberately so. One can argue that it is the lack of an interdisciplinary approach that places us in the situation where many medical devices come up short, both in terms of usability and accessibility.

15.1.1 Never the Twain Shall Meet

Medicine and rehabilitation, though related, have traditionally been separated philosophically and pragmatically, with less-than-optimal sharing of information relative to patient care. Likewise, human factors engineering has struggled for many years to get its "foot in the door" with respect to the health care and medical device domains. Until the FDA mandated in 1997 that human factors and usability be considered by designers, its application was relatively scattered and limited to hospital-based problems (e.g., anesthesiology workstations) and a smattering of issues that had received notice in the media because of their serious and obvious consequences for patients (e.g., radiation therapy overdoses, medication errors). In turn, although one would think that human factors specialists would be sensitive to the needs of people with disabilities and the elderly in design, this is not always the case.

Philosophical differences have often hampered progress in establishing the interdisciplinary mindset necessary to achieve quality in design. In the 1980s, for example, the small group of Human Factors and Ergonomics Society (HFES) members with interests in human factors and rehabilitation was searching for a home among the society's technical groups (TGs). They had been a part of a technical group called Medical Systems and Rehabilitation, but the group had evolved in such a way that its primary interest was medical error, and the human factors involved in rehabilitation were relegated to a back seat. Likewise, when the group considered merging with the Aging Technical Group, it encountered philosophical resistance. The Aging TG was interested only in healthy aging and did not want to embrace disabilities and rehabilitation as part of its scope.

Yet, all of these disciplines are intertwined when it comes to the design of medical devices, particularly as medical devices migrate to the home, where their primary users are not trained medical personnel, but laypersons — and often older laypersons who have one or more disabilities. For example, a diabetic patient monitoring her glucose at home may struggle to read the glucometer display because of a visual impairment that could be age-related or associated with the diabetes. To design accessible and usable medical instrumentation, we need to understand aging, disabilities, and the limitations of the human factors knowledge currently embodied in design standards and guidelines.

15.1.2 The Limitations of Standards and Guidelines

There are many medical device standards. The Association for the Advancement of Medical Instrumentation (AAMI), in particular, sponsors many equipment-specific standards committees that are developing design standards for everything from sterilization equipment to dialysis machines to infusion pumps. Many of these standards are developed with little or no consideration of human factors issues. In some cases this may be appropriate; in others, it is not.

AAMI currently has one human factors process standard (ANSI/AAMI HE-74) [1], which lays out the process for incorporating human factors and usability in medical device design. The AAMI Human Engineering Committee is working on a second standard (intended as ANSI/AAMI HE-75), which provides specific human factors guidelines for the design of medical devices (see Chapter 16 of this book). At present, neither of these documents overtly addresses accessibility, though they cover usability, and the design data they include may not always be appropriate for a user population that is older or that has a significant number of members with disabilities.

Generally speaking, much of the hard data incorporated in human factors and human performance standards and guidelines comes from studies in which the subjects were, largely, young healthy males. Further, many of these studies were conducted at a time when the population was, overall, younger than it is today. Such data cannot be applied unthinkingly to products designed for a population of users that do not have these characteristics. The typical home medical equipment user, for example, is an older female who may have age-related or other disabilities.

Wendy Rogers' human factors group at the Georgia Institute of Technology recently made the case that all empirical papers published in Human Factors should be required to state the age range and age distribution of study participants, so that designers can judge the applicability of the data and results to the population for whom they are designing [2]. Standards data and guidance based on a fairly narrowly defined user group may end up disaccommodating a majority of users who differ significantly from that group by virtue of age or skills and abilities.

But surely human factors and human performance data has been collected specifically with respect to the elderly? This is quite true but, unfortunately, for many years it was being presented and published in venues in which it was unlikely to be seen or noticed by designers or standards developers. This situation has changed to some extent recently, and books such as *Designing for Older Adults: Principles and Creative Human Factors Approaches* [3] and *"Extra-Ordinary" Ergonomics: How to Accommodate Small and Big Persons, the Disabled and Elderly, Expectant Mothers, and Children* [4] are starting to present human performance data about the elderly, as well as people with disabilities, in a form that resonates with designers. Such sources could become the basis for national and international design guidelines and standards.

Finally, the medical device community is just coming to grips with incorporating usability and human factors in design. Accessibility has not yet risen to prominence in design discussions regarding medical instrumentation. However, this is not to say that it should not be, or that it could not be, considered relatively easily. Standards related to accessibility abound — both general guidance and detailed sector-specific guidance — that could be adapted for use in the medical instrumentation domain.

15.1.3 The Escalation of Accessibility Standards Work

Since the passage of the Americans with Disabilities Act, Section 508 of the Rehabilitation Act, and Section 255 of Telecommunications Act, the standards world has been deluged with standardization efforts related to accessibility. So much work is ongoing internationally in this area that a Special International Standards Organization/International Electrotechnical Commission (ISO/IEC) Working Group on Accessibility (SWG-A) was formed in early 2005 for the express purpose of cataloging the various efforts and monitoring the quality of work products produced by the standards bodies. In the area of Information Technology alone, 11 ISO Technical Committees and 19 subcommittees are working on accessibility standards. In addition, other Standards Development Organizations (SDOs), including the International Telecommunications Union (ITU), the Institute for Electrical and Electronic Engineers (IEEE), and the European Committee for Standardization (CEN) are involved in accessibility work, as are groups such as the Consumer Electronics Association (CEA), and the World Wide Web Consortium (W3C). Significant nation-specific efforts have been identified in Japan, U.K., Norway, Sweden, Spain, Canada, Australia, and the U.S. No doubt, the wheel is being reinvented in a number of these activities. Existing and developing accessibility standards range from general guidance in areas such telecommunications services, software user interfaces, Web design, visual displays, and graphical public information symbols to very specific product guidance (e.g., closed captioning systems, ATMs, voting machines, and tactile markings on consumer products).

Of special interest to those involved in human factors work is the commitment of ISO Technical Committee 159 — Ergonomics to ensure that accessibility is considered and incorporated, as appropriate, in all ergonomics standards. This is significant because the work of ISO TC 159 goes beyond information technology and software to virtually all products, systems, and services.

15.1.4 Accessibility Meets Usability in Standards

What is the difference, if any, between usability and accessibility? There is a distinct lack of agreement as to definitions of accessibility. In the ISO software user interface draft standard (ISO CD 9241-171), under development by ISO TC159 SC4 WG5, and expected to be released as a Draft International Standard (DIS) in the spring of 2006, *accessibility* is defined as "usability of a product, service, environment or facility by people with the widest range of capabilities," a definition in which "usability" is integral. Not everyone agrees with this, including many standards developers from the U.S. (see also Chapter 8, Chapter 25, and Chapter 26 of this book). As a consequence, in the U.S. version of this same standard (HFES 200.2), developed by the Human Factors and Ergonomics Society HFES-200 Committee, the term "accessibility" is left undefined, so the U.S. standard will be considered as "harmonizing" with the ISO standard, without the U.S. accepting the ISO definition of accessibility. The extent to which systems considered to be accessible must also have a high degree of usability remains a topic of discussion. To some extent, the international definition of accessibility closely parallels definitions of universal design, which is also considered a problematical construct by many designers, especially those whose focus is highly complex technical systems and equipment. It should be noted that both the U.S. and international versions of the standard contain the same definition of *usability* — "extent to which a product can be used by specified users to achieve specified goals with effectiveness, efficiency, and satisfaction in a specified context of use."

15.2 INTERNATIONAL ACCESSIBILITY STANDARDS EFFORTS TO WATCH

Because many of the medical devices designed today will be used by a broader spectrum of the population than was the case in the past, especially as devices migrate to the home environment, medical device developers need to make use of accessibility data and guidelines that incorporate solutions and approaches to making devices accessible for elderly users and people with disabilities. In addition, the home environment differs in several significant ways from the hospital environment, so designers must take into account the context of use in order to make devices accessible to home users.

15.2.1 Selected Key Standards Activities

15.2.1.1 Software Accessibility: ISO 9241- 171 and ANSI/HFES 200.2

Because many of today's medical devices include software user interfaces, the two aforementioned standardization efforts in the U.S. and internationally (HFES 200.2 — *Human Factors Engineering of Software User Interfaces — Part 2: Accessibility* and ISO 9241-171 — *Ergonomics of Human-System Interaction — Guidance on Software Accessibility,* respectively) should be of interest to device developers. A draft version of HFES 200.2 is already available from the Human Factors and Ergonomics Society [5], and this document has been enhanced significantly since its publication in May 2000. This U.S. document served as the basis for a parallel ISO effort, with a draft standard now being prepared for balloting as ISO 9241-171. Hundreds of hours have been spent ensuring that the U.S. and international versions of the software accessibility standard are harmonized to the greatest extent possible. The latest versions of HFES 200.2 and ISO 9241-171 will be balloted as formal draft ANSI and ISO standards, respectively, within the first half of 2006.

These documents each contain over 100 guidelines relevant to software accessibility, which are grouped into the following categories:

- Input/output alternatives
- Labeling of interactive user interface elements

- User preference choice and perseverance
- Special considerations for accessibility adjustments
- General control and operation guidelines
- Support for acccssibility
- Alternative input options
- Keyboard focus
- Keyboard input
- Pointing devices
- General output guidelines
- Visual output (displays)
- Text/fonts
- Color
- Window appearance and behavior
- Audio output
- Speech input and output
- Text output of audio (captions)
- Media and dynamic content
- Online documentation and help
- Tactile output

The documents explicitly exclude the design of assistive technologies, but contain guidance for providing the operating system and application "hooks" to accommodate the use of and provide compatibility with such technologies to achieve accessibility.

The HFES-200 Committee is currently seeking people and organizations interested and affected by this standard to serve on the canvass committee that will review and vote on the HFES 200.2 document. Individuals interested in receiving the draft and providing input, or working with the HFES-200 Committee, may do so by contacting the chair, Paul Reed (psreed@att.com).

15.2.1.2 General Accessibility Guidance for Systems, Services, and Consumer Products — ISO TR 22411

As noted previously, ISO TC159 — *Ergonomics* has made a commitment to ensure that the needs of populations of people with disabilities are considered in all of the standards it produces. As evidence of its commitment, TC159 established a Working Group (WG2) — *Ergonomic Requirements for People with Special Needs* — directly under the TC159 Committee structurally, as opposed to placing it under one of its subcommittees. ISO TC 159 WG2 has a broad mandate — to consider people with disabilities and activity limitations in the design guidance provided for virtually all products, systems, and services including, of course, medical devices. The convener of WG2 is from Japan, which is not surprising, given that the Japanese are facing ergonomic issues associated with the severely rapid "graying" of their population. In 2003, 19% of Japan's population was over the age of 65 (nearly double the 1985 proportion), and the proportion is expected to rise to 26% by 2015 [6]. In contrast, approximately 12% of the U.S. population is over the age 65, and the proportion is expected to increase to 20% by 2030 [3]. Japan is finding that many changes are necessary in the design of nearly everything to ensure that Japan's elderly citizens can function independently and use products, services, and systems just as easily as its younger citizens do.

The basis for the work in ISO TC159 WG2 is ISO Guide 71 (identical to the European CEN Guide 6 — *Guidelines for standards developers to address the needs of older persons and persons with disabilities*) [7]. This document provides a framework that standards developers can use to ensure that the products, services and systems addressed by their standards will be accessible. It accomplishes this via a series of tables that lay out the ergonomic factors relevant to four broadly described human abilities categories (sensory, physical, cognitive, and allergy) for each of seven aspects of design usually covered in standards:

- Information, labeling, instructions, and warnings
- Packaging — opening, closing, use, and disposal
- Materials
- Installation
- User interface, handling, controls, and feedback
- Maintenance, storage, and disposal
- Built environments (buildings)

In the tables, the four disability categories, labeled human abilities, are further broken down into subcategories:

- Sensory — seeing, hearing, touch, taste/smell, balance
- Physical — dexterity, manipulation, movement, strength, voice
- Cognitive — intellect/memory, language/literacy
- Allergy — contact/food/respiratory

As an example, the ergonomic factors listed in Table 5 of CEN Guide 6, which addresses the user interface, handling, controls, and feedback are as follows (each factor is more completely defined in its own clause in the guide):

- Alternative format
- Location/layout
- Lighting/glare
- Color/contrast
- Size/style of font
- Clear language
- Symbols/drawings
- Loudness/pitch
- Slow pace
- Distinctive form
- Ease of handling
- Surface temperature
- Logical process
- Surface finish
- Nonallergenic/nontoxic
- Acoustics
- Fail-safe

Although ISO Guide 71 (CEN Guide 6) identified the issues relevant to design for older users and people with disabilities and provided a framework for considering them, it did not provide any design guidance or data, *per se*, that could be placed in standards to assist developers. That tall order is the charge of ISO TC159 WG2, which is producing a technical report (TR 22411 — *Ergonomic Data and Ergonomic Guidelines for the Application of ISO/IEC Guide 71 to Products and Services to Address the Needs of Older Persons and Persons with Disabilities*) laying out general ergonomic principles and data related to the skills and abilities of people with disabilities and the elderly. This is intended to be used by standards developers to ensure that accessibility is fully addressed in their standards.

The framework established by ISO Guide 71 is by no means perfect, and its flaws are becoming more apparent as WG2 continues its work on the technical report. In particular, the area of cognitive skills and abilities is not sufficiently detailed or complete. For example, intellect/memory and language/literacy are the only subcategories, and they are general. The topic of attention is not addressed, and this is an important omission, given the number of individuals who have attentional deficits that can impact their use of products and services. Nevertheless, ISO recently declined to revise Guide 71, and indicated that the document should continue to serve as the basis for the development of accessibility guidance, including the work of WG2. ISO Guide 71 is not well known in the U.S., perhaps because it is not readily available. However, interested readers can access its identical European counterpart at http://www.tiresias.org/ guidelines/guide6.

In effect, the task of ISO TC159 WG2 is to fill in the cells of the tables of ISO Guide 71 with ergonomic principles and data that standards developers can use in establishing detailed design standards that address accessibility concerns for a particular product, service, or system. With respect to the tables in ISO Guide 71, some of these cells are easily filled with information because their content has been studied widely, and data exist from many prior studies and other standards documents. This is particularly true, for example, in the case of built environments, where numerous standards and regulations already exist throughout the world to ensure that buildings are physically accessible to people with disabilities. In other areas (e.g., packaging, maintenance), however, there is little design-related data and information beyond what is contained in existing ergonomic standards. In many cases, these standards were established without consideration of special populations, including older adults.

Thus, a pressing need exists for design-relevant data and research results from studies of older people and people with disabilities for inclusion in ISO TC159 WG2's TR 22411 and, in the future, other sector-specific design standards. Participation is needed from more subject matter experts and additional countries in the working group. Because the task of WG2 is so inclusive and broad-based, people with a wide variety of knowledge, skills, and applied experiences will be required to complete the work. (Those who have either data or design guidance that could be contributed to the ISO TC159 WG2 effort are encouraged to contact this author at JDNBonneau@cs.com to become involved in the process.)

15.2.2 Other Accessibility Standards Efforts Potentially Relevant to Medical Devices

15.2.2.1 Human Factors Applied to Medical Devices: AAMI/ANSI HE- 74 and HE- 75

One of the desirable outcomes of the workshop for which this chapter is a product is the specific incorporation of accessibility guidance into medical device standards. The primary candidate document for incorporating such guidance would seem to be AAMI/ANSI HE-75, currently in preparation by AAMI's Human Engineering Committee.

15.2.2.2 A Sampling of Other Accessibility Standards

In addition, many other accessibility standards efforts, some in progress, some complete, may have implications for medical device design now and in the future. The following is a sampling of these efforts.

- ISO 9241-20 (currently being drafted by ISO TC159 SC4 WG6) — *Ergonomics of human system interaction. Accessibility guideline for information communication equipment and services — General Guidelines.* This general standard is intended to set the stage for more detailed standards that will focus on specific equipment and telecommunications services.

- ISO TR 19764 (2004) — *Technical Report on "Guidelines, methodology, and reference criteria for cultural and linguistic adaptability in information technology products."*
- ISO/IEC 18019 (2004) (developed by JTC1 SC7) — *Software documentation guidelines.*
- ISO/IEC TR 19765 (developed by JTC1 SC35 WG6) — *Information Technology.* Survey of icons and symbols that provide access to functions and facilities and improve the use of IT products by the elderly and persons with disabilities.
- ISO/IEC TR 19766 (developed by JTC1 SC35 WG6) — *Information Technology.* Guidelines for the design of icons and symbols to be accessible to all users, including the elderly and persons with disabilities.
- IEEE P1621 — *Standard for User Interface Elements in Power Control of Electronic Devices Employed in Office/Consumer Environments.*
- ANSI/International Committee for Information Technology Standards (INCITS) 389 to 393 — *Universal Remote Console.* All five of these documents are parts of a protocol to facilitate operation of information and electronic products through remote and alternative interfaces and intelligent agents, including a universal remote control (see also Chapter 28 and Chapter 27 of this book).

15.3 CONCLUSIONS

There may be many challenges and barriers to incorporating accessibility guidelines and best practices in the design of medical devices, but there are also many opportunities. Both within the U.S. and internationally, a significant amount of work is currently focusing on accessibility across many design domains — telecommunications, software, the Internet, building design, electronic products, home appliances, and others.

For some aspects of design, rich data sets and research results pertaining to older adults and populations of people with disabilities (e.g., wheelchair users) are available to inform design and provide a basis for design standards. For other aspects, the existing data are limited. Therefore, there is work to do such as, (1) collect design-relevant data, (2) analyze and utilize that data in the development of accessibility guidance, and (3) apply that guidance in the design of medical instrumentation. It will take the joint efforts of device manufacturers and developers, the government, human factors specialists, and specialists on disabilities and aging to improve the accessibility of medical devices and instrumentation.

Many medical devices are still poorly designed from both usability and accessibility perspectives. Nurses struggle to replace infusion sets in infusion pumps and to program these pumps accurately. Both patients and caregivers struggle to read instructions on medical devices because of small font sizes and poor contrast between text and background. This situation has been tolerated within the culture of health care, in which it has been assumed that trained medical professionals would learn to use the equipment, of necessity, no matter how poorly it was designed. Now that many medical devices, some of them complex, are becoming consumer products, being placed in the hands of lay users, i.e., patients and lay caregivers, this situation can no longer stand. We have an obligation to ensure that medical devices are both usable and accessible to the entire population of potential users — or at least as close to that as we can achieve, in order to ensure safe and effective use.

REFERENCES

1. Association for the Advancement of Medical Instrumentation (AAMI), Human Factors Design Process for Medical Devices (ANSI/AAMI HE74:2001), AAMI, Arlington, VA, 2001.
2. Nichols, T.A., Rogers, W.A., and Fisk, A.D., Do you know how old your participants are? Recognizing the importance of participant age classifications, *Ergonomics in Design*, 11(3), 22, 2003.

3. Fisk, A.D., Rogers, W.A., Charness, N., Czaja, S.J., and Sharit, J., *Designing for Older Adults: Principles and Creative Human Factors Approaches*, CRC Press, Boca Raton, FL, 2004.
4. Kroemer, J.H., *"Extra-ordinary" Ergonomics: How to Accommodate Small and Big Persons, the Disabled and Elderly, Expectant Mothers, and Children,* CRC Press, Boca Raton, FL, 2006.
5. Human Factors and Ergonomics Society (HFES), ANSI/HFES 200.2 — Human Factors Engineering of Software User Interfaces — Part 2: Accessibility [Canvass version], HFES, Santa Monica, CA, May 2000.
6. Japan Aging Research Center Web site (http://www.jarc.net/aging03oct.index.shtml) October, 2003.
7. International Standards Organization (ISO), ISO Guide 71: Guidelines for Standards Developers to Address the Need of Older Persons and Persons with Disabilities, ISO, Geneva, 2001.

16 Human Factors Standards for Medical Devices Promote Accessibility

Michael E. Wiklund

CONTENTS

ABSTRACT

This chapter provides a perspective on human factors standards for medical devices with special consideration of accessibility. A perspective is provided by reviewing the evolution of these standards for medical devices. This is followed by consideration of the relationship of human factors standards to accessibility and, especially, to the determination of the intended users for the product. It is suggested that current standards can best be described as sympathetic to accessibility concerns, but not focused on them, and that a companion set of guidelines on making medical devices accessible would be valuable.

16.1 INTRODUCTION

Today, there is a broad-based and reasonably energetic movement to reduce the number of use errors involving medical devices, particularly the kind of misuses that lead to patient injury and death. Many people attribute the movement to the Institute of Medicine report in 2000 titled "To Err Is Human," [1] which estimated that medical error in the United States alone was killing as many as 98,000 people each year. The report made national headlines and stimulated numerous initiatives, including the development of design standards intended to reduce the rate of use error.

However, use-error specialists would assert that the movement really started in the late 1970s when the hazards associated with anesthesia delivery systems came to light. As Peter Carstensen, the U.S. FDA's human factors team leader explained at a recent Association for Advancement Medical Instrumentation (AAMI) conference [2], anesthesia delivery systems of that era were fraught with human factors shortcomings that were killing thousands of people per year. The government and industry responded by establishing standards that required a considerable number of user interface design enhancements for anesthesia delivery systems (see Figure 16.1).

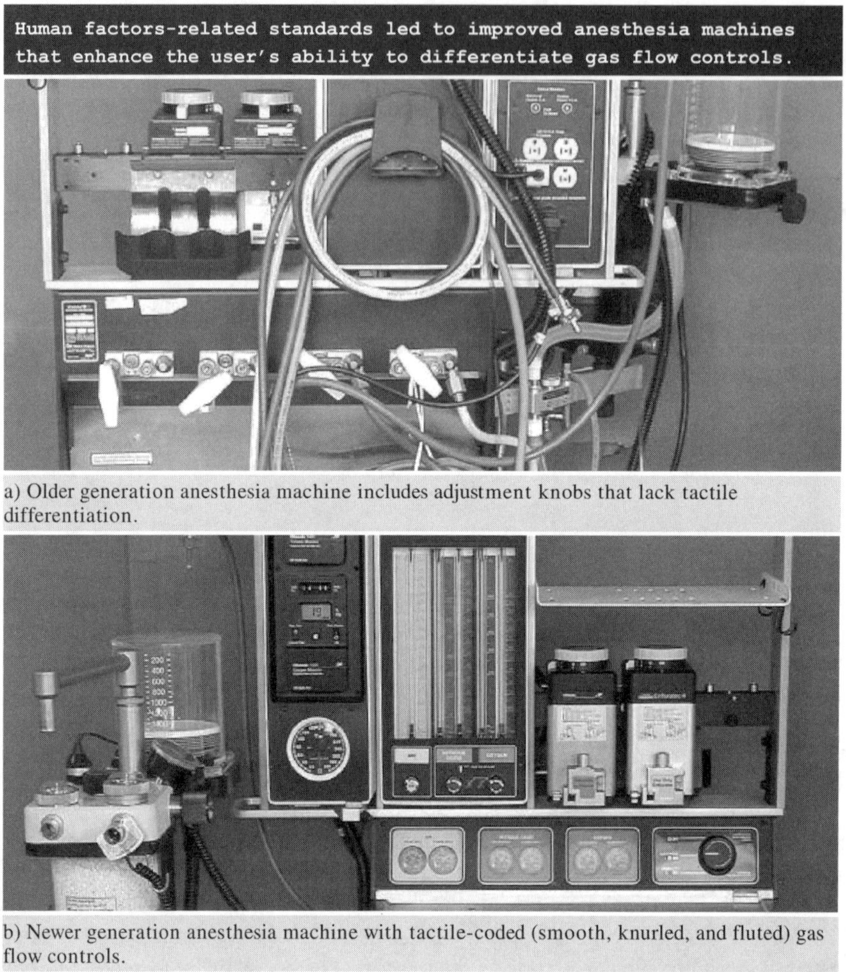

a) Older generation anesthesia machine includes adjustment knobs that lack tactile differentiation.

b) Newer generation anesthesia machine with tactile-coded (smooth, knurled, and fluted) gas flow controls.

FIGURE 16.1 Comparison of (a) older anasthesia workstation design and (b) newer anesthesia workstation design. (From http://www.pemed.com, courtesy of PEMED).

Following the development of new standards for anesthesia equipment, AAMI introduced its first human factors standard for medical devices (AAMI-HE-1988, Human Factors Engineering Guidelines and Preferred Practices for the Design of Medical Devices). This, and subsequent updates (notably AAMI HE48-1993, also titled Human Factors Engineering and Preferred Practices for the Design of Medical Devices) have led some manufacturers to take a more user-centered design approach and reduced the number of user interface design defects. Presumably, this methodological change has improved device safety, although nobody has collected the data and performed the requisite analyses to prove it. Still, anecdotal evidence suggests that medical devices are becoming safer and easier to use as manufacturers invest more resources into applying human factors standards in device development.

In addition to improving safety and ease of use, the influence of human factors standards on manufacturers' design processes also appear to have increased the accessibility of some medical devices. But as this chapter discusses later, overall progress toward usable and accessible medical devices has been slow. Although some medical devices now reflect contemporary user interface design and are more accessible, a disturbing proportion of new devices still have significant shortcomings, which becomes apparent if one performs an informal review of new devices found in hospitals and other medical care settings (see Table 16.1). Troubling to those on the front lines of

TABLE 16.1
Examples of Devices with User Interface Design Affordances vs. Shortcomings and Their Effect on Accessibility by Health Care Workers and Laypersons

Examples of Devices with User Interface Affordances	Examples of Devices with User Interface Shortcomings
Hospital bed equipped with a mechanism to raise and lower the mattress, making it easier and safer for patients to get into and out of bed	**Patient monitor** that displays information using text and numerals that are small or light colored and that middle-aged and older caregivers with presbyopia (blurred vision at near points) have difficulty reading without putting on their reading glasses
Hemodialysis machine incorporating step-by-step instructions for use so that caregivers and patients who treat themselves have less to remember	**Surgical stapler** that requires users to squeeze an actuation lever firmly to shoot a staple, making it uncomfortable to use, if not injurious
Open MRI scanner featuring a larger moving stretcher and opening that ensures access by large individuals, as well as lessens feelings of claustrophobia	**Nurses' central workstation** with a fixed height keyboard that lacks a wrist support and, therefore, may cause repetitive motion injuries
Defibrillator with voice commands that help guide laypersons with varying literacy skills, and who are in a stressful situation, through a rescue procedure	**Laser eye treatment machine** that emits a high-frequency (for example, 4000 Hz) alarm signal that is inaudible to older individuals (particularly men) who have presbycusis (loss of hearing associated with aging)

the usability and accessibility movements, these shortcomings could have been avoided by taking an enlightened design approach — no miracles are required.

16.2 EVOLUTION OF MEDICAL STANDARDS

Human factors standards for medical devices have evolved considerably, but glacially, over the past couple of decades. AAMI's first human factors standard read more like its source document — a military standard titled MIL STD 1472, Human Engineering. Fortunately, AAMI's latest releases are better tailored to ultrasound scanners, infusion pumps, and hospital beds than to radar consoles, tank dashboards, and guns. For example, AAMI HE48:1993 covers classic human factors topics, such as controls, displays, software navigation, alarms, warnings, and many others with a medical technology emphasis. For tutorial purposes, it also provides an introduction to human factors and a human factors design process overview. Although AAMI has automatically withdrawn this standard because it is more than 5 years old, it remains a valuable and sought after resource for user interface designers.

ANSI/AAMI HE74:2001, Human Factors Design Process for Medical Devices, is a partial replacement for AAMI HE48:1993. It outlines a user-centered design process that is closely linked to the FDA's design control process (see Figure 16.2). The newer standard describes a process that fulfills the FDA's requirement for manufacturers to first determine user needs and requirements for new devices, develop design solutions that meet established design principles, and then verify and validate that final designs actually meet user requirements. Accordingly, the FDA has endorsed the standard as an appropriate guide for manufacturers responding to the agency's quality system regulations pertaining to human factors. Written by a committee of consultants, manufacturer representatives, and medical specialists with a strong interest and/or formal training in human factors, this document calls for developers to establish a properly scaled human factors program whenever they develop a new or substantially revised medical device. The committee took care to recommend a range of affordable human factors activities (see Table 16.2) that are suited to the development of products as simple as a syringe and as complex as a diagnostic scanner.

After AAMI released the standard in 2001, the International Electrotechnical Commission's Human Factors Committee adapted it and released it as IEC 60601-1-6: Collateral Standard:

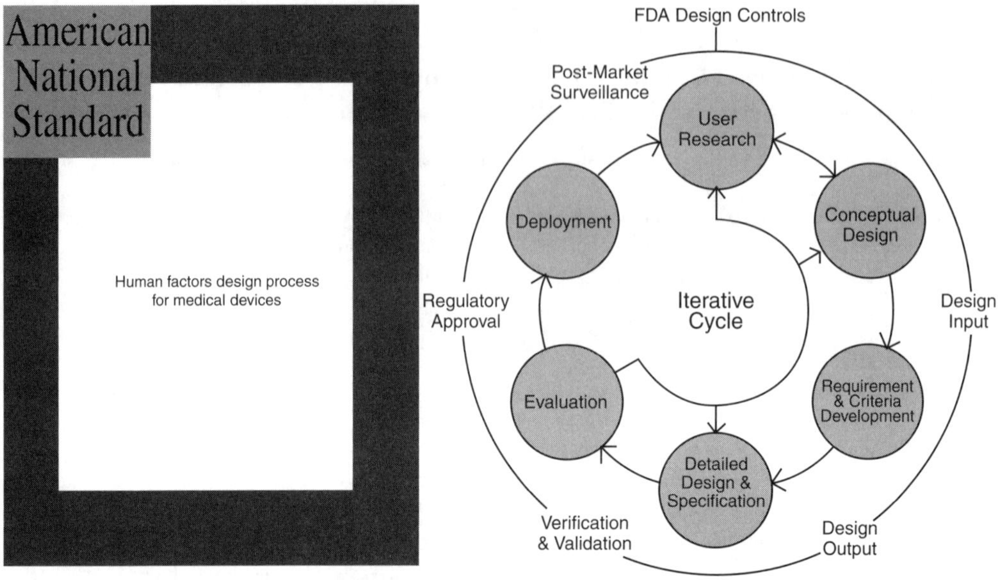

FIGURE 16.2 AAMI HE74:2001 is available for purchase at the Association for the Advancement of Medical Instrumentation's Web site (www.aami.org). The standard includes the above illustration showing the relationship between a user interface design process and the FDA design controls. Courtesy of Association for the Advancement of Medical Instrumentation.

Usability, Analysis, Test, and Validation of Human Factors Compatibility. In effect, this international standard calls for the worldwide application of human factors in the development of electrical medical equipment.

Presently, AAMI is completing work on a companion to AAMI HE74:2001. It will provide extensive design guidance, complementing the previously published design process guidance. Dubbed AAMI HE75:20XX, the document will have an encyclopedic quality that permits one-stop shopping for user interface design tips.

Some of the standard's sections, notably the home health care and hand tools sections, promise to provide a fair amount of accessibility-related guidance as a natural extension of human factors-related guidance. Also, the section on anthropometry and biomechanics will provide product designers with the data necessary to accommodate people with a wide range of physical characteristics and abilities.

16.3 RELATIONSHIP OF HUMAN FACTORS STANDARDS TO ACCESSIBILITY

Most design professionals would agree that human factors and accessibility have considerable overlap but are not synonymous. Human factors excellence benefits just about everybody, including people with disabilities, in many cases. But, designers focused on making devices user-friendly are not always focused on accessibility *per se*. More often, their focus is on device safety, effectiveness, and appeal. Their user research and device evaluation efforts may not extend to individuals with disabilities. For example, a dozen nurses might participate in the evaluation of a patient-lifting mechanism, but the sample might not include someone with hip osteoarthritis or an elderly caregiver who may use the device at home. Therefore, many opportunities to enhance accessibility are lost (see also Chapter 18). In the past, this type of oversight was more common, because device designers did not envision or intend their devices to be used in the home by a layperson.

TABLE 16.2
Common Human Factors Activities That Occur during Product Development

Sample of Human Factors Activities Prescribed by AAMI's Human Factors Design Process Guide	
User profiling	Developing detailed descriptions of people who are likely to use a device, including typical users and, perhaps, a few atypical users whose needs are also worthy of consideration in the design process, such profiles or personas that help design teams set goals and evaluate design alternatives
Task analysis	Decomposing user interactions with devices into a series of discrete steps, such as assimilating information, analyzing information and forming an action plan, taking action, and receiving feedback; such analysis provides insights helpful to developing effective user interface solutions
Anthropometric analysis	Collecting data on the size, movement, and strength of human beings and using it to develop and evaluate the physical suitability of design solutions; an anthropometric analysis helps to determine if individuals who vary widely in terms of their physical characteristics and capabilities can interact with a device in a comfortable, effective manner
Heuristic analysis	Having several human factors specialists evaluate the same design solution in accordance with established human factors design principles, and then comparing their results and drawing a consensus regarding design strengths and opportunities for improvement (in order of priority)
Usability testing	Having representative device users perform key (frequent, urgent, and critical) tasks with a preliminary, refined, preproduction, or production device in order to document task performance and/or identify design strengths and opportunities for improvement

Often, improved accessibility is a serendipitous byproduct of human factors' work. Designers who focus explicitly on human factors and accessibility sometimes refer to their work as universal design, which aims to create solutions that work well for everybody, disabled or not. Unfortunately designers who take an intense, universal design approach are uncommon. Often, they are individuals who have trained in both industrial design and human factors and choose to champion the cause of accessibility (see also Chapter 6).

Current and planned human factors standards for medical devices do not really qualify as universal design standards. In other words, accessibility is not a prime focus. However, a more ergonomic or usable product often facilitates use by people with disabilities. For example:

- An infusion pump that uses large numerals to indicate the flow rate enables nurses to read the rate from across a room (see Figure 16.3a). The large numerals also facilitate reading by individuals with poor vision, such as diabetics with Cataracts, who might use the device at home.
- A blood glucose meter that requires a minimal number of button presses, which is optimal for people with Parkinson's disease or severe arthritis (see Figure 16.3b).
- A home pregnancy test device that uses large graphic symbols in place of ambiguous indicators (such as colors) to display a test result might be considered more usable, appealing, and accessible than previous generations of home pregnancy tests (see Figure 16.3c). Accordingly, current and future human factors design guidelines are sure to make medical devices more accessible, even if accessibility is not an explicit goal.

At a minimum, human factors standards call for designers to define users and users' needs, as well as use environments. As a result, designers learn more about the needs of people with disabilities, which, in turn, may lead to more accessible designs.

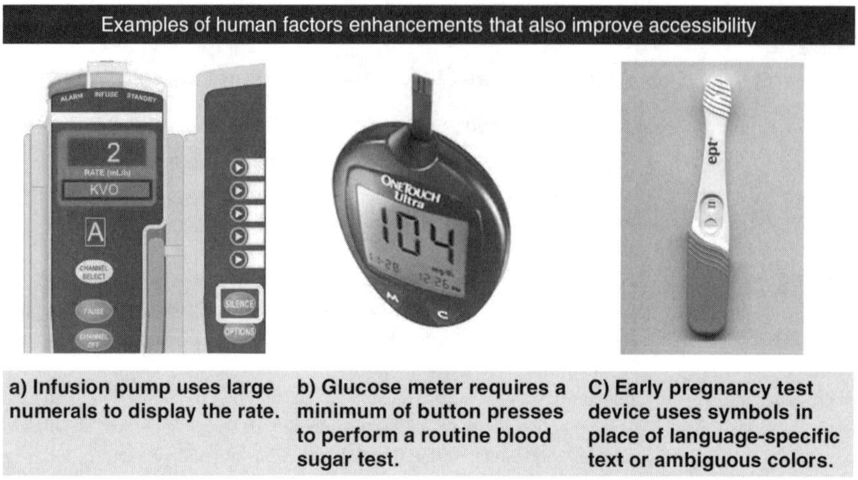

FIGURE 16.3 Diverse medical devices that incorporate design features that benefit all device users, not just those with disabilities. a) Infusion pump uses large numerals to display the rate. (From http://alaris.choc.org/graphics/channel_advisory_kvo_silence.jpg, courtesy of Cordinal Health Inc.,) b) Glucose meter requires a minimum of button presses to perform a routine blood sugar text. (From http://www.hearmore.com/, courtesy of LifeScan, Inc.,) c) Early pregnancy test devices uses symbols in place of language specific text or ambiguous colors. (From http://brockster.com/baby/eptpos588w378h.jpg, courtesy of Brock Wood.)

16.4 DESIGNER PRIORITIES

Arguably, designers spend little time thinking about accessibility — unless people with disabilities make up a large component of the device's user population — because they are consumed by so many other goals related to device functionality, manufacturability, and marketability, such as:

- Controlling costs by reducing the number of case parts
- Shielding internal components from the effects of electromagnetic energy
- Maximizing battery life while minimizing a device's weight
- Making the device enclosure look appealing to the intended users

In small companies, the same designer who has one-shot molding techniques on his/her mind, may also be responsible for the user interface. Consequently, and with few exceptions, special considerations, such as accessibility and human factors receive late and limited attention by individuals who may know little about the subject. That is why designers, who can carve out some time to focus on human factors and accessibility, seek a single source of guidance. In lieu of practical guidelines, designers must resort to using their judgment, which often means meeting their personal needs and preferences; a recipe for human factors and accessibility flaws.

16.5 PROMOTING CHANGE

The human factors community has worked for decades to reverse the pattern of human factors design negligence. The term negligence is chosen here because the medical industry is widely regarded as a laggard — when compared to other industries — in terms of embracing good human factors practices. The same can be said about the industry's approach to accessibility.

For various reasons related to safety assurance and business objectives, the power, aviation, and consumer products industries have been more progressive when it comes to human factors. Their progressiveness is evidenced by enhanced power plant control systems, advanced glass cockpits, and iPods. Arguably, these industries and others are a decade ahead of the medical industry and have lessons to share about promoting change.

These industries teach us that it sometimes takes a major disaster or intense marketplace pressure to produce change. The power industry's impetus was the accident at the Three Mile Island nuclear power plant. Aviation has drawn on a string of airplane crashes and black box data. The consumer products industry has evolved rapidly owing to intense competitive pressures and the success of companies like Apple Computer (computer equipment manufacturer) and Oxo (kitchen/home goods manufacturer). Some people say that the medical industry has not experienced a meltdown or crash of sufficient proportion to motivate rapid change. For some reason, the aforementioned deaths because of device-related use error have been perceived differently. Perhaps, this is because the events have occurred one at a time in hospitals, clinics, ambulances, and peoples' homes around the world, rather than at a single location on a single day.

To motivate change in the absence of a pivotal disaster or a marketplace revolt, AAMI and FDA cosponsored a 1998 conference on human factors in medical device design. The well-attended conference served a primarily remedial purpose, teaching human factors philosophy and methodology to members of the medical device development community. AAMI conducted a follow-up conference on human factors this past summer (2005). During both conferences, presenters advocated a human factors design process and ascription to established human factors guidelines.

At the more recent AAMI conference, some presenters emphasized the safety benefits of human factors, citing ways in which better design could have prevented tragic deaths. Others emphasized the marketing and economic advantages, describing good human factors as the earmark of successful companies and a key to profits.

However, FDA presenters made the most compelling argument in favor of investing in human factors. They described human factors as a regulatory mandate. They pointed out that companies that ignore human factors in design are essentially breaking the law. The legal argument was a wake-up call to an industry that has viewed FDA's human factors requirements with skepticism, wondering if the agency would actually take enforcement action.

Until recently, the medical device community has responded sluggishly to the new quality system regulations and the associated user interface design control process — a process that requires manufacturers to verify that their products are well suited to the intended users.

> GMP: Design validation shall ensure that devices conform to defined user needs and intended uses, and shall include testing of production units under actual or simulated use conditions…[3]

Given the choice of a "carrot-or-stick" approach to motivating change, FDA chose the carrot. In numerous public presentations, it encourages industry to focus more attention on human factors, noting that good human factors is good business. Apparently, the FDA assumed that companies would see the wisdom of adopting a human factors approach and that more aggressive action would not be required.

Several years following the regulatory change, many medical device companies are still in the discovery as opposed to application phase of adopting a human factors approach. Therefore, the FDA now speaks more frequently about the consequences of nonconformance:

- Delays in the regulatory approval process (510(k) or premarket approval) owing to human factors concerns about a new device — for example, the FDA may be concerned that older users may not be able to hear or effectively respond to a device alarm.
- Citations arising from field investigations of a manufacturer's design process — for example, if a company does not conduct usability testing of prototype devices, it may lack evidence that users can perform life-critical tasks in certain situations.
- Postmarket recalls or required design changes due to the discovery of human factors problems with safety implications — for example, user interface design shortcomings

may lead device users to make the same mistake, leading to patient injury or death and a device recall.

The FDA routinely refers medical companies to AAMI's human factors standards as the best guides for planning and implementing a human factors program. As such, the documents are having a strong influence on design practice.

Finally, the industry seems to be making an accelerating transition to user-centered design. This comes just in time as an increasing number of medical devices are migrating from clinical environments and use by trained professionals to nonclinical environments, where they may be used by laypersons with physical or cognitive disabilities.

16.6 CONCLUSION

As stated earlier, good human factors is not synonymous with accessibility. That said, medical devices designed with human factors in mind should be incrementally more accessible than those that are not. However, devices reflecting good human factors engineering for use by the general population may still pose obstacles to people with disabilities.

Today's human factors standards for medical device design can best be described as sympathetic to accessibility concerns, but not focused on them. Therefore, a companion set of guidelines on making medical devices accessible would be quite valuable. Ideally, such guidelines would complement AAMI's and IEC's existing human factors guidelines, so that designers working in small medical companies have an easier time developing integrated design solutions and producing designs that are both usable and accessible. Someday, such guidance might bring the world more devices that are safe, effective, usable, and appealing to use by people who may or may not have their sight, hearing, or mobility. Paradoxically, accessibility guidelines are not readily accessible to today's medical device designers. The void needs filling.

REFERENCES

1. *To Err Is Human: Building a Safer Health System* (2000). Institute of Medicine, National Academy Press, Washington, DC.
2. *2005 AAMI Conference: Human Factors, Ergonomics, and Patient Safety for Medical Devices*, held in Washington, D.C., June 28–30, 2005.
3. Medical Devices; Current Good Manufacturing Practice (CGMP) Final Rule, Quality System Regulation, 21 CFR Parts 820 – Medical Device Quality System Regulation. 820.30 of Title 21, of the Code of Federal Regulations ("21 CFR"). 21 CFR 820.30, Subpart (g) Design Validation. The revised GMP Regulation was released by the U.S. Food and Drug Administration as a final rule on October 7, 1996. The regulation became effective June 1, 1997.

17 Designing Accessible Medical Devices

Ron Kaye and Jay Crowley

CONTENTS

ABSTRACT

There are many issues and challenges involved in designing accessible medical devices. This chapter introduces the problem and provides a framework for addressing issues that include carefully defining intended users, developing accessible design strategies, and evaluating safety and risks in device use. It also provides some specific considerations for accessible device designs and the role of medical device use environments.

17.1 INTRODUCTION

This chapter discusses the general issues involved with designing medical devices to be accessible to people with physical, sensory, or cognitive disadvantages that previously would have prevented them from using medical devices. These disadvantages are manifold and addressing them may represent a variety of potential modifications to medical device user interfaces. Further, designers of medical devices are required to consider the varying needs of users, a practice consistent with designing safe and effective medical devices for any population of users. Preventing or controlling for unintended use error is an essential part of this consideration of user needs. Achieving accessibility may require modifications that are disability-specific, or more general modifications intended to support multiple disabilities. In some cases, accessibility modifications have the potential to improve performance for the general population as well. Limited guidance and few specific examples for accessibility in medical devices indicate that further research and development is called for.

17.2 DEFINING THE USERS OF ACCESSIBLE MEDICAL DEVICES

Medical device features promoting accessibility have not yet become widespread. Assuming that medical devices can be modified to accommodate them, there are currently potential users who could benefit from being able to use devices but are prevented from doing. Accessible devices cannot realistically be made to address each and every disabled user with a given modification in design. *Universal design* concepts (see Chapter 6) are not well articulated, known, or applied in the medical device industry nor are their impact on medical device use or customer acceptance understood. Accessible medical device designs are limited to a degree by technology available for interface enhancements. Other limiting factors are lack of precedent, perceived need, marketing considerations, and overall priorities of the medical device technology producers.

17.2.1 Defining Users in Terms of Need for Accessibility

A device that is easy for one person or a certain group to use safely and effectively might present problems for another person or another group. All users need devices that they can use safely and effectively, so to assure that these needs are met, it is necessary to understand the abilities and limitations of a variety of intended users.

The first consideration is a definition of the user and their needs. Overly general or vague descriptions of users with disabilities are inadequate for specific device design efforts. Good intentions tend to discourage discussion of abilities and lack thereof in the context of accessibility in a quantitative or even an ordinal sense. Rather, the term is discussed more in a qualitative fashion describing "different" kinds of abilities. This lack of information on specific needs of users with disabilities, causes difficulties in articulating specific possible measures that can be taken in the design of medical devices for them.

There are various definitions of "accessibility." For instance, the Merriam-Webster dictionary defines *accessible* as "the quality of being reachable, within reach, or easy to deal with" [1]. The glossary of this book contains these definitions of *accessibility*:

1. Ability to access the intended use of a product or service for which there is a possibility of benefit.
2. Usability of a product, service, environment, or facility by people with the widest range of capabilities.

The definitions are overly broad and when considered in the context of medical devices (or any kind of device) design, they are essentially synonymous with a further dictionary definition of usability: "the extent to which something is capable, convenient or practicable for use" [1]. For medical devices, simply providing access in this sense may not be sufficient to ensure a good outcome, and due to the inherent risks associated with medical devices good outcomes are clearly desirable. Careful consideration of the possible risks associated with modifying or creating novel designs and providing access to new kinds of users is warranted.

There is more to the implication of accessibility here, which comes into focus in the following account regarding degrees of accessibility:

> There are degrees of ability to access a product or service, potentially both at the level of the individual and the level of the total population. Proposed scales include degree of difficulty (up to impossible), and degree of handicap (up to fully handicapped). The former is commonly used in accessibility guidelines; the latter is used in ISO-IEC draft standards.

What we are discussing in this chapter is the issue of intentionally designing medical devices such that persons with some kind of disability are more able to use them.

Returning to the glossary of this book, we find the following definitions of *handicap*.

1. A disadvantage resulting from an impairment or disability that limits or prevents fulfillment of a role that is normal for the affected individual.
2. Barriers which people with disabilities encounter in environment. The gap between a person's capabilities and demands of environment. People are not handicapped by their disability all the time. Wheelchair users are not handicapped in an environment where there are accessible routes and pathways.
3. Anything that may interfere with the accessibility of interactions between users and systems.

These definitions differ in their focus, starting with a descriptive definition of a person's physical limitations followed by views that shift the focus to ways an environment or systems has been designed, resulting in its becoming a barrier to the individual with physical limitations. In the latter cases (definitions 2 and 3), the existence of the handicap is essentially defined by characteristics of the environment. Simply put, if the environment is properly engineered — and this conceivably includes medical devices being engineered — the handicap essentially ceases to exist because that person can interact normally in that environment or with that technology.

Finally we should consider the perspective provided by the definition of *accessibility metrics,* which is the motivation behind the approach described in Chapter 22.

> Measures or scores aimed at estimating the degree of accessibility of a product, typically as a collection of scores that represent accessibility for different general groups of activity limitation, impairment, or disability. The metric typically takes into account both design features and anticipated task procedures.

There are many kinds of physical, motor, and sensory conditions that handicap people with respect to using medical devices. We can expect entire texts and extensive research dedicated specifically to accessibility issues for blind device users; in fact much has been accomplished for blind people, including some accessible medical devices. As indicated by the need for accessibility metrics as defined earlier, within each type of disability, there are actually varying degrees of disability, not to mention potential combinations of disabilities. Therefore, nominally disabled users such as blind users will likely require different device design accommodations based on the extent of the disability.

Consideration of each kind of disability in turn and its relevance to medical device design is beyond the scope of this chapter. Designers of medical devices are encouraged to consider the extent of the various needs of users [2], and in practice this is consistent with designing devices well. The general issues involved with making medical devices more accessible to users necessitates the understanding that this may apply to specific design enhancements to support a specific disability or that such enhancements multiple disabilities and may support? improve performance for the general population of non-disabled users as well.

17.2.2 User Populations that Need Accessible Devices

It is convenient to refer to the group of users who use a given device as its *user population.* It is then helpful to describe the user population with respect to the it's abilities and limitations of its members. For any device, the abilities and limitations of the user population might be relatively uniform. On the other hand, the user population might contain subgroups that have significantly different abilities. Examples that medical device designers often deal with are whether users are young or old, home users or professional health care providers. Fatigue, stress, medication, or other temporary mental or physical conditions can temporarily affect ability levels of device users.

For the general user population, important characteristics include [3]:

- General health and mental state (stressed, relaxed, rested, tired, or affected by medication or disease) when using the device
- Physical size and strength
- Sensory capabilities (vision, hearing, and touch)
- Coordination (manual dexterity)
- Cognitive ability and memory
- Knowledge about device operation and the associated medical condition
- Previous experience with devices (particularly similar devices or user interfaces)
- Expectations about how a device will operate
- Motivation
- Ability to adapt to adverse circumstances

For disabled users, the above considerations apply, as well as the following:

- What is the nature of the disability?
- Does the user have more than one disability?
- How will these disabilities impact the use of a given device, and does it put at the user at a disadvantage?
- How many potential users have this disability?
- What is known about how users function?
- Is it conceivable that a device could be designed such that it can be used safely and effectively by these users?

17.3 ACCESSIBLE MEDICAL DEVICE DESIGN

17.3.1 Medical Device User Interface

The user interface of a medical device includes all components of a device with which users interact while using it, preparing it for use (e.g., calibration, setup, and unpacking), or performing maintenance (e.g., repairing, and cleaning). It includes hardware features that control device operation such as switches, buttons, and knobs and device features that provide information to the user such as indicator lights and displays and auditory and visual alarms. The user interface also includes the logic that directs how the system responds to user actions including how, when, and in what form information (feedback) is provided to the user. An important aspect of the user interface is the extent to which the logic of information display and control actions is consistent with users' abilities, and expectations.

Increasingly, user interfaces for new medical devices are computer based. In these cases, interface characteristics include the manner in which data is organized and presented, control and monitoring screens, screen components, prompts, navigation logic, alerting mechanisms, data entry requirements, help functions, keyboards, computer mice, and pointers. The size and configuration of the device are important parts of the user interface, particularly for handheld devices. Device labeling, packaging, training materials, operating instructions, and other reference materials are also considered part of the user interface.

The purpose of the user interface is to facilitate the safe and effective use of the device. An important concept pertaining to issues of user interface, safety in use, and accessibility is *error tolerance*, the user interface quality that prevents or mitigates dangerous or disastrous consequences when an error occurs. Humans make errors. Some kinds of error can be anticipated and are essentially unavoidable — such as inadvertently pressing an adjacent key on a keypad or bumping the keypad inadvertently while doing other tasks.

The application of human factors engineering (HFE) approaches to device design will increase the likelihood that the design is tolerant of errors likely to be made by users. There are many ways to do this. One example to prevent inadvertent activation is the placement of a shield over the button that initiates a beam of radiation. The logic of device operation can also determine its degree of error tolerance. For example, some devices include "interlocks" or mechanisms that prevent a critical process from being initiated without users verifying their intent to initiate it, or those that require extra control steps to be performed before proceeding. In other cases, devices can be designed to do tasks that users do not do well, such as timing required during certain steps in home-testing procedures, remembering setup parameters or test dates, and mathematical calculations. For complex procedures, devices can prompt users to perform the appropriate action at critical points in the procedure.

17.3.2 Accessible Design Strategies

The concept of accessible medical devices relates to the design of the device's *operator interface*, which is composed of device components with which the user interacts, activates, or manipulates (controls), or those that provide a signal to the user such as a beep, a verbal response, a light, or displayed text. It also applies to the users of the device under consideration. In this context, accessibility pertains to the quality of a device–user interface that allows users with certain disabilities to be able to use or access the device. The desire to design accessible medical devices challenges the designer to modify some aspect or aspects of the user interface to accommodate abilities differing from those of the "general" user. The central idea is that some people cannot use a device designed for the general user; however, with some level of design modification, these users will be able to "access" the device.

There appear to be three strategies for accessible device design. These include:

1. Universal design
2. Multimodal design
3. Specialized design for a user group
4. Interface support for a user's assistive technology that provides access

Universal design indicates design that accommodates to the greater extent possible the widest range of users, including persons with and without disability. Specific guidelines that would apply to medical devices have not yet been established. General human factors processes, involving use testing to include users with certain disabilities could help designers understand device interface features necessary to make the design more "universal" (see also Chapter 16). Such designs might not only be usable but may improve usability and safety for the general user. A case in point can be observed in modifications that have occurred with portable blood glucose meters, users of which, being diabetic, frequently have some degree of retinopathy and/or neuropathy; clinical complications of diabetes that often impair vision and manual dexterity respectively. These disabilities are caused by the very disease that requires the use of that device, thereby causing this user population to be unique in that these disabilities relevant to device use are more prevalent among diabetics. To accommodate them, displays were made larger and easier to read and the application of blood samples to test strips required less coordination. These design characteristics have quickly become *de facto* industry standards and continue to improve, making these devices easier to operate for both diabetic and non-diabetic users.

Multimodal design allows the user to change the "mode" of the user interface to alternative sensory and motor interface modes. People with a disability can often compensate for the disabled sensory or motor ability with another interaction mode in which they are not disabled. This approach may be used for both information display and control of a device. Specific examples for medical devices are uncommon, but prevalent and serious concern for medical devices in general is the complexity of the user interface even without multimodal design characteristics. Inherent in this strategy is a potential for decreased performance by the general user due to increased complexity of the interface.

Specialized designs are intended to address a specific disability, such as a "talking" device for a blind user. These are not intended for the general user. A general user may be able to use the device but would likely be able to perform better with a device that is not designed specifically for a user with a disability. Safety concerns for medical devices with specialized design would necessitate careful testing with individuals who represent users with the disability, designed to determine if adequate, safe performance with the device is achievable.

Interface support for assistive technology is reflected in the section Functional Performance Criteria, Subpart 3 of the federal accessibility standards for electronic and information technology (E&IT), which became a final rule in 2001 in implementation of Section 508 of the Rehabilitation Act Amendments of 1998, in which five of six specifications take the following form [4]:

> At least one mode of operation and information retrieval that does not require user [insert specific disability] shall be provided, or support for assistive technology used by people who are [insert specific disability] shall be provided.

This provides an alternative path to accessibility that could be considered for certain types of medical devices.

As further developed in Chapter 8, all of these are potential accessible design strategies for products such as E&IT devices, as outlined in the federal accessibility guidelines issued by the U.S. Access Board [4]. These guidelines may provide future applicability to medical devices.

17.3.3 Evaluating Safety and Risks of Device Use

The advantage of providing accessible medical devices must be carefully considered with respect to potential safety-related problems that could arise from their use. For instance, a user might be led to believe that they are successfully using a device when they are not, or a device might be designed such that inadvertent errors are more likely for either the user with disability or the general user. In either case, the ability to simply use the device is not the sole consideration; safety is a central concern.

The safe and effective use of medical devices is primarily determined by the quality of the interaction between the operator and the device. Devices that are well designed consider the capabilities, limitations, and requirements of the user and incorporate appropriate design features to accommodate these.

Understanding and optimizing how people use and interact with technology is the subject of human factors engineering (HFE). HFE considerations important to the development of medical devices include device technology, the capabilities and limitations of the intended users, environment in which the technology will be used, how dangerous device use is, and how critical the device is for patient care. The benefits of applying HFE or *usability engineering* to the device design will produce not only a more appealing product, but also safer devices [3,5,6]. These efforts can ensure that a device design will not allow or, worse, lead the operator to make errors that could cause patient injury or death, or affect the quality of the intended medical treatment in which the device is involved.

Device designers begin by understanding the capabilities of the user population for a given device to ensure that its design is appropriate for that population. The intent is that subsequent design must optimize performance and minimize the potential for error. As a simple example, a device designed for a professional health care provider may be relatively complex, whereas one designed for use by patients or family members in the home should be relatively simple to operate. In each case, a simple device is usually better, but because of the professional's greater knowledge, ability, and the variety of applications of the device, they often need more complex devices and are able to use them.

One of the primary goals of any device design is to limit the risks from hazards that occur from device use (use-related hazards) [3]. The process of designing a medical device for any given population, whether or not the population has certain describable disabilities, is essentially the same. The critical component is to thoroughly understand how a device will be used. This must include an understanding of the following:

- Device users (including capabilities and limitations)
- Typical and atypical device use
- Device characteristics
- Characteristics of the environments in which the device will be used
- The interaction between users, devices, and use environments

Following a thorough understanding of device users and use, specific ways of device use that are likely to result in hazards should be identified, prioritized, and investigated through analysis and testing. In addition to investigating known or suspected problems with device use, testing prototype devices with users can identify ways of using devices that could be hazard-related and were not anticipated by designers. This is important because it is extremely difficult to identify all significant device use problems in advance. After these hazards are understood, they are mitigated or controlled by modifying the device user interface (e.g., control or display characteristics, logic of operation, or labeling).

Use-related problems for medical devices can be roughly grouped by the factors that cause them. Most problems with using devices involve cognitive issues in which the user is confused about how to use the device, misunderstands device output, expects the device to operate other than it does, or intentionally uses the device in ways that it was not intended. Other problems can include difficulties with perceiving device output that is difficult for the user to detect such as displayed text, device status indication, or audible alarms. Still other problems can be traced to operator actions such as inadvertently activating the wrong control, data input errors, etc. Device use problems include the following [3]:

- Devices are used in ways that were not anticipated.
- Devices are used in ways that were anticipated, but inadequately controlled for.
- Device use requires physical, perceptual, or cognitive abilities that exceed those of the user.
- Device use is inconsistent with user's expectations or intuition about device operation.
- The use environment affects device operation and this effect is not understood by the user.
- The user's physical, perceptual, or cognitive capacities are exceeded when using the device in a particular environment.

17.3.4 Specific Considerations for Accessible Device Designs

For devices designed for users with abilities that deviate from the general population, it is essential to understand and describe just how the device will be used. These are a few relevant questions:

- How well will the user be able to perform with this device?
- Will the disabled user operate part or all of the device's capabilities?
- Are there certain tasks that the disabled user should never do and therefore be eliminated through design?
- How have accessibility solutions been successfully applied to other domains?

For example, older users might have difficulty remembering specific sequences for operation, using their hands to do tasks that require fine manipulation, hearing sensing device outputs such as auditory alarm sounds, or seeing information displayed visually. Highly trained and motivated users (i.e., device developers, sales personnel, participants in previous use studies, and expert users) are often much more capable of operating complex devices than typical users. They are also likely to adapt better to unexpected or variable circumstances. Motivated and adaptable users are more likely to take actions to compensate for problems with the design of a device. But, if the same device is placed in the hands of more typical users, unexpected use scenarios possibly resulting in hazards could occur.

Answering the following questions can help identify and describe potential user issues:

- How might the physical and mental capabilities of users affect their application of the device?
- What are the critical steps in setting up and operating the device? Can they be performed adequately by the expected users?
- Is the user or use environment likely to be different from that originally intended?
- Are users likely to be affected by clinical or age-related conditions that impact their physical or mental abilities and could affect their ability to use the device?
- Do any aspects of device use seem complex, and how can the operator become "confused" when using the device?
- Are the auditory and visual warnings effective for all users and use environments?

With proper application of HFE, the design of a device can often be made to compensate for limitations in user ability. For example, diabetics often have some degree of retinopathy (degenerative disease of the retina) resulting in impaired eyesight. These users have difficulty reading the results of blood glucose test kits when the meter displays are very small. Blood glucose meters with small displays were not a good design for this user population. After this problem was understood, subsequent models with larger displays mitigated this hazard.

User experience and expectations are important considerations. Users will expect devices and device components to operate in ways that are consistent with their experience with other similar devices or device interface components. For example, users are likely to expect that the flow-rate of a given substance (such as a gas or liquid flow) will increase by turning a control knob counter-clockwise. Hazards result when an electronically driven device control operates in the opposite direction.

17.3.5 The Role of the Medical Device Use Environments

Use environments for medical devices can vary widely and can have major impacts on device use and use-related hazards. Furthermore, the environment can either exacerbate or reduce the effect that disabilities have on safe device use.

The amount of thinking and concentration a person is required to exert while using a device is called *mental workload*. The mental workload imposed on users by the environment in which they use devices can exceed their abilities to use devices properly. For instance, in an operating room, there could be too many alarms on different devices for an anesthetist to be able to identify the source of any single alarm. Mental workload is often used synonymously with mental "stress." There can be a physical component to workload associated with medical device use (physical workload) that also adds to the stress experienced by the user. Under high stress levels, the user is distracted and will have less time to make decisions, consider multiple device outputs, follow complex operating logic, or physically manipulate device components. Devices that can be used safely under conditions of low stress (i.e., low workload) could be difficult or dangerous to use under conditions of high stress.

Use environments can also limit the effectiveness of visual and auditory displays (lighted indicators, auditory alarms, and other signals) if they are not designed appropriately. If the users cannot understand critically important information, errors are likely. For devices used in noisy environments, the user might not be able to notice alarms if they are not sufficiently loud or distinctive. When multiple alarms occur for different devices or on the same device, the user could fail to notice them or to make important distinctions among them. Similarly, motion and vibration can affect the degree to which people are able to perform fine physical manipulations such as typing on the keyboard portion of a medical device. Motion and vibration can also affect the ability of users to read displayed information.

Important considerations for displays (including visual alarm indicators) and device labeling include ambient light levels, viewing angles, and the presence of other devices in the use environment. If the device will be used in low-light conditions, display scales or device status indicators might not be clear to the user. Some scales will be read inaccurately when viewed from an angle due to parallax or because part of the display is blocked. Other display information can be lost under brightly lit conditions because of insufficient contrast. When certain types of equipment are used in close proximity with other devices, it could be difficult for users to associate visual displays and auditory signals with the corresponding equipment. With too much distraction, important information could be missed.

17.4 CONCLUSIONS

Several chapters in this book address the reality that many current users who desire safe use of medical devices have disabilities and sometimes engage in unsafe activities simply to use these devices. Other chapters document lack of access to certain medical devices by persons because of their disabilities, a clear disadvantage, and suggest that the population of intended users needs to grow. The central question to be answered by the FDA is, "Can the intended users operate the device safely and effectively?" This question applies with equal importance to those who represent a group of "disadvantaged" users using a medical device with enhanced accessibility or the general user using a device without such enhancement. For some existing device types, relatively small efforts could likely be adequate to answer this question, whereas others will require more effort. An operational definition of the user in terms of their abilities and requirements will likely be a challenge in either case. The extent of design and evaluation effort required for a given device is often difficult to estimate accurately prior to beginning the design process. Variability in approach and the amount of effort required is defined by the unique characteristics of devices, their expected use, characteristics of the population of users, and the risks of use-related hazards. Given that modifications causing portable glucose monitors to become more accessible to users with vision and manual dexterity complications of diabetes simultaneously made the devices easier for the general user to operate, the FDA is hopeful that similar benefits will result from enhanced accessibility designs for other medical devices as well.

REFERENCES

1. *Merriam Webster's Dictionary.* Springfield, MA. (http://www.m-w.com)
2. 21 CFR 820.31 Design Controls & C Design Input.
3. Kaye, R. and Crowley, J., Device Use Safety: Incorporating Human Factors in Risk Management, FDA, Rockville, MD, 2000 (http://www.fda.gov/cdrh/humfac/ 1497.pdf).
4. U.S. Access Board, Electronic and Information Technology Accessibility Standards (Section 508), Final Rules implementing Section 508 of the Rehabilitation Act Amendments of 1998, 2001 (http://www.access-board.gov/sec508/standards.htm).
5. Kaye, R.D., North, R.A., and Peterson, M.K., UPCARE: an analysis and description tool for medical device use problems, Advances in industrial engineering theory, applications and practice 8, *Proc. 8th Annual International Conference*, Las Vegas, NV, 2003.
6. Sawyer, C., Do It By Design: An Introduction to Human Factors in Medical Devices, FDA, Rockville, 1997 (http://www.fda.gov/cdrh/humfac/doitpdf.pdf).

18 Letting User Ability Define Usability

James L. Mueller

CONTENTS

ABSTRACT

This chapter addresses the significant differences in perspective on usability between standards makers, designers, and users. A brief synopsis of the development of regulations, the Principles of Universal Design, usability measures, and testing techniques is presented, including context from case studies of businesses with experience in design for users with disabilities. Discussion focuses on tools and techniques for assuring that users have an active role in design development and that the resulting design is as usable as possible for as many people as possible. Two examples of these tools are featured in this chapter: personas for presenting user needs research and a user's guide to selecting a cell phone.

18.1 INTRODUCTION

18.1.1 DESIGNERS ARE NOT USERS

The highest standard of usability is universal design. This term, attributed to architect Ron Mace and increasingly adopted in commercial design, means design for people of all ages and abilities.

Universal design is an unachievable goal, but well worth striving for in the development of products for the general public.

On the other hand, the product development process is usually too brief to allow user testing over such a broad range. In reality, designers often grab the closest users available — themselves. Designers and their clients can only hope that enough real users will find the product usable enough.

These real users include many who are too busy, too distracted, or too fatigued to adapt to designs that do not fit them. Millions more have limitations due to age, illness, or injury that make it impossible for them to adapt.

18.1.2 Principles of Universal Design

Ron Mace and a working group of architects, product designers, design researchers, and engineers collaborated to establish the Principles of Universal Design at the Center for Universal Design [1]. These principles were one of the components of a research and demonstration project funded by the National Institute on Disability and Rehabilitation Research (NIDRR). They articulate the scope of the concept and describe characteristics that make designs universally usable. The subsequent guidelines describe ways to incorporate these characteristics into design. These are provided in Section 3 of Chapter 6.

These principles were intended to help implement design access and usability for people of all ages and abilities. As these principles became the "gold standard" for universal design, the vision of a "seal of approval" evaluation program based on these principles seemed a logical next step.

18.2 MEASURES FOR ACCESSIBILITY AND USABILITY

A number of groups have published guidelines for improving accessibility and usability of various specific technologies, most notably those contained in the Telecommunications Act of 1996 [2]. Other guidelines pertain to telephones [3,4], consumer electronic products [5], accessible Internet Web sites [6], or computer software [7]. Staff at Honeywell, Inc. [8] wrote a set of preliminary guidelines, "Human Factors Design Guidelines for the Elderly and People with Disabilities," which, although incomplete, represented a contribution to the field. Vanderheiden and Vanderheiden [9] developed a set of wide-ranging guidelines and recommendations to improve the accessibility of a wide range of consumer products.

18.2.1 Universal Design Performance Measures

Although considerable effort has been invested in developing tools to measure usability for people of diverse ages and abilities, implementing a practical "seal of approval" program for products remains an elusive goal. The difficulties inherent in measuring usability for people of all ages and abilities were examined in a 3-year field-initiated project at the Center for Universal Design. This project included development of the Universal Design Performance Measures for Products. These 29 performance measures reflect the 7 principles and their guidelines [10].

Initially, five versions of the Universal Design Performance Measures for Products were drafted, each with a different format (e.g., checklist, flowchart, or open-ended questions). These drafts were reviewed in focus groups with 28 consumers with disabilities and in interviews with 18 professional product designers and 12 marketing managers from across the U.S.

The performance measures for products were intended to guide the development of more universally usable new products in the following ways:

- Evaluating product usability throughout its life cycle: packaging, instructions, setup, use, maintenance, and disposal
- Comparing different products or designs

- Developing product testing and focus group methodologies for use with people of diverse ages and abilities
- Promoting the universal design features of products to potential customers
- Identifying universal design features of products for design competitions and award programs

The original intent was to develop a single set of performance measures that could be used by consumers as well as designers, so both groups would literally be working off the same page. However, feedback from project reviewers indicated that this would be inappropriate. Consumers were concerned with issues related to their own personal needs, whereas designers were responsible for addressing the needs of a wide diversity of users concurrently. Each of these groups required its own document. For this reason, two versions of the performance measures were subsequently developed (see Figure 18.1). Each of the two working versions of the Universal Design Performance Measures for products comprised a set of 29 statements (corresponding to the 29 guidelines associated with the seven Principles of Universal Design) that assessed how well a product's design satisfied the principles.

The two documents were reviewed by five external project advisors and pilot-tested by four colleagues who suggested changes, which were incorporated into the documents used in the testing phase. A professional survey designer gave the documents a final review and refined the wording for clarity.

The Universal Design Performance Measures for Products were then tested with consumer households and professional product designers and their households across the U.S. Test participants were chosen to be as diverse a group as possible in terms of age, abilities, race, and geographic location. In order to assess the true universal usability of the measures, the consumer group included 60 households that represented 6 age categories, 36 of which households contained at least one member with an identifiable disability and 24 of which contained no one with a disability. The designer group included 18 households, some containing individuals with disabilities and representing a range of experience with and attitudes toward universal design.

Testing of the Performance Measures with both designers and consumers confirmed that these two groups have fundamentally different approaches to assessing universal design. Designers must seek to meet the needs of the broadest possible market; for them, universal design truly means "design for all ages and abilities." Consumers, on the other hand, define universal design as "design for my age and abilities."

Consumers have a point, of course, but standards and measures have tended to be developed for designers' use only. Because the target population available is so small, can the consumer not just try the design? Why are assessment tools needed by the consumer?

The Principles of Universal Design	Consumers' Product Evaluation Survey	Designers' Product Evaluation Survey
2A. Provide choice in methods of use.	2A. I can use this product in whatever way(s) are safe and effective for me.	2A. The product offers any user at least one way to use it safely and effectively.
2B. Accommodate right- or left-handed access and use.	2B. I can use this product with either my right or left side (hand or foot) alone.	2B. This product can be used by either right- or left-dominant users, including amputees with or without prostheses.
2C. Facilitate the user's accuracy and precision.	2C. I can use this product precisely and accurately.	2C. This product facilitates (or does not require) the user's accuracy and precision.
2D. Provide adaptability to the user's pace.	2D. I can use this product as quickly or as slowly as I want.	2D. This product can be used as quickly or as slowly as the user wants.

FIGURE 18.1 Comparison of wording of the Seven Principles of Universal Design and the Consumers' and Designers' Versions of the Universal Design Performance Measures for Products.

One answer lies in the complexity of the design process. The built environment is obviously intended for usability by people, but there are many other factors to consider, including cost and environmental impact. The final design is always a compromise among these factors. In the end, the user must look out for his or her own needs and make the best choice available.

Another factor is how designers define their intended user. Too often, designers design for themselves, imagining themselves as representative of their customer population. As with doctors who treat themselves, designers who design for themselves have a fool for a customer.

This chapter addresses the significant differences in perspective on usability between standard makers, designers, and users. Discussion focuses on tools and techniques to assure that users have an active role in design development and that the resulting design is as usable as possible for as many people as possible.

18.2.2 Regulations and Guidelines for Accessibility

Over the past 10 years, both the federal government and private industry have invested considerable effort to improve the accessibility and usability of electronic and information technology (E&IT).

Section 255 of The Telecommunications Act of 1996 requires telecommunications products and services to be accessible to people with disabilities. Guidelines for compliance with Section 255 were published in February 1998.

In 1998, Congress amended the Rehabilitation Act to include Section 508, which requires federal agencies to make their E&IT products and services accessible to people with disabilities. The Access Board incorporated the language of the Section 255 guidelines into the accessibility standards they developed for Section 508 of the Rehabilitation Act.

The scope of Section 508 is limited to the federal sector. However, E&IT producers realize that the most cost-effective strategy is to design compliance with Section 508 into products and services for both federal and private customers.

Section 508 went into effect in June 2001. Over time, as the industry and others became more familiar with these standards, inquiries became more technical in nature. This justified the need to develop more advanced technical assistance through partnerships between government and industry such as the Accessibility Forum.

This decade of activity has helped manufacturers to understand the folly of allowing their designers to design for themselves. Some manufacturers seeking to comply with standards and guidelines for accessibility and usability (see also Chapter 15) have turned to user testing (see also Chapter 16 and Chapter 17).

18.2.3 User Testing: Desperately Seeking Usability

User testing can save money on technical support costs and in gaining more business through customer referrals. In pursuit of better usability in design, product developers have begun or expanded their programs of testing by samples of users. Ideally, this testing is done by representative users doing real tasks under realistic conditions.

18.2.3.1 Who Is the User?

First and foremost, project engineers and designers are not representative users. They are far too knowledgeable about the design and too invested in its success. No amount of preparation through unlearning or user empathy can change this. One usability professor at Carnegie Mellon University said he always hired undergraduate rather than graduate students, because they were more likely to remember what it was like to not understand the course material and would be better at explaining it [11]. To paraphrase the old saw about doctors and their patients, those who design for themselves have a fool for a customer.

18.2.3.2 When to Test

Pressures of project budgets or deadlines often cause product developers to postpone consideration of user testing until the end of the project, should budget and resources allow. At this point, however, user testing can do little more than expose problems that would be too expensive or time consuming to correct.

User testing is far more cost effective as an integral component of the project, beginning as early as possible and continuing throughout the design process, when it is most effective to address problems without major cost or delay. For example, "information structure and interaction style of a design can be tested with a non–working prototype by asking representative users to indicate how they would carry out a task given a particular design." [12] For some users, a working prototype may be necessary for effective testing. Users with functional limitations or assistive technologies may need access to a working prototype [13].

18.2.3.3 What to Test

Rather than asking the user to envision how they might complete a task or what they might need, user testing observes the user at work or play and evaluates how the product is used in their lives. User testing begins with a clear definition, situation, or scenario of a task to be completed. Success is measured in terms of how long it takes users to complete the task, the number and consequences of any mistakes, their recollection of what they did, and what they liked and disliked. Scripted instructions and pre- and post-test questionnaires may also be used to gather user feedback [14].

18.2.3.4 Where to Test

User testing may be conducted in the laboratory or on-site in the environment where use normally occurs. The laboratory environment may be set up in-house or at an outside firm to approximate the environment where actual use might occur. Advantages of the laboratory environment are a high degree of environmental control, preselection of testers, and facilities for unobtrusive observation, i.e., cameras and one-way mirrors. However, many influential factors, for example, distractions and natural lighting in the normal environment, cannot be replicated.

On-site testing is the opposite of laboratory testing, though testers can also be carefully selected. Testing on-site makes it possible to observe all tasks and environmental factors that relate to the test. However, on-site testing relinquishes control of these factors, and observation is more demanding and obtrusive. On-site testing may also take longer and present logistical problems of permissions, travel costs, etc.

A third alternative involves recruiting users in the field and conducting testing on the spot. Tester selection is naturally far less controlled, but also far less expensive, without the costs of recruiting, selecting, and scheduling users [15].

An approach that combines some of the advantages of these approaches is remote user testing (RUT). RUT has been used effectively to perform tests of software design over a large volume of users who participate in studies from their real context (home or office). RUT has the capacity to gather rich user experience information from geographically diverse users at low cost [16].

18.2.3.5 User Testing in Context

Testing in the user's real context is especially important with testers who have disabilities. As noted in the testing of a cognitive prosthesis for persons with acquired brain injury at the Wireless RERC, visual and auditory distractions and personal compensatory strategies (including assistive technologies) are instrumental in assessing the usability of the device [17].

The usefulness and usability of this cognitive prosthesis, a commercial PDA with modified software and choices of interface options, was tested through a field exercise. This exercise involved using the device to navigate several blocks from an outpatient center to a local grocery store, purchase several items, and remember to send a message upon return to the center.

Most of the user testers completed a similar warm-up exercise easily in the quiet and orderly environment of the outpatient center's offices. However, once out in the community, glare, weather, traffic, store crowds, and other distractions conspired against the concentration of many testers. Incorrect items were purchased, and other tasks were forgotten. This real-world testing taught lessons that the laboratory setting could not have taught. These lessons were then incorporated into redesign of the device and its software, making them much more effective. Coincidentally, incorporating these changes into a commercial PDA would make it more usable for anyone.

An example is provided in Figure 18.2, in which as a consequence of Duracell's using hearing-aid user testers, increasingly smaller batteries became easier to install.

18.2.3.6 Real Users, Real Context: Users as Test Drivers for Wireless Products

In 2001, the Rehabilitation Engineering Research Center on Mobile Wireless Technologies (the Wireless RERC) was established in Atlanta, GA. Among the proposed deliverables of this center's research and development program was a protocol for determining usability of wireless products, especially wireless telecommunications products. At nearly the same time as the Wireless RERC was founded in 2001, guidelines and technical assistance for compliance with the Telecommunications Act and Section 508 of the Rehabilitation Act began to proliferate. Developing yet another set of guidelines for manufacturers to follow seemed counterproductive. The RERC decided on a different approach.

The Wireless RERC began a user needs assessment project at the outset. This project included both a survey and focus groups. As of this writing, over 1200 people with disabilities have responded to the Survey of User Needs (SUN). About half of these people agreed to join a Consumer Advisory Network (CAN) and participate in product testing, focus groups and other project activities. Twelve focus groups with CAN members of diverse ages and cognitive, physical, and sensory abilities have been conducted.

These data have reinforced the impression that users do not care as much about universal design as they do about design that fits their personal universe. Although they may be experts on their own abilities and limitations, users with disabilities need help in applying that expertise to assess usability in the products and environments available to them.

Lessons learned through the user survey and focus groups were used to create a guide for users to be their own product testers for (in this case) cell phones (see Figure 18.3). It is essentially a guide to test-driving cell phones before purchase.

18.2.3.7 Sitting in on Product Development

The goal of the research being conducted at the RERC on Wireless Technologies is greater usefulness and usability of these technologies for customers of all ages and abilities. Who are better to guide providers of these technologies than the users themselves?

As an example, consider the user described in Figure 18.4. Della has a good point about "sitting in when products are designed." Alan Cooper makes this same point in his book on designing for users, entitled *The Inmates are Running the Asylum* [19]. Cooper describes how effectively personas can engage in the product development process because they are individuals, not faceless numbers. Cooper also points out how dismally a design can fail when users are denied a voice in the product development process.

As Cooper points out, "Personas are not real people, but they represent them through the design process. They are hypothetical archetypes of actual users. Although they are imaginary, they are defined with significant rigor and precision. Actually, we don't so much 'make up' our

Figure 2: Duracell uses Hearing Aid User-Testers - Hearing Aids Get Better; Batteries Get Smaller

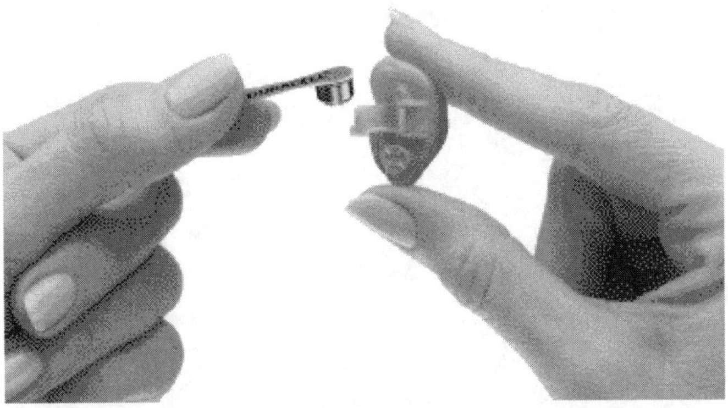

The social stigma attached to wearing a hearing aid has been greatly reduced by the development of less detectable, digital models, some fitting entirely within the ear canal. [18] However, these newer hearing aids require battery changes as often as every week. Arthritis and poor eyesight, compounded with smaller zinc-air batteries, make this weekly chore an ordeal for some users:

> "Oops, I've got it upside down."
> "…can't get the silly box open…"
> "…and my eyesight isn't as great as it should be, either."
> "I feel like an ass."

First introduced for hearing aids in the 1980's, zinc air batteries have become the battery of choice as the power demands of modern hearing aids have increased. To prevent exposure to air before use, zinc air hearing aid batteries are packaged with a small tab that adheres to the battery to create a seal. The tab must be removed to "activate" the battery before insertion. Removing this tiny tab is difficult for seniors with manual dexterity problems.

Duracell saw an opportunity to introduce an innovative package system unique in the market to ease hearing aid battery replacement for consumers. "Duracell was seeking differentiation from competitors who offered "circular-dial" packaging, which made hearing aid batteries difficult to retrieve, load and activate, "says Peter B. Clarke, president and founder of Product Ventures Ltd.

Development of this new package required management commitment to the risks inherent in any new product introduction, including the costs and difficulties of reinventing manufacturing and assembly processes. Duracell and Product Ventures turned to one-on-one interviews and usability testing with senior hearing aid users to guide the development of this entirely new approach.

Clarke explains how user input was gathered and integrated into design development: "We conducted product use focus groups that illustrated the many shortfalls of existing packaging; and we determined that Duracell needed a new delivery system -- not just a new package."

DURACELL EASYTAB was introduced to retail outlets in October 2001. Post-use focus groups confirmed that consumers were elated with the new EASYTAB feature. User-testers of the new package responded with, "Voila," and "Oh, that was easy." In the first month of sales, DURACELL EASYTAB inventory was completely sold out.

The Center for Universal Design. "Duracell Listens to Its Customers". Retrieved on June 22,2005 from: http://design.ncsu.edu/cud/proj_services/projects/case_studies/Duracell.htm

FIGURE 18.2 Duracell uses hearing-aid user testers — hearing aids get better; batteries get smaller.

Figure 3. Cell phone guide - results of testing and development

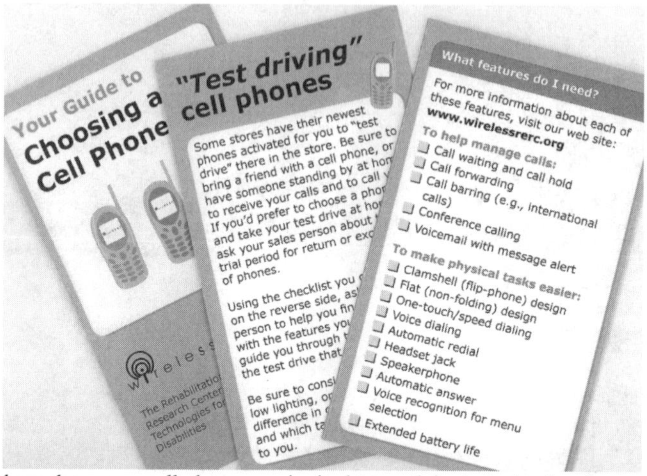

Each CAN member who uses a cell phone was invited to participate in the development of a guide to purchasing a cell phone. Along with this invitation was a 12-question survey about customer satisfaction with their current cell phones, service plans, customer support, and the experience of purchasing this phone. Of the 300 invited, 103 responded. Among the results of this initial survey:

- Nokia and Motorola account for 71% of the brands used (primarily because these phones came free or at significant savings with the calling plan the customer chose).
- 43% have had their current phone for 1 year or less.
- 20% had difficulty carrying their phone
- 14% had negative comments about the display screen; 16% had negative comments about the battery or charger; 16% had negative comments about the process of placing or receiving calls; 22% had negative comments about the voice mail feature; 11% had negative comments about the phone directory and 10% had negative comments about the locking feature (a significant number were unaware their phone had these features)
- 8% were dissatisfied with their purchasing experience, usually because sales staff tended to be too rushed to answer all their concerns.

Testing the "Guide to Choosing a Cell Phone"

Each of the 103 survey participants was then sent a copy of the draft "Guide to Choosing a Cell Phone" and a 5-question follow-up survey to examine how useful this Guide might be to these experienced users. Seventy-seven completed and returned the follow-up survey. The first survey question asked participants to use the Guide's "test drive" to rate the usability of their current cell phone. Results of the "test drive" were similar to the satisfaction with their phones that participants noted in the initial survey: In the initial survey, an average of 16% of respondents noted usability problems. The "test drive" revealed 8% with negative comments about their phone's usability.

Despite their generally positive experiences with their current cell phone, 65% of survey participants felt the Guide would have changed their buying process. Many noted this Guide would be even more important to first-time buyers, especially in making them aware of the array of available features, and specific functions they should try before they buy. Asked if they would like to have this Guide the next time they buy a cell phone, 83% responded positively.

Refining the Guide

Seventy-one percent of survey respondents suggested that no changes should be made to this Guide. However, several suggestions for improvement were made and considered in the final draft. The final version, "Your Guide to Choosing a Cell Phone" is now in print and on the web site of the Wireless RERC: http://www.wirelessrerc.gatech.edu/projects/research/r1_chooseCellPhone.html

FIGURE 18.3 Cell phone guide — results of testing and development.

Figure 4. An example "persona" user: Meet Della

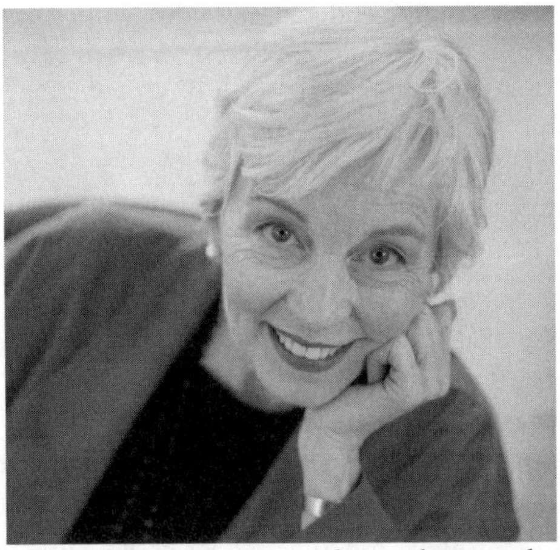

"I'm not a designer. I'm a design customer, and a tough one at that". Della

"I was born in 1938 and have worked all my life. In 1995, I had a mild stroke that limits my strength and coordination on my right side. It doesn't keep me from working though, and frankly the electric scooter I use is faster than I could ever walk before my stroke."

"My point is the huge difference that design makes in my life. And not just me – this is a favorite topic among my coworkers and friends. A lot of the difficulties I've experienced since my stroke, and a lot of the well-designed products I've found, are the same kinds of things that my friends deal with every day, disabled or not. I understand that everyday products are designed to fit the "average" user. But if we're not lucky enough to be "average", we have to adapt to the design. Depending on how well we can adapt, this can be just a minor annoyance or an exhausting, frustrating, even dangerous ordeal. From where I sit (no pun intended), there aren't very many "average" people around anymore."

"For instance, I'm not a techie, but I do carry a cell phone. It's mostly for work, but it's also a safety net. I probably wouldn't travel around nearly so much if I didn't have a way for calling for help in an emergency. My friends with disabilities feel the same way, and some don't have much money to spend on expensive gadgets like this. But there are lots of ways these products could be more usable for everyone."

"It's amazing that products like this can be so advanced, yet still have little problems that seem so easy to solve. I wish I could sit in when products are being designed. It doesn't do a lot of good to point these things out after thousands of them have been made."

Who is Della?

Della is articulate and frank about how designers could benefit from listening to her. But Della isn't just speaking for herself- she's actually one of several "personas" of thousands of people we should be designing for.

FIGURE 18.4 An example "persona" user: Meet Della.

personas as discover them as a by-product of the investigation process. We do, however, make up their names and personal details" [19]. Their photos are purchased from commercial stock photograph suppliers.

Some argue that designers who design for just a few personas are only a little less foolish than those who design for themselves. Their user population is still unrealistically small. Unlike designers, however, personas carefully developed through user research genuinely represent real, substantial user groups.

Della and other personas were developed from customer research that began in 2001 at the Wireless RERC. This research includes a nationwide survey of users and potential users of cell phones and other wireless technologies and focus groups with customers who have cognitive, hearing, physical, or vision disabilities. The research data received from more than 1200 survey respondents and more than 100 focus group participants offers valuable insight into users of wireless technologies who have disabilities. Personas are one of the ways to bring these data to life and to engage in the design process [20].

As real as they seem, personas are not intended to substitute for user research or testing, but rather to introduce us to who potential users may be and how to approach them as design customers. In addition, personas can be used to help designers identify the right users to serve as product testers by modeling the user characteristics they seek.

18.3 CONCLUSION: LETTING USERS DEFINE USABILITY

As a result of a 3-year study of 22 companies, conducted from 1996 to 1999, the Trace Research and Development Center at the University of Wisconsin at Madison (Trace Center) published a "List of Strategies for Facilitating the Adoption and Successful Practice of Universal Design by Consumer Product Manufacturers" [21]. Among these strategies, Trace cited the importance of "a knowledgeable consumer base, where consumers with disabilities readily communicate with companies about their products, offering detailed criticism and suggestions" and "product testing by consumers with disabilities, including recruitment of test subjects" [22].

In its study of 52 companies, conducted from 1994 to 2003, the Center for Universal Design at North Carolina State University learned that direct involvement of customers with disabilities was a central factor for 75% of the companies that had actively sought to meet the needs of these users [23].

In the end, the user's abilities, not those of the designer, define the usability of design. People with limitations due to age or disability have historically been excluded from usability consideration. The good news is that including these populations and the real world in which they live improves usability for everyone. Through tools such as personas and user testing guides and strategies, users of all ages and abilities can take a much more active role in design development than is common in industry today.

ACKNOWLEDGMENT

The chapter has been made possible by funding from the NIDRR of the U.S. Department of Education under grant number H133E010804. The opinions contained in this article are those of the grantee and do not necessarily reflect those of the U.S. Department of Education.

REFERENCES

1. Story, M.F., Principles of universal design, in *Universal Design Handbook*, Ostroff, E. and Prieser, W., Eds., McGraw-Hill, New York, 2001, chap.10.
2. Telecommunications Access Advisory Committee, Access to Telecommunications Equipment and Customer Premises Equipment by Individuals with Disabilities, Architectural and Transportation Barriers Compliance Board, Washington, D.C., 1997.
3. Francik, E., *Telephone Interfaces: Universal Design Filters*, Pacific Bell, San Ramon, CA, 1996.
4. Pacific Bell, A Compilation of Interface Design Rules and Guidelines for Interactive Voice Response Systems (IVRs), Pacific Bell Human Factors Engineering, San Ramon, CA, 1995.
5. Electronics Industries Association and Electronic Industries Foundation, Resource Guide for Accessible Design of Consumer Electronics, Electronics Industries Association and Electronic Industries Foundation, Washington, D.C., 1996.

6. Vanderheiden, G.C. and Lee, C.C., Considerations in the Design of Computers and Operating Systems to Increase Their Accessibility to Persons with Disabilities (Version 4.2), The University of Wisconsin, Trace R&D Center, Madison, WI, 1988.
7. Vanderheiden, G.C., Application Software Design Guidelines: Increasing the Accessibility of Application Software to People with Disabilities and Older Users, The University of Wisconsin, Trace R&D Center, Madison, WI, 1994.
8. Honeywell, Inc., Human Factors Design Guidelines for the Elderly and People with Disabilities (Revision 3, Draft), Honeywell, Inc., Minneapolis, MN, 1990.
9. Vanderheiden, G.C. and Vanderheiden, K.R., Accessible Design of Consumer Products: Guidelines for the Design of Consumer Products to Increase Their Accessibility to Persons with Disabilities or Who Are Aging (Working Draft 1.7), The University of Wisconsin, Trace R&D Center, Madison, WI, 1992.
10. Story, M.F., Mueller, J.L., Montoya-Weiss, M., and Ringholz, D., The development of universal design performance measures, in *Spotlight on Technology: Proceedings of the RESNA '99 Annual Conference*, RESNA, Arlington, VA, pp. 100–102.
11. Retrieved from http://crankyuser.com/user.testing.primer/.
12. Retrieved from http://crankyuser.com/user.testing.primer/.
13. Retrieved from http://accessit.nda.ie/about_user_testing.html#why.
14. Retrieved from http://en.wikipedia.org/wiki/Usability_testing.
15. Retrieved from http://crankyuser.com/user.testing.primer/.
16. Retrieved from http://www.xperienceconsulting.com/eng/servicios.asp?ap=23.
17. Haberman, V., Jones, M., and Mueller, J., Mobile wireless technology for individuals with cognitive impairments: Device analysis and customization, in *Proceedings of the Human Factors and Ergonomics Society 49th Annual Meeting*, Human Factors and Ergonomics Society, Santa Monica, CA, 2005.
18. Hansen, L., New Advances in Hearing Aids, Batteries Enable Better Living, Senior Times, Flash Publishers, Online: http://www.seniortimesonline.com/nov01/stories/110901/hea_1109010021.html. retrieved November 2005.
19. Cooper, A., *The Inmates are Running the Asylum*, SAMS, A Division of Macmillan Computer Publishing, Indianapolis, IN, 1999.
20. Mueller, J.L., Getting Personal with Universal, *Innovation*, Spring 2004.
21. http://trace.wisc.edu/docs/hfes98_barriers/barriers_incentives_facilitators.htm. retrieved November 2005.
22. Retrieved on July 7, 2005 from http://trace.wisc.edu/docs/univ_design_res_proj/udrp.htm.
23. Mueller, J., Case Studies on Universal Design, Center for Universal Design, North Carolina State University, Raleigh, NC, 1997.

19 Macroergonomic and Implementation Issues of Guidelines for Accessible Medical Devices

Pascale Carayon, Anne-Sophie Grenier, and Carla Alvarado

CONTENTS

ABSTRACT

This chapter describes the barriers to the implementation and use of guidelines and other human factors knowledge and skills for the design of accessible medical devices. After describing a generic system design process, we discuss the steps of the design process in which human factors can make significant contribution to improve the usability and accessibility of medical devices. We then describe the elements of the work system of a designer and identify various work system characteristics that can hinder the application of guidelines and human factors knowledge by designers of medical devices. The final part of the chapter provides information on organizational barriers to the implementation of guidelines, such as financial issues, and barriers related to organizational culture and structure.

19.1 INTRODUCTION

The purpose of this chapter is to describe the human factors and organizational issues related to the implementation and use of guidelines for accessible medical devices by medical device manufacturers and their engineers. We distinguish between (1) the use of guidelines by the engineers or designers

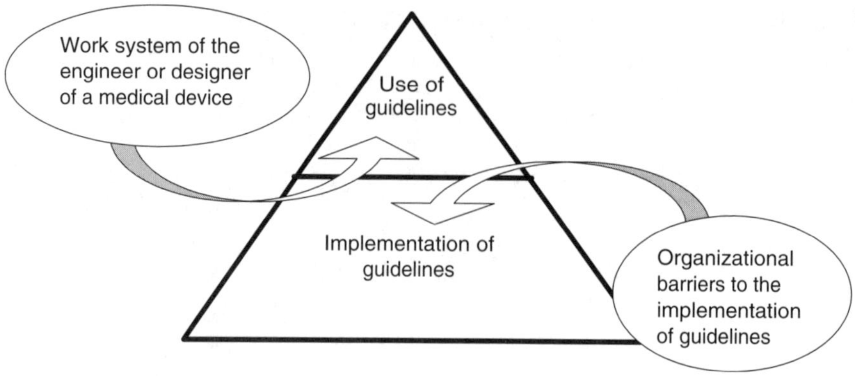

FIGURE 19.1 Pyramid of barriers to the implementation and use of guidelines for accessible medical devices.

of medical devices and (2) the implementation of guidelines by medical device manufacturers. Figure 19.1 represents these two levels by describing the implementation of guidelines as the base that can foster the use of guidelines by engineers and designers. Therefore, organizational barriers to the implementation of guidelines will make it very difficult for engineers and designers to use the guidelines. Once the implementation of guidelines is facilitated at the organizational (manufacturer) level, the use of guidelines by engineers and designers is more likely to occur.

19.2 SYSTEM DESIGN PROCESS

19.2.1 System Design Process

As emphasized by White [1], there is not one best way to describe a design process because "design is universally understood to be a *creative, iterative, decision-making process*" (p. 455). That is the reason why the system design process cannot be depicted as a linear process, but is rather considered as a complex nonlinear process. In order to facilitate the understanding of this complexity, a graphical representation of the system design process is displayed in the form of a flowchart in Figure 19.2, which has been adapted from White [1]. The flowchart describes the different steps the designer has to go through during the system design process. The system design process begins with the user (i.e., defining the user needs) and ends with the user (i.e., delivering the final system design to the user).

The system design process begins with a design problem. Either there is a need for a system, a product or a technology that does not currently exist, or there is a demand for the improvement or redesign of a preexisting system. Human needs and desires have to be evaluated so that they can be transformed and characterized in technical, qualitative, and financial requirements, therefore further clarifying the problem tackled by the system design process. This phase is probably the most critical of the process for two reasons. First, a problem that is clearly defined facilitates the development of potential designs (see also Chapter 8). Second, this phase requires extensive understanding of the users by the designer, which can be a very difficult task (see also Chapter 18).

There are several reasons why the designer may have difficulty in understanding the users' needs. First, the designer has his or her own areas of expertise and experience that are not always fully related to the final system to be designed. For example, a Web site designer might have to design a Web-based medical application. If the designer does not have any medical knowledge or health care experience, the individual's perception of the application may be different from the expectations of the health care personnel who are the end users of the Web-based medical application. The designer may also have a hard time understanding the needs of disabled end users because of the variety of disabilities and their varied impact on medical device design. In any case, the designer needs to understand the customers' requirements. Thus, any potential mismatch of

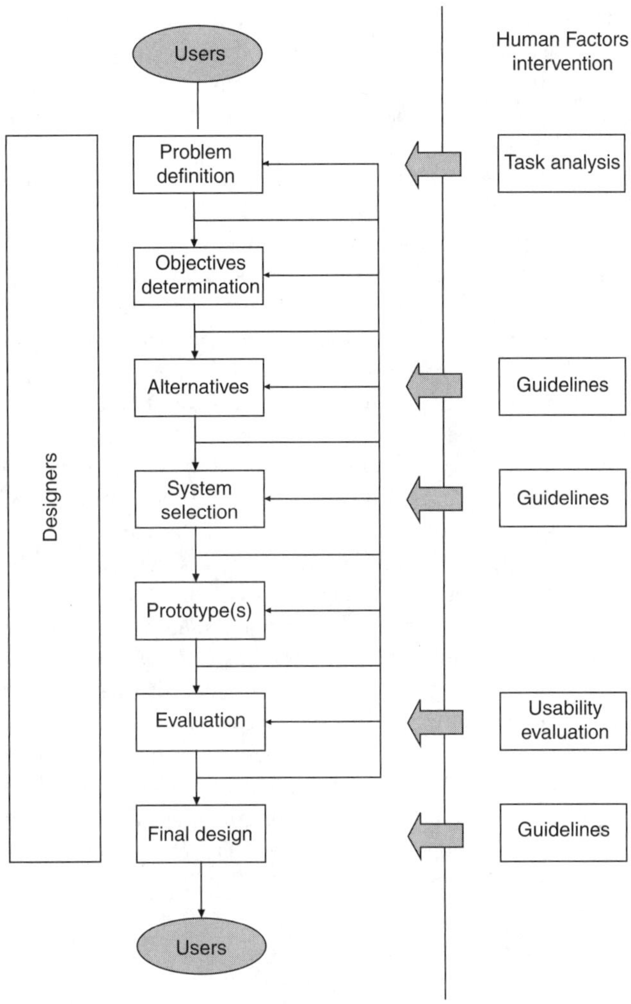

FIGURE 19.2 System design process. (Adapted from White, P.K., Jr., Systems design, in *Handbook of Systems Engineering and Management*, Sage, A.P., Rouse, W.B., Eds., John Wiley & Sons, New York, 1999, pp. 455–482.)

perception needs to be fully understood and addressed at the initiation of the system design process. Second, the designer has to translate multiple users' needs, which can be competing and contradictory, or unclear and even unknown to the user. For instance, the expectations of an experienced nurse regarding intravenous (IV) pump technology may be different from that of a novice. The experienced nurse may have strong beliefs and expectations about what the design should be (e.g., an interface as similar as possible to the IV pump that the nurse is familiar with). The novice, on the other hand, might not have any specific idea of what to expect from the design of an IV pump and, in this sense, would think: "I'll know it when I see it" [2, p. 30].

Once the design problem has been clearly defined, the objectives of the design can be stated. Determining the objectives of the design involves determining performance measures, both qualitative and quantitative, to evaluate the design during and after the design process. Once the objectives of the design are clearly stated, designers can start brainstorming and developing different design alternatives.

The next step is to select the best design alternative by evaluating and ranking the different alternatives against the performance measures. There is no rule about which measures should get priority over the others, simply because design is contingent [3]. Indeed, the performance measures are really specific to the system that is being designed. For example, a blood pressure cuff might have two performance measures: cost and adaptability over the range of users. A design for use with adults might prioritize minimum cost, whereas a design for use with premature babies is more likely to be more concerned with adaptability.

After the best design has been selected from among the various alternatives, one or several prototypes can be developed to evaluate the selected design. Finally, the release of the final design ends the system design process.

At any step of the design process, designers can decide to go back to any of the previous steps; the design process of a system or a technology is continuously evolving. Those iterative cycles are represented by the backward arrows that link to earlier steps in Figure 19.2. Such a process can be characterized as top–down because "design is the solution of a problem" [2, p. 88] as well as bottom–up, as lower levels in the flowchart can feed back information to upper levels.

Different views of the system design process exist. As discussed by Meister and Enderwick [2, p. 3] the system design process is to be differentiated from system development; system development is comprised of the system design process and the continuous testing and evaluation. Some other views such as the one described earlier integrate the iterative feedback loops as part of the system design process [1].

As mentioned earlier, design is contingent because any system design process is fully constrained. Indeed, on top of the operational characteristics of the product, designers have to handle many other constraints arising from various sources: requirements of customers (e.g., personal preferences), demands of clients, capabilities of suppliers, internal expectations of the company (e.g., low cost, minimal delay, and high level of quality), and also legal compliance with federal standards. A number of guidelines for medical devices have been developed, such as those proposed by the FDA (e.g., *Do it by Design* [4] and a set of guidelines tying human factors with risk management [5]) or those developed by the American National Standards Institute and the Association for the Advancement of Medical Instrumentation [6–8]. These guidelines are the direct product of human factors practice and are further developed in Chapter 16. The role of human factors within system design is discussed in the following section.

19.2.2 Human Factors in System Design Process

According to the International Ergonomics Association, "Ergonomics (or human factors) is the scientific discipline concerned with the understanding of interactions among humans and other elements of a system, and the profession that applies theory, principles, data and methods to design in order to optimize human well-being and overall system performance" [9]. Ergonomics should be a priority in system design as well as in the definition of technical requirements or in establishing a safety system. As noted by Ballay [10], the requirements designers have to include functional specifications in their design and also human factors (HF) and usability.

HF is increasingly becoming important in system design in the medical area. Poor design of medical devices can have life-threatening consequences: "Poorly designed medical devices, whether disposable syringes or complex imaging systems, can promote user error and lead to adverse patient outcomes" [11, p. 1484]. In a working environment such as health care, poor designs can not only have negative business consequences but can also harm end users [12]. The harmful impact of poorly designed medical devices may be even greater on disabled end users.

Using HF and ergonomics principles and methods may allow for the creation of better, more usable system designs with fewer bad outcomes. Designing medical systems to be accessible is a natural extension to HF methodology in which consideration is given to users with diverse abilities who could benefit from the intended use of the device. Given that 19% of the general population is classified as having a disability [13], and that for many classes of medical products — especially ones used in the home setting — the user population would be expected to be considerably higher than this, it makes sense to address a diverse group of users (for example, see Chapter 18).

Many HF principles and methods have been developed that can guide designers. HF is slowly becoming an integral part of the design process. For instance, human factors methods such as task analysis can be used to define user needs in a very structured manner, thereby helping the designer to overcome the issues presented earlier. Usability evaluation procedures can be used in assessing a prototype and can streamline the feedback loops. Another example of the determinant role of human factors in system design lies in the numerous design guidelines and standards available to designers. As noted by Chapanis [14, p. 58], "Literally hundreds of published standards and codes constrain engineers and human-factors professionals because they are imposed on designers in some formal way, for example, by legislation, by contract, or by management decree." In some cases, a classic example of legal constraints is accessibility guidelines associated with specific legislation (e.g., see Chapter 15).

Understanding how HF and ergonomics guidelines and standards are applied in system design processes is important. Unfortunately, very often HF is the discipline that gets the last priority in design, if any. Too often, HF guidelines and principles compete with other design requirements such as time, cost, quality, and productivity expectations.

The HF community asks product or system designers to think about products in terms of end users. Similarly, in analyzing the system design process, the HF community should think about the designers as users; the designers are end users of HF guidelines, standards, etc., but in reality, the designers are rarely considered. This mismatch can be extremely detrimental to the design process. Chapanis [14, p. 18] stated this misunderstanding:

> … human-factors data and principles are useful only to the extent that they can be translated into design. Whenever glaring examples are discovered in which machines or systems are poorly designed for human use, there is a tendency to blame the engineer who was responsible for its design. Yet sometimes the fault can be traced to human-factors professionals who could not provide engineers with the kind of information they needed for design. When that happens, the underlying reason often is that human-factors professionals did not understand the design process and how human factors can contribute to that process.

Lack of use or poor implementation of design guidelines cannot be attributed only to the indifference or noncompliance of designers. Barriers to the use and implementation of design guidelines are discussed in the rest of this chapter

19.3 BARRIERS TO USE OF GUIDELINES

The designer may experience a range of barriers to the use of guidelines. In this section, we examine the "work system" of the designer and identify the factors in the work system that may hinder the use of guidelines by the designer. The work system has been conceptualized as being comprised of five elements: the *individual* performing *tasks* using various *tools and technologies* in a *physical environment* under *organizational conditions* [15,16].

19.3.1 Individual Variables

The designers of medical devices may have limited understanding and knowledge about the need for accessible medical devices. There is often a misunderstanding regarding the definition of accessible devices [17]. Designers may think that universal design or the design of accessible medical devices means that the medical device has to be usable by any elderly or disabled person [17]. Universal design is a design practice aimed at ensuring the direct use of products and devices by the largest range of end users and their compatibility with assistive technologies used by older or disabled users. Distinctions between universal and accessible design (which is often tied to specific federal accessibility guidelines) are presented in Chapter 8. The designers' misunderstanding of universal and accessible design may actually contribute to their fear of feeling constrained about their design [17].

Wulff and colleagues [18] conducted exploratory case studies in two engineering design companies that were involved in two distinct projects for designing oil platforms. Data were collected via interviews with designers, supervisors and support staff, and analysis of documents. The majority of designers had limited or no knowledge of HF documents and requirements. Some of the designers knew where to look for HF documents or requirements. Knowledge of HF was enhanced when the designers cooperated or interacted with the HF specialist or had been involved in previous projects with the HF specialist. Designers with little or no knowledge of HF documents and requirements had limited or no perceived awareness of HF.

The AAMI standards clearly specify that the standard "is not intended as a sole source for HFE guidance or as a substitute for human factors expertise" [8, p. 1]. The guidelines can be used to raise the awareness of designers about the importance of HF knowledge, but designers may not have that HF knowledge, and therefore will need to work with HF experts during the design process.

Designers may have limited information processing capacity that hinders their use of HF documents and requirements. This limited information processing capacity may be further reduced when designers experience high workload. The federal and state governments as well as many organizations and expert panels write guidelines. The designer may be faced with information overload in dealing with large groups of guidelines. Making an informed choice as to which guideline fits the intended design is important; and constant comparisons to make sure of guidelines' compatibility is paramount.

19.3.2 Task Complexities

Designers tend to prefer specific requirements to general formulations and recommendations [19]. A specific requirement includes the verb "shall" and a specific design criterion. A general formulation requires the designer to "translate" the requirement and is therefore dependent partly on the HF knowledge and familiarity of the designer. A designer can decide whether or not to apply the requirement; design situations characterized by high workload and time pressure are, therefore, less likely to be situations in which the designer will have the time and resources to apply the recommendation.

Guidelines are often either too general or too specific and, as a consequence, may not be useful in the designer's particular situation. The 1993 AAMI standards [6] included very specific recommendations regarding various characteristics of medical devices, whereas the 2001 AAMI standards [8] used a "performance" approach in which the objectives (e.g., usability of medical devices) are specified and the process to reach those objectives is described (i.e., the HF engineering design cycle).

Guidelines may not address critical issues related to the design of medical devices [20]. Guidelines that are incomplete or not sufficiently comprehensive may discourage designers to use them [20].

Another barrier to the use of guidelines by designers is related to the variety of users for whom medical devices are being designed. The AAMI standards explains that "a user may be a caregiver (e.g., anyone who gives a diabetic an insulin injection); a patient (e.g., diabetics who administer their own insulin injections); or someone who provides support for either a caregiver or a patient (e.g., a diagnostic ultrasound technician)" [8, p. 1]. This variety of users and their varied needs and requirements increases the difficulty of the designer's work. This may be exacerbated with a population of disabled users who have a wide range of characteristics and needs.

19.3.3 Technologies and Tools

Designers use various technologies and tools while performing their design tasks. A key issue in human factors is to ensure the usability and usefulness of technologies and tools and their fit within the overall work system. Burns et al. [21] conducted a series of experiments to examine the usability, usefulness, and viability of HF handbooks. In the first experiment, two HF handbooks were compared; subjects performed various tasks (e.g., searching for specific information in the handbook) and their performance was evaluated (e.g., duration, efficiency of search). One of the handbooks led to higher performance, probably because of its organization; this handbook was organized around application topics as compared to the other handbook organized around a theory of psychological mechanisms. In the second experiment, participants rated the effort of using different information sources. Using their own judgment or talking with a colleague constituted the information source with the least reported effort. Handbooks and other readings had relatively low effort ratings, but their perceived cost associated with finding the information was high. Therefore, designers may prefer to miss information rather than waste their valuable time looking for information in handbooks and other written materials.

Based on the results of these experiments, Burns et al. [21] made four recommendations for improving HF guidance documents:

- Need to contain detailed application-specific information
- Need to understand the needs of designers, the types of HF problems they face, and their strategies and behaviors related to information search
- Need to inform designers about readily available HF documents to help them become more familiar with HF literature
- Need to provide organizational policies and information sources that support designers' search for information

The designer must be aware of how to obtain guideline information. It is not always easy to find guidelines for specific design processes. If the designer does not have access to a technical library or the company does not purchase specific guideline sets, the designer may not have knowledge of or have access to the guidelines. If available, the guideline may not be available to the designer, as the reference document's actual physical location may reside in other areas of the company premises or even other city sites far removed from the designer's location. Additionally, the available guidelines may not be the current, more recently updated versions of the guidelines. Designer access to the Web may resolve some of these barriers, as the Internet search engines may direct the designer to current, electronic versions of many guidelines. However, other barriers to implementation include lack of this electronic access and the knowledge and training to use it.

The quality of guidelines varies considerably. Guidelines can be based on the peer-reviewed scientific literature or just opinions and anecdotal information. Designers may envision selecting the efficacious guidelines a daunting task and fear the repercussions of an improper choice.

As mentioned, the designer is faced with many choices in guidelines selection, and lack of documented guideline validity in similar design uses may be a barrier to guideline adoption. Objectives of a product's design are not always well defined, and this can lead to inadequate or inappropriate guideline selection.

19.3.4 Physical Environment

Designers may be geographically spread, therefore making informal communication and collaboration more difficult. Proximity between designers and HF engineers has been advocated as a way of improving the consideration of human factors engineering considerations in the design process [22].

19.3.5 Organizational Factors

Even if the designer is aware of the HF requirements and guidelines, these requirements and guidelines are not always implemented [19]. Sometimes, use of requirements and guidelines gets sacrificed because of other requirements or time pressures. HF requirements may be dropped during the screening process or during the "bargaining" process. Wulff et al. [19] describes a model of the conflict process that can occur and influence whether HF criteria are implemented in the design process. HF criteria can come into conflict with other design requirements. If this occurs and there is a high degree of HF legitimacy or follow-up by a HF specialist, HF criteria may be partly or fully implemented as long as no other serious obstacles are present.

Burns and Vicente [23] identified three categories of constraints in the design process of a control room for a nuclear power plant: (1) contextual constraints, (2) constraints from parsing and distribution, and (3) constraints from other domains. Contextual constraints relate to the design environment, such as the physical dimensions of an existing space or the anthropometric characteristics of the end user population. A large design problem occurs over a long period of time and is often broken down into small subprojects involving designers with different varying expertise and background. For instance, a designer making a change in one part of the system could influence (and constrain) the design of another part of the system. A range of other domains can create constraints on the design process. The domains can be represented by the different groups involved in the design process, such as ergonomists, engineers, implementers, customers and managers [23]. For instance, other designers may have different guideline selection criteria and needs. Designers rarely work in isolation but must negotiate their design priorities with those of other designers so that the final solution is at least feasible from all perspectives [23].

19.4 BARRIERS TO IMPLEMENTATION OF GUIDELINES

There are external barriers to the implementation of guidelines that are related to organizational factors. Potential external barriers include factors such as organizational culture regarding use of "outside the organization" plans, focusing only on guidelines addressing accuracy and reliability rather than usability, and financial disincentives to guideline use (e.g., delay in product-design-to-market time and increased design-associated costs).

Unfortunately, a gap exists between the information contained in published guidelines and the knowledge and information that are necessary for implementation [24]. Use of guidelines is supposed to make the design process easier to implement and to maintain agreement with previously taken design decisions, but using guidelines can be fairly difficult [25]. Guidelines may be difficult to locate within an organization. Information provided in guidelines is subject to the designer's interpretation. Guidelines can be unclear, paradoxical, conflicting and not always based on the current, scientific peer-reviewed literature. The person using guidelines must have a clear idea about the design objectives and must have the ability to decide whether the guidelines are applicable or not.

The following barriers to guideline implementation are expanded upon from Nicole and Abascal's discussion of using accessibility guidelines [25]:

- Financial costs associated with guideline purchase and use: Although often expensive, electronic reference texts and guidelines minimize the need for physical storage and provide an immediate means of providing access to users. But designers still need access to printed copies of guidelines, and the costs of providing this access are not insignificant. Organizations often consider only the direct costs of guideline purchase and not the future design costs associated with not using the applicable design guidelines. According to Vanderheiden and Tobias [17], any additional costs (e.g., costs associated with guideline purchase and guideline implementation) may be difficult to justify because of internal and external pressures related to limited resources.
- Rapid change in technology making it difficult to keep standards and guidelines up-to-date: Another factor that prevents the use of standards and guidelines is included in a report from the Center for Devices and Radiological Health supported by the Food and Drug Administration, which states that "it is difficult for standards and guidelines to stay current with changes in technology that influence interface design" [5, p. 18].

Guideline application may increase design, materials, and manufacturing costs. Therefore, top management's decisions may influence the designer's use of specific guidelines. "Time to market" is often critical to the product's market share. The design team and the marketing team are often in conflict about the use of guidelines if it slows the commercial availability of a product. Often a seemingly small, cosmetic change in a medical device submitted for FDA review will require an additional review for premarket clearance if a change is made to the device during the review process. As an example, a designer wishes to change a product's color or density of the print ink to improve low-vision or low-light identification of the device top from the bottom. Manufacturers may fear that the additional FDA process will require a device resubmission, holding up the final review and thus delay the product's clearance for market.

Perrow [22] proposed a model of the context of design that emphasizes the organizational and social structures that influence and can be influenced by both designers and human factors engineers. "... Top management goals and perspectives, the reward structure of the organization, insulation of design engineers from the consequences of their decision, and some aspects of organizational culture" are some of the relevant elements of the organizational and social structure discussed by Perrow [22, p. 524]. These organizational factors may influence the factors considered by designers during the design process, as well as the time, attention, and energy that designers spend on understanding the needs and characteristics of end users.

The customers of medical devices are partly responsible for the lack of consideration of HF in the design process. If top managers get "signals" from their customers that human factors aspects of the medical devices (e.g., usability) are important, they will certainly pay attention to HF. HF will then become part of their perspectives, and usability would be an important goal to achieve. Guidelines can play an important role in this process by formalizing the HF knowledge required to improve the design of medical devices. Therefore, customers have an important role to play in pressuring designers and manufacturers of medical devices to consider HF in their design processes. However, one question arises: how powerful are the customers of medical devices and how likely are they to succeed in pressuring the designers and manufacturers? Perrow [22] describes the example of the air transport industry in which performance failures immediately affect profits and reputation. Therefore, there is much pressure from various parties (e.g., the FAA, the National Transportation Safety Board, and the pilots' union) on the designers and manufacturers of systems to consider HF in the design process. How does this apply to the community of disabled end users? Does this community have the power to influence the designers and manufacturers of medical devices, and the institutions that regulate medical devices' design processes?

Considering HF in the design process may not fit with the reward structure of medical devices companies. Top managers of these companies may see very little value (and maybe high cost) to a system design process in which HF plays an important role. Medical devices that incorporate the latest technologies, that are fast and powerful, etc., may be more appealing to top managers than medical devices that are usable, safe to use, etc. [22] The AAMI standards [8] list a number of "potential payoffs of investing in improved usability":

- Faster time to market
- Simpler user manuals and related learning tools
- Improved marketing
- Increased sales
- Reduced customer training and support requirements
- Extended market life
- Clearer compliance with regulatory requirements

We do not know to what extent top managers of medical device companies actually understand or perceive the benefits to be gained from a design process that incorporates HF principles and methods.

Designers may not have any opportunity to know and understand the consequences of their decisions to the users of the medical devices. In many companies, the designers are isolated from the marketing staff and have no contact with customers. Some medical device companies have begun to establish a system for gathering feedback from their customers. Whether this feedback actually reaches the designers of the medical devices is unclear.

Top managers can do much to motivate and encourage designers to consider HF [22]:

- Close proximity between designers and HF engineers
- Requiring that designers learn about HF, e.g., joining the HF group for a "tour of duty"
- Inviting HF engineers to meetings in which design specifications are discussed
- Disseminate information about the contributions of HF engineers
- Informal recognition of the importance of HF engineers

Vicente [26] described a case study of radical change within a PCA pump manufacturing company leading to the adoption of a HF approach for product design. Several factors, including a new leadership and a perception of poor organizational performance, contributed to this change. This case study clearly demonstrates the importance of top management in setting the "right" organizational structure and culture for encouraging and motivating designers to take into account HF in the design process.

19.5 CONCLUSIONS

It is important not only to develop valid guidelines by sound methodology but also to ensure the implementation of evidence-based design recommendations. Guidelines provide an opportunity for users to improve products, expand evidence-based universal design knowledge, and reduce variation in product design. HFE and a systems approach should be used to facilitate guideline implementation by identifying and removing barriers to implementation. Potential activities include awareness-raising initiatives, wide dissemination of guidelines, and using electronic publishing to improve the accessibility and availability of guidelines to designers. Additionally, designers are not often members of sales or marketing departments. Designer interaction with sales, marketing, and finance will help to develop a business case for implementation of appropriate standards and guidelines in product research and development, thus overcoming one of the largest barriers to guideline implementation by designers.

REFERENCES

1. White, P.K., Jr., Systems design, in *Handbook of Systems Engineering and Management*, Sage, A.P., Rouse, W.B., Eds., John Wiley & Sons, New York, 1999, pp. 455–482.
2. Meister, D., Enderwick, T.P., *Human Factors in System Design, Development, and Testing*, L. Erlbaum, Mahwah, NJ, 2002, p. 247.
3. Clegg, C.W., Sociotechnical principles for system design, *Applied Ergonomics,* 31, 463, 2000.
4. Sawyer, D., Do It By Design — An Introduction To Human Factors In Medical Devices, Washington, D.C., 1996, p. 47.
5. Kaye, R., Crowley, J., Guidance for Industry and FDA Premarket and Design Control Reviewers — Medical Device Use-Safety: Incorporating Human Factors Engineering into Risk Management, U.S. Department of Health and Human Services, Food and Drug Administration, Center for Devices and Radiological Health, Division of Device User Programs and Systems Analysis, Office of Health and Industry Programs, Washington, D.C., 2000, p. 33.
6. ANSI/AAMI, HE 48: Human Factors Engineering Guidelines and Preferred Practices for the Design of Medical Devices, Arlington, VA, 1993, p. 88.

7. ANSI/AAMI/ISO, 14971:2000: Medical Devices — Application of Risk Management to Medical Devices, Arlington, VA, 2000, p. 27.
8. ANSI/AAMI, HE 74:2001: Human Factors Design Process for Medical Devices, Arlington, VA, 2001, p. 38.
9. IEA, The Discipline of Ergonomics, retrieved October 6, 2005 from http://www.iea.cc/ergonomics/.
10. Ballay, J.M., An experimental view of the design process, in *System design: Behavioral Perspectives on Designers, Tools, and Organizations*, Rouse, W.B., Boff, K.R., Eds., North-Holland, New York, 1987, pp. 65–82.
11. Weinger, M.B., Pantiskas, C., Wiklund, M.E., Carstensen, P., Incorporating human factors into the design of medical devices, *Journal of the American Medical Association,* 280, 1484, 1998.
12. Lin, L., Isla, R., Doniz, K., Harkness, H., Vicente, K.J., Doyle, J., Applying human factors to the design of medical equipment: Patient-controlled analgesia, *Journal of Clinical Monitoring and Computing*, 14, 253, 1998.
13. U.S. Census Bureau, American FactFinder, retrieved November 20, 2005 from http://factfinder.census.gov/servlet/QTTable?_bm=y&-geo_id=01000US&-qr_name=DEC_2000_SF3_U_DP2&-ds_name=DEC_2000_SF3_U&-_lang=en&-_sse=on.
14. Chapanis, A., *Human Factors in Systems Engineering*, John Wiley & Sons, New York, 1996, p. 332.
15. Smith, M.J., Carayon-Sainfort, P., A balance theory of job design for stress reduction, *International Journal of Industrial Ergonomics,* 4, 67, 1989.
16. Carayon, P., Smith, M.J., Work organization and ergonomics, *Applied Ergonomics*, 31, 649, 2000.
17. Vanderheiden, G., Tobias, J., Barriers, incentives, and facilitators for adoption of universal design practices by consumer product manufacturers, in *Human Factors and Ergonomics Society 42nd Annual Meeting*, Santa Monica, CA, 1998, p. 584.
18. Wulff, I.A., Westgaard, R.H., Rasmussen, B., Ergonomic criteria in large-scale engineering design — I. Management by documentation only? Formal organization vs. designers' perceptions, *Applied Ergonomics*, 30, 191, 1999.
19. Wulff, I.A., Westgaard, R.H., Rasmussen, B., Ergonomic criteria in large-scale engineering design — II. Evaluating and applying requirements in the real-world of design, *Applied Ergonomics,* 30, 207, 1999.
20. Bogner, M.S., An introduction to design, evaluation, and usability testing, in *Ergonomics in Health Care and Rehabilitation*, Rice V.J.B., Ed., Butterworth-Heinemann, Boston, MA, 1998, p. 231.
21. Burns, C.M., Vicente, K.J., Christoffersen, K., Pawlak, W.S., Towards viable, useful and usable human factors design guidance, *Applied Ergonomics*, 28, 311, 1997.
22. Perrow, C., The organizational context of human-factors engineering, *Administrative Science Quarterly,* 28, 521, 1983.
23. Burns, C.M., Vicente, K.J., A participant-observer study of ergonomics in engineering design: how constraints drive design process, *Applied Ergonomics,* 31, 73, 2000.
24. Shiffman, R.N., Michel, G., Essaihi, A., Thornquist, E., Bridging the guideline implementation gap: a systematic, document-centered approach to guideline implementation, *Journal of the American Medical Informatics Association*, 11, 418, 2004.
25. Nicole, C., Abascal, J., *Inclusive Design Guidelines for HCI*, Taylor and Francis, New York, 2001, p. 285.
26. Vicente, K.J., What does it take? A case study of radical change toward patient safety, *Joint Commission Journal on Quality and Safety*, 29, 598, 2003.

20 Reducing Error and Enhancing Access to Home Use of Medical Devices: Designing from the Perspective of the Home Care Provider

Marilyn Sue Bogner

CONTENTS

20.1 INTRODUCTION

Although error in health care has been in the literature for nearly half a century [1,2], it was not until the report on medical error by the Institute of Medicine (IOM) that attributed 44,000 to 98,000 deaths to medical error [3] that the topic became a pressing issue for the public, Congress, and the health care industry. Those numbers essentially were based on retrospective chart reviews of hospitalized individuals. Errors in ambulatory and home care settings were not included, so the 44,000 to 98,000 annual deaths are not representative or even suggestive of the total incidence of adverse events in health care.

Because there are no data for the number of deaths or for the other adverse outcomes of serious injury and prolonged need for medical care attributable to home care error, its magnitude can only be conjectured. Regardless of the incidence, the current and future aging of the population with the attendant chronic conditions and disabilities, the ever increasing reliance on home care, the deleterious affect of error on the well being not only of the home care recipient but also the care provider, and the absence of ready assistance to counteract the impact of an error mandate that concerted efforts be instituted to reduce error and enhance access to assistive and home care medical devices.

To that end, the following discussion considers the nature of error and its relevance in home care by and for elderly and disabled people, briefly presents a heuristic tool — a conceptual model and worksheet for addressing error, and describes how that conceptualization of error can drive the design of assistive and medical devices such that they can be used safely and effectively in home care by and for those populations.

20.2 ERROR

The following discussion may seem overly detailed to some readers; however, the details are given because the conceptualization of error presented, though firmly grounded in research, is different from what is typical, particularly when considering health care error.

20.2.1 Error Defined

Although the topic of error in health care has severe financial consequences and is laden with emotion, there is little unanimity in its definition. Health care error is defined in the IOM report as "The failure of a planned action to be completed as intended (i.e., error of execution) or the use of a wrong plan to achieve an aim (i.e. error of planning)" [3]. Errors have been differentiated into technical errors reflecting skill failures, judgmental errors that involve the selection of an incorrect strategy of treatment, and normative errors that occur when the larger social values embedded within medicine as a profession are violated [4]. Errors also have been described in terms of the aspect of health care in which they occur, such as errors of missed diagnosis, mistakes during treatment, medication misadministration, inadequate postoperative care, and mistaken identity [5].

It is acknowledged that this is not an exhaustive list of definitions of error in health care; however, it is sufficient to illustrate the attitude that is pervasive in definitions of health care error and in nearly all discussions of patient safety — that the care provider is the sole cause of the error and the attendant adverse outcome. Although the focus has been professional health care providers, the attitude pertains to lay care providers. Implicit in that attitude is that errors are caused by carelessness, inattention, and negligence. In keeping with that attitude, efforts to reduce the incidence are focused on the care provider as is apparent in the thrust of the IOM report on error-reporting systems.

20.2.2 Error Reporting

The IOM report advocates that error reporting systems can address and reduce the likelihood of errors in health care by serving two functions: "They can hold providers accountable for performance, or alternatively, they can provide information that can lead to improved safety" [3]. The performance being addressed is providing care in which an error associated with an adverse outcome occurred. Accountability apparently is considered as an end unto itself presupposing that the provider is the source of the problem and by holding the provider accountable, patient safety will be enhanced.

20.2.2.1 Provider Accountability for Error

Error reporting for accountability programs that ask the provider to report any error he or she committed, such as "Dr. Kildarc lacerated Mrs. Patient's liver," provides information about who did what. Additional information sometimes is requested such as time of day and location of the incident; nonetheless, the information collected is who did what. The care providers typically are reluctant to report error because of litigation or disciplinary consequences. The blame culture has been decried, yet when the only cause of error identified is the care provider, then he or she is the only target for blame, hence the blame culture is perpetuated by the emphasis on provider accountability. This can have a particularly negative impact in home care because the care provider typically is a family member or another person who is emotionally connected to the patient and who would be especially devastated by committing an act that is considered an error with an adverse outcome. This is not to absolve the care provider from a role in committing an error, for without a doubt, that person committed the act associated with an adverse outcome. Indeed, if provider accountability reporting is effective, then the blame culture may have credence.

A recent CNN report [6] stated that 195,000 deaths occur annually in hospitals — deaths caused by the care the patients receive. This is far greater than the 100,000 deaths extrapolated from the Harvard Medical Practice Study (HMPS) [7], or the 44,000 to 98,000 preventable deaths stated in the IOM report [3]. The increase in reported deaths due to errors might indicate increased sensitivity to error; however, this seems unlikely given the difference between the 195,000 in the CNN report and the highest estimate of preventable deaths — 100,000 from the HMPS — is 95,000. The specifics of the error reporting programs are varied and geographically diverse so there is little basis to attribute the absence of success to those considerations. Determining the effectiveness of error reporting for provider accountability in reducing the incidence of error is an empirical issue, that is, one to be addressed through experience and research. Fortunately such information is available.

20.2.2.2 Research Findings for Provider Accountability

Shortly after the publication of the IOM report, Congress created the Agency for Health care Research and Quality (AHRQ) and appropriated $50 million per year for 5 years to fund research to reduce the incidence of error by 50% at the end of that time. November 2004 marked the fifth anniversary of the IOM report; a workshop was convened by the Commonwealth Fund to learn of the impact of 5 years of research and other efforts on the incidence of error. Various presenters at that workshop stated in various ways that patient safety is on the right track but the efforts to attain the 50% reduction in error not only did not meet that goal, but the impact of those efforts on error is negligible [8].

The Reuters news service described the information presented at the workshop: "... five years after the IOM report, little data exist showing progress and researchers are still debating not how to save lives, but what to measure" [9]. One presenter stated that "a little bit of progress has been made in U.S. hospitals since 1999, but the difference is not striking" [10]. He went on to say that many states and private health systems require health workers to report medical errors or near misses in which a patient is put at potential risk, but researchers still have not figured out what to do with the reports once they have them.

Although the presenters at the workshop stated that more money, greater cooperation from the medical community, and legislation to protect data from being used in malpractice litigation would expedite progress toward the goal of 50% reduction in medical errors, the lack of progress from the 5 years of efforts very likely indicates that the data gathered, the who did what for provider accountability, do not provide the necessary information to reduce error in health care. One need look no further for an alternative to the who did what approach than the second function of error reporting stated in the IOM report " ... provide information that can lead to improved safety" [3].

To provide that information, it is necessary to identify what needs to be improved; to accomplish that, it is necessary to understand what an error is — the nature of error.

20.2.3 The Nature of Error

The previously quoted definitions of error describe the procedures and aspects of health care in which an error occurs; however, there is no definition of what happens in the process of committing an error — the key to understanding the nature of error. Interestingly enough, the definition is implicit in the consideration of error — error is an act performed by a person that for the purpose of this discussion has an adverse outcome such as death, serious injury, or need for extended treatment; an act is behavior, so error is the result of behavior.

20.2.3.1 Error as Behavior

Because a person commits the error act, that person typically is considered as the sole source of the act. This is accurate and yet incomplete and misleading because an act, by being a behavior by the individual, reflects the impetus for such behavior, which is not solely the volition of that person [11,12]. Centuries of empirical research and theory in the behavioral and physical sciences as well as millennia of philosophical writings attest that behavior, whether of a person or a particle, is a function of the characteristics of that entity and the context in which the behavior — the act — occurs. This has been substantiated albeit inadvertently by the absence of findings that can be implemented to reduce the incidence of error from the research on provider accountability funded by AHRQ and others. Rather, the lack of findings supports the approach grounded in research and theory that to effectively address error it is necessary to consider the context of the error behavior. Given the complexity of the context in which health care is provided including the home and other noninstitutional settings, this may seem to be an insurmountable task; however, results from research on error by industries other than health care provide a simple, powerful approach.

20.3 CONTEXT SYSTEMS APPROACH TO ERROR

Factors in the context in which a person functions influence that person's behavior and as such are involved in error [13,14]. A persuasive argument for considering context in adverse outcomes is stated regarding aviation accidents: "Without full information concerning the context and environments in which accidents occur, it is not possible to understand their genesis and how to take rational steps to prevent future accidents" [15]. Thus, to understand why a care provider committed an error so that rational steps to prevent future adverse events may be taken, it is necessary to address factors in the context in which the error occurred.

20.3.1 Error Research

Research on error conducted by the nuclear power, manufacturing, aviation, and other industries identified categories of environmental factors associated with error [16–18]. The categories that are analogous across industries are applicable to health care with the slight modification that the entity upon which actions are taken, i.e., the product of the endeavor, is a patient rather than a widget or nuclear power plant. Each category is comprised of interacting factors, a system of factors that can impact the task performance of providing health care in a way that results in an error.

20.3.2 Context Systems

It is to be noted that the term *systems* in this discussion refers to categories of factors that affect the individual care provider at the time of providing care. This is not to be confused with the common use of system in discussions of health care as referring to the health care system, which is of dubious accuracy because the various aspects of health care do not interact — a primary characteristic of a system. The context systems in this discussion are the interacting factors that affect the home care provider and only those that affect him or her directly or indirectly.

The systems and examples of factors in each of the categories in terms appropriate for health care are *the patient* (the product of the industry) with personality, psychological factors such as anxiety, and physical characteristics that include weight and frailty, physical mobility and dexterity, cognitive and perceptual acuity in addition to the presenting health problem; *the means of providing care* (the tools for performing a task) such as a medical device together with its physical dimensions and technological sophistication as well as cognitive workload; *the care provider* (the worker) with hard-wired human constraints that include limited perceptual acuity, cognitive functioning including knowledge, heuristics, memory, and anticipation that is affected by stress and fatigue, limited capacity to retain and manipulate units of information, and anthropometric characteristics of height and handedness. Those three categories constitute the nuclear care providing system that is ensconced in a broader context comprised of additional systems of categories of factors identified by industry error research.

The additional five categories with examples indicating the range of factors that can come into play in home care are *ambient conditions* of illumination, temperature, noise, altitude, dust, pet hair; *the physical environment* with placement of medical equipment, room size, clutter, electrical outlets, ventilation, size of bed, availability of water; *the social environment* of other care providers and personnel, professional culture, family members, children, ethnic culture and religion; *organizational factors* such as workload, hours worked, reports, policies for caring for uninsured persons, organizational culture, integrating providing care into work, school and other schedules, medical equipment rental, pharmacies; and *legal-regulatory-reimbursement-national culture factors* that include threat of litigation, regulatory constraints, reimbursement policies, and national cultural mores.

The categories of factors are hierarchical nested systems represented by concentric circles (Figure 20.1). The innermost circle contains the nuclear care providing system of the care provider, the care recipient, and the means of providing care. This system also can represent the special case of self care in which the patient and the care provider are the same individual. The other five systems are nested in the order described in the preceding two paragraphs from the closest to the care provider, the context system with the most direct impact that can be relatively readily

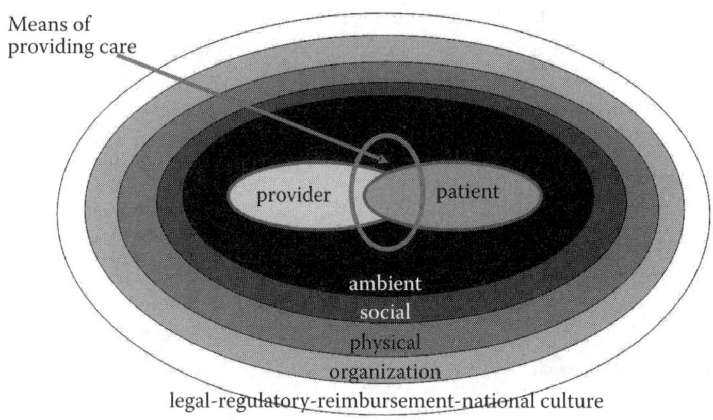

FIGURE 20.1 Context systems of factors that influence behavior. The nuclear care-providing system of the care provider–care recipient means of providing care is nested in the context of the system of ambient conditions. Those systems are affected by the systems of factors in the physical environment context, which are affected by the individuals in the context system of social factors — individuals that by moving the nuclear care-providing system change the context, hence the factors affecting them. Those systems are affected by the factors in the organizational context, which are affected by the overarching context of the legal, regulatory, reimbursement, and national culture factors. Changes in the factors in any context can affect the factors in the other contexts.

changed — that of ambient conditions — to the most difficult to change and furthest removed from the nuclear care providing system — that of the legal-regulatory-reimbursement-national culture factors.

The context systems representation of the factors that can impact the home care provider might be difficult to remember, and because of that, difficult to integrate into everyday consideration of error. As the representation of circumstances that come together to cause an error, the lining up of the holes in slices of Swiss cheese [19], and the various factors that affect performance as layers of an onion [16] have been helpful in conveying concepts of error, the context systems of factors that influence behavior (Figure 20.1) are represented as an artichoke, with the circles of the leaves of the artichoke being analogous to the context systems and the person affected by factors in those systems, the care provider, as the center, the heart of the artichoke (Figure 20.2).

The artichoke representation underscores the critical point of the context systems approach model, that the context systems to be addressed when analyzing an error or in designing an assistive or medical device for home care are those with factors that affect the specific care provider — the individual whose behavior, whose use of assistive and medical devices — is the target of consideration. The interaction of the context systems of an individual can be illustrated by imagining what occurs when the artichoke is squeezed strongly with considerable pressure: the outer leaves, the outer context systems contact or influence the inner ones and ultimately affect the heart of the artichoke — the care provider. When the pressure is sufficiently great, the behavior of the care provider can be so determined by contextual factors — a situation that is not uncommon in home care — that he or she can be considered as "artichoked."

20.3.3 Value of the Context Systems Artichoke Approach

When determining why an incident occurred, the representation of systems encourages consideration of each of those systems for factors that affected the care provider. This is important in countering the "stop rule" — the tendency for people, in seeking to explain why a situation occurred by backward chaining of possible causes, to stop when a plausible, easily explained cause is identified [20]. In health care, the explanation that triggers the stop rule typically is the care provider who committed the error. The context systems approach by determining why the act was committed goes beyond the care provider to consider factors in other systems. Thus, this context systems conceptualization of error is an ordered approach to understanding complex phenomena of error behavior — a systems approach. A simple heuristic tool — a worksheet — can be used to identify factors that contributed to an error [21].

20.3.3.1 Worksheet Tool

A simple tool can assist in eliciting and documenting context system factors that have affected a care provider so as to contribute to error behavior. Once identified, those factors can be addressed to reduce or eliminate their error-inducing impact. The worksheet tool also can be used in designing devices for use in home care by prompting consideration of factors in that setting to be addressed and accommodated by the design.

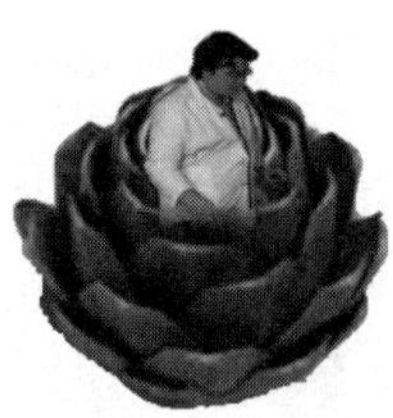

FIGURE 20.2 Context systems affecting the provider.

Briefly, the worksheet is the list of the context systems, each with a blank line beside the name where factors that have or are suspected to have contributed to an error are noted. For example, in misreading the display of a monitor, the ambient condition of dim light is a likely factor as is the equipment surrounding the display that hampers direct vision. The use of the worksheet when designing a home care device is discussed subsequently.

20.4 ERROR BY DESIGN

Often, if not typically, medical devices are designed by individuals who have had minimal or no experience using medical devices or providing health care — for this discussion, providing care in the home. Because of this, designers are limited in their understanding of what is necessary to safely provide health care amid the myriad of factors in a home that can challenge the use of medical and assistive devices — conditions that can lead to if not provoke error. Home care providers not only are not trained, but often are older individuals who are affected by multiple medications and accompanying side affects as well as the perceptual, manual dexterity, and other physical changes that are associated with aging. Such factors affect the provision of care not only of another individual but also in self care when the care recipient and the care provider are the same person.

20.4.1 Self Care

Self care by aging individuals and persons with disabilities is of particular concern because by being both care provider and recipient without an external moderator of the impact of that care, impairment from an error in the use of a medical or assistive device compromises future care, which contributes to other errors and additional impairment of the provider's/patient's condition. Thus, a degenerative cycle is created that most likely will result in an adverse outcome. Because of the chronic nature of physical disabilities, the effects of aging, the many diseases treated in the home, and the relative isolation of the lay care provider from sources of assistance in using the devices, it is imperative that assistive and medical devices be designed to be used safely and effectively in self care that can be conducted in a variety of settings as well as in home care.

20.4.1.1 Examples

1. A simple example of error by design that is pervasive in self care and in home care is one that provokes falls in the bathroom: the placement of the toilet tissue holder that is not in easy reach of the potential user [22]. This requires the individual to lean or swivel to reach the tissue; persons with a short reach and those whose reach is compromised by disability or injury and/or those whose sense of balance is compromised by medication may lean so far as to fall. The reader can verify this error by design condition by observing bathrooms in homes and in facilities for people with disabilities. Had the bathroom designer used the context systems worksheet and, as prompted, considered at least the physical characteristics of a home care patient and the physical environment, such an error-provoking design might not have occurred. It should be noted that in considering the context systems of the worksheet, it is important to design for a worst case scenario such as a small frail elderly person with limited reach who is unsteady from medication. If such a person can function in the situation then others who are not so compromised will be able to do so without error.
2. Many devices used in home care are powered by electricity. In designing such devices so they can be used safely and effectively for home care by elderly and disabled people and by those caring for debilitating chronic conditions, the use of the worksheet tool can focus the designer's attention on conditions in the context that must be accommodated by the device design. Many people age in place — that is, they remain in the home they purchased 50 or 60 plus years ago. The wiring in that home most likely has not been replaced, so

the electrical outlets cannot accommodate the three-pronged plugs nor can the power supply accommodate the power demands of the devices. In addition, the home has no back-up power supply, so when a power outage occurs, the device functions on the battery for whatever short duration that it is operational. There is no manual means on the device to generate power. This error in design could rapidly cause an adverse event. It is to be noted that some portable radios can be powered manually and devices to manually generate power for cell phones are available — manual power generation is feasible.

3. The value of using the context systems artichoke worksheet when designing devices is apparent when considering the ubiquitous assistive device of crutches. The characteristics of the individual in need of assistance who may be elderly and living alone with minimal upper body strength are challenged by the use of the device with the results of sore shoulders, arms, and very likely back pain. Nonetheless crutches are preferred to a wheelchair, given difficulty in accessing bathrooms due to the size of the door and in transporting the chair from one locale to another. A person using crutches for an injury or surgery may not heal as expected. This can be the result of aggravating the wound or injury by putting weight on the limb to engage in activities of daily living such as transferring food from the freezer to microwave to table because it is not possible to carry anything and walk with crutches. Thus, when the physical environment context for use of that assistive device is considered, it becomes apparent that the error of putting weight on the injured extremity is provoked by the design — the crutches need to be designed so that an object can be carried while walking with them.

Using the worksheet when developing the design of a device is of vital importance because the context systems of physical environmental factors in which a device is to be used can determine not only how but also if the device will be used. A device that may be readily used by elderly and disabled people in a physical therapy department or clinic may not be usable in a home setting. For example, walking with crutches on a level nonslick surface may be doable for an elderly or disabled person; however, walking down a ramp that has a slope such that the person's body is thrust forward making it difficult to walk at a measured pace with crutches or to maintain one's balance can provoke a fall that might be considered as resulting from misuse of the device. Devices for use in home care must be designed with respect to the range of situations in which they could be used. To do this, the perspective of the user, including his or her perspective of contexts in which the device will be used, must drive the design of home care devices.

20.5 HOME CARE USER PERSPECTIVE DRIVEN DESIGN

Designing medical devices from the perspective of actual care providers — not the device designer's concept of the providers' perspective — not only can reduce the likelihood of error in the use of home care devices by special populations such as elderly individuals and people with disabilities but also enhances access to such devices by those populations. Access to a device is precluded when it is not functionally viable for those most in need of its use — those most debilitated by age, disability, and chronic disease. How does a designer learn the perspective of those who use medical and assistive devices in home care? From the device users themselves, an approach that has been quite successful in addressing patient care issues [23].

The Pittsburgh Regional Health Initiative (PRHI) has found that those who are closest to a problem know the most about it and have useful suggestions on how to alleviate it [23]. In other words, care providers know from experience the influence of the various aspects of the context (the systems of the artichoke, including their own characteristics and the device design) on the way they use the device. With respect to the design of assistive and medical devices for home care, the stage can be set for obtaining the perspective of the user by casually watching him or her interact with the device in typical home or field settings such as grocery. When the observer notes awkwardness in an aspect of use, he or she asks the user about it and how it might be improved — the names of the context systems from the worksheet can be used as prompts to obtain as complete a reply as possible. This can continue until the user believes and the observer concurs that all problem aspects of the device have been addressed. Use of self care devices as well as caring for another person should be observed in as many settings as possible to ensure maximum problem identification. This should take place with most articulate and most debilitated of the target populations to design for the worst case scenarios.

Information useful in designing devices to prevent errors also can be gleaned by considering near misses — errors that almost happened, but at the last moment were avoided, and hazards, potential errors, accidents waiting to happen — conditions that are not associated with an adverse outcome. It should be noted that an error can have an innocuous outcome or no outcome at all; however, typically errors that are noteworthy are those associated with adverse events.

20.6 IMPLICATIONS

The population is aging with concomitant increases in chronic illness and compromised perceptual and physical abilities. Hence the need for health care by those populations as well as by individuals who are disabled through disease, combat, or accident will increase to a pressing societal necessity in the foreseeable future. The cost of health care is escalating, with hospital care becoming focused on acute illness, surgery, and emergency care, such that care that previously was provided in hospitals by health care professionals has been relegated to the home. Often medical devices designed for hospital or clinic use by trained health care providers also are relegated to the home to be used by lay care providers.

In the past, home care was provided by a stay-at-home wife or maiden aunt; however, there are few such individuals in these early years of the 21st century. Home care is provided by those who are not employed outside the home — typically an older, retired spouse or sibling of the person with the health problem or the individual engages in self-care typically of a chronic condition. Thus the stage for error is set — individuals whose abilities may be compromised by age, illness, and medication side effects endeavor to provide care, often in a home setting that is not amenable to the use of technologically sophisticated medical devices.

When the demands of a task exceed the abilities of the person expected to perform it, as in home care, error ensues. To avoid error and enhance access to medical devices by those involved in home care (people who may be elderly, disabled, or have chronic diseases) the devices must be designed to be used safely and effectively by the most frail of the potential users in the most basic home setting. Designing a device to be used by home care providers without accommodating for the conditions of the context in which the device will be used is inviting misuse, error, and adverse outcomes.

To effectively design devices for home use it is necessary — indeed, it is mandatory — that the perspectives of the actual users of such devices and their perspectives of the use context in their homes be obtained and accommodated by the design. Once the device prototype is developed, it should be placed in worst case situations, and the access and ease of use explored and assessed. The prototype should not be used to actually provide care if that could potentially harm the patient. The prototype could and should be tested by actual severely disabled users in simulated worst case scenarios and the perspectives of the users on the device design obtained. The systems context worksheet can be used in discussing the ease of use of the device so that all aspects of the context can be explored — for example, if the warning lights and alarms are apparent to the user, the extent to which the device fits in the physical environment of the home and if the device settings can be safely changed in the midst of conversations.

Considering the role of context systems in provoking error and in designing a medical device for general use and particularly for home care, necessitates a change in the paradigm for addressing error. Typically the paradigm of health care error has been that the person, the care provider, is the sole source of the error. The time has come and the evidence is available to consider error for what it actually is — a behavior that reflects the interaction of the individual with factors in the environment — the context systems. The implications of such a paradigm change is that medical and assistive devices used in home care would be designed to accommodate all aspects of the user's perspective of the systems of the context of use and by doing so use error would be reduced and access to those devices would be enhanced for home care of the elderly and disabled.

REFERENCES

1. Safren, M.A. and Chapanis, A. (May 1, 1960), A critical incident study of hospital medication errors — part 1, *Hospitals, J.A.H.A. 34*, 32–66.
2. Safren, M.A. and Chapanis, A. (May 16, 1960), A critical incident study of hospital medication errors — part 2, *Hospitals, J.A.H.A. 34*, 54–68.
3. Kohn, L.T., Corrigan, J.M., and Donaldson, M.S. (Eds.) (1999), *To Err is Human: Building a Safer Health System*, Washington, D.C.: National Academy Press.
4. Bosk, C. (1979), *Forgive and Remember: Managing Medical Failures,* Chicago, IL: University of Chicago Press.
5. Gibson, R. and Singh, J.P. (2003), *Wall of Silence: The Untold Story of the Medical Mistakes That Kill and Injure Millions of Americans*, Washington, D.C.: Lifeline Press.
6. CNN.com, Study: Hospital Errors Cause 195,000 Deaths, July 28, 2004.
7. Leape, L.L., Brennan, T.A., Laird, N., Lawthers, A.G., Localio, A.R., Barnes, B.A., Hebert, L., Newhouse, J.P., Weiler, P.C., and Hiatt, H. (1991), The nature of adverse events in hospitalized patients, *New England Journal of Medicine, 324*, 377–384.
8. Commonwealth Fund (2004), See website Commonwealth Fund/Quality Improvement/Patient Safety/*Quality Matters*: November Newsletter, http://www.cmwf.org
9. Zwillich, T. (2004), *Little Progress Seen in Patient Safety Measures*, Washington: Reuters Health Information, November 4, 2004.
10. Wachter, R. (2004), Patient Safety Five Years After *To Err Is Human*. Commonwealth Fund web site/ Quality Improvement/Patient Safety/Quality Matters: November 4 Newsletter, http://www.cmwf.org
11. Bogner, M.S. (1994), *Human Error in Medicine,* Mahwah, NJ: Lawrence Erlbaum.
12. Bogner, M.S. (2004), Understanding human error, In Bogner, M.S., Ed., *Misadventures in Health Care: Inside Stories*, Mahwah, NJ: Lawrence Erlbaum, pp. 41–58.
13. Bogner, M.S. (2004), *Misadventures in Health Care: Inside Stories,* Mahwah, NJ: Lawrence Erlbaum.
14. Bogner, M.S. (2002), Stretching the search for the "why" of error: The systems approach, *Journal of Clinical Engineering, 27*, 110–115.
15. Billings, C.E. (1997), *Aviation Automation: The Search for a Human-Centered Approach*, Mahwah, NJ: Lawrence Erlbaum.
16. Moray, N. (1994), Error reduction as a systems problem, in Bogner, M.S., Ed., *Human Error in Medicine* Hillsdale, NJ: Lawrence Erlbaum, pp. 67–92.
17. Rasmussen, J. (1982), Human errors: a taxonomy for describing human malfunction in industrial installations. *Journal of Occupational Accidents, 4,* 311–333.
18. Senders, J.W. and Moray, N.P. (1991), *Human Error: Cause, Prediction, and Reduction*, Mahwah, NJ: Lawrence Erlbaum.
19. Rasmussen, J. (1990), Human error and the problem of causality in analysis of accidents, *Philosophical Transactions of the Royal Society of London, 337*, 449–462.
20. Reason, J. (1990), *Human Error,* New York: Cambridge University Press.
21. Bogner, M.S. (2000), A systems approach to medical error, in Vincent, C. and DeMol, B., Eds., *Safety in Medicine,* Amsterdam: Pergamon, pp. 83–100.
22. Chapanis, A. (January 1996), Perspective: Musings from a Hospital Bed, *Ergonomics in Design,* pp. 35–36.
23. Pittsburgh Regional Healthcare Initiative (October 2005), PRHI Executive Summary, www.prhi.org.

21 Use of Problem-Solving Tools of TRIZ to Address Equipment Design for Home Care

John W. Gosbee

CONTENTS

ABSTRACT

Design problems complicate the many efforts to move complex health care equipment into the home setting, where users have a greater diversity of abilities. Many design solutions to these problems are a compromise, rather than breakthrough thinking. TRIZ, which consists of design problem-solving techniques and invention-related data, is one likely approach to breakthrough design. TRIZ may help resolve equipment design issues for home care, including how to think out strategies for providing access for persons with diverse abilities. Moreover, many TRIZ techniques can be used hand in hand with human factors engineering techniques such as usability testing.

21.1 INTRODUCTION

When hospital systems, with high complexity and many resources, are moved into the home setting, with its lower complexity and fewer resources, design problems often sabotage the result. Additionally, intended (or unintended) users in this setting many have a greater diversity of abilities. These problems reach new heights when some companies move very complex health care operations into the home (e.g., home hemodialysis). In many cases, the proposed solutions to these problems are a compromise, such as developing a slightly simpler version of the system than that used in hospitals, rather than "breakthrough thinking." In this chapter, an approach called TRIZ is developed, which has potential for resolving issues in equipment design for home care.

21.1.1 What Is TRIZ?

TRIZ is a Russian acronym for Theoria Resheneyva Isobretatelskehuh Zadach, which can be translated as the "theory of solving problems inventively." TRIZ was formulated and said to be a discovery by a talented patent examiner for the Russian navy, Genrich Altshuller [1]. Altshuller originated much of his principles and techniques after studying 200,000 Russian patents during the early 1900s. He recognized that technological systems described in these patents followed predictable patterns. He postulated that using this information could help improve the efficiency of technical evolution. One key aspect of many patents was that problem-solving principles seemed to follow certain trends or themes. Altshuller continued to develop and teach these ideas with others for the next several decades.

TRIZ consists of design problem-solving techniques and invention-related data. TRIZ is one likely approach to embrace or more fully resolve issues for equipment design for home care, including how to think out strategies for providing persons with diverse abilities with access to products to which there would be benefit. Moreover, many TRIZ techniques can be used hand in hand with human factors engineering (HFE) techniques such as usability testing.

21.1.2 Aims of This Chapter

This chapter provides overviews of the main TRIZ concepts and tools, such as "ideality," using all resources, design contradictions, and the invention matrix. It then provides examples from TRIZ literature (there are few medical ones). Several conceptual examples of home medical devices or systems and TRIZ are provided. This is followed by a discussion about how data from usability testing and other HFE methods could be a "feeder system" for the TRIZ techniques. Finally, the role of HFE methods as evaluation techniques of the TRIZ-inspired designs is developed.

21.2 THE ESSENCE OF *TRIZ*

TRIZ can be conceived of as a thinking strategy and a family of tools [2]. The thinking strategy is almost always useful in solving (at least) design problems. The family of tools each has strengths and weaknesses. Therefore, the understanding and efficient application of tools varies depending on the problem type or setting.

Basics of TRIZ include:

- The idea that systems (through inventions) evolve toward ideality
- Moving to ideality by taking advantage of resources within the system
- Resolving or embracing design contradictions as they evolve — not compromising
- Inventive principles can be summarized and presented in a contradiction table

21.2.1 Concept of Ideality or "Ideal Final Result"

This concept seems simple, but most people find it difficult to state the ideal final result clearly. It is hard for people to state how their real goal can be accomplished unfettered by past design constraints. It is hard to conceive of how to do the task with fewest resources. Many developers, engineers, or scientists have put many hours into solving a wrongly or incompletely stated problem. Ideality is about restating the problem so that the useful functions are maximized and harmful functions minimized.

21.2.1.1 Ideality Examples

An everyday example might be to travel from home to work using no energy or no money. A medical example is the problem of mechanical ventilation to a patient with high cervical spine injury. One step towards an ideality statement might be to provide a mechanical ventilator that needs no electrical power source. An even more ideal statement would be to attempt to get the person's blood oxygenated and carbon dioxide removed with no invasive tubes, unfettered, and with no power.

21.2.2 Resource Checklist

Because innovators who want to reach ideality need to use more and more existing resources, it is a crucial activity to develop a comprehensive list of these resources [3]. Then, one can use this resource listing as a checklist when creating new design ideas. Indeed, the full list of resources for even the simplest system can be quite long. For a shoe, the list of physical objects includes laces, sole, and eyelets. Fields would include static electrical field, a small magnetic field, and gravity. Information resources would be existence of smell or not and whether the shoe is dirty or not.

21.2.2.1 Example of Resource Checklist in Action

One example in TRIZ literature is trying to think of the ideal way to remove the cores from a million green bell peppers [2]. Hand-carving and core-removal machines exist, but require many external resources. What resources does the pepper have that could help remove the core with minimal or no external resources? Most people would list seeds and water inside the pepper … which can be heated up to pop off the core and stem of the pepper.

21.2.3 Design Contradictions

Embracing — Not Compromising — Design Contradictions: Most design problems arise when trying to meet the needs of the user (customer), but then reality creeps in [2]. The balance between wanted and unwanted characteristics is termed *design contradictions* in TRIZ literature. For example, an item needs to be made of strong material, but making it stronger might increase the less desirable characteristic of weight. A vehicle needs to have good fuel economy, but the customer also wants faster acceleration and larger size. An organization might want open office space that is conducive to collaboration, but also quieter closed office space for phone communications. Or, a homeowner desires security, but also a welcoming appearance and easy access for the family members.

After a lifetime of suggestions to compromise with our family, coworkers, and friends, we all compromise reflexively. The approach and tools in TRIZ are aimed at embracing or resolving the contradictions, not simple compromise. The designer has the mindset of creating new rules or parameters, not meeting in the middle. The engineer has rules of thumb for handling typical types of contradictions, not half-way methods that take away from functionality.

21.2.3.1 Specific Nonmedical Example of Design Contradictions

If your company wanted every employee to bring exercise weights on travel (via airplane), they might decide you need a 20-lb weight to exercise fully. Upon asking, they find out most employees want to carry only 2 lb. Compromise dictates an 11-lb weight that satisfies neither group. If a person addresses this contradiction, they might find that a water-filled exercise weight exists for travel. The weight is now light during transport, heavy when lifting for exercise.

21.2.3.2 Design Contradictions in Home Health Care

There are many design contradictions in home health care. Given that many tools and work products were merely moved from hospitals (many resources) to homes (fewer resources), one might expect any existing contradictions to be worsened. These are four examples:

1. The ability to use existing holes in people without "using," or clogging, those holes.
2. Making sure pertinent diagnoses and treatment plans of the person receiving home care are clear and obvious to caregivers, while making the medical data "invisible" (anonymous) to preserve confidentiality.
3. Making the infusion pump easy to program and manipulate for some, but hard to tamper or inadvertently change settings by others.
4. Providing several readable (large font) warnings and information on the medication container, but the container is small for portability.

More on these examples and discussion of how to use TRIZ approaches will follow below.

21.2.4 TRIZ Contradiction Table

A seemingly ready-to-use tool is a TRIZ contradiction table that purports to catalogue many of the patterns of invention [2]. The table consists of 40 innovative principles listed in the cells of the table with 39 engineering parameters in the rows (feature to improve) and columns (undesired result). When analyzing the design or manufacturing problem, the concept is to fit the problem into this intimidating matrix.

It is beyond the scope of this chapter to describe this table more fully or how it might apply to home care equipment design.

21.2.5 TRIZ Separation Principles to Address Design Contradictions

The concept of separation principles can help an innovator work through and address the contradictions in the design process. The list of principles is "separation in time," "separation in space," "separation between parts and the whole," and "separation upon conditions." A design contradiction is cars on two roads that intersect cannot be in the same space at the same time. Examples in many cities of how they have addressed this contradiction include

- Separation in time → stop lights
- Separation in space → overpass
- Separation between parts and the whole → a rotary intersection
- Separation upon conditions → a drawbridge

21.3 CASE STUDIES OF HOME CARE EQUIPMENT AND TRIZ

There are few references when searching the research literature about applying TRIZ to any aspect of health care. Using "TRIZ" as a search term in PubMed reveals one partially applicable reference [4], which focuses on the use of TRIZ to design a safer knife for industrial workers. Searching the Internet (e.g., Google) reveals more TRIZ and health care activity, but a cursory review shows the sites to be private consultant groups — and even the short description of this chapter on the planning Web site. Given no direct examples in literature, conceptual examples will be used to illustrate TRIZ separation principles.

21.3.1 Example #1

Use existing entryways in the body for therapy without clogging them. More specifically, depending upon a breathing tube in the trachea–larynx connected to mechanical ventilation, but wanting the ability to speak through the same trachea–larynx. Separation in time could be demonstrated by intermittent removal of the tube for short stints of speech. Separation in space and time could be putting the breathing tube through a hole in the neck to bypass the larynx, but allow air to occasionally exhale out through the larynx for speech (e.g., Passy-Muir valve) [5].

21.3.2 Example #2

Making sure pertinent diagnoses and treatment plans of the person receiving home care are clear and obvious to caregivers, while making the medical data "invisible" (anonymous) to preserve confidentiality. For example, if caregivers need to know during home care that a person is at risk for falling due to neurological changes secondary to diabetes, large signs could alert them. However, privacy dictates that diagnosis be protected (hidden) to the extent possible. Simply put, this means medical advice that is obvious, yet hidden.

A simple design might be to consider separation in time, where a characteristic is present at one time and absent at another. Perhaps information can be present only when health care personnel are present using electronic signage. Another design might take advantage of separation in space, where a characteristic is present in one place and absent in another. A possible design could be "bluer" lights that illuminate text on signs (e.g., "dark lights") are turned on when providers are present. But the same text is not visible with normal home lighting.

21.3.3 Example #3

Making the infusion pump easy to program and manipulate for some, but hard to tamper or inadvertently change settings by others. A design idea might take advantage of separation in space, where a characteristic is present in one place and absent in another. For instance, a plastic cover on a hinge could be lowered over the front of the infusion pump to cover buttons when not in use. Switch covers such as this are used in industry and in hotel conference room thermostat controls.

21.3.4 Example #4

Providing several readable (large font) warnings and information on the medication container, but the container is small for portability. Using separation in space, the label print could be made "larger" by using a small magnifying glass (plastic) attached to the container. Applying separation of condition, where a characteristic is high under one condition and low under another, one could imagine a "pull-out" extension of the printed material. Thus, the information display space is larger when being read, but smaller when carried in a pocket or purse.

21.4 RELATION TO USABILITY AND HUMAN FACTORS ENGINEERING METHODS

21.4.1 Usability Testing as a "Feeder System" for TRIZ

Data from human factors engineering methods applied to home care devices consist mainly of design issues to be fixed or user needs that have gone unmet [6,7]. Usability testing, for example, often reveals problems with existing products related to confusion, inadvertent misuse, and errors that would likely lead to adverse events. During usability testing, it should emphasized that there is a need to use a diverse pool of subjects for testing to ascertain user needs.

As a design team starts to use TRIZ techniques, they will find that many TRIZ-related data is hard to find or hypothesize (e.g., brainstorm). The team will likely need the following specific data from usability testing, such as:

- Information about true user needs to create a better list of contradiction dyads and clearer ideality statements
- Listing of usability flaws, which are often the specific data needed to frame the all-important design contradiction statements
- Fuller understanding of the user environment and interaction with other systems, which provides a more comprehensive inventory of all available resources

21.4.2 HFE Methods and TRIZ-Inspired Designs

Once an innovative idea has arisen from TRIZ methods, it still needs to be evaluated to know if the designers have paid attention to human limitations and characteristics. For the most part TRIZ tools are silent about how and when to do iterative testing of prototypes. Also, prototypes arising from TRIZ processes need to be evaluated in complex settings for usability at various stages — just as any product development process [8,9]. Of note, usability testing does not just happen in large medical product companies; hospitals that have redesigned work areas have used this method [10].

21.5 CONCLUSION AND RECOMMENDATIONS

TRIZ consists of design problem-solving techniques that many have touted for breakthrough thinking in design — innovation. TRIZ is one likely approach to embrace or more fully resolve issues for equipment design for home care, including strategies that could enable more individuals to access and safety use such equipment. TRIZ methods could help break the patterns of older devices that are not as accessible or usable as they could be. Moreover, many TRIZ techniques should be used hand in hand with human factors engineering techniques such as usability testing.

REFERENCES

1. Altshuller, G., Altov, H., and Shulvak, L., *And Suddenly the Inventor Appeared*, Technology Innovation Center, Worcester, MA, 1996.
2. Clark, D.W., *TRIZ: Through the Eyes of an American Specialist,* Applied Innovation Alliance, West Bloomfield, MI, 2002.
3. Rantanen, K. and Domb, E., *Simplified TRIZ: New Problem Solving Applications for Engineers and Manufacturing Professionals*, CRC Press, Boca Raton, FL, 2002.
4. Marsot, J. and Claudon, L., Design and ergonomics: methods for integrating ergonomics at hand tool design stage, *Int J Occup Saf Ergon*, 10, 13, 2004.
5. Kaut, K., Turcott, J.C., and Lavery, M., Passy-Muir speaking valve, *Dimens Crit Care Nurs*., 15, 298, 1996.
6. Gosbee, J.W. and Gosbee, LL., *Using Human Factors Engineering to Improve Patient Safety*, Joint Commission Resources, Oakbrook Terrace, IL, 2005.
7. Gosbee, J.W. Conclusion: you need human factors engineering expertise to see design hazards that are hiding in "plain sight!" *Jt Comm J Qual Saf*., 30, 696, 2004.
8. American National Standards Institute, Association for the Advancement of Medical Instrumentation, Human Factors Design Process for Medical Devices (ANSI/AAMI HE74:2001), Arlington, VA, 2001.
9. U.S. Food and Drug Administration, Human Factors Implications of the New GMP Rule: New Quality System Regulation that Apply to Human Factors, Washington, D.C., 1998.
10. McLaughlin, R.C., Redesigning the crash cart: usability testing improves one facility's medication drawers, *Am J Nurs.,* 103, 64, 2003.

22 Development of the Medical Equipment Device Accessibility and Universal Design Information Tool

Roger O. Smith, Kris Barnekow, Melissa R. Lemke, Rochelle Mendonca, Melinda Winter, Todd Schwanke, and Jack M. Winters

CONTENTS

ABSTRACT

The chapter reports on the early development of the medical equipment device accessibility and universal design information tool (MED-AUDIT). The MED-AUDIT is a software-based assessment system that incorporates innovative measurement strategies to quantify and score the accessibility of medical devices by breaking down scoring categories into strategic measurement categories. The MED-AUDIT embeds three domains of measurement constructs (functional tasks, device features, and impairments) into two versions of the MED-AUDIT. One version targets use by accessibility/universal design experts and the other targets accessibility/ universal design novices. Both demonstrate an ability to quantify accessibility. Studies to validate the instruments are underway to verify their reliability and validity.

22.1 INTRODUCTION

Medical instruments are not inherently accessible for people with disabilities. Designers and engineers do not typically create medical devices with all populations in mind. Consequently, people with disabilities encounter difficulties using medical instruments in physician's offices, outpatient clinics, hospital rooms, surgical procedures, nursing homes, and even with self-administered health procedures for use at home [1–5]. Examples include wheelchair users who may not be able to climb up on top of a physician's exam table, individuals who are blind who cannot use a standard syringe, and individuals who are dyslexic who cannot read instructions to follow a medical-related procedure.

People with disabilities often do not receive equitable health care [6–7]. One quotation from an individual with a disability stated, "Throughout my pregnancy so far, they don't know how much weight I've gained, because they don't have a platform or sitting scale. They didn't monitor my weight at all" [8]. Another patient with a disability responding to treatment received in the dentist's office stated, "When I go to the dentist, I just remain in my chair" [9]. Other examples of in accessibility of various types of medical devices are provided in Chapter 2 and Chapter 1 of this book.

The answer seems simple. Engineers and equipment designers must be encouraged to develop medical instruments that are accessible by all individuals, including people with disabilities. The problem, however, is not so simple. Designers are not typically familiar with people with disabilities (Chapter 18 of this book). Plus, no guidelines exist that directly address how to design medical equipment for populations of users that include people with disabilities. Designers would have an easier time if they had examples. However, very few examples of accessible equipment are available as prototypes.

Ideally, we would have measures of accessibility to use as we examine medical instruments to identify and determine the severity of the accessibility problem. Such an instrument would have multiple benefits, including the following:

1. An access measure would serve as a tool for designers to compare different designs to optimize the accessibility of a new medical device.
2. Such a measure would allow researchers to identify exact levels and profiles of accessible needs for different types of disabilities and for different types of devices.
3. If a reliable and valid measure were available, a threshold and standards could be generated to assure equitable treatment and equitable access to medical procedures by people with disabilities.

22.2 SPECIFICATIONS OF AN ACCESSIBILITY MEASURE

An accessibility measure must meet a number of measurement criteria. Some criteria are general functional goals of such an assessment. Others are important methodological criteria necessary for the implementation of any acceptable evaluation system. Specifications of an accessibility measure are assumed here to include at least the following seven characteristics.

1. The measure must quantify accessibility. The measure must be more precise than a qualitative discussion and subjective comparison of accessibility characteristics. Numerical scores must be objective to optimize its usefulness. In the area of validity, the accessibility measure must demonstrate construct, consequential, content, predictive, and concurrent validity.

2. Scores must relate to many major impairment types. People with disabilities have a wide variety of functional impairments. People with disabilities include people with sensory impairments such as those who are hard of hearing, deaf, blind, or have low vision impairments. Motor impairments are also a type of functional impairment that often affects individuals with limb amputations, paralysis, or overall body endurance fatigue or weakness. Individuals who have intellectual/cognitive impairments also have expressive or comprehensive language impairments, or memory problems. Lastly, many individuals have behavioral or mental impairments that can cause safety issues. Each of the groups represents a large population [10]. An accessibility measure must be inclusive and examine the accessibility of medical devices for a wide variety of functional impairment types.
3. Scores of such an instrument must delineate between essential and desirable accessibility features. Some features of the medical device are required. Without the feature an individual with disability may not be able to use the device at all. On the other hand, some features can be helpful for someone with disability, but not necessarily essential for basic use of the device. An accessibility measure must delineate and produce essential and desirable accessibility scores. As terminology about accessibility can be confusing, for the purposes of this chapter we will operationally call the construct of essential access, "essential access," and the concept of desirable access, "nonessential access."
4. Measures must assist designers by identifying problem areas in their designs. If an accessibility measure only produces an outcome score it might be helpful to compare one device to another. However, part of the goal of an accessibility assessment targets medical instrument designers. Consequently, such a measure must have a diagnostic function. The assessment should "drill down" to identify specific design issues so a designer can reconfigure, reengineer, or remodel the conceptualization to improve on the product design.
5. The accessibility measure must produce scores that make sense for public review. An accessibility measure cannot be so esoteric that only individuals who are highly trained or specialized can understand what scores mean. For example, an accessibility measure must provide a "percent" accessibility score or some other number meaningful to a wide spectrum of individuals interested in medical instrument and medical procedure accessibility.
6. One of the most daunting design criteria for an accessibility measure is that the scores must be credible, robust, and consistent when used by different raters, or from individual to individual. In terms of test and measurement theory, an accessibility measure must be reliable and valid. This includes a number of reliability criteria such as inter-rater reliability, test/retest reliability, and internal consistency.
7. Lastly of course, an accessibility measure must be practical to use in terms of time, training required, and cost.

22.2.1 Is a Measure of Accessibility for Medical Instruments Really Necessary?

Today, designers do not have sufficient accessibility and universal design expertise to design medical instruments for appropriate application with a wide range of people with disabilities. Designers, policy makers, and consumers need to be able to compare and discriminate between the effectiveness of designs in terms of accessibility. These constituents also cannot depend on the goodwill and intuitive best design of engineers and instrument developers. Whereas most designers are altruistic and truly wish the best for people with disabilities, their charge for designing medical devices must also be practical and cost-effective. Many people with disabilities fall at the extremes of a normal bell curve that captures various characteristics of the overall population. Consequently, when a medical device developer designs for individuals who meet the 5th to the 95th percentile of characteristics such as abilities or anthropometrics, a larger proportion of people with disabilities are typically left out.

Related to this are orphan medical technologies that are created and developed because they are needed by relatively small populations of individuals, normally produced by relatively small manufacturers and small businesses (i.e., often at a higher cost to the consumer). Creating accessible designs, particularly when expertise is not contained in-house, becomes an additional expense which is not today practical for the R&D teams in small businesses. Although all design teams need to have resources and better tools to design more accessible and effective medical devices, the need for such resources magnifies for the small businesses and small R&D teams.

22.2.2 If We Had a Magic Wand ...

In the best of all worlds we would have an accessibility scale that would score a device from 0 (as a terrible design and no one can use it) to a score of 100 (equaling the perfect design that anyone could fully use). Obviously, in between would be the range of scores in which the higher the score the better, but scores in between would also identify specific design problems and provide recommendations as they are revealed. Figure 22.1 illustrates an imaginary, perfectly designed accessibility scale.

Some people say that we cannot measure accessibility. Their apprehension is well grounded as reliably and validly measuring accessibility is indeed a challenge. There are several reasons for this doubt and challenge.

In the rehabilitation and disability fields we have identified the extreme variability of people with disabilities for many years [11]. Virtually infinite numbers of types of people with disabilities exist, ranging from someone who cannot grasp a device, to someone who has a body tremor and cannot sit still, to a person who cannot see, to a person who has tactile defensiveness and cannot tolerate contact with foreign materials, to a person with a behavioral problem who cannot cooperate with unfamiliar people or procedures, to a person who is so tall that they cannot fit in virtually any standard positioning device. How to create a measure that can decipher the accessibility of a device, given the extreme diversity of abilities of individuals, is certainly daunting. People with disabilities are extremely complex as individuals and even more complex as a population.

Measuring accessibility is also challenging because of the fact that many thousands of medical devices exist that serve many diverse functions. Medical devices range from small visual scopes requiring a high degree of manual and sensory skill to MRI systems that include complex calibration and instrumentation, substantial training for use, and a specialized environment. There are often dozens of medical devices within certain product classes that represent alternatives for purchase. This large number of medical instruments poses a challenge for anyone who might attempt to measure accessibility across them.

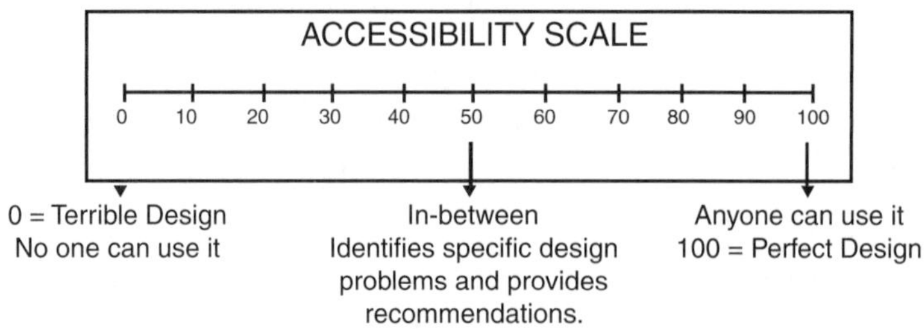

FIGURE 22.1 Universal design scale. **Summary:** The ideal scale to measure the accessibility of medical devices would be a universal design scale from 0 to 100 with 0 indicating a terrible design and 100 indicating perfect design and all values in between indicating design problems with recommendations provided. **Details:** This diagram shows a universal design scale marked on a straight line from 0 to 100 with intermediate values marked in the center in increments of 10. An arrow points down from 0 indicating terrible design, which means no one can use it. Similarly an arrow points down from 100 indicating perfect design, which means that anyone can use it. Lastly, an arrow points down from the numbers in between 0 and 100 indicating that there are specific design problems and provides recommendations.

Further complicating assessment, individuals who need to access medical devices perform three distinctive roles: (1) People with disabilities can be clients or patients who are receiving the medical procedure and would be recipients of the medical instrumentation; (2) people with disabilities may serve as the practitioners or technicians for running and interpreting the medical instrumentation; and (3) medical instruments may be used by individuals that serve both the client and the practitioner role, as self-administered medical procedures using self-administered medical instruments. Ideally, an accessibility measure would delineate the user perspective from which it is measuring, and enable the assessment of accessibility from each perspective that makes sense for the given type of medical device.

As mentioned previously, accessibility is complex. Some accessibility features are essential, even for turning on or off a machine. If an individual cannot turn a device off or on, it may be fundamentally inaccessible. On the other hand, some device characteristics permit more efficient or more comfortable use, but are not requirements. An effective accessibility measure must be able to discriminate between these two levels of accessibility. Chapter 8 and Chapter 25 of this book develop these two definitions of accessibility, the first from the perspective of accessible design specifications vs. the more general approach of accessible design optimization, and the second by scoring accessibility barrier events by degrees of difficulty where the most difficult is impossible (implying inaccessible).

Lastly, but certainly not easiest, the full range of reliability and validity characteristics must be tested and be sufficient for an accessibility measure to be appropriate for use. Test and measurement methodologists commonly cite 6 to 12 types of desired reliability and validity. So, only the most optimistic might think that creating a reliable and valid measure of accessibility for medical instruments would be feasible. However, though there is no "gold standard" for accessibility of medical devices and there are considerable challenges, there is a functional alternative: the federal accessibility guidelines for accessible design, which are concrete technical and functional performance criteria for areas that do have overlap with certain classes of medical devices, most notably the standards for electronic and information technologies; see also Chapter 8 and Chapter 15 of this book.

22.3 THE MED- AUDIT

The medical equipment device accessibility and universal design information tool (MED-AUDIT) confronts this challenge by using an innovative elegant measurement approach. By harnessing simple computer-based dynamic questioning, the MED-AUDIT prototypes multidimensional sets of questions that adapt to the wide variability of functional impairment populations, types of medical devices, and environments where devices are used.

22.3.1 MED- AUDIT Objectives

There are three primary objectives of the MED-AUDIT project. The first is to develop a reliable and valid quantitative assessment tool to measure the relative accessibility of medical instruments. The second is to create a resource for medical equipment designers to identify design problems in terms of accessibility for people with disability. The third is to investigate concepts about of how to best measure successful accessible and universal design [12]. The project hopes to demonstrate conceptual and practical methods for approaching the assessments of accessibility and universal design.

The MED-AUDIT audiences include four primary groups. The first are product designers as mentioned previously. The second group includes consumers of medical devices. Individual consumers may ask for a MED-AUDIT score or description in order to understand how accessible a given medical device might be before they arrive for a medical procedure or select a product for purchase. The third audience for the MED-AUDIT is accessibility consultants. Although we do not expect every medical equipment designer to become an expert in accessible and universal design, key experts who currently serve as accessibility consultants for architectural design or consumer product design may want to expand their expertise into medical equipment accessibility design. New accessibility consultants in the area of medical equipment design may also be necessary. The MED-AUDIT could serve as an important assessment resource and tool for their consultation and evaluation. Lastly, important MED-AUDIT audiences are regulatory and policy stakeholders. In order for us to better understand what accessibility thresholds and design criteria should be met for standards, regulation, or formal policy, we need a reliable and valid measure of accessibility. The MED-AUDIT, if it can be demonstrated as such a successful assessment, can provide data for the regulatory and policy stakeholders for determining appropriate criteria to enable people with disabilities access to medical instrumentation and medical procedures.

22.3.2 Two Versions of the MED- AUDIT

22.3.2.1 The Black Box System Version

The Black Box System Version (Figure 22.2a) has domains that are expert mapped so it contains the background and training of disability, universal design and accessible design. Expert knowledge is hidden within several arrays that link multiple dimensions of medical device use by people with disabilities. This version is designed for individuals who may not have the background or experience designing for people who have disabilities. The rater scores the MED-AUDIT on a simple scale to identify device tasks and device features [13]. The expert map running in the background links the device tasks and the device features to impairments of people with disabilities. Thus, the Black Box Version serves as a simple functional expert-mapped system.

22.3.2.2 The Expert User System Version

The Expert User System Version (Figure 22.2b) of the MED-AUDIT requires the designer to integrate an understanding of device tasks and features with universal design concepts and disability impairments as they score the MED-AUDIT questions [14]. Thus, the users of this version an expected to have a substantial background and training about impairments that people with disabilities encounter as well as universal design strategies.

22.3.2.3 Concurrent Development of Versions

During this development phase of MED-AUDIT, these two versions accompany each other. Each targets different levels of expertise and backgrounds of potential medical device evaluators. Currently, we remain unsure which of these approaches will be most sound or even if one of these is preferred, as they appear to be complementary. Three possibilities exist: (1) the Black Box System Version works best, (2) the Expert User System Version works best, or (3) both versions work best for different accessibility assessors or aims. Consequently, for the time being, we are developing and testing both versions to determine which of these three possibilities emerges as the best alternative for the MED-AUDIT approach [15,16].

22.3.3 Computer- Based Question and Scoring Structure: Trichotomous Tailored Branching Scoring (TTSS)

The MED-AUDIT applies a scoring system developed in the 1980s and 1990s that led to the OTFACT software distributed by the American Occupational Therapy Association. The scoring structure provided a unique elicitation and prompting method for the scorer [17]. Fundamentally, TTSS uses a trichotomous response: 2 = no problem, 0 = total problem, and 1 = partial problem. With a 2 or 0 score, the TTSS algorithm moves to the next major category of questions. Alternately, if the 1 is scored, the TTSS breaks down the category into subcategories and requests more detailed information from the rater. In this way, TTSS provides several specific scoring and measurement advantages. First, the trichotomous scoring is cognitively simple, resulting in increased response reliability and scoring speed [18]. Secondly, TTSS provides efficient branching, only asking detailed

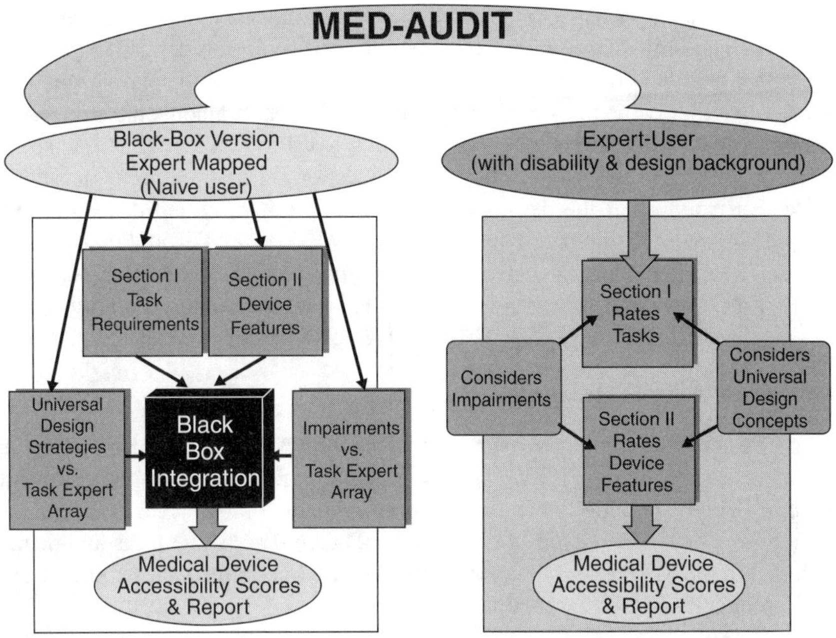

FIGURE 22.2 MED-AUDIT — conceptual flowchart. **Summary:** This flowchart depicts the conceptual models of two versions of the MED-AUDIT instrument. The chart illustrates the difference between versions A and B. **Details:** The figure displays a flow diagram of Sections I and II for the Black Box Version and Sections I and II for the Expert User Version of MED-AUDIT. At the top of the page there is a large umbrella shape, which has MED-AUDIT filled in it that serves as a title for the figure. Below this there is one oval for the Black Box Version and one oval for the Expert User Version. Arrows indicate that the Black Box Version has four components placed in gray boxes: Sections I labeled "Task Requirements," Section II labeled "Device Features," Universal Design Strategies vs. Task Expert Array and Impairments vs. Task Expert Array. Each of these feeds into a central three-dimensional black box via arrows that integrates these components to give accessibility scores for medical devices with respect to different disabilities. Lastly, the black box has an arrow pointing out to an oval titled "Medical Device Accessibility Scores and Reports." The Expert User Version has two components: Section 1, which rates tasks and Section 2, which rates device features. Each of these has two boxes connected to them by arrows labeled "Considers Impairments" and "Considers Universal Design Concepts." This indicates that the expert user version considers universal design concepts by asking if each task and feature is easy and safe and it considers 13 different impairments: Hard of hearing, deaf, low vision, blind, expressive communication, comprehension disorders, other cognitive disorders, sensitivity impairments, mental and behavioral impairments, lower limb impairments, upper limb impairment, head, neck and trunk impairment, and overall body impairment. Both of the main components of rating tasks and rating devices have an arrow to an oval titled "Medical Device Accessibility Scores and Reports." The figure illustrates that the Black Box Version is different than the Expert User Version, and this illustrates the conceptual difference between versions A and B.

questions when they are needed [19]. This also increases the rate of responses and allows the feasible inclusion of many more detailed questions as irrelevant questions are not asked. We know from measurement theory that the more questions that are asked, the more reliable the ultimate score. Thirdly, whereas TTSS provides a fundamental trichotomous set of options, the anchors that accompany the scales are flexible and intentionally can vary in construct. For example, in the MED-AUDIT, one response set of anchors includes, 2 = requires task, 0 = does not require task, and 1 = somewhat requires task. Later, in the same scoring structure, an entire second dimension of questions includes a response set in which 2 = includes feature, 0 = does not include feature, and 1 = somewhat includes features.

Figure 22.3 provides representative screen shots of question layouts based on the OT FACT software interface. The branching outline resides on the left, with the description of the question placed in the upper right and the legal responses (trichotomous scale) display in the bottom right of the screen. Lastly, TTSS, due to its branching and its inclusion of a nonapplicable legal response creates a customized set of questions for every particular assessment [20]. Thus, each device being scored by the MED-AUDIT may have a customized question set that only asks questions specific for that device. For example, if the device is fundamentally an alarm and does not have moving parts or any control system manipulated by the user, the MED-AUDIT would branch around all of the tasks and all the features related to controls or adjustability of components. However, the MED-AUDIT would probably include questions that relate to alternative alarm output of displays such as audio, visual, and tactile displays. The MED-AUDIT prompts this detail.

22.3.4 The MED- AUDIT Taxonomy

The Black Box System Version and Expert User System Version of the MED-AUDIT include a significant number of categories in their respective taxonomies. These taxonomies drive the TTSS question structure. The taxonomies were developed through an iterative team process that involved extensive literature review and organized discussions. Thus, many of the tasks and device feature concepts included in the MED-AUDIT taxonomies are based upon relevant published literature in other areas of product design and accessibility.

22.3.4.1 Black Box System Taxonomy

The current draft of the Black Box System Version includes about 800 distinct questions, 200 under task procedures and 600 under device features [13]. These questions are arranged in a convention of hierarchal outline with roman numerals in major headings broken down five or six levels for the taxonomy. Table 22.1 provides excerpt categories from the taxonomy.

The outline structure provides the branching options from level to level. With this taxonomy, the largest number of questions is associated with device function. Through the logic of branching, parts of the taxonomy that are irrelevant for a give type of device are naturally bypassed. Also, because of branching, the actual questions become more targeted, thus requiring less expertise and conceptual synthesis on the part of the user. The largest number of questions for which a scorer might need to respond equals the total number of categories. The minimum number of questions for which a scorer might need to respond equals the number of parent categories.

22.3.4.2 Expert User Taxonomy

The current draft of the Expert User System Version includes about 700 questions, although these are based on only 16 core questions, 12 related to task procedures and 4 to device features, as they repeat for each of 13 impairment areas (see Table 22.2) [14].

Note that in comparison to the more specific and narrow questions for the Black Box Version, these involve more integrative concepts and thus more rater expertise. Each of these 16 are scored for both "easily/flexibly" and "safely" categories, and each is administered for up to 13 impairment categories that are listed in Subsection 22.3.5. For this version there is no hierarchical branching, with all 32 questions responses asked for any impairment category that the user chooses to address.

22.3.5 Summary Scores

For the Expert User System Version, the summary scores are created by totaling the trichotomous scores generated in the OTFACT base platform. These currently present for 13 different impairment types [21]:

1. Hard of hearing
2. Deaf

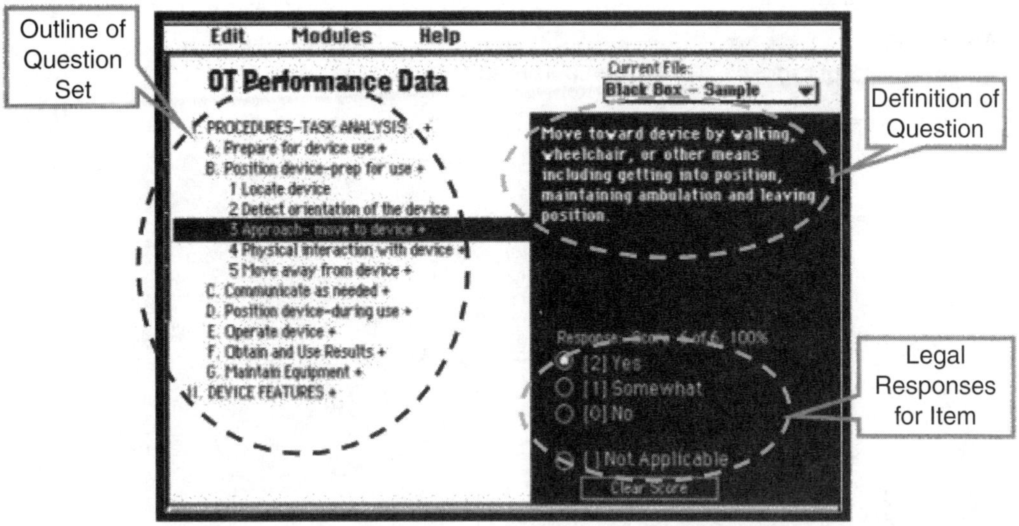

FIGURE 22.3 General description of the MED-AUDIT interface. **Summary:** The slide shows the outline of the Black Box Version with the response sets and the description of each question. **Details:** The photograph is a snapshot of the Black Box Version of the MED-AUDIT as it appears in OT FACT. The interface has a black and white colored background with the outline of the questions on the white background to the left and the description of each question with the response choices on the black background on the right. As one goes through the questions the question being considered at that point is highlighted in black. At the same time, to the left the description changes as the question changes. The response choices appear below the description of the question. The MED-AUDIT uses a trichotomous response scale known as TTSS (Trichotomous Tailored Sub-Branching Scoring). This allows the question set to be customized to the device being assessed. In this case, there are three response choices: "2 — Yes," "1 — Somewhat," and "0 — No." In addition there is a "Not Applicable Response."

3. Low vision
4. Blind
5. Expressive communication impairment
6. Comprehension disorder
7. Other cognitive disorder
8. Sensitivity impairment
9. Mental and behavior impairment
10. Lower limb impairment
11. Upper limb impairment
12. Head, neck, and truck impairment
13. Overall body impairment

The Black Box System Version, on the other hand, integrates relative weights from a hidden matrix in which tasks required for using the medical device are correlated to medical device features. Additionally, device features are correlated to functional impairments of users. This assessment between the device features and user impairment provides the critical design connection between the device and disability. Figure 22.4 highlights a component of the Black Box calculations describing the role of the "usability importance matrix," which defines the relationship between the required tasks of the device and the device features. This figure also highlights the applications of the "accessibility importance matrix," which defines the relationship between the medical device features and user impairments. Through this logic, the MED-AUDIT maps the device task requirements to the user impairments.

TABLE 22.1
Category Excerpts for the Black- Box Taxonomy

I. Procedures-task analysis
  A. Access help to understand device use
  B. Perform general preparation
  C. Communication between client and others
    1. Client communication
    2. Practitioner communication
      a. Explain practitioner role
      b. Check with client about needs
      c. Predict needs of client
      d. Ask to clarify needs of client
      e. Offer choices among options
      f. Ask for suggestions
      g. Confirm if process makes sense
      h. Confirm if results make sense
      i. Communicate with others
  D. Position person/device in prep for use
  E. Reposition person/device during use
  F. Operate device
    1. Manipulate controls of device
    2. Obtain information from display
    3. Integrate operation of device
  G. Administer appropriate dosage
  H. Leave device after use
  I. Sanitize, dispose and replenish
  J. Obtain and use results
  K. Maintain equipment

II. Device features
  A. Accessibile environment where used
  B. Overall device features
  C. Component specific features
    1. Positioners and supports
    2. Grips and grab bars
    3. Rails
    4. Steps
    5. Conduit
    6. Measuring device
    7. Control groupings
    8. Component control types
      a. Pushbutton controls
      b. Keyboard controls
        1) Avoids auto-repeat
        2) Depressed/undepressed indication
        3) Activation feedback

(Continued)

TABLE 22.1 *(Continued)*

- 4) Minimum travel distance
- 5) Size
- 6) Activation force
- 7) Tactile reference keys

c. Membrane key controls

9. Displays
10. Alarms/warning signals

TABLE 22.2
Category Excerpts from the Expert User Taxonomy

I. Hard of hearing
  A. Procedures-task analysis
    1. Communicate as needed
      a. Access help information
      b. Communicate with practitioner
    2. Select, understand, and learn to use
    3. Position self/device in preparation
    4. Position self and device during use
    5. Operate device to accomplish tasks
      a. Manipulate controls of device
      b. Obtain information from displays
      c. Integrate info. for device use
    6. Obtain and use results
      a. Easily/flexibly
      b. Safely
    7 Maintain device/prepare for next use
  B. Device features
    1. Assembly and disassembly of parts
      a. Easy to do
      b. Safe to do
    2. Positioners and supports
      a. Easy to adjust
      b. Safe to adjust
    3. Labeling and documentation
      a. Easy to understand and use
      b. Promotes safe use of device
    4. Integrated controls and displays
      a. Easy to operate
      b. Safe to operate
II. Additional impairment categories repeat

	Blind	Low Vision	Upper Body Mobility	Lower Body Mobility	Reading Disability	Cognitive Processing Problem	Across Disability Weighted by Prevalence
Essential Access	75%	85%	30%	40%	80%	95%	70.85%
Non-essential Access	60%	90%	20%	20%	80%	90%	64.86%

FIGURE 22.4 Example of MED-AUDIT reports. **Summary:** Illustration of the score report generated by the MED-AUDIT software. **Details:** This slide depicts the score reports that will be generated after a respondent has scored the questions on the MED-AUDIT. It will show the AUDIT scores for different impairment types, the AUDIT scores for tasks essential to use the device (accessibility) as well as tasks nonessential to use the device (usability). There is a table with three rows and eight columns. The top row lists the six different impairments: blind, low vision, upper body mobility, lower body mobility, reading disability, and cognitive processing problem, as well as a score across disability weighted by prevalence. The first column had the titles for scores for accessibility as well as usability. The scores were as follows: blind: accessibility — 75% and usability — 85%; low vision: accessibility — 85% and usability — 90%; upper body mobility: accessibility — 30% and usability — 20%; lower body mobility: accessibility — 40% and usability — 20%; reading disability: accessibility — 80% and usability — 80%; cognitive processing problem: accessibility — 95% and usability — 90%. It also shows the average accessibility and usability scores across disabilities, which is accessibility — 70.85 and usability — 64.86.

22.3.6 MED- AUDIT Reports

The MED-AUDIT is in the early feasibility developmental phase. Consequently, the reports are modeled and have not yet been fully empirically evaluated. We anticipate MED-AUDIT reports to portray the following information:

1. Audit scores listed for each impairment type.
2. Audit scores highlighting the tasks that are essential to use the device (basic accessibility).
3. Audit scores identifying tasks that are not essential to using the device (usability).
4. Provide summary scores. One possible portrayal of these scores may resemble Figure 22.4.

A 0% in the accessibility score would indicate that someone with that type of disability would have no access to that device; 100% would signify that that type of disability would have no problem using that device. Because the basic accessibility scores are required scores, anything short of 100% would indicate that certain people with disability would have an extremely difficult or impossible time using that particular device. On the other hand, the usability score does not wield the same 100% requirement to be accessible. Basically, the usability score reflects that 100% would be the most usable and zero would mean it would not be very usable. Poor usability, however, would not indicate that an individual could not function with the device. It just means they might take longer, it might not be efficient, or they might need special strategies to complete the task.

22.4 FUTURE DIRECTIONS

The MED-AUDIT is in its feasibility testing phases. Once both the Black Box System Version and the Expert User System Version platforms have been completed, early testing and revision of the software is planned. Some validation of the MED-AUDIT needs to assure that the scores have meaning. We also have reliability studies underway.

The potential impact of the MED-AUDIT has multiple directions. If the MED-AUDIT is as successful as early indicators seem to suggest is possible, it can provide a quantitative measure for each impairment type providing both essential and nonessential access scores for a particular device. Not only might the scores be helpful for comparing one medical device design with another, the process of evaluation itself informs the designer what types of features and what types of tasks are causing accessibility issues. The result from this process provides specific information to the designer for targeting redesign to improve the medical device function. Once found to be reliable and valid, medical instrument design consultants can use MED-AUDIT assessment to contribute to their "bag of resources" as they consult with industry around accessibility and usability of medical instruments.

Successful quantification of accessibility scores may also directly help consumers. Individuals with impairments can examine scores of different devices or potentially score these alternative devices themselves. These scores may help inform the consumer the difficulty level they could expect when using the device or even whether the device is minimally accessible for their use.

Lastly, successful MED-AUDIT scoring can provide a mechanism to collect research data for determining what levels and what criteria might be recommended as fundamental for accessibility across different disability groups [14]. This potentially could provide criteria for development of medical device accessibility guidelines or even standards. Even if such specific accessibility thresholds cannot be accumulated, providing accessibility and usability information (e.g., in product certification or labeling) could be a substantial benefit to consumers for their own decision making.

ACKNOWLEDGMENT

This work is supported by the Rehabilitation Engineering Research Center on Accessible Medical Instrumentation, funded by the National Institute on Disability and Rehabilitation Research (NIDRR) of the U.S. Department of Education under grant number H133E020729. All opinions are those of the authors.

REFERENCES

1. Grabois, E., Nosek, M.A., and Rossi, D., Accessibility of primary care physicians' offices for people with disabilities, *Archives of Family Medicine, 8*, 44–51, 1999.
2. Sanchez, J., Byfield, G., Brown, T.T., Lafavor, K., Murphy, D., and Laud, P., Perceived accessibility versus actual physical accessibility of healthcare facilities, *Rehabilitation Nursing, 25*(1), 6–9, 2000.
3. Veltman, A., Stewart, D.E., Tardiff, G.S., and Branigan, M., Perceptions of primary healthcare services among people with physical disabilities — Part I: access issues, *Medscape General Medicine, 3*(2), 2001.
4. Young, M.E. and Ellen, G., Managed care experiences of persons with disabilities, *Journal of Rehabilitation, 67*(3), 13–20, 2001.
5. Mendonca, R., RERC-AMI R3 Resource Document: Measuring Accessible Medical Instrumentation: Annotated bibliography, January 2005, available at www.r2d2.uwm. edu/rerc-ami/r3resources.html.
6. Becker, S.A. and Berkemeyer, A., Rapid application design and testing of web usability, *IEEE Multimedia, 9*(4), 38–46, 2002.
7. Reniscow, K.A., Schorow, M., Bloom, H.G., and Massad, R., Obstacles to family practitioners' use of screening tests: determinants of practice? *Preventive Medicine, 18*, 101–112, 1989.
8. Nosek, M.A., Young, M.E., Rintala, D.H., Howland, C.A., Foley, C.C., and Bennett, J.L., Barriers to reproductive health maintenance among women with physical disabilities, *Journal of Women's Health, 4*(5), 505–518, 1995.

9. McClain, L., Medrano, D., Marcum, M., and Schukar, J., A qualitative assessment of wheelchair users' experience with ADA compliance, physical barriers, and secondary health conditions, *Topics in Spinal Cord Injury Rehabilitation, 6*(1), 99–118, 2000.
10. Vanderheiden, G.C., Thirty-something million: should they be exceptions? *Human Factors, 32*(4), 383–396, 1990.
11. Smith, R.O., The science of occupational therapy assessment (guest editorial), *Occupational Therapy Journal of Research,* 12, 3–15, 1992.
12. Pizur-Barnekow, K., Lemke, M.R., Smith, R.O., Winter, M., and Mendonca, R., Measuring accessibility and universal design of medical devices: the medical equipment device-accessibility and universal design information tool (MED-AUDIT), *Proceedings of the RESNA 2005 Conference*, Atlanta, GA, June 2005.
13. Lemke, M., Winter, M., Pizur-Barnekow, K., Mendonca, R., Schwanke, T, Winters, J., and Smith, R.O., RERC-AMI R3 Resource Document: Black Box MED-AUDIT (Medical Equipment Device-Accessibility and Universal Design Information Tool) Taxonomy, 2005, available at www.r2d2.uwm.edu/rerc-ami/r3resources.html.
14. Lemke, M., Winter, M., Pizur-Barnekow, K., Mendonca, R., Schwanke, T., Winters, J., and Smith, R.O., RERC-AMI R3 Resource Document: Expert User MED-AUDIT (Medical Equipment Device-Accessibility and Universal Design Information Tool) Taxonomy, 2005, available at www.r2d2.uwm.edu/rerc-ami/r3resources.html.
15. Mendonca, R., Assessing the Usability of the MED-AUDIT, Master's thesis, University of Wisconsin-Milwaukee, WI, 2005.
16. Mendonca, R., Assessing the usability and the reliability of MED-AUDIT, *Proceedings of the 29th Annual Great Lakes Biomedical Conference, Biomedical Informatics: Applications, Achievements, and Frontiers*, The Milwaukee Chapter of IEEE EMBS, Racine, WI, 2005.
17. Smith, R.O., Sensitivity Analysis of Traditional and Trichotomous Tailored Sub-Branching Scoring (TTSS) Scales, University of Wisconsin-Madison, WI, 1993.
18. Smith, R.O., OTFACT application in mental health, in *Assessments in Occupational Therapy Mental Health: An Integrative Approach*, Drummond, A.E., Ed., SLACK Incorporated, Thorofare, NJ, 1999, pp. 289–308.
19. Smith, R.O., OTFACT: multi-level performance-oriented software with an assistive technology outcomes assessment protocol, *Technology and Disability, 14*, 133–139, 2002.
20. Smith, R.O., Pizur-Barnekow, K., and Rust, K.L., Missing in action: products and technology for medical services, *Proceedings of the 11th Annual NACC Conference on ICF: Mapping the Clinical World to ICF*, Rochester, MN, 2005, available at www.icfconference.com/Abstracts.html.
21. Winter, M. and Lemke, M., RERC-AMI R3 Resource Document: MED-AUDIT Impairment Categories: Working towards mapping AMI usability, January 2005, available at www.r2d2.uwm.edu/rerc-ami/r3resources.html.

23 Access to Medical Instrumentation: The Role of Web Accessibility

Judy Brewer

CONTENTS

ABSTRACT

Web accessibility plays a key role in accessing information, training, and technical assistance in medical instrumentation. This chapter examines accessibility barriers in Web-based information about medical instrumentation and in the interface of medical devices. It explores the cross-disability impact of these barriers on medical professionals with disabilities, consumers, and caregivers, and introduces resources and solutions to address these barriers. Finally, it considers research and policy actions that may increase the ability of medical professionals, consumers, and caregivers to benefit from accessible Web interfaces supporting their use of medical instrumentation.

23.1 OVERVIEW

The objectives of this chapter are to highlight areas where Web accessibility is key to improving accessibility of medical instrumentation, and to introduce Web accessibility guidelines and technical solutions that can be valuable resources in improving the accessibility of medical instrumentation for people with disabilities.

Section 23.2 of this chapter introduces the relevance of Web accessibility to medical instrumentation. Section 23.3 examines the key role that the Web plays in accessing and mastering medical instrumentation. Section 23.4 provides background on Web accessibility and an overview of guidelines and technical resources in the area of Web accessibility. Section 23.5 describes considerations related to the implementation of accessibility solutions, and research and policy steps that could promote a more accessible interface to medical instrumentation.

23.2 INTRODUCTION: RELEVANCE OF WEB ACCESSIBILITY TO MEDICAL INSTRUMENTATION

There are several primary areas of relevance of Web accessibility to medical instrumentation. Information, instructions, training, and technical assistance for diagnostic and therapeutic devices are, in some cases, Web-based, whether the devices are for use in a medical setting or in an independent living setting. In some cases, the interface to medical instrumentation is itself Web-based (for instance, in some telehealth systems).

The accessibility — or lack thereof — of Web-based interfaces to information about medical instrumentation, and to the instrumentation itself, can affect medical professionals who may have disabilities. It can also impact on healthcare consumers with disabilities, and on caregivers who may have their own disabilities.

Authoritative sources of information on the use of medical instrumentation, for instance, information from a device manufacturer, vendor, or relevant medical professional, is the first level of consideration when ensuring accessibility of these resources. However, peer exchange of information on managing medical conditions is increasingly supported by medical institutions, such as hospitals and rehabilitation centers in Web-based fora moderated by medical professionals, and it also occurs in Web-based fora sponsored by peer organizations, such as independent living centers.

23.3 WEB ACCESSIBILITY AND MEDICAL INSTRUMENTATION

23.3.1 Medical Professionals, Consumers, and Caregivers

Accessibility of medical instrumentation can be an issue for people with disabilities who are medical professionals (e.g., Chapter 3), for people with disabilities who are consumers of medical care (e.g., Chapter 2), and for people with disabilities who are caregivers for consumers of medical care. Although the interface to the majority of medical instrumentation is not Web-based, the Web plays a key role at several stages in the use of medical devices.

Medical professionals may need to use the Web to:

- Schedule appointments for services involving medical instrumentation for their patients
- Get updates on instructions related to medical instrumentation
- Access online training and technical assistance from vendors of medical instrumentation products
- Access patients' electronic health records, including results from procedures involving medical instrumentation
- Use or provide a Web service with integrated medical instrumentation or other telehealth capabilities

Medical consumers and their personal caregivers may need to use the Web to:

- Schedule appointments for services involving medical instrumentation
- Obtain instructions essential for preparing for an examination or procedure
- Learn about what to expect during a diagnostic procedure

- Access results of diagnostic procedures involving medical instrumentation
- Update sections of their electronic health record
- Access a remote medical device or service via a telehealth system

23.3.2 Web- Based Information on Medical Instrumentation

The Web is rapidly changing the face of healthcare services. Medical professionals may now need to use the Web to schedule procedures for their patients and to access examination or laboratory results. In some cases, they may also find that they can access the latest training on use of specific devices via online training available on the Web. They may have the option or be required to provide services related to medical instrumentation via a Web-based telehealth system. If these systems are not designed to be accessible, medical professionals with a variety of disabilities may be impeded in their ability to carry out their job functions.

Sometimes, consumers must also now use the Web to schedule appointments for procedures involving medical instrumentation. Increasingly, they are referred to the Web as the primary source for information on what to expect during a diagnostic procedure in order to save time that a medical professional might otherwise spend explaining the procedure to them. Consumers may also need to use the Web to access timely instructions on how to prepare for a procedure such as crucial dietary or medication changes in advance of certain CT scans.

If a patient has complications following a diagnostic procedure, including those involving medical instrumentation, their first line of reference, before contacting medical personnel, may be the Web site of the healthcare facility where the procedure was conducted. Some users of telehealth systems may be able access their examination results over the Web. If these systems are not designed to be accessible, consumers and/or caregivers with a variety of disabilities may be unable to access information that may be important to maintaining their health.

With today's medical technologies, people are increasingly using complex technologies for treatment and rehabilitation outside of medical settings and in the regular course of independent living activities. In some cases, important information is available on the Web regarding how to manage equipment as diverse as digital hearing aids, infusion pumps, G-tubes and J-tubes, heart monitors, biofeedback devices, and rocking beds. For people with print disabilities, such as visual disabilities, dyslexia, or without the use of their hands, paper-based instruction manuals are likely to be of limited use. However, access to documentation via the Web, if designed with Web accessibility in mind, can be both accessible and useful to them.

23.3.3 Misconceptions about Disability and Medical Instrumentation

Neither medical professionals nor those who design equipment for medical professionals are immune to the same stereotypes about disability that the general public holds. In some cases, this can adversely affect the design of medical instrumentation and/or access to information about medical instrumentation.

For instance, many people hold the misconception that disabilities come only singly or only in logical combinations related to a single medical condition. Designers might therefore surmise that an insulin infusion pump for a person with diabetes must be usable by someone with a visual impairment, as diabetes can cause visual impairment. But the same designer might not account for the possibility that an infusion pump for administering insulin, chemotherapy, pain medication, or nutritional support may also be used by someone with an impairment of hearing, mobility, or memory, or any combination of those and other conditions.

Similarly, medical professionals and designers of medical equipment may hold the misconception that certain disabilities essentially confine one to the home, especially when they involve complex medical equipment for ongoing treatment or life support. For instance, designers and vendors of portable ventilators may imagine these being used only in carefully controlled settings in the home, or possibly the school or workplace; whereas the user of a portable ventilator may be busy figuring out how to run the ventilator off car batteries while camping in the woods on vacation, then sharing that information over the Web with other interested users of portable ventilators [1].

In the first case, one can see the need for cross-disability design even in situations where a device is designed for a specific medical condition. In the second case, one can see how a consumer might want access to as much information as possible about the operation of the device from the device vendor, in a reliably accessible format — as well as from other users of the device, so as to continue living a full life.

23.4 WEB ACCESSIBILITY GUIDELINES

23.4.1 Overview of the Web Accessibility Initiative

In 1997, the leading standards organization for the Web, the World Wide Web Consortium (W3C), launched the Web Accessibility Initiative (WAI) [2] in order to develop technical solutions, guidelines, evaluation resources, education and outreach, and to coordinate with research and development to increase the accessibility of the Web, for people with disabilities. These objectives further W3C's goal of promoting universality of the Web.

The early Web showed the potential for greatly increased access to information for people around the world, as well as the potential for digitized information to be accessible to more people than existing print-based information. As the Web became more complex and included information in a variety of media and technical formats to be displayed on an ever-increasing range of devices, it became more challenging to ensure accessibility of the growing number of formats and information environments for people with disabilities.

WAI's access to the latest developing Web technologies at W3C ensures review of new Web technologies to identify potential accessibility problems at a stage when they can still be corrected. In addition, WAI's being situated within W3C ensures that the development of guidelines and educational resources is informed by leading Web experts.

23.4.2 Current Issues and Resources in Web Accessibility

An increasing amount of information about medical research, health care, assistive technology, durable medical equipment, as well as medical instrumentation has become available in recent years over the Web. During this time, there has been considerable progress in the Web industry on awareness of the need for Web accessibility, extensive supporting provisions built into core Web technologies, and implementation of support for production of accessible Web content by Web authoring tools and evaluation tools.

The three guidelines that WAI has produced have become the basis for laws and policies in many countries around the world. In addition, WAI is currently developing a second generation of guidelines that will address more advanced Web technologies, and be more understandable, more easily implemented, and more testable.

23.4.3 Barriers and Misconceptions

Accessibility of the Web applies to a broad range of disabilities and can be accommodated in a variety of ways, including the following:

- *Visual:* descriptions for graphics and video; properly marked-up structures such as tables or frames; interoperability with assistive technologies such as screen readers
- *Auditory:* captioning for audio; supplemental illustration; alternatives to voice-operated portals

- *Movement:* interoperability with assistive technologies such as voice recognition, different types of keyboards and input devices
- *Speech:* alternatives to voice-activated portals
- *Cognitive*: clear and consistent navigation; supplemental illustration; appropriate language level
- *Neurological:* clear and consistent navigation; no flickering or strobe designs

Some misconceptions about Web accessibility stem from designers' unfamiliarity with disabilities in general. For instance, some people may not realize that there are different degrees of visual impairment, hearing loss, loss of mobility or dexterity, and cognitive and neurological disability; they may think of blindness, deafness etc., as an all-or-nothing proposition. In not being aware of the possible gradations of ability, designers may underestimate the numbers of people likely to benefit from accessibility solutions.

Designers may, likewise, overlook the need for people with some disabilities to rely on multiple strategies for optimal access. For example, someone with low vision may rely on a combination of a screen magnifier, plus a screen reader with synthesized speech and/or refreshable Braille output. An accessible Web interface must support all of these options at once. This can be achieved through use of W3C/WAI guidelines that ensure support for a full range of cross-disability requirements.

A misconception that seems specific to the area of Web accessibility is that the only people with disabilities impacted by barriers on the Web are those with visual disabilities. This misconception at times influences choices by Web designers, particularly among those new to Web accessibility, leading to promotion of text-only Web sites as an accessibility solution. In fact, text-only sites are not a good solution even for people with certain kinds of visual disabilities, as they may rely on images in an enlarged form; nor is it a solution that works well for people with some cognitive and neurological disabilities, or for some deaf individuals.

23.4.4 Integrated Web Accessibility Solutions

Accessibility solutions for Web accessibility work must be integrated into core Web technologies. For instance, a multimedia specification such as Synchronized Multimedia Integration Language (SMIL) must be able to carry captions for audio and descriptions of video. This is relevant for training materials for medical instrumentation, because training materials are often presented in an audiovisual format. With technologies such as SMIL, training in rich media formats can now be delivered over the Web and still be accessible.

Integration of accessibility solutions into mainstream Web sites and software is also important. As the majority of Web accessibility solutions also benefit Web users without disabilities, all users benefit from accessibility solutions if the solutions are integrated into mainstream sites. For instance, separation of content from presentation through the use of Cascading Style Sheets (CSS) is a key principle of accessibility; but use of CSS also helps ensure that Web content will display effectively on any kind of device, such as a Web-enabled mobile phone, which someone might use to quickly confirm a question about usage of a particular medical device.

23.4.5 Guidelines for Accessible Web Content, Authoring, and Browsing

The need for accessibility of Web-based interfaces to medical instrumentation can be addressed by using existing Web accessibility guidelines. W3C/WAI has produced three guidelines as W3C recommendations (Web standards). These are the Web Content Accessibility Guidelines 1.0 (WCAG 1.0) [3], which address the accessibility of content on Web sites; the Authoring Tool Accessibility Guidelines 1.0 (ATAG 1.0) [4], which explain how to develop software for producing accessible Web content; and the User Agent Accessibility Guidelines 1.0 (UAAG 1.0) [5], which explain how to ensure the accessibility of browsers, media players, and other software used for accessing Web content.

These three guidelines address the complete range of cross-disability requirements, and are complementary. Web authoring software that conforms to ATAG, in turn, makes it easier to produce Web content that conforms to WCAG and which can be accessed by browsers and media players that conform to UAAG.

All three WAI guidelines include general design principles, specific checkpoints, and/or success criteria, and an extensive array of supporting techniques. The provisions in each are also divided into three priority levels. Policy makers, managers, or designers can therefore select between a basic level of accessibility, a more comprehensive level of accessibility, or an extended level of accessibility.

Advanced versions of the Web content and authoring tool guidelines (WCAG 2.0 [6] and ATAG 2.0 [7]) are currently under development, and will address more advanced Web technologies. These advanced versions are also designed to be more understandable, easier to implement, and easier to test for conformance; and they will be accompanied by extensive technical material to support their implementation.

23.5 RESOURCES AND ACTIONS NEEDED

23.5.1 Issues Affecting Implementation of Web Accessibility

While there has been extensive adoption of Web accessibility standards in the U.S. and worldwide, awareness of the need for Web accessibility and progress on implementation are still slow in some fields. Sometimes, this because of a lack of commitment or training, but at other times, it is still owing to a basic lack of awareness that accessing Web-based resources can be a barrier for people with disabilities. Thus, promoting wider awareness of the need for Web accessibility in the field of medical instrumentation is an important first step.

W3C/WAI has developed a variety of educational and implementation support materials, which can be used as is, or can be adapted for a specific field, such as medical instrumentation. For instance:

- "Developing a Web Accessibility Business Case for Your Organization" [8] provides information on social, technical, financial, and legal factors, which can be customized for a particular field or organization.
- "Policies Relating to Web Accessibility" [9] can help in identifying existing obligations for accessibility.
- "Implementation Plan for Web Accessibility" [10] walks a project manager through the steps needed to develop an accessible design and ensure ongoing conformance with Web accessibility guidelines.
- "Curriculum for Web Content Accessibility Guidelines" [11] provides online instruction in developing an accessible Web site.
- "Evaluating Web Sites for Accessibility" [12] provides instruction and resources for assessing a site's conformance to accessibility guidelines.

These, and other resources, are available from the WAI home page at http://www.w3.org/WAI.

23.5.2 Research on Baseline Awareness and Conformance

In order to more accurately assess the extent of promotional activities and technical assistance that may be needed in the field, it would be instructive to have a more precise baseline regarding the current level of conformance to Web accessibility guidelines of Web sites relating to medical instrumentation. At the same time, one could assess the current extent of Web-based interfaces for information, training, and technical assistance relating to medical instrumentation, and measure the trend for increased Web-based interaction through telehealth systems.

It might also be interesting to assess whether using a Web-like interface might increase the learnability and/or usability of some types of medical instrumentation, given that the Web interface has become one of today's most common design paradigms. Easy learnability by consumers and/or their caregivers can be a critical factor in ensuring effective operation of medical instrumentation in independent living settings.

23.5.3 Policy Development Specific to Medical Instrumentation

In the U.S., Section 508 of the Rehabilitation Act obligates the federal government to ensure that electronic and information technology it procures meets accessibility requirements as stated in the Section 508 regulations. These include accessibility of Web content as described in Section 508 subsection 1194.22, which is based on W3C/WAI WCAG 1.0. In addition, the Americans with Disabilities Act has generally been interpreted as applying to the Internet and the Web, with respect to state and local governments and places of public accommodation.

Clearer policies describing the need for accessibility of Web-based interfaces to medical instrumentation may be helpful in focusing attention and resources in this area. Issues to consider in any such policies would include harmonization with existing standards, as harmonized standards help build a unified market for supporting applications. This unified market can accelerate development of authoring and evaluation tools, which support content production and conformance testing to a common standard, thereby more rapidly leading to an accessible environment in which to learn about and use medical instrumentation essential to maintain the quality of life.

REFERENCES

1. Panzarino, C., Camping with a Ventilator, in *Access Expressed! Very Special Arts Massachusetts News*, January–April 2001, Vol. 11, No. 28, retrieved January 30, 2006 from http://www.accessexpressed.net/articles.php?table=articles&id=142& pageNumber=1.
2. WAI Web site http://www.w3.org/WAI/.
3. Chisholm, W., Vanderheiden, G., and Jacobs, I., Eds., Web Content Accessibility Guidelines 1.0 (WCAG 1.0), W3C Recommendation, World Wide Web Consortium (MIT, INRIA, Keio), May 5, 1999, http://www.w3.org/TR/WCAG10/.
4. Caldwell, B., Chisholm, W., Slatin, J., and Vanderheiden, G., Eds., Web Content Accessibility Guidelines 2.0 (WCAG 2.0), W3C Working Draft, World Wide Web Consortium (MIT, ERCIM, Keio), November 23, 2005, http://www.w3.org/TR/WCAG20/.
5. Treviranus, J., McCathieNevile C., Jacobs, I., and Richards, J., Eds., Authoring Tool Accessibility Guidelines 1.0 (ATAG 1.0), W3C Recommendation, World Wide Web Consortium (MIT, INRIA, Keio), February 3, 2000, http://www.w3.org/TR/ATAG10/.
6. Richards, J., Treviranus, J., and May, M., Eds., Authoring Tool Accessibility Guidelines 2.0 (ATAG 2.0), W3C Working Draft, World Wide Web Consortium (MIT, ERCIM, Keio), November 23, 2005, http://www.w3.org/TR/ATAG20/.
7. Jacobs, I., Gunderson, J., and Hansen, E., Eds., User Agent Accessibility Guidelines 1.0 (UAAG 1.0), W3C Recommendation, World Wide Web Consortium (MIT, INRIA, Keio), December 17, 2002, http://www.w3.org/TR/UAAG10/.
8. Henry, S., et al., Eds., Developing a Web Accessibility Business Case for Your Organization, World Wide Web Consortium (MIT, ERCIM, Keio), September 19, 2005, http://www.w3.org/WAI/bcase/.
9. Henry, S., et al., Eds., Policies Relating to Web Accessibility, World Wide Web Consortium (MIT, ERCIM, Keio), February 14, 2005, http://www.w3.org/WAI/Policy/.
10. Brewer, J., Horton, S. et al., Eds., Implementation Plan for Web Accessibility, World Wide Web Consortium (MIT, INRIA, Keio), October 22, 2002, http://www.w3.org/ WAI/impl/.
11. Letourneau, C. and Freed G., Curriculum for Web Content Accessibility Guidelines, World Wide Web Consortium (MIT, INRIA, Keio), March 17, 2000, http://www.w3.org/WAI/wcag-curric/.
12. Abou-Zahra, S. Ed., Evaluating Web Sites for Accessibility, World Wide Web Consortium (MIT, ERCIM, Keio), November 8, 2005, http://www.w3.org/WAI/eval/.

Part IV

Considerations in Emerging Trends and Technologies

24 Technology for Full Citizenship: Challenges for the Research Community

Katherine D. Seelman

CONTENTS

ABSTRACT

This chapter envisions technology for citizenship using medical devices as an example. Objectives include the following: (1) identify the who and how of the medical device resource and user systems in order to develop strategies for education, communication, and change, (2) stimulate sociotechnical studies that encompass factors internal to the technology development process such as design and external factors such as markets, and (3) generate examples of problem areas for future research. This chapter applies a model of technology development used by the U.S. Congress' now-defunct Office of Technology Assessment (OTA) to identify, organize, and analyze the who and how of the medical device allocation and user systems. The medical device resource system is analyzed using critical theory, which focuses on psychosocial, economic, and political factors that crystallize into social organization. A legacy of discrimination in product development is explored in terms of barriers to mainstream markets, market incentives and disincentives, human factors in design, safety and efficacy regulatory criteria, inclusion and exclusion criteria in clinical trials. There is a dearth of disability-related sociotechnical studies of corporate and government decision making. These studies should be conducted and embedded in a broadly conceived engineering research agenda.

24.1 INTRODUCTION AND BACKGROUND

> ... The functional capacities required of men and women by the current organization of a social life have not been decreed by natural law. [1]

In 1985, Harlan Hahn wrote a seminal article in which he observed that the shape of social life for a person with a disability is controlled by prevailing norms and cultural values. At the time, disability was widely regarded as being caused by medical conditions. Accessible buildings, transportation, and information were not widely valued as important factors in explaining disability. Today, Hahn might use lack of access to and usability of medical devices as an example of a social factor not widely valued in explaining disability. The medical device industry and regulators have not incorporated people with disabilities in their typical, average consumer profile [2]. Consequently, patients and professionals with disabilities, as well as caregivers cannot use many devices important to their health, economic, and employment well-being.

24.1.1 Objectives

This is a "thought piece" with the expansive goal of envisioning technology for citizenship, rather than technology to meet more limited goals related to cognitive, mobility, or sensory function or education and employment. Medical devices are an important case study. The purpose of this chapter involves the following objectives:

- Explore medical device literature and the product development process in the U.S. in order to identify the who and how of relationships within and between the medical device resource system and the user system that may constitute opportunities for participation leading to change
- Stimulate further sociotechnical studies of technology for people with disabilities
- Generate examples of problem areas that suggest future research directions

The mainstream medical device resource system involves market forces, regulation, and legislation. Consumer subpopulations of concern are patients with disabilities, healthcare practitioners with disabilities, and laypersons serving as caregivers in the home and community. The access and user requirements of each group may vary by function and location. Not all users of concern in this paper may conform to the typical, average profile of consumers in mainstream market, suggesting a resource problem in finance and expertise. Some people with disabilities and caregivers can use most mainstream medical devices, suggesting a problem for those doing disability market analysis.

Although key policy issues in medical device technology include safety, efficacy, quality, and evaluation as well as access, usability, and equity, this article will emphasize access, usability, and equity issues. Accessibility means that a medical device can be used effectively and for the same purpose by a person with a disability, as by a person without a disability. Usability means the efficiency with which a user can perform required tasks with a product. Equity means fair distribution of resources. Measures of usability and eventual standardization are derived from the functional characteristics of well-defined user populations. These measures are necessary for design, testing, and evaluation of actual devices or interface controls. The technical configuration of devices and controls for medical instruments and diagnostic equipment, such as mammograms and stethoscopes, is the province of engineering and outside the scope of this chapter.

24.1.2 Approach

24.1.2.1 Critical Theory

Hahn's observation that social organization is not caused by nature suggests the need to identify human determinants for the production and distribution of inaccessible and unusable medical devices. This article applies critical theory [3] to an analysis of the medical device technology development and diffusion process. Critical theory approaches technology through analysis of social, political, economic, and other factors that are crystallized into social organization. Feenberg (2002), for instance, citing examples of the design process and technical codes, identified the social potential of technology as a key factor in its transformation [4]. Stephanidis cites two policy variables, legislation and standardization, as catalysts for change [2].

24.2 DEVELOPMENT AND DIFFUSION MODEL

This article adopts the model of development and diffusion framework used by the U.S. Congress' now-defunct OTA in its 1982 study of technology for people with disabilities, because it provides a useful description of the process. The weakness of the approach lies in its focus on innovation rather than existing technology. The framework is useful in capturing and organizing the who and how of the technology development and diffusion process. The who and how of the process involves actors and their activities, access and equity policy issues, and potential strategies for solutions. The stages of the process are open to various designations such as R&D, evaluation, diffusion, and use. Accessibility and usability, actors, and issues may be located in different stages of the process.

Applying a model of medical technology development and diffusion to medical devices is fraught with complications. The emphasis in this article will be on identifying resource and use problems generated by mainstream market forces, regulation, and legislation. Mainstream and assistive technology (AT) market characteristics differ in consumer profiles, size, market configuration, and financing. On the one hand, AT products are often orphan technologies with small fragmented markets of 200,000 or under and characterized by high production costs and ill-defined consumer profiles that effectively preclude widespread manufacture and sales. Development and diffusion of AT are often highly subsidized by the government, and intervention by third party payers is common [6–8]. Mainstream medical technology products for the average typical user are characterized by a market, which is the global leader in medical device innovation [9]. The medical device industry is heavily invested in R&D activities and is a dynamic, profitable, and highly competitive global industry. To the question of "who" can adopt, internalize, and further develop user interfaces for all and "how," Stephanidis rejects both the AT and mainstream options [2]. He envisions a third option, nonmarket institutions, which will be further explored in Section 24.3.

24.2.1 Legacy of Discrimination

Barriers to medical device development and use are indicative of a legacy of discrimination. The disability community has a history of being segregated from the mainstream of society. Many disability programs showed lags as they evolved during different periods in disability policy development and on the dual tracks of segregation and the mainstream. The Social Security benefits requirements that restrict work and the Ticket to Work and Work Incentives Improvement Act that provide incentives for work are examples of dual-track lags in employment policy. This dual-track lag pattern is also evident in the research, development, and diffusion process where AT products have entered the process late sometime to compensate for lack of universally designed mainstream products. It is beyond the purview of this paper to address the question of whether or not people with disabilities would benefit or lose from maintaining a separate AT marketplace [10]. However, access to accessible medical devices that are developed in the mainstream market is assumed to be a benefit.

Medical device allocations involve legislative and regulatory policy as well as market forces. Legislation is an important driver of change. Legislation, such as the Americans with Disabilities Act and Section 508 of the Rehabilitation Act, has influenced other industries to adopt strategies to make their products more accessible. However, medical device development and diffusion involve the often arcane social organization and rules of science, technology, and bureaucracy. Nonetheless, examples of change in the science and technology decision arenas that have been highly beneficial to people with disabilities exist, but have not been well studied. Rehabilitation engineers, as change agents, have been instrumental in the technology standards process. Medical and technical experts have served as change agents often combining their efforts with disability advocates as in the disability community's long involvement with the Federal Communications Commission [11,12]. During the Clinton presidency, disability issues related to information technology were incorporated in the president's science and technology goals for the nation [13–15]. The role of the change agent is an important consideration in the process of participation and intervention in medical device technology development and use.

24.2.2 Research Directions

The resource allocation and user systems as currently configured have funding, expertise, and structural barriers to participation and intervention. There is a need to generate economic, social, management, and policy studies of the characteristics of the medical device resource allocation and user systems. This article will generate ideas for future research directions. A research agenda can be developed that is nested into the larger field of engineering in which sociotechnical studies most appropriately fit. Rehabilitation engineering has a history of involvement in technology transfer, market structure, and private and public sector relationships [5,8]. The 1999 Workshop on Home Care Technologies for the 21st Century, organized by bioengineers, identified many of the challenges in the medical device industry [16].

24.3 SELECTED LITERATURE REVIEW

This section selects and reviews some of the relevant topical areas in sociotechnical literature. It does not review the studies conducted by the rehabilitation engineering research centers (RERC), such as those generated by the RERC on accessible medical instrumentation. Even a cursory review and annotation of selected social literature relevant to medical devices can highlight needs and gaps. The disciplines represented by these studies can inform future research directions.

24.3.1 Science, Technology, and Society/Policy

The study of the social dimensions of technology has been the province of science, technology, and society/policy studies (STS/P) [17]. STS/P studies assume that human agents make social rules about the development and use of technology [18,19]. STS/P research has utilized both empirical and critical theory methods of inquiry. Technology and social impact assessments will be addressed in the next section. Critical theory is widely used in disability studies and feminist studies, which have generated health technology and AT studies [20–23]. A new paradigm of disability has emerged that integrates health into a model of disability that emphasizes participation and community integration. The new paradigm makes the development and diffusion of accessible health technology and settings more pressing [10,24].

24.3.1.1 Technology Assessment and Diffusion

Technology assessment is a form of policy analysis designed to provide information on the range of effects of a technology, e.g., social, ethical, legal, political, economic, technical, and psychological effects [5]. U.S. Congress' Office of Technology Assessment (OTA) reports, most of which are available on the web, provide examples of highly useful, if at times dated, studies of medical technology assessment. OTA's 1978 report entitled "Assessing the Efficacy and Safety of Medical Technology" lays out policy options as well as explores the concepts of efficacy and safety [25]. The 1982 study of technology for people with disabilities [5] and the 1985 study of technology and aging [26] are important examples of studies targeted to the populations of concern in this article. The 1982 study generated a series of sociotechnical case studies of AT products and processes.

Diffusion research has evolved over time. The focus of classic diffusion research was initially on adoption by the individual with a bias in favor of innovation [27]. The concept of *relative advantage* [27] continues to be extremely useful in calculating economic profitability, social prestige, and other benefits as factors in the degree to which an innovation is perceived as better than the one it succeeds. More recent diffusion research has turned to organizational, economic, and political theories of decision making applied to market competition, regulation, and decisions processes and patterns by diverse groups often within health organizations [9]. Burns and Flam, among others, have put forward the interesting idea that for each and every market there is a unique political economy [18]. Examples of the mainstream diffusion and adoption of wheelchairs, accessible scales, and examining tables (such as their adoption by Magee Hospital in Pittsburgh) invite research attention.

24.3.2 Social Study of Health Technology

The social study of health technology is frequented by many disciplines including management, industrial engineering, marketing, medical sociology, economics, organizational analysis, and policy studies. Studies of the diffusion of mainstream health technology that explicitly include people with disabilities are rare or most probably nonexistent. In one study of mainstream technology in American health care, technology for people with disabilities is referred to as *orphan technology* [9]. There is considerable overlap in orphan technologies and AT literature, which is extensive especially in the U.S., Europe, and Japan. This literature often highlights the economic, esthetic, and other advantages of moving AT into the mainstream [6–8,10]. In a 2001 study of the market diffusion process for AT products, the authors indicate the continuing need for a separate AT industry because of the failure of mainstream manufacturers to embrace the principles of design for all in their consumer products [28]. However, Kyoyo-Hin Foundation [29] in Japan provides an example of commitment to implementation of universal design in response to sharp increase in the aging population.

24.3.3 Human Factors, Universal Design, and User Interfaces for All

It is not within the purview of this article to address human factors or ergonomics, design and standards, and other technical dimensions of engineering. Human factors focuses on how human beings interact with the devices they use [30]. Human factors in AT are not always identical to factors considered in the development and use of mainstream consumer products, the design for which is guided by the profile of the typical, average consumer. The significance of the inclusion of human factors in the design process cannot be overestimated. Human factors, design, and engineering psychology data are crucial to the development and implementation of criteria for fair, accessible, and usable evaluation and testing by such federal agencies as the U.S. Food and Drug Administration (FDA). The fields of engineering, design, and policy are challenged to develop further a product paradigm that bridges users with and without disabilities.

The medical device resource allocation system has the potential to incorporate some of the visionary approaches of universal design and user interfaces for all into a new paradigm for engineering. Universal design or *design for all* is a relatively new concept of design that recognizes and attempts to accommodate the broadest range of human abilities (e.g., see Chapter 6). The *user interfaces for all* literature has emerged from human–computer interaction. It provides examples of both the technical and the social dimensions of engineering. It communicates a vision "... of an approach for the development of computational environments catering for the broadest possible range of human abilities, skills, requirements and references" [2]. The literature also provides a roadmap for integrated, accessible, and useable environments for everyone by attacking assumptions about typical users, business contexts, and desktop computing [2].

The literature also makes a contribution by locating AT in the development and diffusion process. It typifies AT as re-active, because AT development responds to technology concerns late in the process, and thus the resulting devices may be obsolescent. Proactive technology involves efforts to build access features and therefore user input into a products from conception and design through targeted development. To bring interfaces for all into the market, Stephanidis opts for nonmarket institutions, such as the National Science Foundation (NSF) to fund, promote awareness, as well as establish directives, legislative acts, and standards for ensuring the diffusion of technology and its adoption by industry. Although an appropriate mission for NSF, the policy barriers are formidable. Stephantidis sees the need for future efforts focusing on accessibility and standardization (for a review of ongoing activities in the area, see Chapter 15). The challenges to making this vision a reality becomes more apparent in the next section, which concentrates on stages in technology development and linkages between resource and user systems.

24.3.4 Summary

This selected literature review with annotations suggest the need for a more comprehensive review of sociotechnical studies that can inform the study of accessible and usable medical device development and adoption. These studies may be empirically-based research efforts in disciplines such as technology assessment, organizational theory, and public policy that can address resource allocation, decision making, and cultural norms in industry, regulation, and legislation. Studies could explore factors important in change in bureaucratic and regulatory rules for participation and intervention. Targeted case studies of the mainstream and the AT design processes at the R&D and diffusion stages would also be useful. Targeted studies of market size, configuration, and behavior is an ongoing need. Disability studies and related feminist studies can generate analysis of the user experience. Finally, well-respected science policy research centers, such as the Institute of Medicine, are potential sources of studies of equity and access in medical device resource allocation.

24.4 STAGES IN THE DEVELOPMENT AND DIFFUSION OF MEDICAL TECHNOLOGIES

24.4.1 Research and Development and Diffusion and Adoption Process

Diffusion of medical technology is the process by which technology enters and becomes part of the healthcare system [9]. The process involves a balanced relationship between the resource system and the user system. A lack of balance has social consequences and distributional effects that become issues or dimensions of conflict [18].

Research, development, and diffusion and adoption of medical devices are points on a continuum with many feedback loops and overlapping stages. The process is complicated, and the stages in the continuum often do not involve the same skill sets, methods, and goals [5]. Figure 24.1 depicts a classic model of diffusion for medical technologies showing an S-shaped curve. With different theories, such as diffusion studies of decision making in health settings, the model's

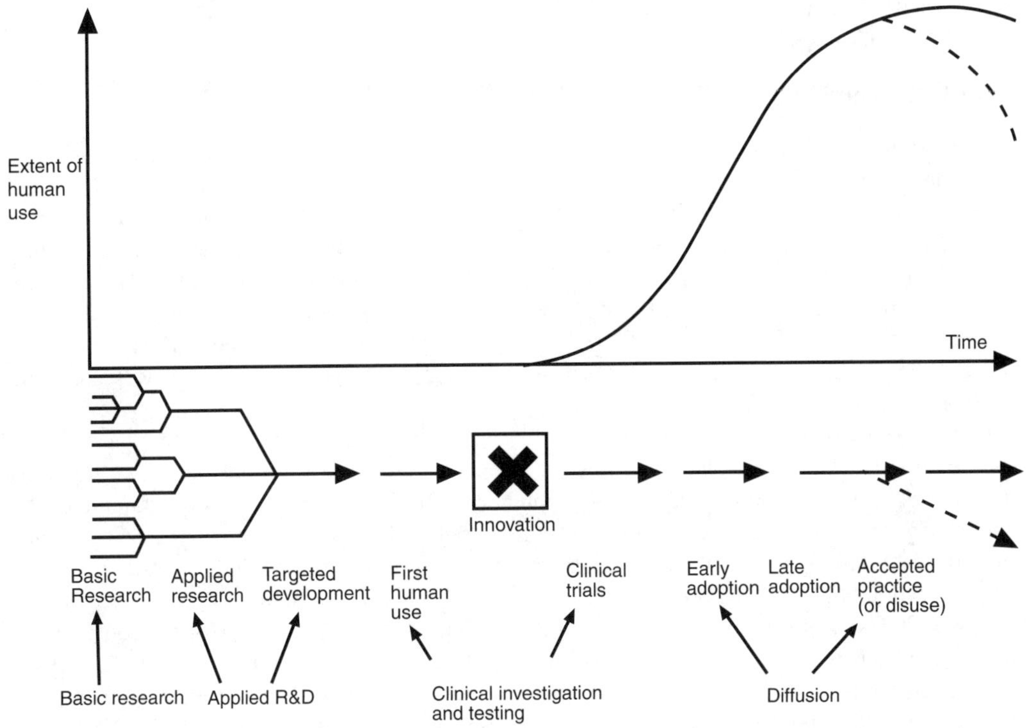

SOURCE: Office of Technology Assessment, *U.S. Congress, Development of Medical Technology: Opportunities for Assessment* (Washington, D.C.: U.S. Government Printing Office, August, 1976.

FIGURE 24.1 Model of diffusion for medical technologies.

S-shaped curve would take on a different configuration. However, the stages of development in the classic model used by OTA continue to be useful.

24.4.2 Actors, Issues, and Policy Considerations

An exploration of each of the stages in the development of medical technology suggests a concentration of somewhat discrete groupings of actors, issues, and policy considerations. These actors, issues, and policy considerations are of considerable interest to the medical device industry as reflected in industry trend analysis. Trends in the medical device industry routinely identify as important for monitoring purposes, regulation, purchasing (group purchasing organizations), and reimbursement [31]. The industry recognizes as among key trend makers, regulators such as the FDA, reimbursers such as the U.S. Centers for Medicare and Medicaid Services (CMS), state attorney generals involved in antitrust violations, and the attitudes of the general public.

The FDA has a basic mission in regulation of the safety and efficacy of medical devices. Issues deemed important enough to monitor by the FDA include the following: (1) changes in health system, (2) device customization, (3) home/self care, and (4) social factors such as activist patients and consumers and aging patient populations [32]. In its 1998 analysis of trends, the FDA met with representatives of the following four groups: investors and manufacturers, physicians and other direct health care providers, institutional payers and reimbursers, and patients and consumers. The FDA may be focusing its more recent efforts on devices for children, as a recent Institute of Medicine study found the FDA lacking in oversight of medical devices for children [33]. There also have been efforts to integrate human factors approaches with risk management into the design process for medical devices [34,35] (see also Chapter 17). Regulation is a ubiquitous presence throughout the process.

24.4.3 Stages in the Development and Diffusion of Medical Devices: R&D and Evaluation

24.4.3.1 Research and Development (R&D)

Investors and physicians may hold the financial and prestige resources at the R&D stage, but researchers are the knowledge resource necessary to do the work. Industry and government are active in support of medical device R&D. Basic research may involve precompetitive and even collaborative efforts among research institutes and consortia. Basic research receives funding support from private and public funders, including the National Institutes of Health (NIH), the NSF, and the Department of Defense (DOD). Applied research is more the province of either the private sector or in the case of AT, the National Institute on Disability and Rehabilitation Research's (NIDRR) RERC and the Department of Veteran Affairs' (DVA) Rehabilitation Research and Development Centers (RRDC).

Issues identified as important to success in this stage include: (1) availability of finance capital, (2) competition in the marketplace, (3) severity and urgency of medical problems, and (4) activist patients and consumers and aging patient population [9]. R&D for AT may be stimulated by personal, economic, social, and political incentives but is funded to a large degree by public nonprofit sources, which are subject to policy cycles and scrutinized for reimbursement potential.

The location of technology transfer in the R&D and diffusion continuum is open to speculation. Technology transfer efforts involve transfer of basic research to the private sector for commercialization and also using existing know-how for new applications [27]. Universities and federal R&D labs, such as the National Aeronautics and Space Administration (NASA), use existing know-how and apply it to different applications including those involved with disability [27]. The federal laboratories, however, do not have a disability research mission [36].

The mainstream R&D phase is dominated by finance investors and technical experts, whereas public sector R&D may also include those who do cost-effective analyses of the use of public funds. Unlike rehabilitation engineering, the mainstream organizational culture and norms of basic and even applied research do not seem to support user involvement. These norms present a significant barrier to the introduction of human factors methodology and approaches, such as universal design that would influence the design process to represent the range of function common to people with disabilities (see also Chapter 18). The role of the researcher as change agent becomes more important. Publicly funded basic and applied research and technology transfer provides another potential opportunity for intervention and participation in legislative committees and other policy and planning arenas.

24.4.3.2 Targeted Development and Evaluation

Regulators and evaluators internal to the industry or to federal agencies have intense involvement at this precommercialization stage. The FDA criteria and approval process for medical devices dominates this stage. The DVA and the Department of Defense (DOD) also do evaluation and testing studies. The purpose of the evaluation process is to assure economically sound resource allocation and cost containment, as well as protecting the health and safety of the public. This is the stage in which issues of safety and efficacy are of great concern. Safety is a judgment of the acceptability of risk in a particular situation [9,25] (see also Chapter 17). Efficacy may be understood to mean the probability of benefit to a population. Both are relative concepts, because no technology is completely safe. The population affected is a key factor, because risks correlate to age and condition.

Methods of evaluating technology used by the NSF, NIH, and the private sector include case studies, consensus development, randomized controlled trials (RCT), and economic analysis, as well as metrics that measure safety and efficacy. Of these methods, according to Cohen and Hanft, only case studies and consensus development, which may focus on specific technologies, are concerned with social, ethical, and legal dimensions of medical devices. For many years, RCTs discriminated against women and minorities who were not regarded as average, typical subjects. Women's health groups and Congress brought pressure on the NIH and the FDA to address these biases. Apparently both NIH and FDA complied, but the FDA took less aggressive action [9].

The targeted development stage, like the R&D stage, is dominated by experts and also involves determinations of usability. However, examples of successful intervention are evident. Activities of women's health interests inside and outside of government, coupled with an NIH director with a women's health research agenda, resulted in significant changes in NIH and even FDA practice. Increased participation and intervention in NIH and FDA was the result of women's movement, bureaucracy, and Congressional influence to change evaluation processes, including case studies and consensus conferences and even randomized clinical trials and related metrics.

24.4.4 Stages in the Development and Diffusion of Medical Devices: Diffusion and Adoption

24.4.4.1 Evaluation, Manufacturing, Marketing, and Diffusion into the Health System

This is the commercialization phase in which new ideas are put into a form to meet the needs of potential adopters. Capitol investors, manufacturers, reimbursers, physicians, and other medical personnel, as well as consumers are important actors in this stage. Evaluation studies are now directed more to feasibility and probability of adoption, such as business and technical feasibility, technical R&D, product R&D, market testing, commercial production and marketing, and government policies. New products ideas are sequentially reduced as they pass through initial R&D screening tests, evaluation and into marketing, manufacturing, and adoption. Economic profitability, social prestige, procurement and purchase, and third party payer's benefits are important issues at this stage.

Marketing and manufacturing are driven by perceptions of consumer demand by the private sector and government. Technical manufacturers are particularly interested in medical device adoption practices of hospitals and providers of health insurance and payment systems. They are also interested at the state level in the antitrust experience of group purchasing organizations.

Consumers, often patient advocates, can be effective in bringing a product to the marketplace. Diffusion may reach a high rate soon after the technology becomes available because of lack of suitable alternative technology combined with a desperate patient population and providers with no other treatment options. This pattern has been termed *desperation reaction model* and may occur even in the absence of efficacy or safety studies [25].

As indicated previously, the medical device marketplace for consumers with disabilities is characterized by small markets, high production costs, and ill-defined consumer profiles. Although needs exist for accessible and usable medical devices, the OTA (1982) listed a number of additional disincentives to marketing and manufacturing AT including the following: (1) add on costs of design for production and (2) costs of assuring that technology meets functional, technical, reliability, and safety requirements [25]. Acknowledging that technologies that have potentially high social benefits do not have resource capabilities, the OTA recommended: (1) demographic and market research, (2) low-cost loans or grants, (3) tax incentives, (4) studying European systems, and (5) contracting arrangements [25]. The OTA's recommended package of benefits to promote business investments also included arrangements for government as a purchaser and establishment of testing and evaluation centers suitable for use by people with disabilities.

The diffusion and adoption stage has important implications for accessibility because of decisions about procurement and purchase of medical devices. This stage involves diverse groups of stakeholders and consumers. Successful intervention in the mainstream marketplace is largely a matter of economics. Successful interventions may also be possible through civil rights and other legislations, such as the application of section 508 of the Rehabilitation Act to the procurement and purchase practices of the DVA and DOD. Antitrust action may be possible, especially in those states that have certificate of need (CON) programs that control health technology capacity [9].

24.4.5 Other Actors, Issues, and Strategies

24.4.5.1 Agencies

The U.S. Congress OTA, once the leading federal agency responsible for studying the range of effects of technology, closed in 1995. Others agencies are more peripherally involved, such as the Government Accountability Office (GAO) and the Center for Practice and Technology Assessment in the Agency for Health Care Policy and Research (AHCPR). The GAO reports have addressed shortcomings in the science and technology arena including shortcomings of RCTs [9]. The AHCPR has assisted CMS in health care coverage determinations [9].

24.4.5.2 Legislation

The Orphan Drug Act passed in 1983 by Congress has attracted the attention of AT researchers and policymakers [9,10,19,36]. The Orphan Drug Act provides manufacturers with development incentives in the form of research grants, a 50% tax credit for expenses, an expedited review process, and 7 years of market exclusivity to the first company to reach the market with a new drug. These incentives have significantly increased the development of orphan drugs. An Orphan Technology Act might provide relief to consumers and manufacturers in the AT marketplace.

24.4.5.3 Capacity Building

Science, engineering, and medicine (STEM) has not attracted people with disabilities into its ranks commensurate with population size [37]. The NSF and the NIH have begun to remedy this situation through studies and support for researchers with disabilities. STEM curricula may also require adjustment to address the new paradigm needs for health access and usability; examples of educational materials and approaches related to embedding accessible and universal design into engineering curricula, funded primarily by NSF, is provided in Chapter 8. Engineering science currently may focus more on process. Training future engineers, including engineering researchers, with sensitivity to human factors, quality of life, and accessible design are important potential change agents [38]. These researchers would bring human factors skills and commitment to the R&D process and serve as change agents.

24.5 CONCLUSIONS AND RESEARCH DIRECTIONS

Realization of a vision of technology for all citizens may be linked to the emergence of an engineering paradigm that complements the integrative paradigm of disability [10,24]. The disciplinary engineering matrix would integrate the beliefs, values, and techniques of human factors, especially human factors and related quality of life work in AT, universal design, and user interfaces for all. This paradigmatic shift in engineering will need resource support. The NSF, with some appropriate activities by NIH, is the appropriate organizational arena in the U.S. for basic engineering research that can be transferred and translated into more practical problems by and for the RERCs and the RDCs. Cynics may reject this vision because of the difficulties in marshalling the financial and political resources to make it a reality. However, the vision and its practical potential to save public resources associated with the costs of aging may well stimulate members of Congress to provide NSF with funding and guidance that would include user participation. A preliminary study by the Institute on Medicine may be a stimulant to generating further resources.

As the political scientist Harland Hahn observed, social organization is not decreed by natural law. Irrespective of the realization of emerging paradigms, the rehabilitation research community has a responsibility to build capacity in the social and behavioral sciences, statistics and demographics, economics, social thought, organizational theory, and business-related disciplines to engage in sophisticated, empirically based, and qualitative sociotechnical studies. Sociotechnical studies are appropriate to an expanded notion of engineering. Although these studies must maintain the technical base of technology, they can isolate social factors inherent to technology and the context of technology development and diffusion. Disability studies has an important role to play for people with disabilities just as feminist studies has for women. Disability studies can conduct experientially based studies of medical devices. Disability studies should be further stimulated to engage with STS/P in theories and methods that address science and engineering culture and the social construction of technology. A well-designed literature synthesis would be a very helpful first step in identifying what has been done.

The challenges associated with meeting the needs of people with disabilities in mainstream and AT markets are not new. The problem of defining the consumer market may be confounded by the reluctance of the aging and disability communities to count the other in their numbers and policy goals. However, the need to bridge mainstream and AT efforts has been made more pressing as technology becomes the arbiter of life's most precious resources including personal relationships, community integration, health, voting rights, employment, and education.

A study of the Orphan Technology Act would probe its political feasibility and the appropriateness at the R&D stage of introducing an incentive package to increase the availability of assistive technology. At the R&D and evaluation stages, studies may identify behavioral, policy, and organizational variables that have influenced Congress, regulatory agencies, and research institutes to change their rules, practices, and criteria for participation. The NIH and FDA's engagement with the women's health community may serve as a case study. Studies can be useful that focus on the activities of successful expert change agent interventions within bureaucracy and consumer change activities usually located outside the bureaucracy. At the diffusion stage, studies are needed of procurement and purchase decisions by the DVA, DOD, and state and local group purchasing organizations.

REFERENCES

1. Hahn, H., Introduction: disability policy and the problem of discrimination, *Am. Behav. Sci.*, 28(3), 297, 1985.
2. Stephanidis, C. (Ed.), *User Interfaces for All: Concepts, Methods and Tools,* Lawrence Erlbaum, Mahway, NJ, 2001.
3. Guba, E.G. and Lincoln, Y.S., Competing paradigms in qualitative research, in *Handbook of Qualitative Research,* Denzin, N.K. and Lincoln, Y.S., Eds., SAGE, Thousand Oaks, CA, 1994, chap. 6.
4. Feenberg, A., *Transforming Technology*, Oxford University Press, New York, 2002.
5. U.S. Congress Office of Technology Assessment, Technology and Handicapped People, Washington, D.C., 1983, retrieved on October, 2005 from http://www.wws.princeton.edu/ota/.
6. U.S. Department of Commerce, Technology Assessment and the U.S. Assistive Technology Industry, Bureau of Industry and Security Office of Strategic Industries and Economics, Washington, D.C., 2003, 1–107, retrieved October 2004 from http://www.bxa.doc.gov/DefenseIndustrialBasePrograms/OSIES/DefMarketResearchRpts/assisttechrept/.
7. European Commission, Access to Assistive Technology in the European Union, European Commission Directorate-General for Employment and Social Affairs Unit E. 4, 2003, 1–188.
8. Rehabilitation Engineering Research Center on Technology Transfer, Symposium on the state of the science and practice of technology transfer, *Journal of Technology Transfer*, 28(3/4), August 2003.
9. Cohen, A.B. and Hanft, R.S., *Technology in American Health Care: Policy Directions for Effective Evaluation and Management*, University of Michigan Press, Ann Arbor, MI, 2004, p.65.
10. Seelman, K.D., Universal design and orphan technology: do we need both?, *Disability Studies Quarterly*, 25(3), Summer 2005.
11. Peltz-Strauss, K., personal communication, 2005.

12. Seelman, K.D. and Schmeler, M., Operation wheeler dealer: CMS crackdown on wheelchairs highlights tensions between health and disability policy, *Disability World,* 23, April–May 2004.
13. Seelman, K.D., IT R&D: incorporating accessibility for people with disabilities, President's Information Technology Advisory Committee, National Coordination Office for Information Technology Research and Development, May 18, 2000, National Coordination Office for Information Technology Research and Development, available at http://www.itrd.gov/ac/pitac-18may00/accessibility/assess-seelman.pdf, May 20, 2002.
14. Seelman, K.D., Meeting the needs of people with disabilities through federal technology transfer, U.S. House, Committee on Science, Hearings on Assistive Technology, Washington, D.C., July 15, 1997. (Y4.SC12:105/26), available at http:// www.house.gov/science/seelman_7-15.html, May 20, 2002.
15. Seelman, K.D., The information age: participation challenges and policy strategies to Include people with disabilities, in Proceedings of the World Health Organization Collaborating Centre Seminar: Creation of an Inclusive Society in an Advanced Information and Communications Society, November 6, 2003, Tokorozawa, Saitama, Japan.
16. Winters, J. and Herman, W., Workshop on Home Care Technologies for the 21st Century, Food and Drug Administration, Rockville, MD., April 7–9, 1999, retrieved from http://www.eng.mu.edu/wintersj/HCTWorkshop.
17. Jasanoff, S., Markle, G.E., Petersen, J.C., and Pinch, T., Eds., *Handbook of Technology Studies,* SAGE, Thousand Oaks, CA, 1995.
18. Burns, T.R. and Flam, H., *The Shaping of Social Organization: Social Rule System Theory with Applications*, SAGE, Thousand Oaks, CA, 1987.
19. Seelman, K.D., Science and technology: Is disability a missing factor?, in Seelman, K.D., Albrecht, G., and Bury, M., Eds., *Handbook of Disability Studies,* SAGE, Thousand Oaks, CA., 2001.
20. Seelman, K.D., Trends in rehabilitation and disability: transition from a medical model to an integrative model, *Encyclopedia of Special Education, accepted 2005 for* 2006.
21. Gill, C.J., The last sisters: disabled women's health, in Ruzek, S.B., Olesen, V., and Clarke, A., Eds., *Women's health: complexities and differences*, Ohio State University Press, Columbus, OH, 1997.
22. Kailes, J., Health, Wellness and Aging with a Disability, retrieved on October 2005 from http://www.jik.com/hwawd.html.
23. Daly, J., Guillemin, M., and Hill, S., Eds., *Technologies and Health: Critical Compromises,* Oxford University Press, Melbourne, 2001.
24. World Health Organization, International Classification of Functioning, Disability and Health, World Health Organization, Geneva, Switzerland, 2001.
25. U.S. Congress Office of Technology Assessment, Assessing the Efficacy and Safety of Medical Technologies, 1978, retrieved on October 2005 from http://www.wws.princeton.edu/ota/.
26. U.S. Congress Office of Technology Assessment, Technology and Aging in America, 1985, retrieved on October, 2005 from htttp://www.wws.princeton.edu/ota/.
27. Rogers, E.M., *Diffusion of Innovations,* New York, Free Press, 1995.
28. Normie, L. and Gavrish, A., Market diffusion processes for assistive technology products, 2001, in Marincek, C., Buhler, C., Knops, H., and Andrich, R., Eds., *Assistive Technology — Added Value to Quality of Life* (AATE'01), IOS Press. Washington, D.C., pp. 701–709.
29. Kyoyo-Hin Foundation, Kyoyo-Hin White Paper 2001, retrieved on October 2004 from http://kyoyohin.org/eng/index.html.
30. King, T., *Assistive Technology: Essential Human Factors*, Allyn and Bacon, Boston, MA, 1999.
31. Greenfield, P., An Introduction to the Medical Device Industry, Clinica reports, CBS931, 2004, retrieved on September, 2005 from http://www.pjbpubs.com/cms.asp?pageid=1762#Executive.
32. U.S. Food and Drug Administration, Future Trends in Medical Device Technology: Results of an Expert Survey, April 8, 1998, retrieved on September 2005 from http://www.fda.gov/cdrh/ost/trends/toc.html.
33. Institute on Medicine, IOM Report Reveals Inadequate Oversight of Medical Devices for Children, retrieved on October 2005 from http://www.pedaids.org/ latest_news_IOM_u.18.05htm.
34. Sawyer, D., Do It By Design: An Introduction to Human Factors in Medical Devices, retrieved on 2005 from http://www.fda.gov/cdrh/humfac/doit.html.

35. Kay, R. and Crowley, J., Guidance for Industry and FDA Premarket and Design Control Reviewers — Medical Device Use-Safety: Incorporating Human Factors Engineering into Risk Management, retrieved on October 2005 from http://www.fda.gov/cdrh/humfac/1497.html.
36. Brandt, C.D., Availability and accessibility of the nation's research infrastructure: the transfer of assistive technology by federal laboratories, *Journal of Technology Transfer*, 28(3/4), 197–205, 2003.
37. U.S. National Science Foundation, Women, Minorities, and Persons with Disabilities in Science and Engineering 1998, National Science Foundation, Arlington, VA, NSF 99-338, 1999.
38. Yamauchi, S. and Satoh, T., Assistive engineering as a new discipline, International conference Montreal, 1996, 107–109.

25 Future Possibilities for Interface Technologies that Enhance Universal Access to Health Care Devices and Services

Jack M. Winters

CONTENTS

ABSTRACT

Human–technology interfaces are going through an evolutionary transformation, one that is likely to impact on future medical device interfaces. This chapter reviews technical trends in interfaces, especially as related multimodal interaction. This is followed by consideration of approaches for enhancing universal access to health care devices and services, where universal access is assumed to include barriers of distance and cost as well as direct accessibility of the interface. Such approaches include considerations of the procedural nature of most use of health care devices, recognition of the distinctions between accessibility and usability and how this can impact on access, and a trend toward approaches that emphasize personalized interfaces.

25.1 INTRODUCTION

At a workshop in 1999 on home care technologies for the 21st century, many health care and policy experts expressed the sense that society was on the verge of a paradigm shift towards consumer-driven health care [1,2]. Although the momentum has perhaps slowed, seeds for change remain, such as our aging society and remarkable technological advances. There are many possible actors and paths that could lead to such transformation, and it could take many forms. Technology transfer specialists often refer to conceptual "forces" that can "push" and "pull" to yield change. One technical push is the continued advances in information technologies that are promoting greater interconnectivity and interoperability, which may inevitably cause the medical device industry to ride this wave and adapt its product lines. A possible society push is that research investments combined with relatively new laws and guidelines will cause enhanced access to and usability of certain types of products and services by people with diverse abilities and economic status. A market-driven consumer pull is that as baby boomers age they will demand better and more convenient access, likely resulting in a greater focus on usability testing of products. Still another force is a potential obstacle that is nonetheless also an opportunity: the multifaceted social pull to bring down spiraling health care costs. In reality all of these dynamic processes have benefits, and evolutionary change can take many forms.

Such converging trends provide a window of opportunity for systems change that could impact the degree of universal access to health care products and services. But will this evolutionary process yield products that are more accessible for persons with disabilities and older adults? It is difficult to tell. The nature of an evolutionary process is that often some individuals can be left behind, especially those with less power or ability to adapt. If we are not careful, many individuals might not have the opportunity to participate in, and thus benefit from, a consumer-driven paradigm shift. It is certainly not automatic. Framing the questions and questioning the frameworks may be necessary.

This chapter addresses a narrow window within this health care challenge: the evolutionary trends in interfaces, specifically as related to promoting accessible medical instrumentation. This framing of the challenge reflects a bias: as often suggested by authors of chapters in this book, many of the key challenges and opportunities rest with issues related to human–technology interfaces, issues with both a social and technical dimension. Along with Chapter 24 of this book that provides the vision from a societal and policy perspective, and Chapter 26 that provides a perspective of the trends and challenges from a technical and business perspective, this chapter is intended to help set the conceptual stage for discussions on emerging trends and future directions.

This chapter also reflects part of the mission of the Rehabilitation Engineering Research Center on Accessible Medical Instrumentation (RERC-AMI), specifically as related to anticipating future trends and selecting strategic opportunities for demonstrating possibilities for more accessible health care interfaces. Examples are given in Chapter 27 and Chapter 28 of this book. But these are just examples, constrained by the reality of limited resources that can be invested in such activities. To help envision the broader possibilities that are the scope of this chapter, consider the following scenario:

> Imagine it is the year 2010. An elderly couple lives at home, the husband with stroke-induced disability and high blood pressure, and the wife with severe arthritis that affects hand function plus mild diabetes that includes a degree of visual impairment. He's a retired engineer and manager who is quite goal-directed, though seemingly more and more absent-minded. He follows a computer-assisted rehabilitation therapy

that bears similarity to the vision described in Chapter 27. His "universal gym" of arm and leg exercise technologies adjust settings based on his recent history of performance as well as his mood and aims, as interpreted from his answers to several questions initiated by the system.

An interface is established when he's in their family room and says, "OK, healthy time." The picture-in-picture of his HDTV then functions as his health/performance monitor. In the primary picture he typically views the interactive game he's playing, a sports event (especially when doing more routine and "boring" aerobics) or, occasionally, his brother or daughter or his remote therapist or a nurse. Typically his interactive games are played remotely against his brother or daughter, with the sound off when he plays against his brother unless he wins, and the sound up and video available in the picture-in-picture when he plays against his daughter; this all adjusts automatically as a default. He also is prompted to record his resting heart rate and blood pressure each morning and evening, using a system that automatically stores and uploads this information, and even adjusts the dose of his blood pressure medication and sends reminders if he forgets to take the pills.

His wife uses a similar system, but typically chooses to use it in full talking mode. Her glucose monitor also talks with her, as well as transparently communicating with her personalized health record. Something (she's not sure what) sends reminders to her wristwatch to take blood glucose level measurements, and something else provides her with an appropriate dose of insulin that can be automatically administered without her needing to use her hands. She also uses her husband's exercise system to provide gentle stretching exercises to her hands and feet, and head-neck, typically during the commercials while she and her husband are watching TV. To her husband's chagrin, she also insists that all of the "wireless technology stuff" stay in the family room. The exception is when her daughter calls, during which the system automatically works everywhere within range; indeed, this even extends to carrying on three-way hands-free conversations that often continue during walks, or four-ways when one of the grandkids is on.

All aspects of the preceding vision are technically feasible. Indeed, many are already possible, especially in innovative countries such as Japan that seem more ready to embrace ubiquitous technology that is assistive. Although there are technical challenges, such as reliable integration of products across diverse product lines and from different companies (challenges of reliability and interoperability), most of the challenges reside at the human–technology interface, an interface that is typically two-way. As the preceding example suggests, a human brings a diversity of abilities, preferences, experiences, aims and moods to this interface. And humans can change, sometimes within seconds, sometimes over the course of years. The interface technology, to be effective in delivering the intended uses of the device and have it be embraced by its owner, would ideally adapt to this dynamically changing partner that it is designed to serve.

Here we also assume that by 2010, there will be leadership within our larger community which will insist that, as much as possible, society move toward the vision that all members of this community have access to the intended use of all products. Right now there are just a few select domains where accessibility is required; for the U.S., this specifically applies to architectural design, transportation systems, and electronic and information technologies (E&IT). These domains could, and should, include medical devices. Such a new playing field, as long it is level through use of well-defined rules, should satisfy companies. Indeed, for the medical device industry in which the client base for many products includes a disproportionately larger number of users with disabilities, it makes special sense — for many products such policy opens up larger markets, both nationally and internationally. It would also stimulate the type of commercial environment that enables creative designers to innovate.

So with these presuppositions, where are we? Of the many paths toward improved access to the intended use of products, most can be categorized into one of the following two alternative strategies:

- Design the interface using approaches motivated by universal design (UD), i.e., "design for all" strategies (e.g., Chapter 6 and Chapter 8 of this book).
- Personalize (customize) the interface based on the abilities and preferences of a specific user or the user's agent (e.g., Chapter 26, Chapter 27, and Chapter 28 of this book).

Undoubtedly some colleagues will disagree with this simplification, because it views these as fundamentally distinct approaches (despite some procedural overlap). This battle has a long history within the rehabilitation community, as assistive technologies and universally designed products each make the most sense within the context of addressing certain real challenges. The accessibility-oriented laws of the U.S. bear this out, and thus it is acceptable for a product to either be directly accessible (often called *direct access*) or to provide an interface for a user's personal assistive technology that provides them with roughly equivalent access to the intended use of the product or service (called *compatible access*). Specifically, the E&IT Accessibility Standards maintained by the U.S. Access Board [3] include, under Subpart C — Functional Performance Criteria, a collection of guidelines of the following form (§ 1194.31):

> At least one mode of operation and information retrieval that does not require [user sensory or motor ability] shall be provided, or support for assistive technology used by people who are ...

Furthermore, from this author's perspective the Web Content Accessibility Guidelines represented a paradigm shift towards personalized interface design by formalizing requirements such as text equivalents with the specific intent that a user's assistive technology or user agent can provide an accessible interface (see Chapter 23 of this book for a broader perspective). From the perspective of access, the two strategies cannot become one, as much as well-intentioned people might try. Given the product diversity among the roughly 30,000 devices within the health care field, it is suggested that both approaches need to be proactively pursued and nurtured if universal access is to become a reality.

In this chapter Section 25.2 reviews current technology trends as related to interfaces, with emphasis on anticipated emerging technologies that have the potential to change the landscape for certain areas of health care interfaces and health care practice. This does not imply that such changes will occur, but simply that from a technical perspective there are opportunities for significant impact.

Section 25.3 then proposes conceptual foundations for framing the problem. Specifically, it develops a broader perspective for considering future possibilities for interface technologies that move toward universal access to health care procedures. Note the use of the word *access*. This chapter is not about universal usability, but about the civil right of access to the intended use of a product or service, to a degree that is readily achievable. Here "readily achievable" is a hard-to-see line, drawn in the sand of difficulty to access, that can (and should) shift as technology enables greater inclusiveness and flexibility in use.

Because this chapter is about future possibilities, there are no results or discussion sections, as the future must still evolve. Instead, there is a future directions section that considers a few product categories that the RERC-AMI's national consumer survey (Chapter 2 of this book) revealed contain considerable barriers to access. For these, some future priorities and directions are suggested.

25.2 BACKGROUND: TECHNOLOGICAL TRENDS IN INTERFACES

The word *interface* seems so simple. Yet it is complex, largely because humans are complex, adaptive creatures. Humans are so adaptive that despite the design of the interface for many products often almost an afterthought, being certain types of products still succeed financially. In such cases users simply adapt to it, if they are able. Yet in the year 2005, it was well understood that subtle considerations in interface design can make or break a product, or even a company. Indeed, a past statement by Microsoft's Bill Gates that the future is in the human–technology interface now seems obvious. Well-designed interfaces add value to a product. Companies such as Microsoft or Nokia would not dream of putting a product on the market without first having it go through usability evaluation, including testing with intended users.

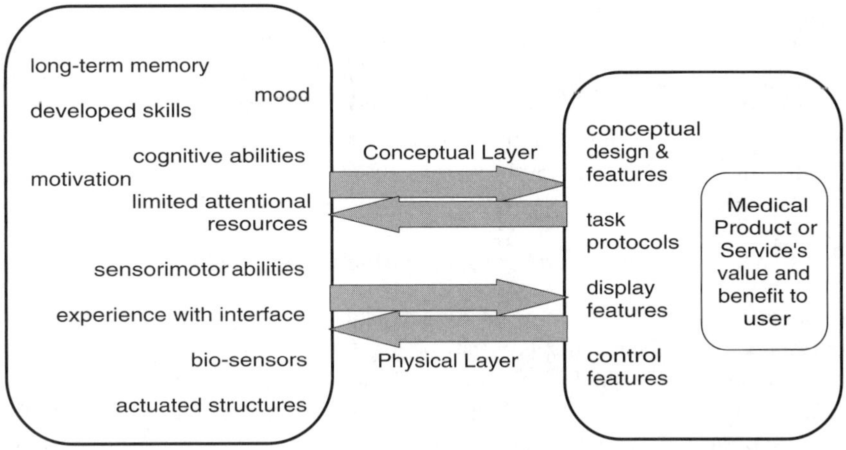

FIGURE 25.1 A systems representation of human–technology interfaces. The human is represented as having sensorimotor capabilities that often include sensors and actuators that support alternative strategies for completing a given subtask, attentional resources that include short-term memory and adaptation, cognitive abilities, and longer-term memory that stores adaptive learning. The medical product is assumed to be used in a procedural way. Using a computer analogy, this interface is conceptualized as including both a lower-level control/display interface (physical layer) and a middle-level conceptual motivational interface (conceptual layer).

In this section, we outline alternative technologies and emerging technological trends for interfaces, using a systems input–output conceptualization of the interface, as is presented in Figure 25.1. Notice the assumption of two layers — a physical layer and a conceptual layer.

25.2.1 Trends in Physical Layer Interfaces

25.2.1.1 Physics of the Physical Layer: One- Way and Two- Way Interfaces

Scientifically, interfaces in the physical world can be inherently two-way (e.g., physical contact between a human and device) or one-way (e.g., sound waves triggering a multistage mechanical process within the inner ear that cause signal changes in sensory neurons). Interfaces can be viewed as transmitting power or information, depending on the "impedance" across the interface. If it is reasonably matched, interaction is usually viewed as a two-way power transfer, whereas if it is dramatically mismatched, one-way information (a signal) is transferred.

Interfaces involving physical contact, for instance between the hand and device, are often inherently two-way unless the device impedance is either really high (e.g., pushing against a wall) or really low (pushing against air). Such interfaces exist in physical space, and have locations and orientations. One example is hand tools. With experience and practice, the body can often discover such two-way interfaces to the point where they can become an almost subconscious extension of the body. This is the extended physiological proprioception (EPP) concept that was first proposed by Simpson [4], which although originally applied to body-powered upper extremity prostheses, also applies to use of products such as a tennis racquet, a pencil, or many machine tools. It turns out that the key criteria are: (1) that a pair of signals (e.g., a force–velocity pair, whose product is mechanical power) cross the interface, (2) that the mechanical behavior on the other side of the interface be predictable so that it can be discoverable by the neuromotor system, and (3) that there be enough richness in the interaction so as to assist this discovery process. The result can be wonderful — a technology that is assistive, functioning essentially as a subconscious extension of the body. Similarly, other types of well-designed physical interfaces are subconsciously forgotten, for instance forgetting that one is sitting in a comfortable chair or wearing a hat. Thus, a well-designed two-way interface becomes subconscious; either it is used as a subconscious extension of self, or its existence is forgotten. The most effective designs exhibit both features.

One-way information transfer interfaces are also common and, indeed, more commonly the subject of analysis. Often, these are integrated into a signal pair that includes one-way information in both directions. If information is being transferred from the device to the human without human intervention, we often call it a display. With this definition, displays can take many forms, the most common of which is visual. If information is being transferred from the human to the device, we often call it a *control*. Controls can also take many forms.

25.2.1.2 Display Technologies for Sensory Input and Cognitive Use

A *display*, defined broadly, provides information that can be sensed and subsequently perceived as information. At the physical layer, displays may be perceived through use of senses such as vision, hearing, touching, or even smelling. Each of these modes has their strengths and weaknesses. The visual system excels at both spatial and temporal processing of signals, but optimum sensing requires the use of eye movements to foviate on an area of interest (see Chapter 10 of this book). The auditory system extracts both magnitude and frequency content from an acoustic signal and is especially effective at temporal recognition. Tactile sensing includes limited spatial and temporal resolution and is best for displays transmitting a few bits of information.

Visual displays take too many forms to fully review here, but a few key trends [5] are:

- Flat panel displays that are replacing CRT displays, with better luminescence and reduced cost
- Low-cost LCD panels, including lower-cost paintable flexible displays
- Heads-up displays and eyeglass displays that can be worn by a user and project a virtual display of various sizes and increasing resolution
- Virtual environment enhancements such as three-dimensional displays that improve perceptual visualizations and augmented realities that project objects

Of special note is that some are mobile (e.g., display on PDA device) and wearable (heads-up and eyeglass displays) and that the trend has been toward better clarity at reduced cost. These seem especially suitable for future use in personalized interfaces.

Also available for enhancing vision are augmentation devices and magnifiers/ telescopes. These are normally applied as an assistive technology that is personalized to an individual, similar to how eyeglasses are used by a person who uses them only occasionally. However, they could also be integrated into universally designed products (e.g., display magnifier integrated into an exercise ergometer).

Finally, and perhaps most importantly, improved video compression algorithms such as MPEG 4 and bandwidth, such as cable modems, are setting the stage for more universally transmittable video [2]. This especially has applications for personalized interfaces. One particularly important vision is that of universal wall monitors that could be used on the fly to display text and images from mobile devices in larger size.

Auditory displays also continue to improve in terms of technological capabilities, and specifically in terms of flexibility for use. Wireless technologies, especially built on the Bluetooth or WiFi standards, can now reliably transmit an audio signal to a very small earpiece from a PDA, cell phone, or household device. Furthermore, improved compression algorithms combined with the iPod digital music phenomenon are resulting in a considerable variety of consumer options.

Both text-to-speech and speech recognition technologies continue to improve, with clearer (and more personalized) synthesized voice and a better rate of speech recognition (see also Chapter 10 of this book). Trends such as home networking and W3C (World Wide Web Consortium) standards activities (see Chapter 26 of this book) for speech will make personalized audio display and speech control more and more ubiquitous within the home and office environment. Advances are also occurring in personal mobility/orientation/navigation devices.

Kinesthetic feedback displays enable a user to sense forces applied by a device, with the primary cases of interest involving computer mice (vibration) and joysticks (vibrations or actual applied forces); these are used extensively for the UniTherapy technology described in Chapter 27 of this book). Other examples include Braille displays, duplicators, and embossers.

One final point relates to the trend toward use of mobile devices for health care, applications including use of cell phones. For such devices displays are very small, and often a tradeoff has to be made between navigation and information content or controls per screen (see Chapter 28). It is interesting that because of such challenges, the W3C groups on device independence, accessibility, and multimodal interfaces have recognized a need to combine expertise, because users of mobile devices essentially have capability limitations similar to disability [6]. Thus, there are reasons well beyond disability for considering multimodal displays.

25.2.1.3 Control (Action) Technologies for Manipulation and Expression

Most of these technologies in some way sample information that is based on neuromotor expression that causes muscle activity, and in turn causes skeletal motion that is expressed at a body endpoint such as the hand. Common modes of such expression include the hand, foot, mouth, and head, and gestures of the arms, head, lips, or face. Another possibility, currently at an early research stage, is the use of indirect brain control to operate switches or move external objects.

There have been continued advances in a range of interface technologies that sense human motor abilities, including the following:

1. Direct-actuated and operated input technologies:
   - *Mouse and joystick/gamepad technologies:* Although most of the capabilities of these technologies have existed for some time for more expensive virtual reality and teleoperator systems, there have been advances, especially for wireless mice that enable mouse control by movement of the hand or a device (such as a virtual tennis racket) in the hand in physical space or by an optical pointing device on a screen. Currently, the primary application has been high-end virtual game therapy, but the number of potential applications is high (e.g., see Chapter 27 of this book).
   - *Keyboard technologies, including special keyboards:* Most keyboards are operated by the hand. These range in size from large to miniature, gentle touch of key to keys requiring greater excursion or force, and from integrated into portable devices to wireless units to foldable fabrics to projected on a tabletop. A variety of specialized keyboards also have been proposed that include keyboard shapes intended to promote good ergonomic postures and minimize repetitive motion disorders, keyboards that sense finger forces without significant motion, and head- or eyegaze-operated keyboards. It is expected, however, that keyboard operation may be less common in the future.
   - *Glove technologies:* The primary motivation for the glove technologies that matured in the 1990s was high-tech virtual reality applications. The more expensive systems measure many degrees of freedom of hand movement and finger forces. Lower-cost ones use fairly crude technologies and have not really caught on.
2. Motor expression recognition technologies:
   - *Speech recognition:* These technologies have been around for a long time, with early use by persons with disabilities. But the systems continue to improve, with fewer recognition errors and lower costs, suggesting that speech recognition could become appropriate as an alternate modal control. This represents a critical component of the multimodal suite.

- *Pen-based handwriting recognition:* Advances in handwriting recognition coupled with a greater variety of digital pen and pad/tablet interfaces represent intriguing technologies for both text entry and as controls. These would seem well positioned for many medical device applications as an alternative modal control.
- *Gesture recognition:* These technologies have used mostly image-based recognition approaches, transducing hand, arm, body, and facial movements and using them to control switches and for text input. It is difficult to see how this could be reliably used for a medical device, but perhaps as switches for positioning.
- *Lip recognition (augmented with acoustic information):* Although intriguing, such technologies do not seem particularly viable for medical device applications.
- *Biometric recognition:* There are many advances in this area, as related to personal identification. Technologies include fingerprint, retinal scans, and voice recognition. These have considerable potential for medical devices, both for personal access and security and as a way of adding robustness to the device interface, for instance, by helping the device recognize a person and adapt its display and control interface strategy to the user's abilities and preferences. It is especially relevant for personalized interfaces.

25.2.1.4 Two- and One- Way Positioning and Orienting Interfaces and Tools

The RERC-AMI's national consumer survey shows that many accessibility barriers relate to positioning and orienting of individuals relative to medical equipment (Chapter 2 of this book). There are no new technological trends to report, except to note the following (1) advances in load-history-dependent materials that are used for cushioning, (2) the greater availability of antigravity mechanisms that can be operated with little or no external power, and (3) the trend toward exam tables/chairs/beds with more accessible features (most commonly attained by the "brute force" approach of increasing the device power requirements and the cost of the equipment by adding motors to address more degrees of freedom such as table height or the angle of a seatback).

Of note is that powered operations normally involve one-way control switches, and do not use EPP. Such approaches may add to accessibility and improve access when cost is not a barrier. But the negative is that the user becomes an observer of an open-loop control operation (to them) rather than an interactive operator. However, there are alternatives that could in principle be applied to medical equipment. One alternative would be to augment human power, similar in concept to power steering for a car; this can be designed to follow EPP principles, but can get expensive. Another option of potentially moderate cost is to compensate for gravity by creating an antigravity potential energy field through the use of strategically placed springs and DC magnets; such strategies are being used, for instance, in newer weight-training equipment.

25.2.2 Conceptual Layer Interfaces

The human–device interface is much more than physical. Indeed, often the focus of a usability analysis is what is here called the *conceptual interface* — that part of the interface that intangibly connects to the perceptual, cognitive, motivational, and adaptive part of the human user. In a recent best-selling book called *The World is Flat* by well-known author and syndicated columnist Thomas Friedman, one of the overriding themes was that technology is about to change how people interact with products and each other to a degree that is unprecedented in history. Access barriers such as distance will break down, and products and services will be accessible to consumers in new, creative ways. This implies opportunity and also suggests that companies that do not adapt may be left behind. It also suggests the importance of outside-the-box thinking about the interface as a means for interaction within an increasingly flattened world where technical access should improve and, importantly, the (conceptual) interface takes on increasing importance. It is particularly hard to imagine medical monitoring technologies and approaches not changing dramatically, especially products or services that target clients in the home setting.

The number of emerging software technologies and standards that are taking up the challenge of supporting more conceptual and intelligent interfaces is staggering and will not be reviewed here. Two other chapters in this book address many of these trends — Chapter 26 on software trends for interface standards and Chapter 27 on integrated treatment of personalized interfaces connecting to Web-based services. Here we briefly highlight some key trends:

- Decoupling and modularizing of physical and middleware layers in information technology standards, promoting greater product interoperability and leveraging investments, and enabling innovation at the physical layer as well as the conceptual layer
- Continued growth in computing power (memory times speed), and in the development of smaller devices
- Networking and interface standards that promote ubiquitous and distributed computing
- Emergence of a international computing language for expressing structure and concepts (XML) that can used as a base to establish consensus protocols and guidelines to be used by the technical community interested in accessibility
- Emergence of the semantic Web standard for structuring more natural interaction between human and machine, which among other applications can promote access for persons with cognitive disabilities and performance enhancement for individuals with many forms of activity limitations (see also Chapter 23 and Chapter 26 of this book)
- Advances in intelligent systems, specifically intelligent agents and intelligent assistants

Historically, medical products that employ E&IT interfaces tend to have about a 3 to 5 year lag in adoption of technology standards. For instance, many medical device companies are just starting to explore USB connectivity. One interesting question in this context is, "In an increasingly flat world where creative innovation can find a worldwide market, are medical device companies and their regulators ready to handle a world of devices that are more modular, interoperable and operate with more intelligent conceptual interfaces?"

25.3 METHODS: APPROACHES ENHANCING ACCESS TO HEALTH CARE

Given the breadth of emerging technologies described in the previous section, it is clear that future designers of devices that enhance access to health care products and services are going to have an ever-richer variety of interface technologies from which to select. This includes both at the low-level physical layer and the more conceptual and motivational middle layer. The potential is certainly there for enhanced access. How does one make a selection from these varied technologies?

25.3.1 Classifying Procedural Use of Health Care Devices

To develop accessible interfaces, it is worthwhile to start by understanding how a device and its interface participate in the health care process. The interface is part of an encounter that involves the device and at least one user.

25.3.1.1 Recognize Overall Reasons for a Health Care Encounter

Classic aims for a health care encounter include the following:

- Obtaining or gathering information on health status (e.g., diagnosis and health assessment)
- Assisting with providing a procedural service (e.g., dental or eye exam)
- Providing therapy of (assumed) therapeutic benefit (e.g., physical therapy)

This is not a perfect classification as there can be overlap (e.g., a dentist provides a procedural service that includes use of diagnostic tools such as x-rays and then provides a form of therapeutic intervention). Use of an assistive technology within the context of health care also often integrating into a procedural framework. The interface takes many forms, in part because there are many goals for health care procedures. More specifically, there is often a goal-directed sequence of tasks.

25.3.1.2 Recognize Roles for Entities Participating in a Health Care Encounter

One of the most thoroughly thought-out representations of the health care encounter involves the scheme used by Health Level 7 (HL7), a mature international standard for health care messaging and informatics that is used extensively for interoperable communication of health care information. Figure 25.2 summarizes the basic structure that is implemented in the XML-based HL7 version 3.0. The key concept is that "an *entity* in a *role participates* in an *act*," where there is extensive significance within an object-oriented structure for each of the four emphasized words. Each of these terms is carefully defined as follows:

- *Entity* — The physical objects in health care, which are nouns that can represent a person, place, or thing (e.g., device).
- *Role* — Ascertains the part that entities play as they partake in health care acts; roles for individuals range from physician to patient and include caregiver, and roles for devices range from an entity measuring blood pressure to an exam table.
- *Act* — The health care actions or activities, a verb. An act relationship can be used to "bind" a series of acts.
- *Participate* — Instances of an "entity-in-a-role" performing an act [7].

Notice that an entity can include an individual with disability. This person can participate in roles such as a patient or consumer. Thus a patient or a consumer refers to the person only in the context of a certain role. Until a role is established, it is not possible to participate in an act.

In this formalism, when an individual uses an interface to a medical device, both the person and the device are participating in its use (e.g., act sequence) from the context of their roles. The interface is part of the entity called *device* and is critical to its role in the encounter and to the form of the participation. The advantage of this construct is its clarity, which was developed over a multiyear consensus process and has stood the test of having been used for millions of reimbursable encounters in health care settings.

25.3.1.3 Recognize the Strengths of Tools Available for Analysis

The chapters of this book provide a plethora of viable approaches for evaluating and designing interfaces for medical equipment. We see effective use of ergonomics (Chapter 11 in this book), human factors engineering (Chapter 16 in this book), UD (Chapter 6 and Chapter 8 in this book), usability and accessibility evaluation (Chapter 13 in this book), accessibility evaluation (Chapter 22 in this book), and accessibility standards (Chapter 15 and Chapter 23 in this book). One could add human performance analysis and perhaps cost-benefit analysis. Each approach has its own procedures and tools associated with design and evaluation of health care interfaces. All have strengths, and, indeed, all have, over time, extended their field to encompass a range of interface issues. Thus, although ergonomics may have a primary focus on the biomechanical study of work, the approach

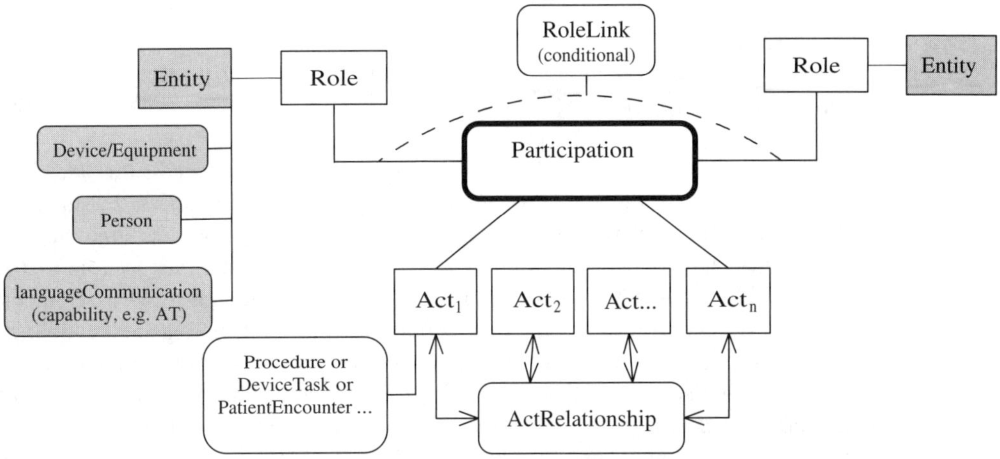

FIGURE 25.2 Model of health care procedures based on the Reference Information Model (RIM) of the international Health Level 7 (HL7) standard that is used for medical messaging (e.g., for communication between products, for documenting billable activities and procedures). In this model, an entity describes the physical objects in health care, such as medical devices and people. They only participate in health care acts in the context of a role, which ascertains the part that an entity plays. An act is a health care action or activity, and an act relationship provides the binding for a series of acts that often constitute a procedure.

extends to visual displays and cognitive considerations. Similarly, UD concepts are positioned to include aspects of usability and accessibility analysis.

So what to use? It depends on the aims of the analysis. A good starting point is human factors engineering, because that is the FDA's frame of reference (Chapter 17 of this book), and it provides a good frame of reference for addressing safety and user error. A useful analogy is the diversity of religious faiths, which suggests there are many paths toward the aim of enlightenment. But as with religions, subtleties in the different approaches in fact may result in different solutions. In this next section the context for this analysis is emphasized by perceiving the light at the end of the tunnel — universal access.

25.3.2 Framework for Understanding Universal Access

Universal access was purposely used in the title of this chapter despite having become a controversial, hard-to-define concept. To the U.S. Federal Communications Commission (FCC), it relates to the rights of access to telecommunications services across distance. To the disability community, it is a sort of combination of the valued concepts of accessibility and UD. To standards bodies that have agreed to disagree on precise definition of the term *accessibility* and therefore often do not define the term, it can range from being an all-inclusive term meaning everyone and everything (which then threatens becoming meaningless) or a targeted conceptual framework that can be used once its dimensions are defined.

So the key challenge seems to be to define the dimensions of universal access — the types of barriers that are to be overcome to enable access by the largest number and greatest diversity of people. In this case, we are concerned with access to products that deliver or support health care interventions and assessments. Three barriers, and their associated domains, stand out:

1. Barrier of access to an accessible interface, i.e. one that will enable a user to have access to the intended use or benefit of a health care intervention or assessment capability
2. Barrier of distance, which ranges from challenges related to position and orientation of a person relative to a nearby product within their local environment to challenges due

to larger distances of geographical separation between an individual and beneficial products or services
3. Barrier of access because of economic status, which for the present purposes meaning serious consideration of the cost of a product

For the present purposes, we will use an operational definition of universal access that addresses these three important domains of interest — the ability of all persons to fully access the intended uses of a product or service for which there is potential benefit from the health care intervention or assessment; the barriers relate to the accessibility of the interface across distance and the barrier of cost. The word "service" is included because so many health interventions and assessments require access to a trained health professional. This definition has an interesting implication: an interface that adds accessibility features by increasing its cost may or may not have increased its degree of universal access. It also implies that a product with some accessible features but without distance-aware support can have a lower degree of universal access than a product with fewer accessible features but with greater means for supporting access across distance or personalized interfaces. These implications might be controversial and subject to discussion, but they seem consistent with policy research within the disability community, such as reviewed in Chapter 24 of this book.

25.3.2.1 Product Access and Acceptance through Designing for Abilities

It has already been mentioned within the context of conceptual interfaces (Subsection 25.2.2) that a key part of interface design involves taking advantage of the abilities of the user. Here is a list of abilities to consider for characterizing an interface, some targeting the human and some the communication technologies that are behind the device interface:

1. Accessibility (ability to access)
2. Usability (ability to use effectively)
3. Reliability (ability to depend on)
4. Interoperability and cooperability (ability to work with other entities)
5. Learnability (ability to learn)
6. "Safeability" (ability to safely access for intended use)

These represent the classic "big five" abilities plus a new term, *safeability*. Each of these could be viewed as being the most important, depending on the purpose of the analysis. For instance, a product regulatory body such as the FDA would be expected to care most about product safeability, especially in the context of its usability and reliability. Safety and human err is also an important societal issue [8]. Practitioners typically care foremost about reliability. The disability community cares about all of these, but the one that stands out is accessibility, which has been the push within this community in terms of civil rights and laws. The educational community cares especially about learnability, and it is instructive to consider the six principles for accessible learning that form the framework for consensus online learning accessibility guidelines maintained by the IMS Global Learning Consortium [9]:

1. Allow for customization based on user preference
2. Provide equivalent access to auditory and visual content based on user preference
3. Provide compatibility with assistive technologies and include complete keyboard access
4. Provide context and orientation information
5. Follow IMS specifications and other relevant specifications, standards, and guidelines
6. Consider the use of XML

Notice the emphasis on personalized learning interfaces. Brewer (Chapter 23 of this book) makes the case that Weblike interfaces might increase learnability for certain types of medical instrumentation.

As an RERC, the RERC-AMI's first constituency is the disability community. Hence accessibility must be our first priority. (It is even in our book's title.) But it is tricky. On the surface, one might think that it is possible for a design to reasonably satisfy all of these criteria. In reality, however, although more often than not there is clear synergy between these concepts, there are clear cases of conflict. For instance, designing for accessibility may lower usability for some or even most people, and potentially reliability and interoperability. Interestingly, the RERC-AMI's national survey results suggests that individuals care strongly about safe use as well as accessibility (Chapter 2 of this book), and video-based identification of biomechanical access barriers tend to trend closely with identification of safety events (Chapter 14 of this book).

There are approaches for dealing with all of these criteria under one umbrella. The most logical approach is to use the tool of fuzzy logic — a theory and associated collection of technologies that are made for reasoning of this type. This helps explain why, starting with commercial products from Japanese companies during 1980s, many billions of dollars' worth of products such as cars and washing machines have embedded fuzzy controllers. These fuzzy systems add robustness to their products because this type of logic-based framework approximates the reasoning of human experts. It is a technical tool that can be used to formalize the concept of relative importance i.e., degrees of membership. For this reason, the accessibility and preferences taxonomy that our group is developing (see Chapter 28 in this book for an early activity) is recognizing that there can be degrees of abilities and preferences.

Finally, human abilities evolve, especially as a user becomes more experienced with an interface. Abilities include short- and long-term memory, cognition, and skill acquisition. A novice user of a device brings different abilities to the encounter than an experienced user.

25.3.2.2 Distinctions in Dimensions of Accessibility and Usability

When those involved in designing and evaluating devices think about making a product more accessible, it is nearly habitual to think in terms of enhancing usability. But the paths for maximizing accessibility and maximizing usability often diverge. Although they are often synergistic, optimizing an interface for accessibility (ability to access, and benefit from use) may (and often should) yield different solutions than optimizing for usability (ability to use). This is often not apparent because the abstract ultimate consequences — universal access and universal usability — tend to converge because both use words such as *all* or *everyone*.

Figure 25.3 represents an attempt to explain this difference. At a core level, the domains differ. One cannot assume a monotonically increasing relationship between these two. There are many classic examples. For instance, the Access Board's ADA Accessibility Guidelines [3] include requirements for including design features (e.g., multimodal options) that can make an interface more complex and potentially harder to use. At the level of the individual, a person who has previously lacked access may receive so much benefit from access to a product or service that they may be more than willing to put up with otherwise poor usability. Alternatively, someone with access may prefer greater usability, perhaps even if it denies access to others. Indeed, one of the missions of the RERC on Telecommunications Access is to look out for technological innovation that benefits many but may eliminate previous access for a few (e.g., people with hearing impairments).

Both accessibility and usability can be applied to the needs of an individual or a population. Both are amendable to approaches based on task procedure analysis or design feature analysis, which happen to be the two core pillars of the MED-AUDIT tool that the RERC-AMI is working on as an accessibility metric (Chapter 14 and Chapter 22 of this book).

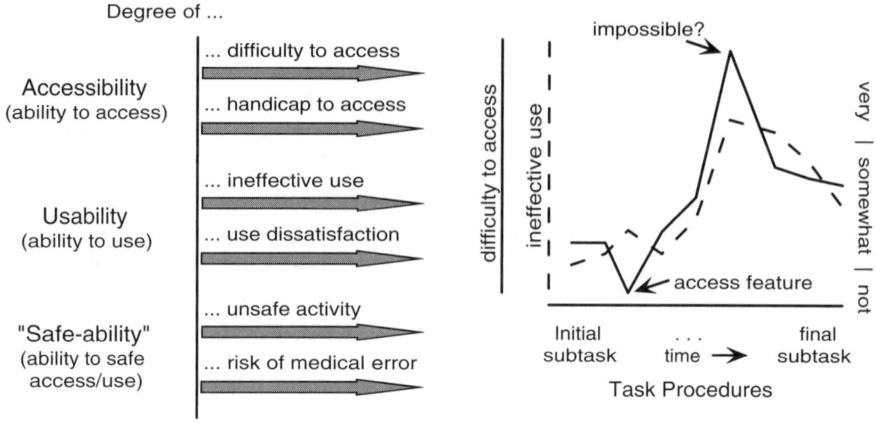

FIGURE 25.3 Possible dimensions of representation, here two each for accessibility, usability and safe-ability. Each is not black-and-white, but rather there are degrees. On the right is a conceptual example showing two of the six dimensions overplotted, with a time axis that represents healthcare task procedures associated with use of a device. This is somewhat similar to how the Mobile Usability Lab (see Chapter 13 in this book) is used to capture events that are mildly difficult, difficult or impossible for a subject. Notice that on the "difficulty to access" domain, an "impossible" event means the device is not accessible for that person; it is a nonlinear effect. Notice also that an event marked by use of an accessibility feature caused complexity and less effective use. Overall, in comparison to the "difficulty" domain the "ineffective use" domain is more integrative of the whole task.

For individuals, there can be degrees of both accessibility and usability, but with several distinctions, some shown in Figure 25.3b. From the perspective of a task analysis approach, if any subtask during use is impossible, the product cannot be accessed for its intended use and the degree of accessibility is zero for that person. In contrast, a usability analysis may find that it is partially usable by that person. People have remarkable adaptive capabilities, and if an individual finds a creative solution to overcoming a difficulty and thus accesses the intended use of the product, then the product is accessible, perhaps to a large degree, for that person. But from a usability perspective, it might be an awful design. If the person needs to use a device feature to obtain access to the product, as long as they can achieve the intended use, then the product is accessible, though there may be degrees of difficulty to access that are worthwhile to evaluate; that is, there may be degrees of usability of an accessibility feature.

It is not always obvious how to determine a population effect from individual effects, or from device effects. Consider the following possible use of "bins" to establish subgroups of the whole population. How would the following be ordered?

1. Considerable difficulty with one essential feature, but no difficulty with all other essential and nonessential features and subtasks
2. Difficulty with most essential features, but able to use and complete task
3. Difficulty with a few essential features, and alternative strategies (one requiring an assistive technology) can be successfully used but with great effort

The order depends largely on the domain being used.

As pointed out in Chapter 18 and Chapter 24 of this book, a population is really a collection of individuals whose traits need to be defined carefully. It is the developers or evaluators who determine the population, either implicitly or explicitly, by how they choose to approach the problem of identifying the characteristics of the intended users. Ideally, they represent a diverse range of abilities and opinions. For a population, there can be a collection of design features that may be required so as to reasonably accommodate these intended users. Accessibility guidelines try to extend the size of the population of intended users to include everyone or nearly everyone. Furthermore, as developed in Chapter 8 of this book, federal accessibility guidelines include statements such as the following:

> Provide one mode that is operable without: pointing, vision, fast response, fine motor, simultaneous action, speech, presence of body parts.

Perhaps the clearest distinction between accessibility and usability comes with how standards bodies treat the two concepts (and not how they define them). Accessibility guidelines permeate many recent standards activities and tend to take the form of a design features approach, e.g., in the form of a checklist (see Chapter 15 of this book). Engineers tend to like such guidance as it provides concrete design specifications. But the result can be accessible products that may or may not be usable. Usability standards and human factors standards tend to focus primarily on processes and practice techniques that shape designer strategies and user performance (see Chapters 16 and 17 of this book).

25.3.2.3 Whenever Feasible, Design for Abilities and to Extend Proprioception

Many human–device interfaces work despite the limitations of the designer. For instance, kids who are really engaged in playing video games can learn virtually any mapping that the game designer employs between game functions and the joystick or gamepad controls. This reflects the remarkable capacity of human to learn and adapt. For instance, humans have the potential capability to:

1. Excel at pattern recognition
2. Adjust to or even find alternative interfaces
3. Use redundancy that is built into their system (e.g., many more muscles than joint degrees of freedom, more joint degrees of freedom than endpoint degrees of freedom, massive degrees of sensor redundancy and perhaps central processing structures) to find alternative solutions or discover ways to use multimodal interfaces
4. Have the highest ability to learn of any creature that we are aware of
5. Acquire new skills (over time)
6. Be easily overwhelmed by a novel interface or context

When an individual has functional impairments, they often find that other functional abilities can become enhanced. Examples abound — the blind person with remarkable ability to process sound, the manual wheelchair user with impressive arm strength, or the deaf person with exceptional observational skills.

Consider the combined human–device system. The user and the device both bring abilities to the encounter. When viewed together, it makes sense to enhance overall system performance by taking advantage of available abilities of the human system. For instance, it is typically best for the human to act as supervisor. Yet it is often worthwhile for the human to delegate control for tedious tasks to the device.

Often the user desires consistency, predictability, and control when interacting with a device. Also, the device is often used as a tool, usually in a two-way (bi-causal) contact interface mode. As noted earlier, EPP is a concept that was defined by Simpson [4] based on observations of users of body-powered upper extremity prostheses. With practice, often the device became a true prosthesis, or a part of self, as if the two had become one. The device had essentially become encompassed into the physical apparatus that was under direct neuromotor control and subconscious use, with minimal requirements for attentional resources. EPP can apply to objects such as a pencil, tennis racket, or computer mouse. It is an ideal interface to be strived for that is often overlooked as a possibility.

25.3.2.4 Recognize Alternatives of Universal Design and Personalized Design

As mentioned in Section 25.1, UD and personalized interface design are viewed here as alternative strategies. Sometimes both may be integrated into a strategy for an accessible interface design.

UD describes the characteristics that make a design more universally usable. As noted in Chapter 18 of this book, UD is the highest standard of usability, and represents an unachievable goal for most types of products that is nonetheless worth striving for. In other words, it has ceiling (saturation) effects, depending on the type of product. Key concepts related to universally designed interfaces are integrating redundancy and direct access into operation of the device, not relying on the aid of an individual's assistive technology or user agent.

Personalized interface designs are customized to the abilities and preferences of the user. In contrast to interface redundancy, personalized interfaces emphasize establishing equivalency of modes and compatible access. Specifically, the interface is designed with "hooks" to the user's assistive technology or user agent. These hooks are often based on standardized interface protocols. Motivation for this approach is described especially in Chapter 27 of this book. Interestingly, the examples presented there and in Chapter 28 of this book describe a standard called a user interface socket (UI Socket), which is defined by a collection of XML files that are used to form a presentation mapping between the personalized interface (called a universal remote console) and the target device or service [10]. Such a universal technical interface or socket supports a remapping of the interaction across the human–technology interface (see Figure 25.4). In this sense, it can be viewed as a sort of assistive technology that travels with a person as their personalized user agent interface. This URC interface may itself take advantage of UD concepts, but it also may not need to. One consequence of personalized design is that although it may be less inclusive, such an interface can potentially enable higher user performance. It also can add consistency and predictability for the user. This perhaps explains the learning community's seeming preference for personalized access interfaces, as reflected by the IMS Global Learning Consortium's published principles and guidelines [9].

Technologies related to personalized interfaces, such as those related to personalized medicine, will continue to advance simply because of the magnitude of the commercial investment in the area, especially as related to mobile devices. The W3C's Device Independence Working Group is an example of the degree of interest in industry and the recognition of need for more intelligent interfaces that include multimodal interaction capabilities. This is very promising for future universal access. Intelligent interfaces can be conceptualized into two types [5]: intelligent/user assistants and intelligent/user agents. The main difference between an assistant and an agent is that an intelligent assistant works as an AT that actively assists the client, for example, in performing tasks associated with device use. This can include reminders, functioning as a predictable assistive technology, or providing direct cooperative functional assistance. In contrast, a supervised intelligent agent acts as a broker on behalf of the client, interacting with other entities on their behalf when the activity is discerned to be within the scope of their accepted role [11]. Both have value. An analogy is an effective administrative assistant who has learned when to function in the role of assistant and when to function in the role of agent.

Multi-modal interfaces fit conceptually with either UD or personalized interface design, depending on the context and circumstances. However, rarely is multimodality transparent and, thus, in addition to enhancing accessibility it often adds complexity to the interface. There are also performance tradeoffs between modes, for instance, between sensory modes of visual and audio displays, and between motor modes of hand and speech operation.

Given that individuals with disabilities make disproportionately large use of medical devices and services, how will this impact on future medical device interfaces? Could the medical device

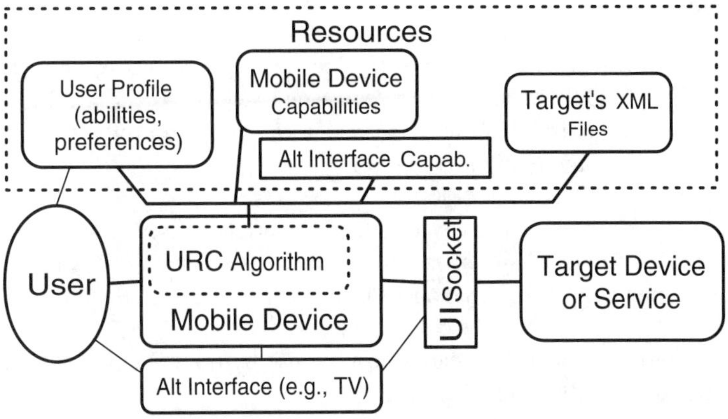

FIGURE 25.4 User Interface (UI) socket as an interface between a URC and a target, here from the perspective of the URC algorithm that must generate an interface. It is assumed that URC algorithm functions as an intelligent agent of the user that often "knows" something about the user's abilities and preferences by reading a user profile resource. It is also assumed that the user has a mobile device (e.g., PDA), but may take advantage of alternative devices (e.g., TV monitor) when they are in range and available.

industry provide leadership in interface innovation or will this generally conservative and late-adopting industry lag behind? And in any case, what might these changes be? What will be the drivers?

25.3.2.5 Recognize That in Striving toward Universal Access, We Cannot Sacrifice Safety or Increase Risk of Use Error

As reviewed in Chapter 3 of this book in the context of practitioner use and Chapter 16 and 17 of this book for device evaluation, statistics show that use error is a major societal challenge. The medical device industry is regulated, and within the U.S. the responsible agency is the FDA, which has been given the charge of evaluating products using the criteria of safety and efficacy. Considering that the eighth leading cause of death in the U.S. is said to be medical error [8], it is apparent that there is a need for study of the "science of people" in the context of interfaces. For many health care products, especially ones used within the home setting, the proportion of intended users with activity limitations or disabilities greatly exceeds the 19% of the general population that has a disability. In considering the possibility of enhancing access to products and noting that accessibility is not the same as usability, what are the risks? This is an important question, one that needs answers.

25.4 FUTURE DIRECTIONS: INITIATIVES AND OPPORTUNITIES

The title of this chapter indicated a focus on future possibilities for interfaces that enhance universal access to health care devices and services. It has been suggested that the designer of the future is going to have considerably more options to consider and, furthermore, the conceptual framework and the selected design and evaluation methodology will impact on her or his choices. It has also been emphasized that given the considerable variety of roles for health care devices and services, many types of solutions should be expected. Finally, a definition of *universal access* was proposed, which suggested that in addition to accessible interface features, cost and distance should be considered.

With this as a context, several future possibilities are put forward for consideration, with an emphasis on areas of major need, as reflected by results of the RERC-AMI's national consumer survey (Chapter 2 of this book).

For exam tables, exam chairs, and beds, consider the following:

- Mechanical "gravity-assist" that minimizes power requirements by the human through potential energy fields operating at the device interface
- Mechanical "power-assist" that uses EPP, with force-assist and velocity matching (where F is force and v is velocity at an interface):
- $F_{user} * v_{user} = K*(F_{device} * v_{device}) = (K * F_{device}) * v_{device}$.
- Orientation-assist multimodal cues to help users orient a user to EPP controllers, and URC for a PD interface that serves to control access to the EPP interface while also providing remote control for any non-EPP powered degrees of freedom.

For medical monitors intended for shared hospital use by trained clinicians/technicians under time pressure, consider the following:

- Design a default interface using UD principles but then have a PD interface (e.g., customized remote control, customized voice recognition), so as to improve both performance and shared access (e.g., across distance) to changing settings.
- Encourage PDs with open standards for certain classes of devices, including both for interfaces and for transparent medical informatics, with both supported by intelligent agents.

For health care monitors and infusion products intended for home use and remote support, consider the following:

- Start with an assumption that any such system should include universal access across the domains of interface accessibility, distance, and cost. Also, that home-based monitoring and infusion systems of the future will be primarily mobile devices, continuing a recent trend.
- Design a simple interface using basic UD (which is a bit more involved for infusion systems), augmented by a proactive multimodal PD system that includes a URC interface that can also make use of other available home display devices such as TV monitors.
- Provide proactive telesupport, including automatic remote transfer of monitoring data, interactive reminders, and an intuitive multimedia interface (that supports image transfer, videoconferencing, educational streaming).

For exercise ergometers for home use:

- Proactively incorporate UD principles into the physical apparatus.
- Provide a display/control interface that proactively incorporates multimodal PD that furthermore supports either a built-in modular display (perhaps with virtual reality goggles) or use of alternative display/control (e.g., local TV/computer monitor).
- Provide support for alternatives of possible interest to clients, including telemonitoring, automated storage, tele-encounters, and virtual gaming.

ACKNOWLEDGMENT

This work is supported by the RERC-AMI, funded by the National Institute on Disability and Rehabilitation Research (NIDRR) of the U.S. Department of Education under grant number H133E020729. All opinions are those of the author.

REFERENCES

1. Winters, J.M. and Herman, W., Report of the Workshop on Home Care Technologies for the 21st Century, 1999, Washington, retrieved from http://www.eng.mu.edu/wintersj/ hctworkshop.
2. Winters, J.M., Emerging rehabilitative healthcare anywhere: was the homecare technologies workshop visionary?, in *Emerging and Accessible Telecommunication, Information and Healthcare Technologies,* Winters, J.M., Robinson, C.J., Simpson, R.C., and Vanderheiden, G.C., Eds., RESNA Press, Arlington, VA, 2002, pp. 152–184, chap. 16.
3. U.S. Access Board, Electronic and Information Technology Accessibility Standards (Section 508), http://www.access-board.gov/sec508/standards.htm, also published in the *Federal Register* on December 21, 2000.
4. Simpson, D.C., The Choice of Control System for the Multimovement Prosthesis: Extended Physiological Proprioception (E.P.P.), in *The Control of Upper Extremity Prostheses and Orthoses,* Herberts, P. et al., Eds., 1974, Charles C Thomas, New York, pp. 146–150.
5. Vanderheiden, G.C. and Zimmermann, G., State-of-the-science: access to information technologies, in *Emerging and Accessible Telecommunication, Information and Healthcare Technologies*, Winters, J.M., Robinson, C.J., Simpson, R.C., and Vanderheiden, G.C., Eds., RESNA Press, Arlington, VA, 2002, pp. 95–111, chap. 16.
6. W3C Device Independence Working Group, Device Independence, Accessibility and Multimodal Interaction, http://www.w3.org/2005/04/di_mmi_wai.html.
7. Health Level Seven (HL7) Standards Version 3.0, http://www/hl7.org.
8. Institute of Medicine, *To Err is Human: Building a Safer Health System*, 2000, Washington, D.C.: National Academy Press, p. 287.
9. Barstow C. and Rothberg M., IMS Guidelines for Developing Accessible Learning Applications, Version 1.0, http://www.imsglobal.org/accessibility/accessiblevers/, IMS Global Learning Consortium, Burlington, MA, 2002.

10 International Committee for Information Technology Standards (INCITS), V2 — IT Access Interfaces, ANSI/INCITS 389–393, 2005, http://www.incits.org/tc_home/ v2.htm.

11. Winters, J.M., Wang, Y., and Winters, J.M., Wearable Sensors and Telerehabilitation: Integrating Intelligent Telerehabilitation Assistants with a Model for Optimizing Home Therapy, *IEEE/EMBS Magazine, Special Issue on Wearable Medical Technologies*, 22, 56–65, 2003.

26 Trends to Watch: Trends in Information and Communications Technology That May Influence Developments in Access to Medical Instrumentation

Alfred S. Gilman

CONTENTS

ABSTRACT

This chapter relates trends in electronics and information technology (E&IT) to the future course of access to medical instrumentation. We are looking for ways to bring medical instrumentation to a point where user-adaptable, assured-usable user interfaces are *de rigueur.* We conclude that the Web experience has contributions to make to medical instrumentation, but falls short in some areas. Even combining Web technology (for reaching the user) with medical informatics standardization (of the terms of the business logic of the device), we are left with some gaps. Some approaches that may be advantageous in filling those gaps are suggested.

26.1 INTRODUCTION

This chapter discusses perceived trends in E&IT that are thought to have relevance to the future course of access to medical instrumentation, with particular emphasis on the legacy of lessons learned from the World Wide Web and Web accessibility. It complements Chapter 23 on how insights from Web accessibility could impact on medical interface design, and Chapter 25 on universal access and multimodal interfaces.

We will start by looking back at some history, and then look forward with some conjectures. In between, we will stop to summarize a few of the challenges we face and look around to current technological developments outside the Web or medical instrumentation domains that seem to be of interest.

We conclude that the Web experience has things to contribute to the medical instrumentation application domain, but falls short in some areas. Some of the shortfalls, fortunately, are covered by the superior application-layer modeling emerging in the area of medical informatics and metadata.

Even combining Web technology (for reaching the user) with medical informatics standardization (of the terms of the business logic of the device), we still have a few capabilities of our technology base. If we are to attain a climate of practice in medical instrumentation that routinely delivers adaptable-to-the-user, assured-usable user interfaces, these gaps must be bridged. We postulate some approaches, which may be advantageous in filling those gaps.

26.2 LOOKING BACK

26.2.1 Web Explosion vs. Wireless Web Fizzle

Tim Berners-Lee, the visionary behind the Web, united the reach of the Internet with the actionable allusions of hyperlinking to frame a global commons of information sharing. When the Mosaic browser united this commons with a point-and-click graphical user interface (GUI), the world went wild. Personal computers went from merely an office must-have to a home fixture, and an immense speculative bubble passed over Wall Street.

The personal mobile communications industry, with their cell phones going digital, saw their chance. We also have the digital network in place for that medium. However, users tried mobile browsers once and stayed away in droves. It seems that the hypercontent that was so compelling on the computer was terminally tedious on the phone [1].

From this difference we can take away the following lesson related to human–computer interface (HCI) design: the user's access to information on the contemporary computer screen is embarrassingly parallel. We have little idea where they pick up what cues from the context of what they act on. To sustain user orientation when there is not such an embarrassment of display riches requires a much better articulated dialog structure so that the business-process essentials can be wrapped in an appropriate amount of context coaching such as headings, breadcrumb trails, and navigation links.

The architecture being pursued by the World Wide Web Consortium (W3C) Device Independence Activity recognizes that one can't hide all the variations across client devices in stylesheets, and allow the Web developers to invest in targeted presentation designs for as many flavors of presentation as they wish, in addition to gaining the economies of reuse for the logical primitives common to all flavors. See Subsection 26.4.3.5 for more on this technology.

26.2.2 Blending Presentation Principles in the CSS Cascade

The design of cascading stylesheets (CSS) recognized that interest in the presentation properties of Web content would come from different quarters. CSS uses a systematic cascading algorithm in which the appearance properties of content are determined from multiple applicable stylesheets with the cascading algorithm serving as traffic cop for the style rules. Therefore, the page presentation could blend the interests of, say, an author and a user.

In practice, this has not worked as well as hoped. There are too many interactions in the psychology of perception between the various aspects of style for the feature-by-feature algorithm in CSS to produce a net effect that was not worse than making an overall choice between one designed style profile and another likewise internally consistent profile.

What has proven efficacious, in the main, are two approaches. To deal with incremental, parametric adjustment of the presentation (for example, larger text) the author predesigns a range of stylesheets and gives the user a control in the page that selects from among them (clickable, right there — the formula that made hyperlinks a winner). The other approach is for the user to put their computer in a system-supported high-contrast (with large text) mode and ignore the styling that the author designed. This, for instance, is an option within the accessibility features of the Windows operating system.

Based on this experience with CSS, one is tempted to step back from the idea of the adaptation space as a continuum, or at least to seek a constructive solution along lines similar to that pursued by the W3C Device Independence Activity. Their approach uses a collection of discrete interaction-space templates or morphotypes that, given parametric adjustments such as font size within the presentation of each morphotype, would collectively cover the adaptation-requirements space — not one structure that would flex to address all needs, but a library of structures such that at least one of them would flex to meet each profile of need. For example, the newspaper-format web page organization — with head, foot, two sidebars and an interior main area — is an example of such a morphotype. So is a cell phone with a graphics screen but with only one dimension of list navigation through a three-state rocker switch. Another is an all-audio dialog that can be passed through a vanilla voice-grade telephone line. Another is the EZ Access(R) cluster of interaction features discussed in Subsection 26.4.5.1.

26.3 CHALLENGES WHERE WE ARE

26.3.1 The Style Economy

Modern business theory places great importance on marketing. This includes understanding what motivates buyers and framing offerings that will attract them. The current vogue is that a lot of this has to do with style. The industrial age has reduced many labor-saving functions to commodities;

it is very hard to attract buyers by how clean you wash the clothes when all your competitors wash the clothes as clean as you do.

Not only has technological progress commoditized functional virtuosity, but the technology-enabled trend of unbundling the process of manufacturing products and services has left the value-addition equation very heavily concentrated in a marketing organization that, similar to the Cheshire Cat, is nothing more than the grin; the capital that they control is just the consumer's positive attitude toward a certain perceived sense of style.

Although within the medical enterprise there is a persistent emphasis on function, and promotion revolves around more primitive tools than multipage glossy advertisements in strategic magazines, in the consumer economy where the cost is mostly being driven out of device technologies by mass marketing, the proposition that devices should make themselves operable as remote slaves through an interface not of their devising will face tough sledding.

The general rule will be that marketers or product creators will want to establish a direct connection with their users, and control how their offering appears to these users in every regard. The net effect in the medical device market, and especially in the home health market, can be a growing collection of stovepiped uncooperating interfaces demanding understanding and attention from the user. We will look at some exceptions to this rule in the Section 26.4 that follows. Because this is the general trend in the E&IT economy, we need to look carefully for niche markets where the conditions are favorable for flexible-presentation interface technology to be developed and sustained by the market economy.

26.3.2 No One Ever Went Broke Underestimating the Public

One of the enduring ironies of the usability profession is that productizers must listen to the consumers, but you can't just do what they say. Gregg Vanderheiden of the Trace Center at the University of Wisconsin–Madison consistently says: "You can't ask someone for whom (a user interface) is not working what it has to do for it to work." You can't confirm that it will work for users without users using it; but when it doesn't work, you (not they) have to go back to the drawing board. The user is still the most flexible element in the man–machine system performing the task when it *does* work. As rehabilitation researcher Cheryl Trepagnier has succinctly said, "People *are* adapted."

This relates to a difference between what has been accomplished in terms of accessibility on the World Wide Web and what will be needed in the area of medical and health equipment.

On the Web, the emphasis is on getting the server to deliver content in a form where the presentation of that content can be controlled on the client side, by the user through their browser and assistive technology. The watchword has been user empowerment; getting them enabled to profile the presentation.

In the medical domain, the vendor relationship to the usability of the user interface is not so much one of branding as of liability. If the manufacturer gives the user a confusing or difficult-to-use interface and use errors can be attributed to this, the adverse consequences for the manufacturer may be considerable. The medical instrument takes on a mantle of *in loco doctoris*, an obligation to do no harm. For this chapter, we will assume that leaving the presentation of the user dialog to be entirely at the user's discretion and dependent on their interface-tuning proficiency is too risky for medical equipment.

26.3.3 Out of Sight, Out of Mind

A number of metadata features in HTML, conspicuously the "link" element and the "rel/rev" attributes on hyperlinks, could make significant contributions to the usability of adapted-presentation user interfaces. However, they have been almost totally ignored in practice. Because they never show up and make any evident difference in the routine use of the Web, they are not used.

This experience suggests caution in relying on metadata. Anything that is not going to be obvious in the routine use of an interface, and is supposed to be reliably present, has to be backed by a well-thought-out enforcement strategy. Well-thought-out includes the property that it imposes a light burden on equipment developers.

26.3.4 The Regulation Divide between Medical and ICT Markets

Economic analysis suggests that we can cut the cost of healthcare by doing more to sustain health and thereby have less to do in terms of having to address illness. But our system for payment has a strong "if it isn't broken, don't fix it" bias. So there is a sharply delineated fortress of medical enterprise outside the moat of which is beginning to spring up a market in alternative products that consumers can buy if they believe these products will contribute to their health.

This was a conspicuous problem encountered by the Rehabilitation Engineering Research Center (RERC) on Telerehabilitation [2]. It would save overall cost to move some health care functions to the home, supported by telematic participation by the medical establishment. But this *modus operandi* is not in the code book of reimbursable procedures, and that proves to be a distinct barrier to entry.

What we are left with in looking at access to equipment that contributes to health maintenance is that we will be forced to take different tactics, if not root strategies, in dealing with products developed for regulated and unregulated markets. The market forces on product manufacturers condition their business decisions about interfaces and interconnection rather differently.

In terms of services, we are seeing some creative moves by the payers to reflect the actual drivers of healthcare efficacy. If you have the right health insurance today, you have fee-free access to an advice nurse who will answer your calls [3]. If you have asthma, they won't wait for you to call but will place the call. So although third-party payers are easy to paint as the villains that won't pay for what you want, in some ways they are sound economists prepared to act in ways that will lower outlay experience.

26.4 LOOKING AROUND

This section discusses some relevant technologies. Some are available in products, some are emerging.

26.4.1 Enterprise Applications Value Flexible Presentation

Why are firms investing in the open architecture for rationalized business processes and flexible presentation that is under development in the W3C Device Independence Activity? [4] Because there are business processes that

- Sustain the 24/7 workplace. These functions want to be available both through the office desktop and 24/7 to the personal devices that people on travel take with them.
- Are outside the style economy. These functions conduct business between entities that are already in a long-term committed relationship. They are not trying to lure passers-by into casual contact the way most B2C sites are.

These functions are called *enterprise applications*. They are the busywork of participating in an organization: filing your time sheet; scheduling meetings; planning travel, and the like. They are hosted by the employer and are exercised by employees. Many large businesses have so much of their workforce traveling at any given time that one can't assume access to these functions from their own desk or even from a laptop computer. But the transactions are swifter and surer if the presentation capitalizes on the desktop dialog capabilities when it is conducted from that context.

So the enterprises are committed to diverse access paths, and the infrastructure for cost-effective development and delivery of such applications is a big enough demand to fuel the W3C Activity. Application examples are discussed in the vendor presentations at the W3C Workshop on Device Independent Authoring Techniques [4]. On the whole, the range of presentation options addressed in this community ranges from desktop/laptop down to telephones with character-grid displays. It does not extend to the pure audio dialogs addressed by the W3C's Voice Browser Activity. On the other hand, academic researchers at Carnegie Mellon University have algorithmically generated quite usable voice-only views out of a similar framework [5].

In this market, at least, one finds a systematic architecture for flexible presentation alive and well for economic reasons.

26.4.2 Medical Errors and Records Automation

There is another market where rationalized data and device diversity are being served by XML formats. This has to do with automating the process of doctors writing orders in hospitals [6]. With the automation, the doctor scribbles on his or her personal digital assistant (PDA) rather than (potentially illegibly) on a paper pad. Eliminating the middleman, the data entry clerk who enters the orders into the computer, helps eliminate medical errors. Medical errors have serious consequences and strike a nerve with the public. Both doctors and hospitals will agree that is important.

The presentation is not frozen at the pixel level in these applications, however. Doctors have just too much clout in the medical enterprise for the hospital to tell them what PDA they will carry. So the device-independence practices such as are being published in W3C are practiced in these systems. These systems generally bridge between PDA-level devices including Blackberry, Palm, and PocketPC flavors and personal computers at nurses' stations, so they are not quite so stressed as the desk-to-mobile systems in the device independence market. But because of the strong concern for information integrity, they look better from the data-modeler or schema-writer's perspective.

This approach makes this sort of hospital automation another existence proof for economically viable flexible-presentation technology in the execution of tasks where function is critical and flair takes a back seat.

26.4.3 Technologies for Marshalling Application Resources for Flexible Presentation

26.4.3.1 The Standard, or DAISY, Digital Talking Book

The ANSI/NISO Z39.86-2002 or digital audio-based information system (DAISY) digital format for talking books reflects a success story in the application of Web technology to increase access by people with disabilities to information [7].

Talking books are books produced in alternate formats for people with print disabilities. The standard talking book format was developed by the worldwide DAISY Consortium of libraries for the blind and other interested parties, and has been standardized through the National Information Standards Organization (NISO). It integrates audio and visual objects in various codecs with text and structure in XML formats defined and profiled in the standard. It makes apt use of the synchronized multimedia integration language (SMIL) developed for Web purposes by the W3C to marshal the presentation of audio clips.

Basing this format on XML has radically accelerated the process of converting books where the publisher of the book, for their own reasons, had chosen to base their publishing process on XML, any XML. Although human effort was still required to map the high-level structures in the publishing pipeline to those in the DAISY format, the use of XML technology at the lower level meant that the manual effort for the conversion was reduced, because the standardization on XML had absorbed the detailed manipulations that constitute the preponderance of the conversion effort.

The DAISY book format sets a benchmark for rich multimedia presentations that are broadly accessible. These do not directly address interaction other than for navigation, but the format is oriented to modular extension and hybrids reflecting both document and task wisdom can be contemplated using DAISY as a host format.

26.4.3.2 The Universal Remote Console Standards

The Universal Remote Console (URC) Standards [ANSI/INCITS 389-393-2005, also under international consideration as ISO/IEC 24752] define a framework, which opens up a commons where a user can operate a product or service from another device of their choosing [8–12; Chapter 28]. Neither the user's device nor the product or service that they are operating has to take any account of the design of the other device other than to: (1) have some interoperable means of data communication and (2) follow the provisions of this standard for the export/import of the console connection.

The framework is currently running in concept-validation prototypes developed by multiple parties. It probably has some limitations in the complexity of the service for which it can export an acceptable interface; that is to say, it is clearly a candidate for the fever thermometer, but there may be more attractive alternatives for booking a multileg travel itinerary starting from scratch.

The specifications in the framework concentrate on assuring that there is enough core information for a repurposed presentation of the dialog between the user at their operating console and the product or service they are operating. There is one format for a structural sketch of one presentation not unlike a Web page, and the framework makes provisions for other user interface implementation descriptions (UIIDs) in nonstandard formats, including executable code compiled for a particular remote device, in addition to the public version of the essentials of the dialog.

In terms of the postulated concern in the medical domain for an assured level of usability in adapted interfaces, there is a gap in this standard as it leaves the presentation of the dialog up to the best efforts of the user's device. A simulation environment for demonstration of its use for certain classes of medical devices, called MedURC, is provided in Chapter 28.

26.4.3.3 XForms

XForms [13] is a second-generation forms technology developed by W3C. It resembles the URC standards in assuring the integrity of the business logic of the dialog and leaving the presentation aspects up to the best efforts of others. XForms may have fewer limitations as to service complexity than the URC standards, but on the other hand, it requires the developer to do more of the data-communication layer in the way that it would be done in the wide area network (WAN) context of the Internet. This is not always an obvious choice in the home or even in a hospital.

Like the URC standards, XForms is very good at sustaining the integrity of the business logic, and agnostic about the appropriateness of presentations.

26.4.3.4 XHTML 2.0

XHTML 2.0 [14] is another second-generation technology from W3C. XHTML at level 1, that is XHTML 1.0 and XHTML 1.1, have worked within the functional precedent set by HTML 4.0. XHTML adds well-formed XML syntax, and XHTML 1.1 decomposes the language into a family of modules. In XHTML 2.0, functional changes have been allowed.

XHTML 2.0 seeks to meet the functional requirements of a broad-spectrum Web hypertext format, with a streamlined set of more powerful, recombinant features. XHTML 2.0 incorporates XForms directly within its own namespace, so that writing forms in Web pages does not require a namespace-aware processor.

XHTML 2.0 is still under development. The slow rate of adoption of XHTML 1.0 and XHTML 1.1 in the Web at large does not augur well for its instant adoption as a replacement for everything that has come before. On the other hand, it will, within a reasonable span of time, be a stable specification with competing implementations. Assured-usable medical instrument interfaces will probably be an application that favors using the better-rationalized feature set of XHTML 2.0 over "what the browser will bear" HTML. The XHTML 2.0 advantage is similar to what the DAISY3 book format gains by using second-generation XML technology for its structure and text formats.

26.4.3.5 Content Selection for Device Independence

One of the component technologies under development by the device independence group of W3C is called Content Selection for Device Independence (DISelect) [15]. This is an interesting lowest-level approach to content rationalization. Rather than try to reduce idiosyncratic, idiomatic human expression (natural language and visual cliches) entirely to a canonical form of model data and view transform, it accepts the idea that sometimes all we have to represent an abstract concept is a bundle of alternate representations. Each representation is at a fairly low modeling level, such as a sound file, an image, and, if we are lucky, a textual version.

The DISelect is a computer geek's generalization of conditional compilation, using XML to wrap the content fragments and XPath to capture the inclusion conditions. One has to remember that this format is optimized not for direct representation of semantics to humans but rather for rapid extraction of a tailored presentation by a server after it learns, on the fly, the conditions at the delivery context (client side).

But it does make determining what data fragments substitute for one another, and where the selected one of them goes in the assemblage, a deterministic algorithmic task. And if one is indeed targeting the presentation to a short list of defined interaction-space concepts, it is a commercial technology with competing support that does the job.

26.4.4 Technologies for Presentation Adaptation

26.4.4.1 Semantic Web Accessibility Platform (SWAP)

An aggressive program of cross-disability presentation adaptation is undertaken by the Semantic Web Accessibility Platform (SWAP) [16]. This is a middleware offering. Users browse the Web through an adapting middleware server. Origin servers cooperate with the middleware service as their disability accommodation strategy. Cooperating sites are subjected to an analysis of their Web media usage patterns, and metadata is created binding their house style to SWAP-understood rhetorical-role concepts.

SWAP finesses the large and diverse amount of metadata standardization by housing the transform design and the origin-site style analysis in the same business organization. The system functions whether or not any second organization can understand or will employ the concepts that key the transformations. But it is impressive testimony to what can be accomplished with a dab of analysis and indirection.

26.4.4.2 The IMS Accessibility Specification

The IMS Global Learning Consortium has produced the most fully-developed metadata specification to date for characterizing user needs and preferences to upstream services [17]. It comes out of the educational arena where one key use case is that of an instructor looking for instructional units to collect and compose into a course. In particular, if the instructor encounters one educational resource that is inaccessible to one of the students, the teacher may be in the market for alternate courseware chunks that cover the same learning objectives. The recent motion toward more atomized and articulated learning objectives also contributes to making this market in individual laboratory-experiment-scale courseware units plausible.

The IMS terms for characterizing the actual delivery context as adapted for a given student is very practical, oriented to information that one could collect relatively easily, such as system settings of font, color, ShowSounds, and the like. It does not get to biophysicical measures, such as to the angle subtended at the eye by two neighbor pixels.

Possible limitations of the taxonomy that follow from its domain of origin are a possible bias toward the traditional I/O configuration of a computer in a school. Medical and home-health equipment interfaces do not always resemble a computer in their look and feel. So some further work on the metadata may be in order. But this is clearly a strong baseline from which to start.

26.4.4.3 Multimodal Interaction Framework Rationalizes AJAX

Some industry pundits have started talking about creating Web interaction media with Asynchronous Javascript and XML (AJAX). Meanwhile, pen-based data input is entering the connected personal-mobile device arena through PDAs with phone functionality and phones with PDA functionality.

Aware of how the subtle differences between the interaction capabilities of the early wireless Web phones made developing interactive content very laborious, many vendors involved in the existing interactive voice response (IVR) and Web industries are working under the umbrella of the W3C to come up with a rationalized integration framework for multimodal interaction [18]. The architecture takes interaction modalities as blades and then runs with the composite it has in the current delivery context. It adapts to a wide mix of interaction modalities.

This will be addressed on the server side with Web applications that have *designed* voice-input capability, rather than forcing voice input to emulate the input events of some other device that works in ways ill-suited to voice.

This will provide a platform for the following: (1) using the novel input modalities of voice and ink more readily in adapted interfaces on more devices and (2) experimentation with direct support for a wider range of AT I/O devices rather than always working through an emulation of another I/O device.

26.4.5 Technologies for Broadly Accessible Dialogs

26.4.5.1 EZ Access

The EZ® or EZ Access® access technology from the Trace Center [19] is a system of interaction capabilities and dialog structures mated to these interaction capabilities. It is designed to enable operation with a very broad spectrum of abilities and disabilities.

The system has seen field use in some voting systems and now more widely in the automated postal centers of the U.S. Postal Service.

26.4.5.2 ETSI Generic Commands

On the desktop, the look-and-feel standards promulgated by the operating system serve to make new applications work in a way that the user is prepared to expect.

In IVR systems on the telephone, there is no such look-and-feel autocrat. The industry received lots of complaints of being lost in IVR menus. In an attempt to reduce this source of resistance to the technology, the European Telecommunication Standards Institute (ETSI) conducted a harmonization process to come up with a broadly reusable repertory of command concepts [20]. These concepts have been prescreened by successful use, and their consistent use across applications would further de-confuse users encountering new applications.

If our working hypothesis is that a significant number of medical equipment use errors are the product of user misunderstandings (see Chapter 17), basing dialogs strongly in this vocabulary could contribute to reduced use errors in the field.

26.4.5.3 DiamondHelp

It is widely recognized in HCI that context-sensitive help is more helpful in de-confusing users than old-fashioned "help," which is just a virtual user-manual, neither responsive to the state of the user dialog nor enabled to activate the operations of the application.

The current version of context-sensitive help is still rather limited. Its context awareness is limited to "where you are in the current displayed panel." What you really need to know at any given moment depends on what you are trying to do. Placing the state of the interface in the context of the action sequences that accomplish tasks sheds more light on how to coach the user than this static view.

Analytically, we could describe this as expanding the model referenced in the system's interactive behavior from the state space of the dialog to the trajectory space of the dialog. One example of a technology that takes this extra step is the DiamondHelp system from Mitsubishi Electric Research Laboratories [21].

26.5 LOOKING AHEAD

26.5.1 A Library of Predefined UI- Builder Kits

As suggested above in discussing the disappointing results from blending in CSS, one strategy that might prove fruitful is divide and conquer: divide up the problem space and develop a collection of UI-building kits, each with some flexibility, but where the user or interface adapter has a range of kits to start from. Each kit would include the equivalent of a widget library and composition rules. The usability of a device seeking to offer an adaptable UI could be estimated by creating user interfaces for that device with a) the abstract model provided by the device developer, and b) each of these kits in turn. Usability prognostics applied to the multiple interface mock-ups would give an early indication of the effectiveness of the device's operating logic and the abstract model provided to represent that logic, when subjected to use under a variety of adapted UI conditions. Patient usability gaps in the user-need space could be identified by this process. Vendor-designed interfaces would be qualified both by the general-purpose prognostic screening and by more systematic user testing. Crossover points where the prognostics suggest that a standard morphotype may perform better than the vendor-designed interface would be identified in this process and made available to health professionals identifying equipment for patient use. This would allow the professionals to identify cases where they should suggest the use of equipment-supported settings and/or third-party AT to enhance usability and reduce errors.

26.5.2 Task- Oriented Analysis and Qualification of Interfaces

For individuals with disabilities, high-cost interventions, such as coaching by a rehabilitation engineer or occupational therapist could be managed appropriately, using the facts of the individual case. Rather than saying "Is this *devic*e accessible?" a just-in-time analysis would be performed before the equipment was prescribed to review what the patient was supposed to do with this equipment, together with the patient's customary or hypothesized interface adaptation.

For tasks that didn't get a solid endorsement from the prognostics but had no clear rule-out factors, rehearsal of the therapeutic use with the aid of health professionals, such as a rehabilitation engineer, occupational therapist, or peer counselor could be indicated selectively, focusing on those tasks that appeared to put the patient most at risk.

26.5.3 Mixed Initiative Is the Name of the Dialog Game

In the Web Accessibility Initiative, we have a concept we sometimes call *author proposes, user disposes* [22]. In this concept, the author's strong grasp of the content and concern that it communicates is tapped so that there is a pixel-perfect presentation that has been optimized with some care. On the other hand, for various client-side reasons, a given connection may not be workable with that presentation, so: (1) the message is transmitted in an encoding where the essential content is severable from the presentation details and (2) the user is given functions in the Web client software to reprofile the presentation so that it works [23].

At the 2001 State of the Science meeting for the RERC on Information Technology Access, there was an interesting briefing on forward-looking concepts in user interaction. This presentation resonated with the above accessibility principle in terms of a concept of *mixed initiative*. Past efforts at taking workload away from users by applying machine intelligence had been too presumptive. The path to success was to keep the user making decisions, but offering nominations from the automation segment that got a majority "yes" response, or resolved to an answer with fewer user steps. This is the ergonomic energy that has brought so much economic energy to Google. They committed to "don't be evil" and didn't take away any search findings from the user. This was the same as other search services. What they did better, that made them a winner, was implementing better prognostics concerning which hits the user would prefer to visit. The users found that they completed their tasks after visiting fewer of the hits in the search-report page. This made them a loyal base of users and increased what Google could charge for advertising.

In the client-server Web we have two parties getting together over how the business process is presented. In medical equipment, we have three: the equipment supplier, the clinical care team, and the patient/customer. This nudges us toward an explicitly constraint-programming framework for the interface adaptation engine. In the eventual marketed products, there may be a much more familiar world of XML data and imperative scripts; but for purposes of concept validation, a robust constraint-guided problem-solving engine approach may be the technology of choice.

26.5.4 The Patient's Workbook

Conversation between doctor and patient is a high-cost, high-risk zone. Anything we can do that will make communication more efficacious along this connection will have major health and cost benefits.

Presently, patient education about their condition and treatment plan is mostly transmitted through canned materials prepared by drug and medical equipment makers. Understanding of the medical situation and compliance with care plans could both be improved by creating a tailored patient take-away workbook that contains all the facts of their case on which they have been briefed and helps to guide them through compliance with their instructions.

If the care plan involves medical equipment that they have not used before, or will be using in new ways, part of this take-away workbook could be a learning module for them to be trained in the appropriate use of the equipment that they should now use. The training requirements only increase if the user is going to use an atypical user interface configuration in using the equipment.

Benchmark technologies to draw on in creating accessible and use-error-reducing patient's workbooks would include the DAISY Standard talking book format, the SCORM standard for learning modules, Health Level 7 for the prescribed activities in the care plan, among others [24].

26.5.5 Don't Expect What You Don't Inspect

Access to E&IT today hinges on getting access to information and actions in a software abstraction that is available either directly through the consumer device or through a programmatic interface to third-party software and hardware that the device allows you to add on.

Although this is necessary for access to medical instrumentation, it is not sufficient. For medical information, we need more assurance that the adapted user interface will be usable. This is needed to meet safety demands in the medical enterprise, where consumers are viewed as being at the mercy of the professional participants. For the government to feel that they can assure the safety of devices, an established formal assessment methodology may be necessary (Chapter 17). This will probably take advances in both the per-device management of interface adaptation and per-medical-domain qualification methods for user interfaces with flexibility.

The logic for such an assurance process is not unknown, in terms of the underlying science. There are precedents in both medicine and aerospace. But the principles that are known, if applied with brute force, would still be cost-prohibitive. A knowledge-engineering effort is in order to reduce what is predictable to rote and put it in a form where it can routinely and affordably be applied to evaluation of actual interfaces.

Rapidly and economically qualifying the use-error-retardant qualities of a flexible user interface on a small-volume product will require a formality and automation of the assessment of usability beyond anything we have seen to date. This seems like a stiff challenge. On the other hand, the problem is not as new as it may seem.

In the aerospace industry there are clearly life-safety risks, and computer simulation and operations analysis are used extensively to drive risk out of technological innovations before people have to depend on them. The failure mode analysis and redundancy management disciplines developed in this context are prior art for the logical process of in-silico qualification.

This will have to be adapted to a Web world of interfaces portable across endemic devices. The network-effect energy of the Web made the personal computer a household commodity. On the other hand, in the long term, the personal mobile communications device and the television at the center of the user's perception of their home entertainment hold better cards to remain pervasive and capture the user interface manager/mediator role. But the migration to digital communication and hence the data transmission of the messages to the user appear to be secure.

26.6 CONCLUSIONS

The Web has provided a convincing demonstration of the gains to all that are realized when applications reach their users through a neutral commons. But it does this by being very light in the demands it places on model knowledge or metadata for the data exchanged. Trusted-usable, flexible-presentation user interfaces for medical functions will need better modeling than the ones the Web runs on today. Medical informatics and metadata are in better shape, with relatively strong standards emerging. But medical device manufacturers have yet to embrace the idea that the path to the user should pass through a commons.

We seek to bring medical instrumentation into an operating domain where user-adaptable, assured-usable user interfaces are *de rigeur*. To get there, we can and should build on the legacy of the Web and the foundation of medical informatics. But there is a yet a gap to fill in which we face both challenges and opportunities.

An example challenge is how to structure the business and trust relationships for industrial-strength usability assurance. Doing high-assurance assessments of fuzzy human factors for devices without mass markets would seem to favor outsourcing the activity to specialist businesses. But the contracts, the terms of trust, can't be quite the same as for certification to fire codes; the substance of what is being observed is more statistical in nature.

An example opportunity is a user's workbook that is a take-away from the doctor visit, tailored to their specific care plan. The innovation here would be to combine knowledge of the devices the user is to use and the tasks the user is to accomplish with that equipment. Building on the accessible-by-construction DAISY book format and the IMS accessibility taxonomy for user needs could be implemented with low resistance, because it is a new function without a committed user base that we would be asking to change.

ACKNOWLEDGMENTS

The material presented here would not have been possible without two indirect supporting relationships. One is a history of support from the U.S. Department of Education and National Science Foundation through the research programs of the Trace Center, University of Wisconsin–Madison.

The other is the willingness of the World Wide Web, Web Accessibility Initiative, to entrust the management of some of its efforts to my charge.

REFERENCES

1. Trace R&D Center, Middleware and the eSCaped Web, conference handout for Supercomputing 2000, available at http://trace.wisc.edu/handouts/sc2000/ middleware_and_eSCaped_web/.
2. *Proceedings: State of the Science Conference on Telerehabilitation and Applications of Virtual Reality*, Rosen, M.J. and Lauderdale, D.E., Eds., NRH Press, Washington, D.C., October 12–13, 2001.
3. FirstHelp(R) Nurse Advice Line, more information at http://www.yourmedicaresolutions.com/staying_well/ medicareblue_ppo/firsthelp_nurse.html.
4. *W3C Workshop on Device Independent Authoring Techniques*, St. Leon-Rot, Germany, September 25–26, 2002, Final agenda with links to presentations, available at http://www.w3.org/2002/07/ DIAT/final.html.
5. Nichols, J., Myers, B., Harris, T.K., Rosenfeld, R., Shriver, S., Higgins, M., and Hughes, J., Requirements for Automatically Generating Multi-Modal Interfaces for Complex Appliances, *IEEE Fourth International Conference on Multimodal Interfaces*, ICMI'02. Pittsburgh, PA. October 14–16, 2002. pp. 377–382.
6. The Digital Hospital (cover story), *Newsweek*, March 28, 2005, available at http://www.businessweek.com/magazine/content/05_13/b3926001_mz001.htm.
7. American National Standard Z39.86-2002, Specifications for the Digital Talking Book, available at http://www.niso.org/standards/resources/Z39-86-2002.html.
8. InterNational Committee for Information Technology Standards, Protocol to Facilitate Operation of Information and Electronic Products through Remote and Alternative Interfaces and Intelligent Agents: Universal Remote Console, ANSI/INCITS 389-2005, August 12, 2005, Washington, D.C.
9. InterNational Committee for Information Technology Standards, Information technology — Protocol to Facilitate Operation of Information and Electronic Products through Remote and Alternative Interfaces and Intelligent Agents: User Interface Socket, ANSI/INCITS 390-2005, August 12, 2005, Washington, D.C.
10. InterNational Committee for Information Technology Standards, Information technology — Protocol to Facilitate Operation of Information and Electronic Products through Remote and Alternative Interfaces and Intelligent Agents: Presentation Template, ANSI/INCITS 391-2005, August 12, 2005, Washington, D.C.
11. InterNational Committee for Information Technology Standards, Information technology — Protocol to Facilitate Operation of Information and Electronic Products through Remote and Alternative Interfaces and Intelligent Agents: Target Description, ANSI/INCITS 392-2005, August 12, 2005, Washington, D.C.
12. InterNational Committee for Information Technology Standards, Information technology — Protocol to Facilitate Operation of Information and Electronic Products through Remote and Alternative Interfaces and Intelligent Agents: Resource Description, ANSI/INCITS 393-2005, August 12, 2005, Washington, D.C.
13. Dubinko, M., Klotz, L.L., Merrick, R., and Raman, T.V., Eds, XForms 1.0, W3C Recommendation, October 14, 2003, available at http://www.w3.org/TR/2003/REC-xforms-20031014/.
14. Axelsson, J., Birbeck, M., Dubinko, M., Epperson, B., Ishikawa, M., McCarron. S., Navarro, A., and Pemberton, S., Eds., "XHTML™ 2.0," W3C Working Draft, May 27, 2005 [work in progress], Updates available from http://www.w3.org/TR/xhtml2.
15. Lewis, R. and Merrick, R., Eds., Content Selection for Device Independence (DISelect) 1.0, W3C Working Draft, 02 May 2005 [work in progress], Updates available from http://www.w3.org/TR/cselection/.
16. UBAccess, Semantic Web Accessibility Platform, available at http://www.ubaccess.com/swap.html.
17. IMS Global Learning Consortium, Accessibility Specification, available at http:// www.imsglobal.org/accessibility/.
18. Larson, J.A., Raman, T.V., and Raggett, D., Eds., W3C Multimodal Interaction Framework, W3C NOTE 06 May 2003, available from http://www.w3.org/TR/mmi-framework/.

19. Trace R&D Center, EZ Access®*, available from http://trace.wisc.edu/world/ kiosks/ez/.
20. European Telecommunication Standards Institute, Human Factors (HF); User Interfaces: Generic Spoken Command Vocabulary for ICT Devices and Services, ETSI Standard ETSI ES 202 076 V1.1.2 (2002-11).
21. Mitsubishi Electric Research Laboratories, DiamondHelp: Collaborative Help for Networked Home Products, available at http://www.merl.com/projects/diamondhelp/.
22. Velasco, C.A., Yehya Mohamad, Y., Gilman, A.S., Viorres, N., Vlachogiannis, E., Arnellos, A., and Darzentas, J.S., Universal access to information services — the need for user information and its relationship to device profiles, *Universal Access in the Information Society*, Vol. 3, No. 1, 2004, p. 88.
23. Jacobs, I., Gunderson, J., and Hansen, E., Eds., User Agent Accessibility Guidelines 1.0, W3C Recommendation 17 December 2002, available at http://www.w3.org/TR/ UAAG10/.
24. Advanced Distributed Learning Network, Sharable Courseware Object Reference Model, available at http://www.adlnet.org/scorm/index.cfm.

* EZ® and EZ Access® are registered trademarks of the University of Wisconsin.

27 Emerging Personalized Home Rehabilitation: Integrating Service with Interface

Xin Feng and Jack M. Winters

CONTENTS

ABSTRACT

This chapter addresses the potential for personalized interfaces for medical devices with a specific focus on home-based rehabilitation, which is an area of special need and opportunity. In particular, the focus is on innovative approaches for personalized access to Web-based services, designed in ways that enhance universal access. There are many opportunities for personalizing health care through emerging ubiquitous home environment technology, but there are also barriers to this vision. These are addressed, and possible solutions presented, including the new User Socket Interface/Universal Remote Console standard. An example technology infrastructure is reported, called UniTherapy by our group, that is intended to function as a personalized home rehabilitation appliance.

27.1 INTRODUCTION

As seen in other chapters in this book, there are many technical strategies for enhancing access to medical devices (see Chapter 25 and Chapter 15). Two pillars are approaches that are motivated by *universal design* applied to products (see Chapter 6, Chapter 8, and Chapter 9) and approaches motivated by *personalized interfaces* supported by standards (see Chapter 23, Chapter 26, and Chapter 28). The latter approach seems synergistic with a vision of the future shared by many with a vested interest in *personalized medicine*, ranging from researchers to venture capitalists. This chapter describes the type of emerging technical infrastructure that could make such access a reality for a specific target area: *home rehabilitation*.

Historically, rehabilitative therapy has followed conventional reimbursement protocols, implemented primarily through both inpatient and outpatient programs. These programs tend to be semipersonalized, based on implementing an intervention plan for a specific patient involving an initial diagnosis and prognosis and, hopefully, ongoing assessment of progress. This is especially true for patients who have access to an inpatient phase. But because of limited resources, these programs have become shorter in duration. Patients are also encouraged to make progress on their own, typically while at home, perhaps with assistance from a home caregiver. At this stage, the individual is no longer participating in the role of patient, nor as a consumer of services, because there are none to be consumed.

For certain types of rehabilitation, such as after soft-tissue injuries or orthopedic surgery, this service delivery model often works — the mix of spontaneous healing supplemented by mild interventions is sufficient. Outpatient or home visits, two or three per week, are adequate. But for areas such as neurorehabilitation, there is mounting scientific evidence that suggests this is a suboptimal approach. For instance, for individuals recovering from stroke, evidence that has accumulated related to neural plasticity and brain reorganization mechanisms suggests a need for more intensive and longer-term rehabilitation. This has motivated the development of new approaches toward neurorehabilitation. These alternatives often make use of technologies based on tools from the robotics and virtual reality fields that help automate aspects of the therapeutic process. Studies using the most notable of these approaches have shown positive results. Yet the technologies are expensive, and access is currently limited to small geographic regions of the country. Some research groups, including the authors', are now actively exploring alternative approaches that strive to reduce access barriers such as cost and distance by taking advantage of emerging trends and advances in mass-market electronic and information technologies (E&IT). The trend is also toward more home-centered approaches. But currently, an individual with, for instance, stroke-induced disability lacks access to more personalized interventions.

There are a number of challenges that the authors' group and others face:

- Lack of personalized health care services. No two people are exactly alike, especially when it comes to rehabilitative medicine. However, the paradigm "one size fits all" is still common in rehabilitation, for reasons such as lack of sufficient scientific knowledge of a better alternative, limited resources for therapy and ongoing timely assessments, and a shortage of implementation tools that are engaging or client-appropriate.
- Limited methods for addressing low access of clients to timely services or researchers to timely research data. One possibility is a telerehabilitation link that can provide both patients with rehabilitative services and researchers to subject populations. It helps minimize the barrier of distance, and this enhanced access opens up new possibilities for discovering and implementing optimized intervention strategies across the continuum

of care. Advances in E&IT hold considerable promise for new telerehabilitation applications.
- Lack of effective human–technology interfaces, or in some cases human– technology–human interfaces, especially for an interface that uses the personal computer and emerging E&IT and interface standards to help implement assessment and therapy programs.

This chapter first presents scientific findings in neurorehabilitation research in the last decade, and then state-of-the-art advances in E&IT and human–technology interfaces for the home environment. Finally, a home-based neurorehabilitation platform, which was implemented by the authors' group, is presented as an example.

27.2 BACKGROUND

Consider, for example, a population in which a more personalized form of home-based rehabilitation holds great promise: the over 4 million individuals with stroke-induced disability in America who live with various degrees of functional impairment [1]. Over the past decade, as the duration of reimbursed therapy has decreased due to economic pressures on the U.S. health-care system, individuals have been discharged well within the range of time when even spontaneous recovery can still be expected. The burden for health care services has thus shifted toward outpatient and home visits, in which case distance can be a barrier. Although a challenge, this shift also provides an opportunity. For instance, 100 experts at a workshop on home care technologies for the 21st century strongly recommended a shift toward a consumer-oriented health care system that integrates tele-supported home self-care into the mix [2,3]. However, little is known about outcomes of consumer-oriented health care systems integrating tele-supported home self-care.

Currently, numerous therapeutic techniques for upper-extremity stroke rehabilitation are being implemented in research environments, with much of the excitement initially motivated by the concepts of "learned nonuse" [4] and "forced use" [5]. Subsequent findings show that a few weeks of intensive constraint-induced movement therapy (CI-therapy) can produce significant improvements in limb use for motivated subjects meeting certain poststroke criteria [6].

Other therapeutic approaches, such as robotic-assisted therapy, also have shown that significant improvements in function are possible even years after the initial stroke. Reviews of stroke rehabilitation interventions describe robot-assisted therapy as one of the most promising interventions for upper limb therapy [7]. One of the better known is the MIT-MANUS two-degree-of-freedom manipulator with low intrinsic end-point impedance, now sold commercially, which allows the device to measure free movements as well as guide weak limb movements. It uses simple video games to help engage subjects in therapy, based on a research study showing that after five 1-h sessions per week for five weeks, experimental subjects had greater gains in strength, reduced upper extremity impairment that was still significant in a 3-year follow-up, and greater recovery of functional independence [8]. Another study, with different robotic manipulators and protocol, has shown that compared to conventional sessions, a robot group had larger improvements in a clinical motor impairment scale, strength, and reach [9]. Other studies are exploring virtual reality as a training tool in stroke rehabilitation [10,11]. Virtual reality is computer technology that simulates real-life learning and allows for increased intensity of training while providing augmented sensory feedback.

What are the lessons of these scientific findings? In 2001, a workshop on innovations in neurorehabilitation at Marquette University brought together engineering and clinical representatives from key research groups involved in innovative technological and robotic therapy clinical trials [12]. Some conclusions drawn by the workshop and from a diversity of existing scientific literature are listed as follows:

- For brain reorganization, rehabilitative intervention should be varied, not just repetitive. Changes in motor cortex are driven by acquisition of new motor skills, not simply motor use.
- Most rehabilitation experts agree that motivation has an important role in rehabilitation.
- The best form for stroke therapy, as well as the optimal timing for intervention, remains illusive.
- There is great potential for home rehabilitation when an appropriate support system is available.

To summarize, there is a great need to develop and implement a consumer-centered, alternative therapeutic strategy for neurorehabilitative therapy that can be accepted and adapted for the home environment. For this strategy to work, it is suggested that the technology must fit the user; i.e., it must be personalized to their abilities, preferences, and therapeutic needs. Additionally, the individual user needs access to a support network that includes a practitioner, especially with a view to making timely assessments that can help tune a subsequent intervention protocol. A key challenge relates to how to design such personalized systems that integrate considerations of a cost-effective service with a user-effective interface, as universal access is a function of cost as well as the design of the interface.

27.3 DELIVERY METHODS FOR FUTURE HOME REHABILITATION

27.3.1 TELEREHABILITATION: ADDRESSING THE ACCESS BARRIER OF DISTANCE

As seen in Figure 27.1, the home rehabilitation process has structural similarities to the classic engineering optimization problem [13]. The specific aim is to design an optimal "treatment plan" (algorithm) and to implement this plan as a collection of "therapeutic interventions" (controls). The processes of "diagnosis," "prognosis," and "treatment plan" could be put under the umbrella of "personalized rehabilitation," which means these processes would be customized to an individual's dynamic system and personal demand.

Ideally, the optimal strategy may change based on sampling of interventions (e.g., to check for compliance) and the ongoing status of the person (e.g., making assessments). A telereahabilitation

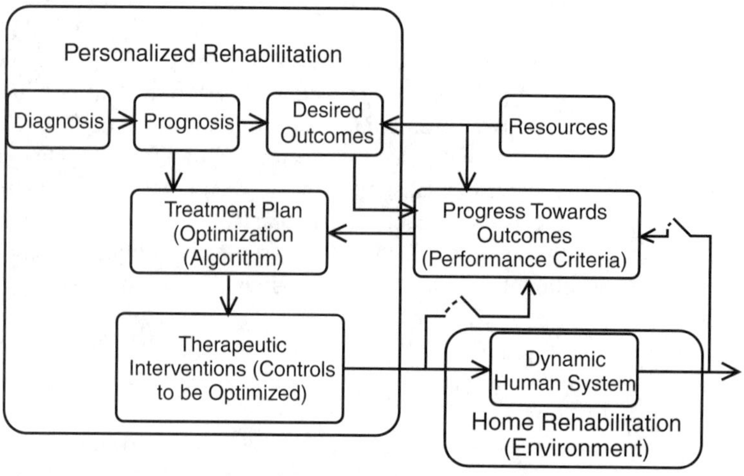

FIGURE 27.1 Overview of the process of home rehabilitation from an "optimization" perspective. A person enters this process with a "diagnosis" (classification) related to a disease or functional impairment (the states of the dynamic human system). This diagnosis results in a "prognosis" (prediction of dynamic human system behavior) and desired "outcomes."

link makes possible better and more frequent sampling of the health and functional status of the person. Consider the conceptual models of telerehabilitation service delivery [3]:

- *Teleconsultation:* standard "face-to-face" telemedicine model using interactive videoconferencing, typically with high bandwidth between sites.
- *Telehomecare:* often uses a telenurse coordinating service delivery, typically with a low- or moderate-bandwidth interactive connection.
- *Telemonitoring:* unobtrusively monitors patient data remotely, with possible interactive teleassessment.
- *Teletherapy:* patient "plays" or "exercises" in the home environment, and therapist has the ability to change settings remotely, based on patient's performance.
- *Telecooperation:* by using the telerehabilitation link, multiple persons can cooperate together to accomplish a goal-directed task. Some experts suggest that this novel model with its kind of team-work activity will enhance the motivation of persons at both ends and thus optimize the rehabilitation outcomes.

Advances in E&IT as well as emergence of ubiquitous computing and smart wearable devices are enabling personalized health care services to be delivered to individuals at any place and at any time. In a ubiquitous computing home environment, computing entities (ranging from sensors, actuators, and devices to Web services and applications) are scattered in different locations and serve people even without their awareness. For example, a wearable health monitoring device can sample one's blood pressure, temperature, heart rate, and so on; the home patient can use some exercise devices, the setting of which can be remotely set by the telepractitioner; Web services can intelligently adjust the exercise plan of the patient.

27.3.2 Personalized Rehabilitation Services

Personalized health care provides medical services that are truly effective for "you." This ensures that health care services provisioned for an individual are customized to his or her prevailing health care needs. With personalized health care, we also have the opportunity to achieve a more "proactive" system, in which disease can be addressed and hopefully prevented at the earliest possible moment, rather than a "reactive" model, in which the emphasis is mainly on diagnosis and treatment [2].

Both a patient and practitioner can benefit from personalized rehabilitation. To achieve personalized health care, in addition to phenotypic and genotypic patient data, many other factors can be considered. Patient data such as an individual's diet, living conditions, device capabilities, and event occurrences should be taken into account. Such personalization factors are known as *context*, which refers to any information that can be used to characterize the situation of an entity (which can be personal, environmental, or computational objects) and the interaction between them [14]. It is well established in the intelligent systems community that a key barrier to intelligent use of information is context awareness; thus, one of the steps to implementing personalized health care is context awareness. For example, in the authors' group a neurofuzzy modeling framework is developed; if carefully designed with sufficient expert knowledge and scientific evidence, it is able to make predictions or real-time estimations of context. The latter is intended to provide awareness of a changing context [15].

27.3.3 Personalized Access through Web Services

The current societal investment in E&IT is unprecedented. It would be advantageous for rehabilitation to take advantage of this multibillion-dollar investment by performing concurrent research that anticipates future mass-market technology developments. There are four basic modes of human telecommunication: voice, video or images, data exchange, and virtual contact.

Telecommunication technology has experienced dramatic growth in the past few years. In August 2005, broadband penetration exceeded 60% in the U.S. among active Internet users [16]. Penetration is even higher for Japan and much of Europe, and growing dramatically in other countries. The wireless network is increasingly able to carry data; currently, in the U.S. it is easy to reach 19.2 KHz data rates, with some phone companies offering about 100 KHz; new mobile tools (e.g., camera phone and Blackberry) are becoming more popular. All these technological advances hold promise as constituting a societal infrastructure for launching novel telerehabilitation applications.

Of special interest is an emerging collection of standards that enable Web services, including services that inherently promote accessibility that are based on top of Extensible Markup Language (XML) and related technologies (see also Chapter 23 and Chapter 26). XML, which was developed by the World Wide Web Consortium (W3C) in 1996, provides a framework for defining markup languages. Beyond XML, "the XML family" is a growing set of modules that offer useful services to accomplish important and frequently demanded tasks [17–21]. More and more modules and tools are available or under development. In the past few years, Web services have emerged as the next generation of Web-based technology for exchanging information and providing services. This growth is being powered by the program-to-program communication model of Web services built on existing and emerging standards such as HyperText Transfer Protocol (HTTP), Simple Object Access Protocol (SOAP), Web Services Description Language (WSDL), and the Universal Description, Discovery, and Integration (UDDI) technologies. The latter three are all XML-related technologies.

A *Web service* performs a specific task or a collection of tasks through an *interface* that describes a collection of business operations that can be accessed through standardized XML messaging by a network [22]. As shown in Figure 27.2, three key processes are involved in this service-oriented architecture: first, a Web service is described using a standard, formal XML language expressed in WSDL, called its *service description,* that provides all the details necessary to interact with the service; second, the service provider then publishes the service with a service directory based on a UDDI specification which will provide the service consumer with information that can be used to directly bind to the service provider and invoke it; and third, on top of the networking layer is an XML-based messaging layer (in SOAP) that facilitates communications between service provider and service consumer. SOAP is an XML-based messaging layer protocol for messaging and remote procedure calls (RPCs).

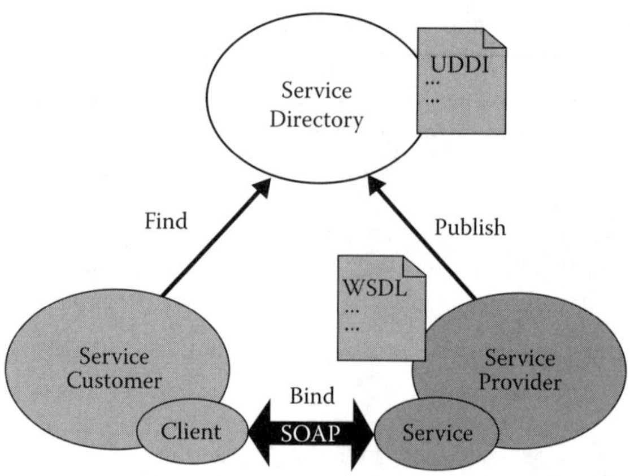

FIGURE 27.2 Web services can be described in terms of a service-oriented architecture. This architecture is set up by three roles and three operations. The three roles are the service provider, the service consumer, and the service directory, and the operations performed on the three roles, or between them, are publish, find, and bind.

So how can the XML-related technologies and a Web-service model benefit home rehabilitation applications? Here are a few compelling reasons to consider:

- *Collaborations:* Using Web services, the business logic of individual systems can be exposed over the Web, and service can be delivered in the standard communication protocol (e.g., SOAP). In the rehabilitation field, this can enable different participants in the home rehabilitation process (e.g., patient, physical therapist, and rehabilitation engineer) to collaborate. For example, a home patient can send his or her vital sign data to the service subscriber, which could be their physical therapist who can adjust their exercise plan, whereas the rehabilitation engineer will be able to update the algorithm used in the home exercise machine based on the latest scientific findings.
- *Easy to access:* Web services published in the UDDI registry and advertised in the WSDL description can be searched by a machine-agent, similar to the manner in which Google searches through Web pages today. Thinking of health care more as a "service," this could profoundly change the medical model used in today's society.
- *Ubiquitous:* Because Web services are provided over the Internet and use existing infrastructure, they are potentially accessible from anywhere. Advances in wireless telecommunication and mobile technologies are speeding this process. Furthermore, because of the standards with which they are developed, Web services respect existing security systems such as firewalls. Further discussion of ubiquitous computing follows in Subsection 27.3.4.
- *Semantic Web:* This emerging vision is "an extension of the current Web in which information is given well-defined meaning, better enabling computers and people to work in cooperation" [23; Chapter 23]. The evolution of the Web into a semantic Web will result in information which is presented in a way that it can be "reprocessed" by an intelligent agent. Searches and activities only performed by Web experts today may be commonplace for everyone with the assistance of intelligent agents [24].
- *Health information standards:* Most of the information standards in different application fields have been influenced by the XML standard. For instance, two examples in the health care field are Health Level Seven (HL7) [25] and Systematized Nomenclature of Medicine Clinical Terms (SNOMED CT) [26]. HL7's domain is to: " ... provide standards for the exchange, management and integration of data ...". The upcoming Version 3 uses only XML encoding.

27.3.4 Personalizing Health Care through Ubiquitous Home Environment Technology

The word *ubiquitous* comes from Latin and means existing universally everywhere, evenly and simultaneously. As shown as Figure 27.3, in a ubiquitous computing home environment, computing entities (e.g., audiovisual systems, intelligent appliances, sensors, and home exercise equipments) are supposed to scatter in different locations and serve people even without their awareness. Many of those entities can be put into one of two categories: sensors or actuators, which are the primary concerns of home rehabilitation applications. Smart wearable devices (sensors) and gaming technology devices (actuators) are used as examples discussed in this section. Home network infrastructure, including both hardware (e.g., wired or wireless network) and software (e.g., middleware platform), provide a platform for sending data between human and environment, and appropriately processing, storing, and presenting such data [27]. Another consideration is that user interfaces of computer entities at home need to be more user-centered and support user preferences [28]. It will be critical to generate human–technology interfaces that are sensitive to a client's capabilities and personal preferences, taking advantages of innovation in universal interfaces, intelligent agents and other state-of-the-art user interface standard technologies.

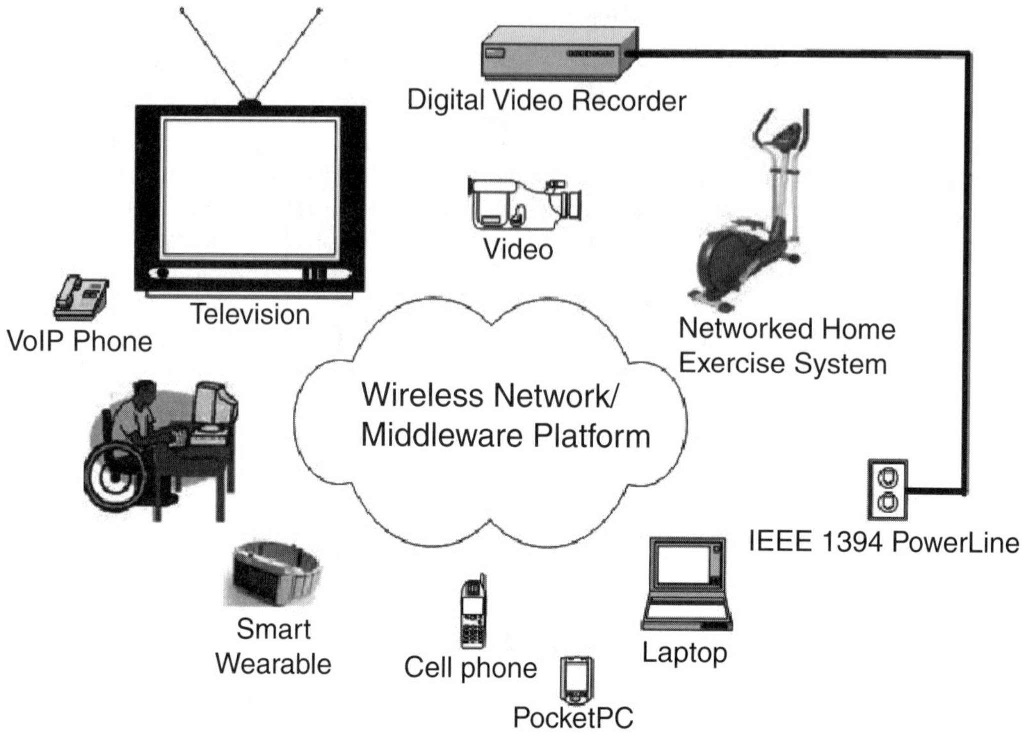

FIGURE 27.3 Conceptual model of a ubiquitous home environment. The intelligent appliances and other computer entities can interact through the home network.

27.3.4.1 Emerging Smart Wearable Health Care Technologies

Today, smart wearable devices are under development to cover the specific needs of several groups of endusers (or consumers); e.g., home telemonitoring for chronic patients, blood composition monitoring and drug delivery for diabetic patients, early disease prevention, and telemonitoring for cardiovascular and pulmonary diseases.

Smart health wearable devices may be attached to clothes, jewelry, or wristwatches, or they may be separately wearable (e.g., a chest belt heart-rate monitor). Generally, a smart wearable personal system should be light in weight and have low power consumption, be reasonably low in cost, easily accessible by an inexperienced user, and be able to maintain a network connection [29].

One of the most critical decisions to be made, in an early stage of device development, concerns the scenarios of use and, consequently, the operation modes and embedded alerting algorithms. Several major issues that have to be addressed in order to satisfy user needs and implemented within the development and validation phase of smart health wearable applications are:

- *Telecommunication:* the link between sensors or link between smart wearable device and health care provider (or through intermediate wireless telecom facility (e.g., mobile phone).
- *Data storage:* a backup data buffer solution is usually necessary, especially because networks are not always available.
- *Human technology interface:* includes the graphical user interface, speech interface, tactile interface, and so on.
- *Patient safety:* relates to potential risks from any electronic or radiation device (e.g, electromagnetic fields).
- *Standardization and interoperability:* smart wearable devices are being developed in a way that precludes communication between them and clinical information systems, which

is undesirable. Structured but open communication standards and messaging protocols would bring subsequent clinical, administrative and research benefits.

- *Biomedical sensors:* A new generation of biomedical sensors is emerging that could generate new approaches for timely diagnosis, ambulatory health care, care at home and at the point of need. These include wearable noninvasive sensors that can be applied in contact with or near to the body (e.g., wristwatch or belt) and measure an impressive number of physiologic signals (e.g., ECG, pulse, blood oxygen saturation, respiration, skin temperature, blood pressure, and CO_2) and activity and movement signals (e.g., EMG, posture, fall, movement, speed, acceleration, and contact pressure). Wearable devices benefit today from significant progress in system integration and miniaturization and can be applied in different body locations.

27.3.4.2 Gaming and Home Exercise

The U.S. gaming industry has continued to grow dramatically over the past decade, with an estimated $13 billion in sales in 2002 [30]. Along with the rapid progress in E&IT, the gaming industry has also involved a suite of novel technologies:

- *Virtual reality:* This has been intensively integrated into the gaming technologies. 3D computer graphics, computer music, and tactile interfaces have been intensively used in enriching the sensation of computer game users. Ironically, this kind of "augmentative interface" idea was originally developed by the rehabilitation community to provide alternative interfaces for disabled users.
- *Wireless access:* Most gaming platforms nowadays can be used as stand-alone computing entities; for example, the latest Xbox platform (Xbox 360) by Microsoft uses three custom IBM PowerPC-based processors with wireless support and can interact with other home appliances (e.g., central storage or media player) in the home network [31]. These gaming platforms with wireless access capability would ideally fit into the ubiquitous home environment.
- *Online games:* A lot of computer game software today is also network accessible; computer game users can log in to internet game servers and either compete against or collaborate with some other user. Online games have become one of the fastest growing segments in the international entertainment industry. For example, popular online games in South Korea are enjoying a four million-strong subscription base [32]. This popularity indicates that gaming technology could be used to motivate users' participation in rehabilitative therapy.
- *Standard interactive ports:* Force feedback devices such as joystick, wheel, mouse, and so on, have been widely used in computer games. Altogether, more than 500 games use force feedback, and more than 100 tactile hardware products are available on the gaming market [33]. Using scientific insights from the robotic therapy field, the authors' group is developing a framework to use force feedback devices in rehabilitation. Although the mechanical power of force feedback devices is limited, it has proven to be effective at providing assistance to hemiplegic patients in initial pilot studies. In addition, the commercial device could easily be approved by regulators (e.g., FDA) as rehabilitation equipment that could be safely used in the home environment [34].

Considering its high availability, low cost, and associated large and motivated user populations with existing accessible communication technology and standards, gaming technology can readily be used as a tool for home rehabilitation, especially using approaches such as computer-assisted motivated rehabilitation (CAMR), because research shows that therapy that proactively considers motivation is more likely to be effective in functional restoration. [35]

27.3.4.3 Home Information Infrastructure: Networking and Middleware Platform

An inherent property for wearable sensors is their mobility. Hence, optimally, they should be able to communicate their measurement data by wireless. Different technical solutions based on network standards (e.g., WiFi or IEEE 802.11 local area network, Bluetooth personal area network, and infrared) have been introduced. In general, there is a trade-off between these options.

TABLE 27.1
Family of Medical Information Bus (MIB) Standards in Object- Oriented Framework [IEEE 1073 Web Site]

P1073.1 provides definitions for information representation and interchange
P1073.2 defines the application profiles which specify protocols and services relevant to the upper three layers of the ISO/OSI reference model
P1073.3 specifies protocols and services for connection and message transport, using existing international standards where possible
P1073.4 addresses the cable-connected physical layer

Middleware for home health care systems comprises both hardware and software — its aim is to provide a platform to which the sensors send their measurement data, which sends control data to actuators, and in which the data is processed further, stored, and presented, or from which the data are further transmitted for central storage. As home networking and, more generically, ubiquitous computing environments are emerging, in order to be affordable and cost efficient, health monitoring systems would also need to support generic platforms (i.e., to interoperate or coexist with other platforms), such as home automation platforms. This is especially true for middleware, networking technology, and user interface devices used for user feedback.

Potentially integrated into this mix are the IEEE 1073 standards, also called Medical Information Bus (MIB), which provide "interconnection and interoperability of medical devices and computerized health care information systems" [36]. As shown in Table 27.1, MIB standards consist of a family of substandards organized in an object-oriented framework. MIB defines nearly all the elements (e.g., information model, communication model, and service access) needed to implement wearable monitoring systems. In the MIB model, this section of the chapter maps to the bottom three layers; more information about the P1073.1 layer is given in Subsection 27.3.4.4.

As an example of a home health care middleware platform solution, the home environment is generally equipped with a server (e.g., a home server) and a local area network, to which the wearable sensors or actuators may discover or control and send data, using different network protocols (e.g., Wireless LAN (WLAN), Bluetooth, X-10, power lines, or infrared). The technology and software issues for health monitoring and other intelligent applications based on an ad hoc LAN concept are being explored in many network communication protocols, including Universal Plug&Play (UPnP), Open Service Gateway initiative (OSGi), Jini (Java/Jini), etc. In these concepts, wearable health-monitoring sensors may be considered as ad hoc networked (mobile) devices, each providing a service to the network (e.g., access to health data). A health care application residing in the network (e.g., running on a home or remote server) receives the data from the sensor and sends the command to the actuator dynamically and takes the necessary actions such as storing, processing, alarming, and giving feedback. The framework provides support for dynamic updates of the sensor and actuator, or other software or intelligent agents as well as management of their mobility (e.g., discovery, control, and communication).

27.3.4.4 Infrastructure for Personalized Interface: Universal Remote Console (URC) Standard and Related Technologies

The vision of ubiquitous computing as "user-friendly computing resources anywhere and anytime," in which services and devices "disappear" into the environment, has already emerged. As discussed in earlier sections, network and middleware technologies are available in the home enviroment, providing methods for seamless discovery, controlling and eventing. However, user interfaces of networked devices and services still must be authored separately for each controller platform. Furthermore, many existing user interfaces are not intuitive and natural for human users; a *personalized interface* needs to be regenerated based on the individual's personal preference and capability.

A standardized but flexible abstract user interface description for target devices (e.g., intelligent appliance) or services (e.g., Web services or software programs) will be required, so that any remote control can connect to discover, access, and control a remote device or service on top of a network communication protocol (e.g., UPnP, Java/Jini, or OSGi). With such an abstract user interface description, a remote control with universal interface capabilities (e.g., speech interface, natural language interface, and tactitle interface) should be able to be supported by various computing devices, ranging from desktop computer to handheld PCs, and so on.

Among many of these efforts to develop a scheme for automatically generating a user interface on a remote control [37,38], the V2 committee within the InterNational Committee for Information Technology Standards (INCITS) and under the American National Standards Institute (ANSI) has developed Universal Remote Console (URC) standards for the discovery, selection, operation, and substitution of user interfaces and options [39]. The purpose of V2's URC standard, which has become an official national standard (ANSI/INCITS 389-393-2005) and is under consideration to be adopted as the international standard, ISO/IEC 24752, is to facilitate the development and deployment of a wide variety of devices (from different manufacturers) that can act as URC's for an equally varied range of devices and services (see also Chapter 28).

As shown in Figure 27.4, the URC standards specify communications between a target device or service that a user selects to access and operate and a universal remote console (URC) that presents the user with a remote user interface through which the user can discover, select, access, and operate the target. The URC is software that is typically hosted on the user's physical device, but a distributed approach is also possible. Communication between the target and URC takes place over a network, the target-URC network (TUN). Interaction between a target and a URC consists of a discovery phase and an optional control phase. The discovery phase initializes the URC to locate and identify all available targets and their sockets. The control phase is the period of time during which a target and a URC initiate, maintain, and terminate a control session. A control session is a connection between the URC and a target's socket, so that the URC controls a functional unit of the target. The user interface (UI) builder in URC will generate the user interface on URC with target information and supplemental resources on the URC, from the target, or from a remote network.

So how can these emerging UI-Socket/URC standards benefit home rehabilitation applications?

- *Universal interfaces:* By using URC, which supports novel interfaces such as speech interface, natural language interface, tactile interface, and so on, the user may apply those interfaces to interact with a URC target that may not support these features.
- *Personalized interface:* One of the important resources URC can use to generate a user interface is provided by User Accessibility Resources, which include both user capability and preference. Thus, a URC can always generate a personalized interface, for example, in the user's native language and with a big font size for a non-English-speaking user with visual impairments.

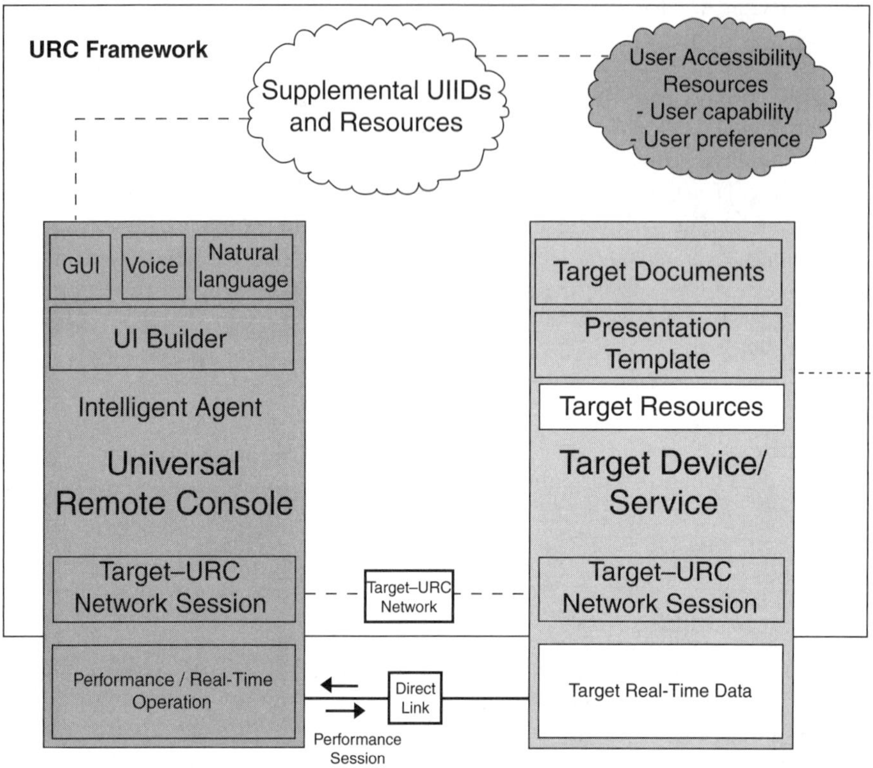

FIGURE 27.4 URC Standards Overall Framework is described within the black frame; outside the framework is an optional performance session. The user interface (UI) builder in URC will generate the user interface on URC with target information (e.g., target document, presentation template, and resources) and supplemental User Interface Implementation Description (UIID) and resources on the network, which is connected to URC by Resource URC Network (RUC); this process is optionally involved with an intelligent agent embedded in the URC. Besides TUN, a performance session may run on Direct Link, which is not necessarily compliant with V2 standards and transfers high-frequency performance data between URC and the target.

- *Device independency:* The URC standard provides a standard mechanism for products to share their functionality with remote controls. A URC could range from a desktop PC to PDA to cellphone. Thus, it allows a manufacturer to support all these and other options without having to create or even predict what the user would like.
- *Intelligent agent programming:* The URC standards allow the intelligent agent to be in the controller. The intelligent agent would allow the user to control home devices in many ways we cannot do today [40]. The Task Model Description (TMD) for an intelligent agent is one of the substandards that the INCITS V2 committee is working on today.

Along with three other RERCs, the Rehabilitation Engineering Research Center on Accessible Medical Instrumentation (RERC-AMI) is a member of the INCITS V2 workgroup and is involved in multiple V2-URC activities. MedURC for medical devices (see also Chapter 28) and interfaces for UniTherapy technology for rehabilitative assessment and therapy (see Section 27.4) are two prototype projects developed by the authors' group; the group is also proposing an accessibility schema to set up a user accessibility profile that a URC can use to create a personalized user interface (as a master's thesis project see also Chapter 28). An outgrowth of this work is the MUPad software tool, which was designed to provide a graphical user interface for generating

UI-Socket/URC compliant XML documents. This assists a developer in generating UI-Socket/URC compliant files for a target device or service without requiring much previous knowledge of the UI-Socket/URC standards (e.g., schema and grammar).

27.4 UNITHERAPY TECHNOLOGY AS A PERSONALIZED HOME REHABILITATION APPLIANCE

As discussed earlier, there is great potential for home rehabilitation when an appropriate support system (both interpersonal and technical) is available. This section presents the development and implementation of a consumer-centered alternative therapeutic strategy for neurorehabilitative therapy: a personalized home rehabilitation framework, called UniTherapy, that supports a rich menu of diverse forms of therapy and assessment, adapted for the home environment.

27.4.1 Conceptual Model

The design of such a personalized rehabilitation framework starts with understanding the user needs, roles, and interactive sequences of each user involved in the rehabilitation process. Three roles are defined as *therapy designer*, *telepractitioner*, and *home user*; more roles can be defined in finer granularity. The therapy designer has full access to UniTherapy's design suite to create personalized intervention protocols for the home user (patient) and, optionally, the telepractitioner, with the protocol able to be refined based on the outcome of timely assessment of the patient's recent progress. All the tasks in protocols can be put into two categories: self-routine tasks, which a home user can run by the individual client, and interactive tasks, in which a telepractitioner will supervise and periodically interact with the home user remotely and evaluate results, with the ability to remotely change the intervention protocol, which depends on the protocol's setting. A home user participates in all aspects of intervention sessions and, optionally, can access his or her own progress and history; positive feedback may improve the user's motivation. A home user does not need to design intervention protocols, although she can design goal-directed tasks herself as part of an intervention. These roles may change over the stages of an iterative rehabilitative process (e.g., a practitioner may assume both therapy designer and telepractitioner roles).

27.4.2 The'rapeutic Devices

One requirement for the home rehabilitation framework is that it should have support for mass-marketed devices that can be used in computer-based therapy and assessment. By supporting the DirectX standard [41], potentially all input devices compliant with the Microsoft Windows or DirectX platform can be used within the UniTherapy framework. For instance, UniTherapy supports force-feedback joysticks, force-feedback driving wheels, various pointing devices (e.g., mouse, trackball, and PDA stylus pen) and Windows keyboards. Some features in UniTherapy, though, are only relevant when using force-feedback devices. UniTherapy also supports customized devices that are compliant with the DirectX standard. For example, the authors' group also has designed a larger, customized joystick device called TheraJoy [42], which is applicable to vertical as well as horizontal arm movements that include the shoulder. UniTherapy also is supporting customized assessment and therapy capabilities for the TheraDrive wheel project [43]. UniTherapy can program a series of force effects such as constant, spring, damper, and inertia on the Joystick via Microsoft DirectX Software Development Kit (SDK). Signal translation is implemented between several types of devices; for example, a utility called "JoyMouse" implemented in UniTherapy can capture a joystick's signal and use it to control the mouse cursor. This provides an accessible way to use a joystick to perform windows goal-directed assessment tasks which are only open to mouse.

27.4.3 Assessment, Therapy, and Telerehabilitation Support

Assessment is a critical component of the framework, important both for evaluation of performance so as to support an iterative optimization process and as a key motivational tool. Assessment tasks include four toolboxes: range of motion (ROM), tracking, system identification, and conventional forms.

- *Working in user ability space:* Range of motion (ROM) maps between the workspace range and the user capability range. This mapping is based on a two-step ROM task that is normally performed upon first use and prompts the patient to draw a circle as big as possible. UniTherapy then fits the data with a rectangle that is used to represent the patient's estimated ROM. This mapping helps ensure that the user can reach most of the space used for subsequent tasks.
- *Tracking:* This has already been widely used in the practice of neurorehabilitation, with the purpose being to assess various aspects of a person's movement capability. UniTherapy supports two categories of tracking tasks: discrete tracking (point-to-point target acquisition) and continuous tracking (pursuit/preview tracking), with different instructions to the patient.
- *System identification:* This enables the therapy designer to design a task that applies predefined force perturbations to the subject and measures their response while under a certain instruction (e.g., "hold" or "relax"). UniTherapy records force data and instruction as input and the subject's movement data as output.
- *Conventional forms:* This toolbox currently includes eight questionnaires instruments (e.g., Barthel Index [44]), which are integrated into UniTherapy as form-based assessment instruments.

Movement data (e.g., position, timestamp, and applied force) are recorded into XML files for subsequent analysis, with the data structure defined by an XML schema. A data analysis module is being developed. Results can be not only displayed in both graphics and report form, but also stored as an XML file with the data structure that is described by an XML schema. The core suite of assessment metrics such as movement time, reaction time, and path error are retrieved intelligently once the data are input into the program, based on input device type (e.g., joystick or wheel), and task type (e.g., discrete tracking, continuous tracking, or system identification).

UniTherapy supports the integration of third-party computer game programs by treating them as add-ins and setting up shortcuts. Therapy Manager in UniTherapy allows the user to add or remove third-party programs and change sequences. Smart Driver, Pong, and Pacman are current arcade-game examples of fun motivation therapy tools in which UniTherapy can run in the background. UniTherapy can get access through DirectX to sampling joystick port signals without affecting the performance of most games, and can provide use history summaries.

A telerehabilitation link between patient interface (PI) and telepractitioner interface (TI), which is supported by TCP/IP network, has been implemented. Both the PI and TI support a view of the patient's performance data in real time. The result can be viewed at both sides in graph and report forms afterwards. As an option, the user at the TI can decide if the patient can participate in the task design phase. Instant messaging (IM) and computer-based teleconferencing is integrated into UniTherapy so that both users at the PI and TI can communicate by audio, video, and text.

27.4.4 Usability and Accessibility Design: Home Rehab Appliance and URC Standard- Related Technologies

The Home User version of UniTherapy is designed and implemented as a multimodal application with a simple user interface that resembles a media player. As shown in Figure 27.5, home users

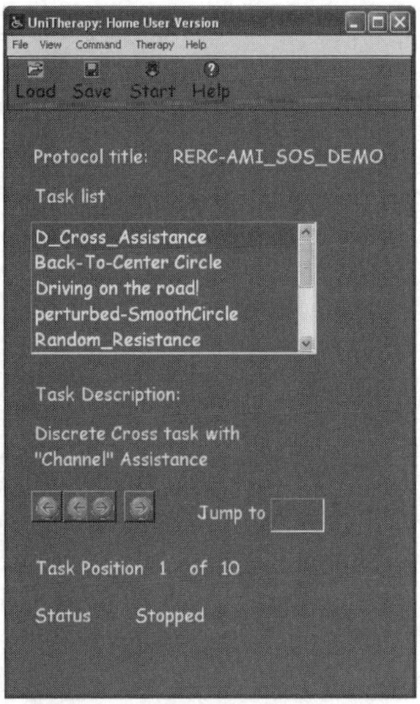

FIGURE 27.5 UniTherapy Home User version: designed as a home rehab appliance resembling a CD-player user interface. A user can navigate through the protocol list and select the task; simple voice commands (e.g., "start," "stop," "next," "previous," or "repeat") are supported, which is implemented using Microsoft Speech SDK; thus the home user can operate via voice command. Certain accessibility features are implemented and are ready to be used for screen-reader application after more evaluation, as planned, based on usability.

can load the protocol predefined by their therapy designer into UniTherapy as they would load a CD into a CD player; the descriptive information such as "protocol title," "task information," and "status" will display information for the home user in a manner that appears simple and intuitive to use. By using the existing telerehabilitation link, telepractitioners or caregivers can supervise the home user in real time. The authors are also investigating integrating user-agent technology into UniTherapy to provide context-awareness help online (e.g., an animated character could provide some simple positive feedback [e.g., "good job!"] to the home user after the goal-directed task is finished).

The Home User version is also compliant with the UI-Socket/URC standards. The authors' approach is to treat UniTherapy as a target service, called *home rehab appliance* and, thus, provide abstract user interface information in standard-compliant documents, which are sufficient for a URC to construct a full-function custom-tailored user interface for UniTherapy on the remote control. A URC prototype running on the PocketPC is implemented and can successfully operate UniTherapy as a remote control; the authors are using the TUN library developed by the Wireless RERC, which is implemented on top of UPnP Remote UI standard, and are gradually adding universal interface support into the URC. An intelligent context-aware UI builder with user capability and preference support is also under development. A critical part of this process is having the user complete a short survey on user accessibility and preferences. UniTherapy's own assessment tools can be used to augment information on a user's performance capabilities. Finally, the authors are developing a generic UPnP control point, which will be embedded into the UniTherapy home user version so that UniTherapy would evolve into an Environmental Control Unit (ECU) for UPnP-compliant home appliances within the home environment.

In summary, an interactive framework for a personalized home rehabilitation appliance has been implemented with a consumer-centered design and CAMR approach. A diverse menu of assessment capabilities are available and can be used together with other services that include a protocol manager and data analysis tool with a telerehabilitation link. UniTherapy has been used as a research platform for rehabilitation and usability studies in three sites in the Milwaukee local area [42,43,46]; the authors received positive user feedback from patients and therapists during initial usability research studies.

27.5 FUTURE DIRECTION

To implement the personalized home rehabilitation model discussed earlier, there is still a lot of work to do. A few key tasks are:

- Additional research and clinical studies, aimed at quantifying the outcome of personalized intervention in home rehabilitation, need to test the hypothesis that personalized interventions will optimize rehabilitation outcomes. The authors are planning to conduct a new research study that will deploy the UniTherapy platform at patients' home sites with telerehabilitation link support, with the hope that the result will provide hard evidence to support the personalized home rehabilitation approach.
- Web services have evolved into a dominant distributing computing model; viewing health care as a service provides new opportunities to collaborate with experts in different aspects of rehabilitation (e.g., physical therapist and rehabilitation engineer), and work together to set up an optimized model that is better tailored to an individual.
- New opportunities and issues are emerging around the UI-Socket/URC standard. For example, the authors' group is looking into creating an accessibility profile for identifying an individual's capabilities and preferences. Another important example is the URC workgroup's emerging Task Model Description, which can be used to build a task model that can be used to control one or more targets or services. The authors are especially interested in how to generate a personalized health care interface that establishes leadership of solutions for accessibility, and in how the home health care devices could interact within a ubiquitous home environment.

In summary, despite some restrictions, personalized health care systems are emerging [47,48]. The authors are developing a universal access platform for personalized home rehabilitation with support by telerehabilitation link; the authors' hope is that in the next few years, an intelligent, personalized rehabilitation appliance will be implemented in the home environment, providing an alternative consumer-centered approach for rehabilitation that has the convenience of home while allowing access to a much larger population who could benefit from transfer of this scientific research.

ACKNOWLEDGMENT

The UniTherapy research project is supported by the RERC-AMI, U.S. Dept. of Education/National Institute on Disability and Rehabilitation Research (NIDRR) grant #H133E020729, and by the Falk Neurorehabilitation Engineering Research Center. The authors thank Michelle Johnson, Edward Maher, and Laura Johnson for using UniTherapy in their research studies, and the V2 community, especially Gottfried Zimmermann and Jeremy Johnson. The opinions expressed in this chapter are those of the authors.

REFERENCES

1. Greshman G.E., Duncan P.W., Stason W.B. et al., Post-Stroke Rehabilitation: Assessment, Referral and Patient Management, Clinical practice guidelines, Aspen Publ., Gaithersburg, 1996, see also http://www.ninds.nih.gov/health_and_medical/pubs/ poststrokerehab.htm.

2. Winters, J.M. and Herman, W., Report of the Workshop on Home Care Technologies for the 21st Century, Technical Report HCTR-10-v1.0, Catholic University of America, Washington, 1999, 96 p., see also http://www.eng.mu.edu/wintersj/HCTWorkshop.
3. Winters, J.M., TeleRehabilitation research: emerging opportunities, *Annu. Rev. Biomed. Eng.*, 4, 287–320, 2002.
4. Taub, E. and Crago, J.E., Behavioral plasticity following central nervous system damage in monkeys and man, in Julesz, B. and Kovacs, I., Eds., *Maturational Windows and Adult Cortical Plasticity*, Addison-Wesley, Redwood City, CA, 1995.
5. Wolf, S.L., Lecraw, D.E., Barton, L.A., and Jann, B.B. Force use of hemiplegic upper extremities to reverse the effect of learned nonuse among chronic stroke and head-injured patients, *Exp. Neurol*, 104, 125–132, 1989.
6. Taub, E. and Wolf, S.L., Constraint-Induced Movement techniques to facilitate upper extremity use in stroke patients, *Top. Stroke Rehabil.*, 3, 38–61, 1997.
7. Reinkensmeyer, D., Lum, P., and Winters, J.M., Emerging technologies for improving access to movement therapy following neurologic injury, in *Emerging and Accessible Telecommunications, Information and Healthcare Technologies*, Winters, J.M., Robinson, C., Simpson, R., and Vanderheiden, G., Eds., RESNA Press, Arlington, VA, 2001.
8. Volpe, B., Krebs, H., Hogan, N., Edelstein, L., Diels, C., and Aisen M., A novel approach to stroke rehabilitation: robot-aided sensorimotor stimulation, *Neurology*, 54, 1938–44, 2000.
9. Lum, P.S., Burgar, C.G., and Shor, P. Evidence for improved muscle activation patterns after retraining of reaching movements with the MIME robotic system in subjects with post-stroke hemiparesis. *IEEE Trans. Neural Syst. Rehabil. Eng.*, 12(2), 186–194, 2004.
10. Adamovich, S., Merians, A., Boian, R., Tremaine, M., Burdea, G., Recce, M., and Poizner, H., A virtual reality based exercise system for hand rehabilitation post-stroke, presence, *Special Issue on Virtual Rehabilitation*, 14(2), 161–174, 2005.
11. Holden, M.K., Dyar, T., Dayan–Cimadoro, L., Schwamm, L., and Bizzi, E., Virtual environment training in the home via telerehabilitation, *Arch. Phys. Med. Rehabil.*, 85(8), E12, 2004.
12. Winters, J.M., Harris, G., Schmit, B., and Scheidt, R., Report of the Workshop on Innovations in Neurorehabilitation. Future Possibilities for Technology-Assisted Neuromotor Assessment and Movement Therapy, Milwaukee, 2001, http://www.eng.mu.edu/ rehab/falk-workshop-sum.htm.
13. Winters, J.M. and Winters, J.M., A telehomecare model for optimizing rehabilitation outcomes, *J. Telemed. E-Health*, 10, 200–212, 2004.
14. Zhang, C., Yu, Z., and Chin, C.-Y., Context-aware infrastructure for personalized healthcare, *The International Workshop on Personalized Health*, IOS Press, Belfast, Northern Ireland.
15. Wang, Y. and Winters, J.M., A dynamic neuro-fuzzy model providing bio-state estimation and prognosis prediction for wearable intelligent assistants, *J. NeuroEng. Rehabil.*, 2005 (in press).
16. The Bandwidth Report, see also http://www.websiteoptimization.com/bw/0509/.
17. W3C, XML Linking Language (XLink) Version 1.0, see also http://www.w3.org/ TR/xlink/.
18. W3C, XML Pointer Language (XPointer) Version 1.0, see also http://www.w3.org/ TR/WD-xptr.
19. W3C, XSL Transformations (XSLT) Version 1.0, see also http://www.w3.org/TR/xslt.
20. W3C, XML Schema Part 1: Structures Second Edition, see also http://www.w3.org/ TR/xmlschema-1/.
21. W3C, XForms 1.0, see also http://www.w3.org/TR/xforms/.
22. Gottschalk, K., Graham, S., Kreger, H., and Snell, J., Introduction to Web services architecture, *IBM Syst. J.*, 41(2), 2002.
23. W3C, Semantic Web, see also http://www.w3.org/2001/sw/.
24. Vanderheiden, G. and Zimmermann, G., State of the science: access to information technologies, in *Emerging and Accessible Telecommunications, Information and Healthcare Technologies*, Winters, J.M., Robinson, C., Simpson, R., Vanderheiden, G., Eds., RESNA Press, Arlington, VA, 2002.
25. Health Level 7 Standard, see also http://www.hl7.org/.
26. SNOMED Clinical Terms (CT), see also http://www.snomed.org/.
27. Korhonen, I., Pärkkä, J., and van Gils, M., Health monitoring in the home of the future: infrastructure and usage models for wearable sensors, *IEEE Eng. Med. Biol.*, 22(3), 66–73, 2003.
28. Winters, J.M., Wang, Y., and Winters, J.M., Wearable Sensors and Telerehabilitation: Integrating Intelligent Telerehabilitation Assistants With a Model for Optimizing Home Therapy, *IEEE/EMBS Magazine*, Special Issue on Wearable Medical Technologies, 22, June 2003, pp. 56–65.

29. Lymberis A., Smart wearable systems for personalized health management: current R&D and future challenges, *Proc. 25th Annu. Int. Conf. IEEE EMBS*, Cancun, Mexico, 2003.
30. Gaudiosi, J., New Systems Give Games New Life, *Video Store*, 23(48), 8, 33, 2001.
31. Microsoft Xbox, see also http://www.xbox.com/.
32. Levander, M., Where Does Fantasy End?, *Time*, June 4, 2001, p. 22.
33. Chang, D., Haptics: gaming's new sensation, *Computer*, 35(8), 84–86, 2002.
34. FDA Center for Devices and Radiological Health, Medical Device Advice, see also http://www.fda.gov/cdrh/devadvice/3132.html.
35. Bach-y-Rita, P., Conceptual issues relevant to present and future neurologic rehabilitation, in Levin, H. and Grafman, J., Eds., *Neuroplasticity and Reorganization of Function after Brain Injury*, Oxford University Press, New York, 2000, pp. 357–379.
36. IEEE 1073 Medical Device Communications Standard, see http://www.ieee1073.org/.
37. Nichols, J. and Myers, B.A., Automatically generating interfaces for multi-device environments, *Ubicomp 2003 Workshop on Multi-Device Interfaces for Ubiquitous Peripheral Interaction*, October, 2003, Seattle, WA.
38. Abrams, M. et al., UIML: an appliance-independent XML user interface language, *WWW8 Conference*, May 1999, Toronto, Canada.
39. American National Standards Institute, (ANSI)/InterNational Committee for Information Technoloy Standards, (INCITS) 389-393 2005 Standard, August, 2005, Washington, D.C., see also http://www.incits.org/tc_home/v2.htm.
40. Vanderheiden, G., Zimmermann, G., and Trewin, S., Interface Sockets, Remote Consoles, and Natural Language Agents: A V2 URC Standards Whitepaper, see http://www.myurc.com/.
41. Microsoft DirectX standard, see also http://www.microsoft.com/DirectX.
42. Johnson, L.M. and Winters, J.M., Target Tracking Patterns Using Rehabilitation Interfaces, *BMES*, 2005 (in press).
43. Johnson, M.J., Trickey, M., Brauer E., and Feng, X., TheraDrive: a new stroke therapy concept for home-based computer-assisted motivating rehabilitation, *Proc. IEEE/EMBS*, San Francisco, CA, 2004.
44. Mahoney, F.I., Barthel, D.W., Functional evaluation: the Barthel index. *Md. State Med. J.* 14, 61–5, 1965.
45. Feng, X. and Winters, J.M., UniTherapy: a computer-assisted motivating neurorehabilitation platform for teleassessment and remote therapy, *Proc. Int. Congr. Rehabil. Robotics (ICORR)*, 4 p, 2005.
46. Feng, X. and Winters, J.M., Progress towards a service-oriented universal access telerehabilitation platform, *Proc. Int. Congr. Rehabil. Robotics (ICORR)*, 4 p, 2005.
47. Koutikias, V.G., Meletiadis, S.L., and Maglavera, N., WAP-based Personalized Healthcare Systems. *Health Inf. J.*, 7(3–4), 183–189, 2001.
48. Yao, J., Schmitz, R., and Warren, S.A. Wearable point-of-care system for home use that incorporates plug-and-play and wireless standards, *IEEE Trans. Inf. Technol. Biomed.*, 9(3), 2005.

28 Progress in Using the Universal Remote Console Standard to Create User-Customized Interfaces for Future Medical Devices

R. Sarma Danturthi, Pawan Shroff, and Jack M. Winters

CONTENTS

ABSTRACT

Most current interfaces for medical devices have single modes for display of information and operation of controls. Such interfaces can be difficult or impossible to use for many individuals with disabilities. This chapter addresses a novel approach for implementing personalized interfaces for health care products that makes use of the User Interface Socket/Universal Remote Console (UI-Socket/URC) suite of national standards. Using this standard, we show how a URC can generate, on-the-fly, personalized interfaces for simulated instances of three strategic classes of medical and exercise devices. Specifically, an algorithm integrates "hints" from standards-complaint XML files that describe the target device and its socket, plus an XML file providing a user accessibility or preferences profile previously obtained through an interactive user survey. Results for nine subjects, including four with disabilities, showed that the subjects could successfully use on-the-fly interfaces and, furthermore, strongly preferred interfaces that were personalized to their abilities and preferences.

28.1 INTRODUCTION

There is a need for interfaces, including those to be used within a home environment, that make medical instrumentation more usable and accessible [1]. One approach for addressing this need is to strive to design interfaces that are based more on the principles of universal design, as discussed in many other chapters in this book (Chapter 6, Chapter 8, and Chapter 18). An alternative is to create personalized interfaces, in which the form of the interface is based on the preferences and abilities of a specific user. With an appropriate infrastructure, a preferred interface that is small enough can then move with the person, functioning as a sort of assistive technology that interfaces with the target device or service to which the user desires access. This especially makes sense as a viable strategy for medical instrumentation with a clear display-control type of interface and not too many signals to display, such as home health care monitors or controls for exam chairs. However, for such a strategy to work, there must be agreed-to specifications — standards — to enable this mapping between a personalized console and the product to which access is desired. Imagine a world in which this personalized device could be used to wirelessly access a multitude of devices at home or work, including medical devices; an approach to meeting such a vision is the topic of this chapter.

This chapter reports on progress by the Rehabilitation Engineering Research Center on Accessible Medical Instrumentation (RERC-AMI) in developing a Medical Universal Remote Console (MedURC). This project falls under Development Program 3 (Emerging and Accessible Health care Technologies) and is the RERC's primary activity related to Project D3.2 (Modality Translation and Cross-Disability Interfaces for Communication), which aims to demonstrate strategic alternatives for user-centered medical monitoring interfaces that enhance accessibility. Specifically, the RERC-AMI proposed to collaborate with other third parties (e.g., other RERCs) to develop approaches for modality translation and to participate in the technical development process for standards and guidelines that help ensure that people with disabilities have access to medical technologies and services.

This chapter is divided into various sections. In the background section, a conceptual framework is developed that provides motivation for this activity. This includes a brief introduction to the current state-of-the-art of interfaces for medical monitoring devices, followed by introduction to the new User Interface Socket/ Universal Remote Console (UI-Socket/URC) national standards (ANSI-INCITS 389-393 [2,3]). This helps provide inspiration for the MedURC demonstration project [4] that involves simulating alternatives for creating user-customized medical device interfaces.

The methods section consists of three parts:

1. Development of standards-complaint XML files for describing certain classes of "target" devices, which represent medical devices examples of implementation of the standard.
2. Development of a URC that generates user-customized interfaces on-the-fly, based on knowledge from having read standardized files about the target's socket and the information from user preferences, in the case presented here, resulting in a compact and effective interface for a device with a display that matches the standard screen size of most PDAs.
3. Finally, implementation of a cross-platform simulation framework that provides connectivity between a Windows-based URC and Internet-based target devices through a standards-compliant socket, thus demonstrating use of these programs that collectively constitute MedURC.

In the last section, examples of results are provided for three categories of target devices: vital sign monitors, exam bed/table/chair controls, and home exercise ergometers. Each of these is based on generalized target files that, if used by companies making products of these areas, could be easily adapted to their product line, thereby making their interfaces more accessible. These are also areas in which medical products are often used in the home or community setting, often by a user population that is likely to consist of a considerably larger proportion of individuals with disabilities as compared to the population as a whole. These are areas in which the RERC-AMI has published technical product reviews [5–7]. Future directions for such multimodal user interfaces are discussed at the end of this chapter.

28.2 BACKGROUND

Because current technological trends change on a nearly everyday basis, standards in the electronic and information technology (E&IT) area tend to involve relatively short development times. In contrast, the medical community tends to lag in adopting trends such as USB drives or Web interfaces for various reasons, including practical considerations such as regulatory, liability, and reimbursement constraints. Currently most medical devices in a clinical setting seem to use proprietary interfaces. Some may follow medically oriented standards such as HL7 (Health Level 7) for medical information exchange or the Medical Information Bus (IEEE 1073), but the reality is that medically related standards tend to progress much more slowly than E&IT standards. Often biomedical technician professionals who must implement and support medical devices have to backtrack in the technology, using newer information technology (e.g., IEEE 802.11 wireless standards) for standard hospital office communication and yet older medical technologies for interfaces [1]. For instance, many, if not most, medical monitoring products still have standard serial port interfaces rather than the now more common USB port (with its higher speed and support for plug-and-play), and most do not support convenient interface features such as remote control. Medical standards tend to take time. For instance, activity on the Medical Information Bus predates wireless standards such as IEEE 802.11 and Bluetooth that are now used in millions of products and a part of our information infrastructure. Several challenges are involved in updating interfaces for medical products. It appears that, often when a new national or international standard is available, the medical community has to form committees to discuss its use, and in the interim, the standard might have become old and ready for another update.

Over the last few years, the V2 Technical Committee of the International Committee on Information Technology Standards (INCITS) has been working with the novel idea of a UI-Socket/URC standard that could work with many devices. The basic idea of UI-Socket/URC is to have a small instrument like a PDA work as a URC for any remotely controllable device in its vicinity. For such intelligent controlling, two different requirements exist. First, the URC should be able to detect a device and, through a discovery process, come to understand the nature of its interface socket, and second, without knowing about the target device beforehand, it should be able to generate for its user an effective interface for the target device. To meet these two requirements, ANSI/INCITS proceeded to design a standard that is now implemented as ANSI/INCITS 389–393:2005, with the process for implementation as an international standard (ISO/IEC 24752) under way. The RERC-AMI is one of four RERCs funded by the Department of Education that have collaborated on this ANSI standard, which became official in August 2005. Unlike other ongoing applications for this UI-Socket/URC standard that target primarily consumer electronics [6], our work focuses on interfaces for introducing this new ANSI standard to strategic classes of medical devices.

28.3 METHODS

28.3.1 Development of Compliant XML Files for Target Devices

The ANSI/INCITS 389-393 collection of standards, commonly referred to as the UI-Socket/URC standard, defines protocols for describing a target's socket and its properties in a form that is useful for a URC [2]. These protocols are described in an universally accepted format of eXtensible Markup Language (XML) files. The core set of target-based files are four in number. They are:

- A user interface socket file (uiSocket) that presents the functions and their properties of the device or appliance (ANSI/INCITS 390)
- A core presentation template (preT) file, which gives abstract hints about how the interface could be presented to the user through the URC, describing possible forms for widgets for each of the socket elements, and for grouping between elements (ANSI/INCITS 391)
- A target description (TD) file through which the target initiates the target discovery process with URCs (ANSI/INCITS 392)
- A target resource description framework (RDF) file for use as an atomic resource by the URC to help generate a concrete interface, for instance, in generating labeling and menu information (ANSI/INCITS 393)

Of all these files, the resource description file tends to be the largest in size, and the presentation file the smallest of the files. Any device with these four files can be available for the URC to detect and control. A URC may also use additional resource files to help build an interface to control the target, for instance, related to user preferences. In other words, once the set of four files (likely three for the international version, as the presentation template is expected to become optional) is available and the URC has access to a functioning socket that it now understands, a URC can recognize a device and automatically construct a user interface for the device to control. It also means that the user interface is dynamically constructed and modified every time the target files are modified for a new session, for instance, by the manufacturer. What follows here is a brief description of each file.

28.3.1.1 Target Discovery: The TD File

The job of URC-target discovery, including identifying the location of the target files, is handled by the target description (TD) file. This XML file is used to announce the socket of a target device to the URC. By reading the TD file, URC is able to know the location of the socket, presentation, RDF files, and other properties derived from those files.

A segment of the target description file is shown in the following listing:

```
<location id="location">
 <geocoordinates>
    <gml:Point srsName="vital-signs">
     <gml:coordinates>10.0, 10.0</gml:coordinates>
    </gml:Point>
 </geocoordinates>
</location>
<locator type="audio" id="audio-locator"/>
<locator type="visual" id="visual-locator"/>
<locator type="other" id="IRPing">
 <extension><rerc:IRPing type="rerc:basicIR"/></extension>
</locator>
```

```
  <dc:identifier
xsi:type="rerc:companyCode">0123456</dc:identifier>

<dcterms:conformsTo>http://www.incits.org/incits392-
2005</dcterms:conformsTo>
  <dcterms:modified>2005-08-12</dcterms:modified>
  <socket id="socket" name="http://www.rerc-
ami.org/V2/Simulation/XMLFiles/V2Required">
   <!-- In the following line, path is relative -->

<socketDescriptionLocalAt>V2Required/VitalSigns.uiSocket.xml</
socketDescriptionLocalAt>
   <category taxonomyName="http://www.unspsc.org">41.11.22.00
</category>
  </socket>
```

In this example, the location element of the file contains the geo-coordinates of the target device. The socket element of the file describes where the socket file reference is available for the URC and also gives the name of the socket file as a local path relative to the referenced location.

28.3.1.2 Describing Attributes of Socket Signals: The Socket File

The User Interface Socket (UIS) is an abstract concept that, when implemented, exposes the functionality and state of a target. As currently implemented in ANSI/INCITS 390, the socket contains four types of members: static elements (fixed constants), variables (dynamic signals), commands (core function from URC as request to target) and notifications (from target to URC). There is expected to be some expansion for the international (ISO) version. We will call the state of each socket element its "signal," and the UIS thus describes the socket signals along with their attributes. A collection of attributes are defined by the standard, and they can identify "secret" signals, signals that "time out," so on and so forth. One can also fix the length of the value of the signal, upper and lower limits of the signal value and the decimal places required for the signal value. Thus, a UIS file, implemented using XML, describes the details of the signals to be displayed on or controlled by a URC as it interacts with the target through its UIS. A segment of socket file is shown as follows:

```
<! - Standard type variable -- >
<variable id="Power" type="xsd:boolean">
<dependency read="true()" write="true()" />
</variable>
<! - Derived type variable. Also see below -- >
<variable id="Heartrate" type="xsd:HRType">
<dependency read="value('Power') = true()" write="false()" />
<!-- heart rate is a readable parameter when the power is
'ON' but it cannot be written to -->
```

```
</variable>
...
...
...
  <xsd:simpleType name="HRType" id="idHRtype">
   <xsd:restriction base="xsd:decimal">
      <xsd:minInclusive value="50"/>
      <xsd:maxInclusive value="150"/>
      <xsd:totalDigits value="3"/>
      <xsd:fractionDigits value="0"/>
   </xsd:restriction>
  </xsd:simpleType>
```

In the above listing, Power is Boolean and Heartrate is a derived type from decimal type. There are upper and lower limits for the Heartrate variable and the total digits are three without any decimal places to display. With the comments given, the dependency part is self-explanatory in both cases.

28.3.1.3 Hints for Interface Generation: The Presentation (PreT) File

The presentation template file, which tends to be the shortest file of the set of ANSI/INCITS standard files, contains abstract "hints" about how a user interface could be presented and describes how the user interface might look. It has reserved words that come from the forms controls within the W3C's XForm recommendation (http://www.w3.org/TR/2003/REC-xforms-20031014/), such as "range," "input," "select," and "select1" which are referred to as *interactors* in the standard. A URC, reading these interactors, knows the appropriate set of "widgets" that are viable for the type of interactor; for instance, as a slider is in the set of possibilities for "range," a textbox for "input," a list box for "select," and a group of radio buttons for "select1." The advantage of using interactors for presentation construction is that the set of viable alternative modes (including audio) for each type of interactor is clearly establsihed, enabling "on-the-fly" interface generation in which the URC algorithm uses some criteria to select appropriate widgets. For the two signals — Power and HeartRate — listed in the XML socket listing of Subsection 28.3.1.2, the presentation file might contain the partial listing as follows:

```
<input id="Power" ref="http://www.rerc-ami.org/
Medical/V2/VitalSigns/Socket#Power" />

<output id="Heartrate" ref="http://www.rerc-ami.org/
Medical/V2/VitalSigns/Socket#HeartRate"/>
```

Here the "Heartrate" signal is described as an "output" interactor because the heart rate is only being displayed over time and cannot be set or modified by the URC. The "input" interactor defined for "Power" informs the URC that the data need to be set by the user for turning power on or off. The on/off Boolean inference itself comes from the socket file.

Another very important part of the PreT standard is the ability to use the "group" definition to connect socket signals which normally should be presented together. These can be layered, and socket signals can belong to more than one group.

Of note is that a core PreT file for a target is currently required by the national ANSI/INCITS standard; based on recent work by the INCITS V2 Technical Committee, it is expected that in future the core PreT may be optional, as most of the this information could also be embedded (though less efficiently) in RDF files, which are described next.

28.3.1.4 Resources for Refining an Interface: The Resource Description (RD) Framework

Resources support URC generation of effective interfaces. The W3C's Resource Description Framework (RDF) / XML recommendation is used to describe resources. There must be one core resource file, called a resource sheet, for each target, and this must contain an "atomic resource description" that includes (or points to) storage of content (e.g., text, sound, image, animation, and video clip) such as help messages and labeling. For instance, it informs the URC about the content of labels that are associated with a socket variable. It also gives details of menu items and their shortcuts called *access keys*, values of the font, units of the parameter and any other information the URC needs to display the socket signal in a full context. For each socket signal, there may be several labels, access keys, unit labels, and the associated font (or emphasis) features for all these labels. A consequence is that the target's RDF can become quite large. However, the basic structure of the RDF is very simple, for instance, with a basic <useContext> node repeating several times in the <aResourceDescription> element of the RDF, as illustrated in the following partial listing:

```
<aResourceDescription>
<AResourceDescription rdf:about="http://www.rerc-ami.org/
Medical/V2/VitalSigns/Socket/
Vitalsigns/VitalSigns-label-en.rdf.xml#heartrate_label">
  <content rdf:parseType="Literal"><span
xml:lang="en">HR</span></content>
  <dcterms:conformsTo
rdf:resource="http://www.incits.org/incits393-2005"/>
  <!-- Socket signal identification here -->
  <useContext>
   <UseContext>
   <elementRef rdf:resource="http://www.rerc-ami.org/
Medical/V2/VitalSigns/Socket#HeartRate" />
   <role rdf:resource="http://www.incits.org/incits393-
2005#label" />
   <languageContext>en</languageContext>
   </UseContext>
  </useContext>
  <!-- Presentation template identifier here -->
  <useContext>
   <UseContext>
   <elementRef rdf:resource="http://www.rerc-ami.org/
Medical/V2/VitalSigns/pret#HeartRate" />
   <role rdf:resource="http://www.incits.org/incits393-
2005#label" />
   <languageContext>en</languageContext>
```

```
      </UseContext>
    </useContext>
  </AResourceDescription>
  </aResourceDescription>
```

Units of the signal and the font size for the units, etc., can be similarly described in other <aResourceDescription> nodes in the RDF. Alternative representations such as images or audio files can also be part of (or pointed to) by RDF files, as can images such as company logos. It should be understood that an RDF file contains and has to describe a set of labels for each of the signals defined in a socket file. For example, for the heart rate there would be at least three components: one for the "HR" label, one for the signal value of heart rate (say 82) and one for the units ("BPM").

For medical monitors, often the value of the signal is displayed in a larger font whereas its name or units use smaller fonts, with such labels surrounding the primary signal in a specified way. Because such a format may be based on human factors approaches by the manufacturer, it might be worth preserving as the "default" for presentation. For this purpose, we have defined a special 3×3 grid plus 10 different parameter values to potentially associate with each socket signal. Each grid cell location (or locations), of potentially variable row and column size and order (for audio presentation), can house a particular feature of the signal, e.g., different font size for labels and the value, inclusion of pictorial or audio icons, etc. We have implemented this convention in several ways, including a more readable version that dosen't use the atomic resource formalism but is still coded with RDF/XML. In addition to enabling near-replication of a manufacturer's preferred approach, this enables flexibility in how a URC may choose to implement the values and "hints" in the RDF files that describe a socket element.

Note that the URC algorithm can also make use of other RDF/XML resources, such as a resource file (or an XML fragment within a file) that describes user abilities and preferences (see Subsection 28.3.2), or a resource that describes capabilities of the remote device to be used (e.g., screen size; whether it supports speech recognition).

28.3.1.5 Summary

In short, the files described in the preceding text form the backbone of the ANSI/INCITS 389-393 standard for the controllable devices. With the help of these XML files, the UI-Socket for a target device or service can be adequately described and made available to a URC. Once a URC is powered on, the basic task of detecting a target device therefore becomes as simple as looking for the set of target description, socket, presentation, and RDF files. Any new target device introduced into the market has to just have these four defining files for a standards-compliant URC to detect and control it. New devices or new models of the same device can be introduced, and old devices can be modified at will by changing the contents of these files.

To introduce medical instrumentation applications of this standard, our primary interest for simulation are three classes of devices for which the RERC-AMI has earlier generated technical reports [5–7]: vital signs monitors that display signals such as heart rate and body temperature, equipment requiring positioning such as exam tables and chairs, and a subclass of exercise ergometers. The three standards-compliant suite of files are intended to encompass the necessary interfaces for most of the devices on the market in these categories. While our primary purpose in creating these files was to demonstrate the potential for MedURC, these files will be made freely available to medical devices manufacturers, thus helping shorten their development cycle if they choose to implement the UI-Socket/URC standard.

The next section describes our specific implementation of a URC from the ANSI/INCITS point of view. This is important because a URC can have a different interface for controlling each target.

28.3.2 Development of a MedURC Interface Generator

Consider the family room of a modern home. As the controllable target devices multiply, the number of remote controls also increases, often with as many as four or more handheld remotes sitting on a coffee table. This picture becomes more complicated when one considers the narrow capabilities for each of these remotes, when advances in intelligent interfaces might suggest that user-centered challenges such as support for different languages (Japanese, Chinese, etc.) are desirable when a person travels overseas. Although there are a number of other approaches to intelligent interfaces [8–10], our approach stems from the basic idea behind the new ANSI/INCITS standard, i.e., one personalized remote control for all the devices available now, one that would also interface with devices to be introduced and purchased in the future. The ANSI/INCITS 389-393 standard illuminates a strategy for enabling mobile devices such as handhelds, conceptualized as universal console, to be used to access devices as diverse as a TV and a medical monitor. The uniqueness and significance of the standard comes from the fact that the URC has no prior knowledge about the target. A compatible target, once detected, gives the URC sufficient information via a few structured XML files and an RDF file to generate an interface that replicates a remote console for controlling the target, as well as displaying strategic information from the target by modes that could include visual, audio, and tactile. This means that the URC has to depend on the content of these files for interface generation and controlling the target device. This section briefly describes the development of a MedURC Interface Generator, an on-the-fly algorithm that can automatically generate interfaces for the three classes of medical devices mentioned previously. This was the focus of a recent master's thesis [11]. The idea is for the user to experience interaction with the simulated target device by using a simulated remote control to observe the status of signals on these medical devices, and/or controlling features of a device such as the angle of a seatback for an exam table.

Part of this objective is also to create interfaces that are as accessible and user centered as possible, based on information about the abilities and preferences of the user. This means that the URC must have access to an additional RDF file, the User Abilities/Preferences Profile file. Our MedURC specification includes, in addition to the ANSI/INCITS 389–393 compliant files to describe the target device, this user-based (vs. target-based) file that provides information on the abilities and preferences of the user. Note that this file is associated with a specific user and is required to be created just once, and it can then be reused for subsequent interface generation with any target. Also, the user preferences can be modified as many times as desired until the user is satisfied with the revised preferences.

A prototype computer program, the Accessibility and Preferences Evaluation Survey, was developed to collect such information about an individual user's abilities and preferences. This program has a simple graphical user interface, with a screen of a size that is convenient for PDA devices such as the pocket PC (which is supported); users (or someone on their behalf) enter information regarding their abilities and preferences, navigating through the various sections of this program by selecting appropriate tab pages. The first section of this program deals with user abilities: users provide information regarding their difficulties, disabilities, or impairments that would affect their ability to use a handheld device or computer interface, a desktop keyboard, mouse, or monitor system. This section itself is further divided into visual impairments or difficulties, hearing and speech impairments, posture and balance challenges, and arm and hand motor coordination impairments. The second section of the program relates to collecting information about users' preferences with respect to user interfaces associated with control and display. In this section, users are provided with options to change settings related to user controls and screen displays such as fonts (type, size, and styles). The user then has the opportunity to iteratively operate the program with their preferences in use, so as to experience what it is like and then interact with the program to make any changes. The user then exits the program when it is felt that the types of choices for interfaces are satisfactory. The User Abilities/Preferences Profile file is usually stored on the URC side.

The prototype MedURC algorithm that uses the UI-Socket/URC standard to construct on-the-fly interfaces is basically programmed to do two different tasks. The first task is to read the group of XML and RDF files that are available to be transmitted by the target. As explained earlier, the target-based XML files basically contain core information and helpful hints for the URC to construct an interface, as well as begin a communication protocol between the URC and the target. Neither URC nor the target device can change the ANSI/INCITS standard XML files, once they are created and used within a given session.

The second task is more challenging: to incorporate the information from the accessibility and preferences file with the data read in first task to construct an optimal interface that suits the particular user — a personalized interface. Because handheld devices are portable with relatively small screens, the amount of information one can display on a handheld device screen is relatively small. If a large amount of information is required to be displayed on these screens the information could become tiny. Alternatively, if the amount of information is large, the number of "pages" to display the information increases, thereby making navigation a necessity. When several pages are added for the user to navigate, even the friendliest interface can be become irritating at times. These are some of the classic reasons why the World Wide Web Consortium (W3C) groups on device independence, accessibility, and multimodal interfaces have recognized a need to combine expertise, as users of mobile devices essentially have capability limitations similar to disability. The User Abilities/Preferences Profile data is used at several stages of the algorithm, with the first being to select each widget from the viable set of possibilities. The URC algorithm attempts to integrate, on-the-fly, all these data, constructing interfaces which should be satisfactory, if not optimal, for the user. This should be the case because user abilities and preferences affect the output of the algorithm and thus the form of the interface. User preferences influence certain aspects such as fonts, font colors, font types, controls, and navigation preferences. They also influence certain choices of controls. Accessibility features available on Windows XP and Windows CE platforms [12] can also be used with our software simulation [4], which is written in C# in the Microsoft Visual Studio development environment [13]. The flow diagram for the algorithm is presented in Figure 28.1. An example of its implementation, for various user ability and preference choices, is presented in Figure 28.2.

The algorithm developed by RERC-AMI attempts to maintain a trade-off and creates a balance between navigation and display. It also places the controls in such a manner as to minimize the number of screens required to display the information and maximize the content per screen. This involves careful calculation of the x- and y-coordinate space for each widget, maximizing the former while minimizing the latter. It also attempts to follow natural grouping and prioritization as suggested by the target's PreT file. To summarize, the algorithm for the MedURC Interface Generator is programmed to read the ANSI/INCITS UI-Socket/URC standard files and the User Abilities/Preferences Profile file and combine them to better suit the user of the URC who is interacting with the target. Subsection 28.3.4 summarizes results of a pilot study [11] that involved human subjects with and without disabilities using various alternative interfaces.

28.3.3 Implementation of a Cross- Platform Simulation Framework

The URC runs on a client machine and communicates with the target device residing on the RERC-AMI Web site. The target device can also be programmed to work on the client machine (in which the URC resides) on its local host Web site with the help of Internet Information Server (IIS). The communication between URC and target happens via a request-acknowledgement method. The ANSI/INCITS standard files always reside on the target (Web) side. Depending on the number of files available, when queried, the target informs the URC of the available devices, and the URC builds an interface for the selected device. An instance of the data being transferred on this communication can optionally be stored on either target or URC side, and the instance file is usually named after the user who logs in. If no username is given, a guest user is assumed.

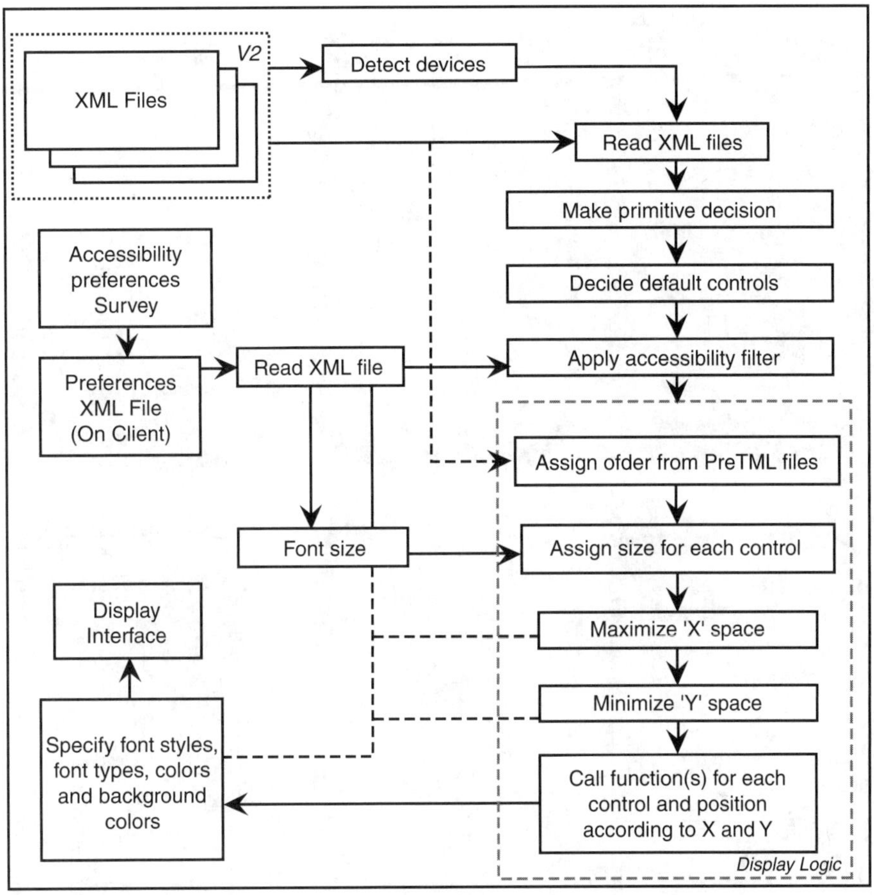

FIGURE 28.1 Flow diagram of the URC algorithm.

Whether a user logs in with a valid username or wants to test the system as a guest, an instance file will be constructed by the target when one is not available. But if an instance file already exists, URC gives the option to the user to load the instance file or start a fresh instance of the target. It should be mentioned here that in this simulation, URC resides on a local computer (Windows XP Professional) and attempts to invoke the target residing on a local or remote host computer with a HTTP protocol. Both programs are coded in C# on WinXP platform, but the target device uses ASP.NET for its communication and simulation protocol, which is summarized in Figure 28.3.

A simple principle is used to implement communication between the URC and the target. When the URC is ready, it allows the user to log in as a registered or guest user, in which case the user can select his preferences and save them. In the next step, when the URC is ready to read or control a target, it sends a query to the target HTTP location (local or remote). The target checks the number of files available in its control and sends the URC a list of devices that are available. In deciding the compatibility, the target looks for a set of four ANSI/INCITS files (Socket, Presentation, RDF, and Target Description) for a device to be made available to URC. As described earlier, the set of four files follow a standard format in name and content. The target sends a list of devices back to the URC as a concatenated string. It is the job of URC to split the long string into individual device names and show them as a list of available devices to the user in the format the user prefers. The user is then allowed to select a target device for controlling. Once a device is selected by the user, the URC sends a query again to the target asking it to open, display, close, and do many other

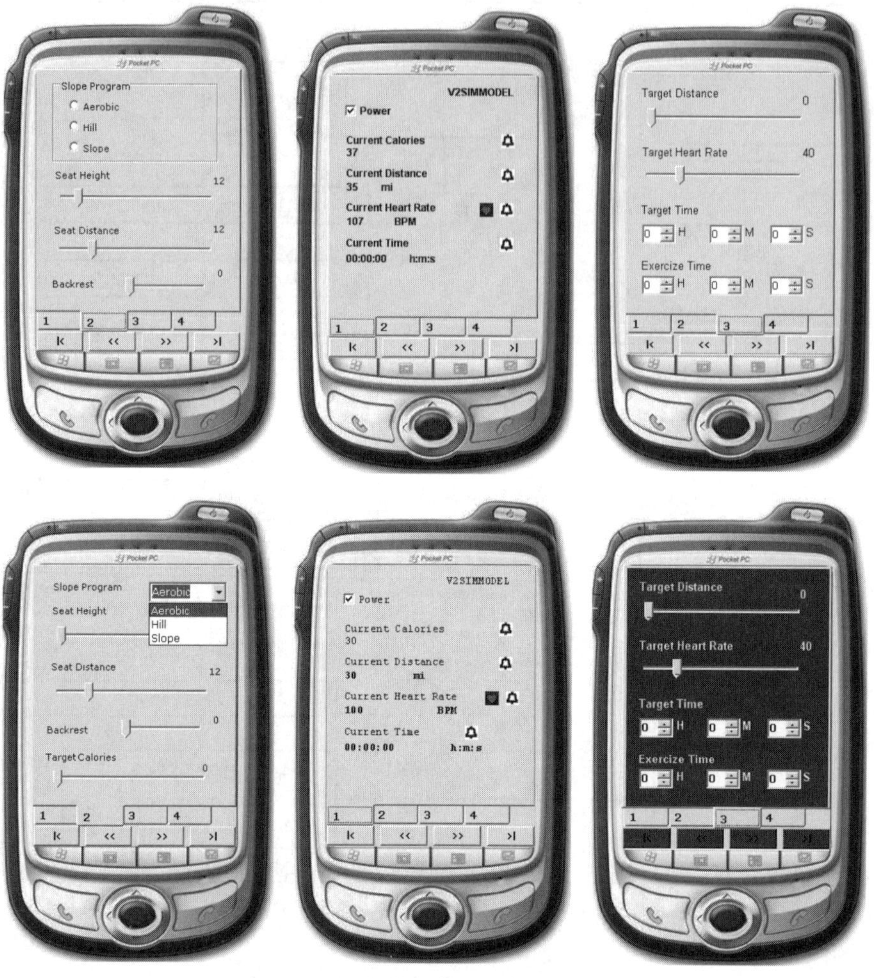

(a) (b) (c)

FIGURE 28.2 Examples of how user abilities and preferences can affect the interfaces that are automatically generated by MedURC here for a screen related to the ergometers target device. (a) Sample interface with radio buttons (top) and with list boxes (bottom) to select from a list of options. (b) Sample interface with Arial, size 11, Bold font (top) and the same interface with Bookman old style, size 11, regular font (bottom). (c) Sample interface with default settings (top) and the same interface with a high-contrast scheme (bottom) for visually impaired individuals.

functions. Once a device is selected and communication established, everything the URC sends is received by the target, and the target is updated immediately. When the URC does not send a query, the target goes on working in its programmed mode, updating itself automatically. In the vital signs monitor, for example, while the URC is not sending any data, the target can update the vital sign values that are randomly chosen. But every time the target is queried, it gives an acknowledgement to URC and gives the status of "all" variables and other entities. These status signals can be populated by URC on its screens as appropriate. If not queried, the target keeps updating those values and does not bother about URC. The target does not concern itself on how the URC populates the data sent by it and how URC sends the next query. The target only looks for a query to come in from a URC. Once a query comes in, current data on hand is sent immediately back to URC. URC can also program a thread to invoke or update the target at regular intervals without user intervention.

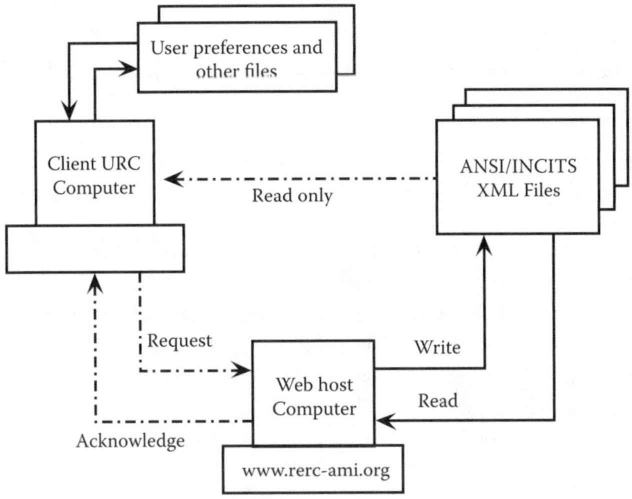

FIGURE 28.3 Communication Protocol between URC and the target host. Solid lines indicate a connection on the same side. Dotted lines indicate cross-platform connection from local client machine to the Web host via Internet.

URC also has the ability to close a target. When the URC sends a request to close a target device, the target closes the currently visible aspx page and reminds the URC that the existing instance of data can be saved. If the save option is selected, the data is saved on the target side. URC can also close the target without saving the existing instance of the data. The query-acknowledgement system of communication is implemented because of the cross-platform programming and to make the device XML files available on the RERC-AMI Web site. Reading those XML files, one can relate to the working mechanism of the ANSI/INCITS standard. A target can also be opened without the intervention of a URC. Typing the target Web site address in the Web browser such as Internet Explorer can display the target device, opening it for a guest user. These Web sites for three different medical devices, RERC-AMI simulated, can be viewed at the following locations:

http://www.rerc-ami.org/V2/Simulation/VitalSigns/TargetOpen.aspx
http://www.rerc-ami.org/V2/Simulation/ExamTables/TargetOpen.aspx
http://www.rerc-ami.org/V2/Simulation/Ergometers/TargetOpen.aspx

To make the simulation more realistic, the Web software includes internal algorithms that vary sensor signals such as heart rate or blood pressure in a reasonably physiologic manner. These are then faithfully updated on-the-fly on the MedURC, communicating only through the open socket between the MedURC executable running in Windows on the local computer and the Web site running an instance of the target, which also houses the standards-compliant files.

As stated briefly earlier, the medical community has accepted the messaging standard as HL7. HL7 in turn involves clinical terms that are used widely and are a part of another standard called SNOMED clinical terms (CT). The RERC-AMI has made every effort to include SNOMED-CT for the vital signs monitors in the simulation environment, extracting these SNOMED CTs for the vital signs signals from the National Library of Medicine's (NLM) meta-thesaurus available on the Web to registered users [13]. This is an attempt to merge the new developments in medicine and technology with the ANSI standard.

Finally, there is no reason why another URC could not interact with our Web page implementation of a simulation environment for target devices. RERC-AMI has made a document available on its Web site for the public, which explains the simple communication protocol and discovery process. Using this document, any user can construct or obtain one's own URC to communicate with the RERC-AMI's target. Similarly, there is no reason why our URC cannot interact with other targets. Indeed, this has already been implemented; our URC implementation can read and use the target files on the www.myurc.org simulation environment supported by the Trace Center [3].

28.4 RESULTS AND DISCUSSION

RERC-AMI research team has demonstrated that the URC and target work in tandem and are communicating satisfactorily. The ultimate aim is to achieve an ideal simulation environment for remotely controllable medical devices such as vital signs monitors, examination tables used in a hospital setting, and exercise ergometers. The progress so far has been very encouraging, and an earlier version of the simulation was successfully demonstrated to the ANSI/INCITS URC committee during a plenary meeting in August 2005 in Washington DC. Figure 28.4 to Figure 28.7 provide examples of MedURC simulations.

28.4.1 HUMAN SUBJECTS PILOT STUDY

To test the MedURC Interface Generator algorithm, a diverse set of individuals, including five able-bodied "normal" individuals and four individuals with functional impairments (including hearing, visual, and hand and motor functioning), were recruited to test and evaluate these generated MedURC interfaces. These enabled the users to use, control, and operate the generated user interfaces for these simulated target devices. To evaluate this algorithm, a set of simple goal oriented tasks were created for each target. Each task sequence was performed four times, once with each of four different interface alternatives:

- *Alternative 1:* default user interfaces
- *Alternative 2:* on-the-fly user interfaces created by taking into account information extracted from the User Ability/Preferences Profile (as stored in XML file) for each user

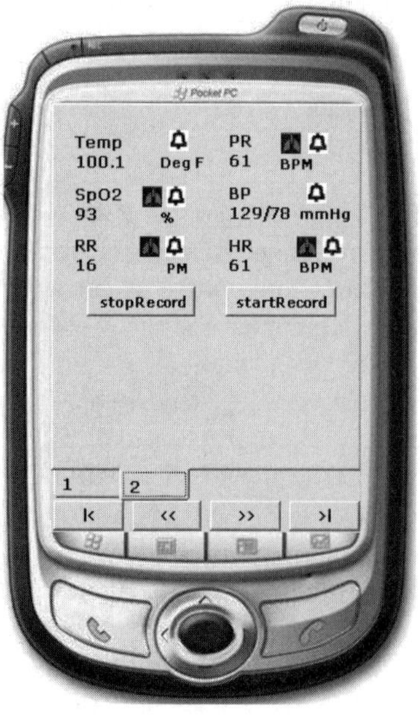

Target Device - Vital Signs

Parameter	Type	Value	Min - Max	Scope	Secret	Sensitive	Timeout
Heart Rate	HRType	99	50 - 150	Global	false	false	false
Body Temperature	TempType	101.9	96 - 105	Global	false	false	false
Pulse Rate	HRType	71	50 - 150	Global	false	false	false
SpO2	Spo2Type	87	80 - 98	Global	false	false	false
Blood Pressure	BpType	113/86	60 - 170	Global	false	false	false
Resp. Rate	RespType	21	5 - 30	Global	false	false	false
Sweep Speed	SweepSpeedType	5500	100 - 10000	Global	false	false	false
Volume	VolumeNumberType	9	1 - 10	Global	false	false	false
Power	xsd:boolean	True	-	Global	false	false	false
Mute	xsd:boolean	False	-	Global	false	false	false
Audio Readout	xsd:boolean	False	-	Global	false	false	false
Start Record	basicCommand	True	-	Global	false	false	false
Stop Record	basicCommand	False	-	Global	false	false	false

Set Notify to TRUE   Set RandomNo to TRUE

FIGURE 28.4 Example showing vital signs monitoring — MedURC screen (left) and target on the Web (right).

- *Alternative 3:* user interfaces created by using only the "preferences" data extracted from the User Ability/Preferences Profile
- *Alternative 4:* default user interface with Microsoft Accessibility features [13], specifically using Narrator, High Contrast, Sound Sentry, Show Sounds and Mouse Keys features which both Windows XP and CE support

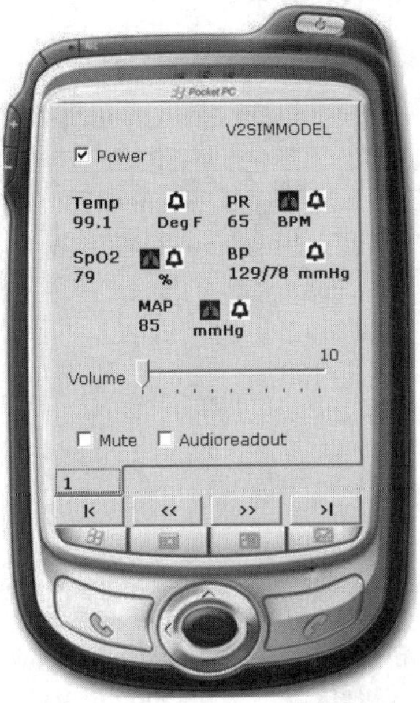

Target Device - CAS 740 Vital Signs

Parameter	Type	Value	Min - Max	Scope	Secret	Sensitive	Timeout
Temperature	TempType	100.0	96 - 105	Global	false	false	false
Pulse Rate	HRType	60	50 - 150	Global	false	false	false
SpO2	Spo2Type	91	80 - 98	Global	false	false	false
BP	BpType	114/63	60 - 170	Global	false	false	false
MAP	xsd:double	80	-	Global	false	false	false
Volume	VolumeNumberType	1	1 - 10	Global	false	false	false
Power	xsd:boolean	True	-	Global	false	false	false

Set Notify to TRUE   Set RandomNo to TRUE

FIGURE 28.5 CAS-740 vital signs monitoring — MedURC screen (left) and target on the Web (right).

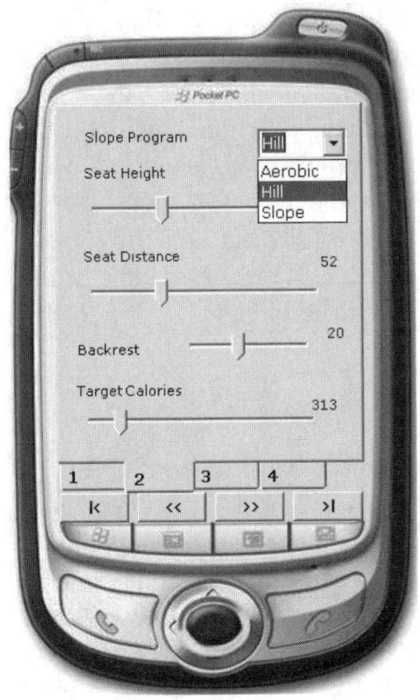

Target Device - Exercise Ergometers

Parameter	Type	Value	Min - Max	Scope	Secret	Sensitive	Timeout
Seat Height (in)	SeatHeightType	23	12 - 72	Global	false	false	false
Seat Distance (in)	SeatDistanceType	12	12 - 72	Global	false	false	false
Backrest (deg)	BackRestType	15	0 - 90	Global	false	false	false
Exercize Time (hh:mm:ss)	TimeType	12:30:00	0:0:0 - 23:59:59	Global	false	false	false
CurrentCalories	CaloriesType	45	0 - 3000	Global	false	false	false
TargetCalories	CaloriesType	300	0 - 3000	Global	false	false	false
CurrentDistance (mi)	DistanceType	1	0 - 50	Global	false	false	false
TargetDistance (mi)	DistanceType	2.5	0 - 50	Global	false	false	false
CurrentHeartRate	HeartRateType	70	40 - 250	Global	false	false	false
TargetHeartRate	HeartRateType	132	40 - 250	Global	false	false	false
CurrentTime (hh:mm:ss)	TimeType	00:00:15	0:0:0 - 05:59:59	Global	false	false	false
TargetTime (hh:mm:ss)	TimeType	00:05:30	0:0:0 - 05:59:59	Global	false	false	false
SlopeProgram	SlopeNumberType	Aerobic	Hill, Aerobic, Random	Global	false	false	false
Volume	VolumeNumberType	6	1 - 10	Global	false	false	false
Power	xsd:boolean	True	-	Global	false	false	false
Mute	xsd:boolean	False	-	Global	false	false	false
Audio Readout	xsd:boolean	False	-	Global	false	false	false
Start Record	basicCommand	True	-	Global	false	false	false
Stop Record	basicCommand	False	-	Global	false	false	false

Set Notify to TRUE   Set RandomNo to TRUE

FIGURE 28.6 Ergometers monitoring — MedURC screen (left) and target on the Web (right).

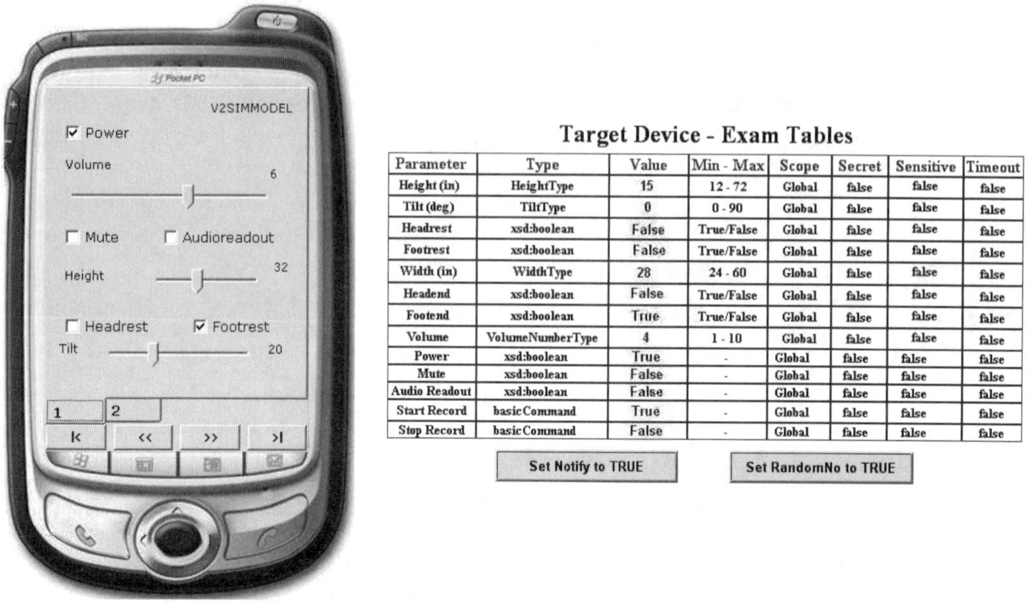

Parameter	Type	Value	Min - Max	Scope	Secret	Sensitive	Timeout
Height (in)	HeightType	15	12 - 72	Global	false	false	false
Tilt (deg)	TiltType	0	0 - 90	Global	false	false	false
Headrest	xsd:boolean	False	True/False	Global	false	false	false
Footrest	xsd:boolean	False	True/False	Global	false	false	false
Width (in)	WidthType	28	24 - 60	Global	false	false	false
Headend	xsd:boolean	False	True/False	Global	false	false	false
Footend	xsd:boolean	True	True/False	Global	false	false	false
Volume	VolumeNumberType	4	1 - 10	Global	false	false	false
Power	xsd:boolean	True	-	Global	false	false	false
Mute	xsd:boolean	False	-	Global	false	false	false
Audio Readout	xsd:boolean	False	-	Global	false	false	false
Start Record	basicCommand	True	-	Global	false	false	false
Stop Record	basicCommand	False	-	Global	false	false	false

FIGURE 28.7 Exam tables monitoring — MedURC screen (left) and target on the Web (right).

These alternative user interfaces were provided to the users randomly, and each subject took 60 to 90 min to complete the set of tasks for the four alternative interfaces. Upon completion, each subject then filled out a questionnaire that used ordinal scales to obtain users' opinions with respect to the difference between the interfaces. The goals of this feasibility study were to determine how well "on-the-fly" interface generation actually works, and whether users preferred a more personalized interface (generated on-the-fly) rather then a default one.

It is interesting that every participant selected different preferences, and subsequently had a different interface for most (if not all) screens. Table 28.1 provides means and standard deviations between the four alternatives for each of the questions (scored on an ordinal scale from 1 to 4) across the entire population of subjects which participated in this study. In addition to the important base finding that robust on-the-fly interfaces are possible and, furthermore, satisfactory, the results clearly suggest that users do prefer a customizable interface that adapts to their abilities and preferences. The trend for almost every criterion is toward a user interface customized to a user's abilities or preferences, rather than a default one. Indeed, for 11 of the 14 categories, either no subjects or only one of the nine subjects felt otherwise. This suggests, at least indirectly, that a personalized interface improves usability and enhances user performance. Results also indicate that the noncontrol population also preferred interfaces customized to their abilities [11].

28.5 FUTURE DIRECTIONS

The ANSI/INCITS 389-393 committee has now proposed this suite of standards to the ISO/IEC for international adoption and, if approved, it is expected to become ISO/IEC 24752. At the same time, improvements are being offered, and the RERC-AMI is concentrating on items such as streamlining the RDF files. Because for more complicated applications such as medical instrumentation the RDF files can grow to a very large size, reducing and compacting the size of RDF becomes necessary. It has also been tentatively decided not to require a core PreT file, which is further focusing our efforts, because both interactors and grouping are critical data for our MedURC Interface Generator algorithm. We are thus implementing use of other RDF/XML alternatives, such as the W3C's Composite Capabilities/Preferences Profile (CC/PP) protocol, see www.w3.org/mobile/ccpp.

TABLE 28.1
Means of Preferences for Alternative User Interfaces under Different Criteria

Interface Criteria	Default UI		Default UI With User Preferences and Abilities		Default UI With User Preferences		Default UI With MS Accessibility	
	Mean	±Std Dev	Mean	±Std Dev	Mean	±Std Dev	Mean	±Std Dev
Ability to see all labels	2.78	0.67	3.56	0.53	3.33	0.50	1.78	1.09
Ability to interpret all information	2.78	0.44	3.44	0.53	3.33	0.50	1.89	1.05
Ability to find all controls	2.89	0.60	2.89	0.78	2.89	0.60	2.11	0.93
Ability to understand status of interface	2.67	0.87	3.00	0.87	2.89	0.78	2.11	0.78
Ability to get feedback	2.56	0.53	3.00	0.71	2.89	0.33	2.00	1.00
Ability to operate controls	2.78	0.83	3.33	0.71	3.33	0.71	2.22	0.67
Ability to operate without mistakes	2.33	1.00	2.89	0.93	2.78	0.97	1.67	1.00
Text/background colors	2.22	1.09	3.22	0.83	3.44	0.73	1.00	0.87
Fonts	2.22	0.97	3.11	0.78	3.11	0.78	1.78	0.83
Font size	2.11	0.33	3.11	0.60	3.22	0.67	2.11	0.60
Organization of controls	2.22	1.09	3.22	0.83	3.00	0.71	1.33	1.22
Ease of navigation	1.89	0.60	2.67	0.71	2.67	0.50	1.22	0.83
Ability to complete task	2.11	0.78	2.56	0.73	2.44	0.73	1.00	0.50
Color contrast	1.89	1.05	2.56	0.88	2.56	0.73	1.22	1.39

Note: Means and standard deviations have been calculated from ordinal scales in which a "4" represents the highest possible score. Notice strong preference for Alternatives 2 and 3, where the interfaces are based on XML information from the accessibility and preferences profile.

Additionally, we are adding MedURC specifications that go slightly beyond the standard, especially, as related to having an ability to more precisely lay out medical monitoring signals in a manner that, as a default, can replicate the professional "feel" and "corporate presence" of existing products as well as fully implement safety features such as alerts. From our perspective, being able to replicate the content and feel of a current device interface is the default from which we can then improve the interfaces as it is personalized to the user, and also acknowledges the human factors efforts within the medical device community (Chapter 15 to Chapter 21) Chapter 27 in this book. For example, for heart rate the display often shows a label as "HR" and the units (e.g., BPM) in smaller fonts and the changing value (of the actual socket signal) in larger fonts, with the value flashing and the monitor beeping if it leaves the desired range. MedURC should start by being able to provide an interface that a usability analysis would deem to be essentially equivalent. As another example, the labeling terminology implemented by RERC-AMI is also consistent with HL7 medical messaging and the SNOWMED clinical terms [14]. Based in part on interaction with INCITS V2 Technical Community, the RERC-AMI is also planning to participate in activities that include integration of HL7/medical data. The opportunity of having a MedURC-like technology that supports both interface generation and health care messaging in an integrated way seems to represent an especially intriguing opportunity.

Part of the beauty of the standards-based URC approach is its flexibility. For instance, as briefly described in Chapter 27, our UniTherapy technology also possesses a suitable set of target files, and our URC interface generator has successfully been used for its simpler home user interface mode, for which such an interface makes sense. The designer of the UniTherapy technology (see Chapter 27 in this book), has also created a program that automatically creates two key files for a target device, the socket and the PreT. Thus, it is becoming easier to add new classes of targets. Although there are no immediate plans to do so, we anticipate that the RERC-AMI is likely to, at some stage, add more classes of health care devices that we support, as well as more formats for each device for the simulation environment. Once the target files are placed on the Web, any URC reaching the Web will see that these are available.

Finally, the RERC-AMI plans to aggressively suggest to the health care and medical device industry that the ANSI/INCITS standard can ideally work in a hospital setting or a homecare medical device. One of the key potential challenges, the regulatory environment, does not seem an overwhelming challenge, although security issues, in particular, need to be worked out.

In summary, it is hoped that this MedURC demonstration project will prove to be an outstanding tool in the coming few years, one that can help launch a new generation of personalized health care interfaces that are not only more accessible and usable, but also enhance user performance because they are more tuned to their abilities.

ACKNOWLEDGMENT

This work is supported by the RERC-AMI and funded by the National Institute on Disability and Rehabilitation Research (NIDRR) of the U.S. Department of Education under grant number H133E020729. All opinions are those of the authors.

REFERENCES

1. Winters, J.M., Emerging rehabilitative healthcare anywhere: was the homecare technologies workshop visionary? in *Emerging and Accessible Telecommunications, Information and Healthcare Technologies*, Winters et al., Eds., RESNA Press, Arlington, VA, 2001, pp. 95–111.
2. ANSI/INCITS 389-393:2005 standard, retrieved from http://www.incits.org/ tc_home/ v2.htm.
3. INCITS V2 web page, at www.myurc.com, 2005.
4. MedURC informational web pages, available at http://www.rerc-ami.org/medurc, 2005.
5. Lemke, M., Johnson, L.M., and Omiatek, E., Tech Report on Exam Tables and Chairs, published by RERC-AMI as TR-AMI-MU-001, 2005, available at http://www.rerc-ami.org/ami/tech/ tr-ami-mu-001_examtables.aspx.
6. Schaning, M., Mundschau, M., Yatco, A., and Omiatek., E., Tech Report on Exam Tables, Chairs and Beds, published by RERC-AMI as TR-AMI-MU-002, 2005, available at http://www.rerc-ami.org/ami/tech/tr-ami-mu-002_monitors.aspx.
7. Omiatek, E. and Mielcarek, L, Tech Report on Cardiopulmonary Exercise Equipment, published by RERC-AMI as TR-AMI-MU-003, 2005, available at http://www.rerc-ami.org/ami/tech/tr-ami-mu-003_monitors.aspx.
8. Rubin, E. and Yates, R.. Designing GUI Applications with Windows Forms, November 2003, www.informit.com.
9. Gajos, K. and Weld, D.S., SUPPLE: automatically generating user interfaces, in *Proceedings of IUI'04*. Funchal, Portugal, 2004.
10. Gohil B., Automatic GUI Generation, Dissertation Bournemouth, University School of Design, Engineering and Computing: Dorset, U.K., April 1999.

11. Shroff, P., Algorithm to Automatically Generate Multi Modal User Interfaces based on User Preferences and Abilities, Master's thesis, Marquette University, Milwaukee WI, 2005.
12. GotDotNet: The Microsoft .NET Framework Community, http://gotdotnet.com/.
13. Microsoft Accessibility, http://www.microsoft.com/enable.
14. National Library of Medicine, UMLS Knowledge Source Server, Meta-Thesaurus, retrieved from http://umlsks.nlm.nih.gov/kss/servlet/Turbine/template/admin,user, KSS_login.vm, 2005.

29 Usability and Access Issues in Telerehabilitation

Linda van Roosmalen

CONTENTS

ABSTRACT

The home health care market is rapidly growing within the U.S., and so is the opportunity for telerehabilitation. Through the increasingly available technology such as wireless sensors, videoconferencing, PDAs, and camera phones, people now have access to products that can assist them in tracking their vital signs, assess their homes on accessibility, control their physical status, and remotely communicate their health information to their health professional from the comfort of their own homes. Telerehabilitation can reduce travel times and health care cost for patients as well as health professionals. This chapter will discuss some of the user and access issues associated with telerehabilitation as a result of patient cognition, mobility, and sensation.

29.1 INTRODUCTION

What does telerehabilitation have to do with "accessible medical instrumentation"? Telerehabilitation has shown to benefit clinicians in providing rehabilitation services to a variety of patients in home settings or other remote care facilities. Telerehabilitation has made health care more accessible for individuals in need of rehabilitation.

Because telerehabilitation is especially useful for patients that are unable to travel, the real benefit of telerehabilitation seems to be for clinicians and patients who are elderly or have multiple limitations or chronic illnesses. State-of-the-art rehabilitation services directed to this population often make use of devices such as vital sign monitors or therapeutic equipment and therapeutic exercises and medication. Patient populations, including elders and those with disabilities, are not necessarily skilled in using these technical medical devices or may be unable to use medical devises due to their cognitive, physical or sensory limitations, as developed in Chapter 2 and Chapter 14. Therefore, accessible medical instrumentation could greatly enhance the use of telerehabilitation for elders and those with multiple disabilities.

One of the barriers introduced by telerehabilitation is distance. Elders and people with disabilities may have difficulty replicating complex training schemes that are prescribed by occupational therapists or physical therapists (OT's or PT's) and need assistance through the presence of a clinician or direct communication. The distance between rehabilitation clinicians and (remote) clients requires the use of interfaces to clearly connect the two. It further requires modes for communication and ways to transfer information between the two parties. While making a connection, communicating, or transferring information between sites, sensory, cognitive, and mobility skills of both the patient as well as the rehab professional is needed. Any limitation in these three areas will affect the availability, accessibility and reliability of telerehabilitation for use by elders and people with disabilities. When introducing technology for use by elders or people with disabilities, problems may arise related to usability, safety, and effectiveness of the interface media used.

The focus of this book is on accessibility and usability of medical instrumentation; there appear to be many comparable issues that affect the accessibility and usability of telerehabilitation, which will be described in this chapter.

29.1.1 Telerehabilitation in Service Delivery

One of the most rapidly growing segments of the U.S. health care market is home health care. To be more cost and time efficient, visits of nurses can be replaced by visits with a real-time video, visits using phone technology, remote tracking of vital signs to check patients health, progress, medication, or other health related data from patients. In addition to communicating health-related information remotely, other areas in which remote information is shared may be in vocational rehabilitation. Another rapidly growing industry is wireless technology, portable technology, digital video, Bluetooth, and devices that can record a variety of vital sign data from people. The availability of this technology has opened the door for telerehabilitation.

Telerehabilitation is often viewed in context with telehealth. Telehealth is an area that has been successfully "practiced" for quite some time (e.g., Chapter 25). One of the reasons that telehealth has become successful is the fact that it has become a mainstream service delivery model. Additionally, telehealth meets specific requirements related to quality of health care and access, acceptability, and cost effectiveness. In a way, telehealth has set the stage for remote rehabilitation service delivery and has provided a means of interacting in a client-centered manner, promoting client autonomy through education and improved communications.

Telerehabilitation is a tool specifically developed for the remote or distance provision or participation in rehabilitation services. Examples include elders or people with disabilities who require rehabilitation services after being discharged from the hospital, people who require follow-up visits to assess progress or meet other rehabilitation needs. Some individuals require instruction from OTs or PTs on the use of assistive technology. Others require a complete assessment of their homes to check the need for modification to ensure accessibility and enable independent living of an individual with a chronic illness or having a disability.

Common practice currently dictates that clinicians as well as individuals with disabilities need to travel regularly to receive or provide the aforementioned rehabilitation services. Because rehabilitation services tend to be based primarily in metropolitan areas, many rural areas are underserved, requiring patients and expert clinicians to travel many miles to remote areas, increasing time and associated costs of rehabilitation professionals providing services in rural areas. Remote rehabilitation (telerehabilitation) between expert rehabilitation professionals and clients offers increased access to specialized services while reducing time and money [1–4]. Because telerehabilitation is still a fairly new method, it is still unclear if telerehabilitation is an optimal solution for the common rehabilitation services that are received by patients to date. This chapter explores these areas of telerehabilitation that may present usability and access issues related to the use of telerehabilitation technologies and services.

Remote rehabilitation service delivery is suggested to increase the efficiency of the rehabilitation professional's time allocated to clients, for several reasons. First, rehabilitation professionals spend much of their time traveling to and from rural areas to visit clients who are unable to travel. Second, when clients have a progressive disability that makes it difficult to travel, remote rehabilitation services would increase their opportunities for successful and quality rehab. Time and costs involved in traveling and accompanying clients by caregivers will decrease when rehabilitation services can be done on a remote basis. Finally, because third party payers continue to decrease therapy reimbursement, follow-up visits, AT assessment time, or other rehabilitation services, remote rehabilitation can ensure a more effective use of time and money for all parties involved. However, these assumptions can only be true if telerehabilitation services are as easy, comfortable, reliable, effective, quick, and affordable as those services that are currently provided face to face.

29.1.2 Research on Telerehabilitation

To make an effective connection between the specialist and the (remote) patient and to provide effective rehabilitation services that have the quality of a face-to-face visit, specific communication technology is necessary to match up with potential patients. Recent and future technological developments in technology that fosters easier remote communication includes improved and more widespread wireless technology, increased World Wide Web availability, the availability of mobile phones, and recorders; upgrades to personal digital assistants (PDAs) and other "smart" technologies now allow remote health data recording and monitoring, distance education, job coaching, remote wheelchair assessments, and remote accessibility assessments as well.

29.1.2.1 Outcome Studies

The following cases show how technology and remote services can be successful in meeting the needs of clinicians and patients at home:

- *Quality improvement with telerehabilitation:* At the Royal, Free and University College Medical School, London, a study showed that "virtual outreach" (remote rehabilitation) reduced the numbers of clinical tests and investigations needed for clients who were consulted remotely. An increase in the number of outpatient visits was also found, and patient satisfaction was greater after the virtual outreach consultation. Implementation of remote consultations may depend on client demand, costs, and the attitude of clinical staff. Also, changes in cost and technology used for remote rehabilitation services may improve the quality of remote consultations [5].
- *Motor skill evaluation:* The McGovern Institute for Brain Research in Massachusetts Institute of Technology, Cambridge, MA, reports on their review of virtual reality (VR) for use with rehabilitation of patients. VR technology was used for individuals with a variety of disabilities, for a variety of purposes. Clients ranged from those having had a stroke to those with acquired brain injury or Parkinson's disease and who receive orthopedic rehabilitation, balance training, and wheelchair mobility and functional activities of daily living training. One important finding includes that individuals with disabilities seem capable of learning motor skills within a VR environment. Movements learned by individuals with disabilities in a VR environment seem to transfer to equivalent real-world motor tasks in most cases [6].
- *Gait analysis:* The department of physiotherapy, University of Queensland, Australia, investigated the accuracy and reliability of Internet-based observational kinematic gait assessment

(low-bandwidth Internet-link (18 kbit/s) and a higher-speed Internet-link (128 kbps)) compared to the traditional assessment (using video recordings). The online assessment was found to be as accurate as the traditional assessment and high intra-rater and inter-rater reliability was shown in the online assessment. The researchers conclude that low-bandwidth telerehabilitation applications are possible via Internet. This means that a larger population can be reached for this type of telerehabilitation service [2].

- *Stroke Neurorehabilitation:* Telerehabilitation has also been applied to individuals who had a stroke to allow independent practice and monitoring of rehabilitation therapy [7]. A Web-based system was accessible using a variety of input devices and included tests, games, and progress charts used in therapy of stroke patients. The Web-based tool was also used to assist in movement and tracking improvements in movement ability of this population [8,9]. Another example is the UniTherapy approach in Chapter 27, which supports a range of computer interface devices for implementing game-oriented therapy and assessment protocols, and includes support for tele-encounters between home users and telepractitioners in which each uses an interface customized to the user's role and abilities.
- *Wound care:* An exploratory study was set up by the Shephard Center [1] to investigate the possibility of managing pressure ulcers via telerehabilitation. A still image video-phone was used to capture a client's wound. Pictures were sent from patient homes to the clinic for evaluation. Because no travel was involved, a weekly assessment of the patients was done on a remote basis. This weekly assessment is often difficult to arrange. Findings of the study demonstrated successful pressure ulcer management via this remote assessment [1]. In another study conducted among 54 Veterans Affairs (VA) patients with lower-limb ulcers or lower-limb amputations, the technical acceptability of information available via a customized telerehabilitation system was determined [3]. Results provide evidence for the telerehabilitation service to have the potential to present sufficient information to experienced clinicians for successful wound management.
- *Home modifications:* Teleconferencing technology as part of the telerehabilitation has great potential for home modification assessment services. A project of the Veterans Affairs Rehabilitation R&D Center in Decatur, GA, focused on the application of tele-video technology to provide remote home assessment services prior to patients being discharged from a specialty clinic in order to improve the independent functioning at home after discharge [4]. Home evaluations were done at home and remotely by two occupational therapists. Results showed that remote telerehabilitation has the potential to be used to evaluate and prescribe modifications of home environments. It can also be used to detect potential accessibility problems of home environments.
- *Memory and attention:* Kessler Medical Rehabilitation Research and Education Corporation surveyed 71 individuals with acquired brain injury to assess their interest in telerehabilitation [8]. Results show that there is interest in telerehabilitation, especially, related to services focusing on memory, attention, problem solving, and activities of daily living. What the study also concluded was that although "telerehabilitation seems to be an appropriate assessment and treatment modality for individuals with brain injury, it will only succeed if those individuals have the interest — and the access — necessary to use new and evolving technologies" [8].
- *Speech therapy:* The Speech–Language Pathology Service in the National Rehabilitation Hospital in Washington, DC found alternatives in maximizing family input in group treatment by providing treatment via telepractice technology in remote settings. Like many other rehabilitation specialists, speech–language pathologists (SLPs) are also often practicing in environments in which they have less time to manage communication impairments of their patients. Telerehabilitation approach enables SLPs to maximize and enhance functional outcomes for their patients [9].

29.1.3 Telerehabilitation Applications and Interfaces

To provide remote rehabilitation services to people with disabilities, the elderly, support groups, students, and others, there is a need for some type of medium to allow communication. By introducing telerehabilitation, a shift is made from face-to-face interaction to remote interaction. This shift is accompanied by an introduction of (one or more) of the following interface media:

- A computer or TV screen with an interactive video of the client's physical therapist, showing patients the "exercise of the day"
- A wireless device that a patient wears and that records movements, medicine intake, vital signs, or activities throughout the day
- A cell phone reminding a patient every 3 h to attend to his or her (cell phone based) "to-do list"
- A video camera with Internet connection to assist with the assessment of someone's seated posture or help assess the accessibility of a patient's home

These examples of interface media require, respectively, eyesight, cognition, hearing, and mobility. Some patients may not have one or more of these capabilities, making a certain remote service impossible or ineffective.

29.1.3.1 Telerehabilitation Services

Potential users of telerehabilitation services are people with disabilities, caregivers, and clinicians involved in telerehabilitation services. Types of disabilities can roughly be divided into the following categories:

- Sensory
- Mobility
- Cognitive

Because the function of individuals with disabilities is very much related to the environment or setting in which people reside, the user environment also needs to be defined. We can categorize potential environments for remote service delivery as follows:

- Nursing homes
- Assisted living communities
- Educational settings (school or home)
- Home settings
- Transitory residences, such as hotels
- Environments in which caregivers are present

Based on discussions held among rehabilitation professionals, the following services were brought forward as being candidates for remote service delivery:

- Health assessment to establish mental and physical limitations
- Follow-up treatment for newly injured clients
- Monitoring and guiding individuals in medical treatment
- Early intervention and follow-up to prevent health issues or secondary complications
- Assistive technology assessment, prescription, evaluation, and training
- Seating and mobility
- Augmentative communication

- Environmental access
- Computer access
- Job accommodations
- Home environment
- Activities of daily living
- Routine inspection and modifications to AT (over time)
- Counseling toward social integration, independent living, education, employment, and client and caregiver support
- Clinical training and education
- Reporting and follow-up planning

Based on information in the field of rehabilitation and from some early entrepreneurs, we know that some technologies work for some individuals and some applications. However, before we can determine if telerehabilitation services are easy, comfortable, reliable, effective, quick, and affordable for all potential user groups, we need more evidence. All potential telerehabilitation applications or telerehabilitation services need to be listed in relation with the types of client categories that would require these applications on a remote basis.

The next factor considers how telerehabilitation technology plays a role in meeting the needs of a variety of clients (and functional capabilities), their rehabilitation needs within their environmental setting.

29.1.3.2 Telerehabilitation Technology

Rapid changes are occurring in the capacity, speed, and quality of communication technologies as a result of the large demand of a fast growing market in need of these technologies. Concurrently, integration of several technologies is also ongoing (digital camera-Web access-cell phone).

The quality of new and evolving video technologies is improving over time. A good example of the current high quality of mobile phone digital images is given by a study conducted at the University of London, department of otolaryngology. This study compared the accuracy of radiological investigations when using a mobile phone digital image [10]. CT scans and x-ray images taken from and transmitted via a mobile phone were compared with examination of the same films on a conventional x-ray. All doctors made the correct diagnosis for every case examined. Such an application is a much cheaper solution compared to conventional telemedicine technology.

The potential for telerehabilitation is created by these technical developments or combinations of them. Unfortunately, rural areas are likely to be the last to benefit from improved technology needed for telerehabilitation. Additionally, because of remote locations, low-income clients and alternative type housing, problems may arise related to the implementation and installation of state-of-the-art telerehabilitation equipment. Other limitations of the current computing and communications infrastructure are cost of equipment, capacity, and availability of the communications channels. Moreover, for wireless technology to be effective and useful in rural areas, bandwidths need to be further increased, video quality needs to be improved, and data capacity needs to be increased.

The Shepherd Center in Atlanta, GA, states that the field of interactive health communication (IHC) is growing because it makes health-related information and services more accessible to people with disabilities [11]. The center also states that it is important to evaluate what the user needs are when developing interactive health communication. The center conducted a 3-year survey among individuals with brain or spinal cord injury. The results show that 73% of the respondents have access to and use computers. The results also show that 68% of the respondents have access to the Internet. The results indicate that tools such as computers and the Internet have good potential to be used for telerehabilitation services [11].

29.2 USABILITY AND ACCESS ISSUES

Telerehabilitation will alter therapists' perceived responsibility over the therapeutic and rehabilitation service. There is no immediate contact between clinician and client and, therefore, reliability of diagnoses and confidence of treatment may be influenced.

Ever-evolving technologies that potentially can be used for telerehabilitation may require training for those who will be using them. Clinicians on both ends of the "communication line" will need to be qualified using these telerehabilitation technologies and need to be knowledgeable on the limitations of certain technologies and their application with a variety of clients and their functional capabilities.

Clinical experts cannot physically feel a client, and visual images may not clearly communicate tremors of a client. Therapists and clinical experts may therefore be less confident in making decisions based on remote assessments. A study conducted by Guilfoyle et al. investigated user satisfaction between a face-to-face assessment vs. an assessment conducted using videoconferencing. The results indicate that a number of issues are related to acceptance of a remote service such as videoconferencing. These issues can be related to the videoconferencing equipment, the videoconferencing environment, and the environment in which the assessments were performed. The results also indicated that most staff preferred a face-to-face format [12].

User issues that relate to rehabilitation are primarily dependent on the type of client that is in need of rehabilitation services and the specific rehabilitation service that is provided for them. Besides that, the equipment necessary to provide the specific rehabilitation services should be accessible to both the clinicians as well as the clients who use the equipment at home.

Technology may effectively provide a specific service remotely, but end up being inaccessible to the client and, therefore, may be discarded or pose a health hazard when used without supervision. The type of technology (e.g., high-speed DSL) needed may also not be available to certain clients, yet. A cell phone reminding an aging individual with a stroke and accompanying memory loss to take her daily medication may be a great solution; however, if the house of the client is located in an area without reliable cell phone reception, the technology is not effective at all times and may therefore be unsafe and unreliable. Further development within existing and new technologies is needed to ensure technology access for a larger percentage of potential users of telerehabilitation.

Besides the technology itself, the devices necessary to support certain types of technology, too, should be made accessible to people in their home. Potential users of telerehabilitation are elderly or individuals with sensory, mobility, or cognitive limitations. Equipment needs the capability to be adjustable to meet personal client needs before that equipment can be used independently at the clients' home. Enlarged buttons, speech recognition, easy-use clues, or adjustments in dimensions are examples to make devices more accessible for the potential users with certain limitations.

Medical products that assist with telerehabilitation services initially require the usage of both a clinician and the client at home. In these situations, the user interface should not only support medically trained users, but it should also be clear to individuals at home how to use that specific device independently and enable telerehabilitation to become a successful service. People who are not technology savvy are often uncertain about using complex technology or devices that were not part of their lives before their introduction. Personal computers, wireless data loggers, and other special equipment that may be used in telerehabilitation may have an associated acceptance barrier and may therefore be more difficult to apply for use with the aging population.

Accessibility of medical and other products or technology used in telerehabilitation plays an important role when dealing with personal acceptance barriers. Lack of experience with more complex new technologies can sustain an acceptance barrier resulting in rejection of the device or technology. The usability and, in some cases, accessibility of technology can be improved by reducing its complexity:

- Reduce the number of device functions or controls
- Less necessary handlings to use device or simple construction
- Hide controls that users at home do not need or use

For instance, a cell phone especially developed for elderly populations only has five buttons with only one function for each button, which makes this device more usable. Whether it is more accessible is an interesting area for research, as reducing complexity may imply fewer features which may imply lack of access for persons who might be able to use the interface if it has those features (see also discussions in Chapter 9, Chapter 15, and Chapter 25).

In designing technology that people at home can use independently, it is important to acknowledge the cognitive limitations of key populations of users who could benefit from the service, learn from it, and redesign interface technologies to provide more effective telerehabilitation services.

Besides age, other factors that play a role in usability and access to telerehabilitation are related to the variety of disabilities and associated functional, cognitive, and sensory capabilities. Some examples include:

- Increasingly complex technology (e.g., taking sharp images with a digital camera and downloading, e-mailing, and communicating them through a computer) involves cognitive skills of sequencing and new procedural memory.
- People with cognitive limitations may experience difficulty when the complexity of technology used increases.
- People with sensory impairments may be at a disadvantage because remote communication may exacerbate already-existing communication limitations (e.g., an individual with a hearing impairment who normally gets speech therapy face to face may experience greater difficulty in communication using speech broadcasted over the Web, or through a phone; individuals with visual limitations may find it more difficult to access or to obtain modified written materials remotely than when face to face).
- People with limited use of their upper extremities may experience difficulty using input devices needed for rehabilitation (e.g., use of joystick).

A review done by the CAIP Center at Rutgers University [13] discussed the advantages and disadvantages of rehabilitation applications of VR. Remote rehabilitation showed significant advantages for individuals with conditions such as post-stroke and musculoskeletal conditions. Patient motivation, online remote data access, and reduced medical costs were some of these advantages. Challenges for the use of VR in rehabilitation were related to the lack of a supportive infrastructure, lack of computer skills of therapists, relatively expensive equipment, inadequate communication infrastructure in rural areas, and patient safety concerns [13].

29.2.1 Other Issues

Telerehabilitation has merit to facilitate improved access to rehabilitation services for individuals who live in remote areas or outside metropolitan areas, resulting in fewer trips to clinics by both patients and clinical personnel. Where once there was a lack of clinical expertise, with the help of a remote connection, specialists can be brought to special cases at a short notice, resulting in financial benefits. Various organizations have demonstrated the cost effectiveness of telerehabilitation in rural areas. However, not much research data can be found related to acceptability, access, and quality of care of telerehabilitation services [14, 15]. Also, according to a study done by Palsbo and Bauer, many patients have not been reimbursed for telerehabilitation services because of the lack of large-scale controlled trials proving clinical and cost effectiveness in telerehabilitation and telemedicine [16]. Besides these issues, there are several other questions that need answered:

- Is information obtained from a remote assessment reliable enough for clinicians to safely prescribe assistive technology to patients?
- How restrictive is an in-state license on the potential of telerehabilitation?
- How can personal health information such as medical history and medication use be transmitted or remotely communicated reliably and confidentially?

- What are the barriers for clinicians and patients of product use of telerehabilitation technologies?
- What types of rehabilitation services and patients benefit from remote service delivery vs. a face-to-face service?
- Are all types of rehabilitation services that are provided remotely equally useful and cost effective?

The Rehabilitation Engineering Rehabilitation Center (RERC) on Telerehabilitation is planning to tackle some of these questions by developing a structural model that incorporates user needs, technology capabilities, outcome data, and an associated research database.

29.3 NEED FOR STRUCTURE: AIMS OF THE RERC ON TELEREHABILITATION

The first RERC on Telerehabilitation was initiated in 1997 by the National Institute on Disability and Rehabilitation Research (NIDRR) of the U.S. Department of Education at the Catholic University and the National Rehabilitation Hospital. In 2004, NIDRR awarded a second RERC on Telerehabilitation to the University of Pittsburgh to build upon the past research and to focus on the following identified research topics:

- Telerehabilitation infrastructure and architecture
- Clinical assessment modeling
- Teleassessment for promoting communication in children with disabilities
- Remote wheeled mobility assessment
- Behavioral monitoring and job coaching in vocational rehabilitation
- Remote accessibility assessment of the built environment

With a focus on these research and development areas, the RERC at Pittsburgh hopes to effectively serve all people with disabilities through the development of methods, systems, and technologies that support remote delivery of rehabilitation and home health care services for individuals who have currently limited local access to medical rehabilitation outpatient and community-based services.

Although research and literature have become available describing the benefits and potential applications of telerehabilitation, there is not yet a widespread used model that describes the boundaries of telerehabilitation. Additionally, there does not seem to be a standard "best practice" for clinicians to successfully use telerehabilitation in its various applications. Finally, a model of telerehabilitation is needed that includes the various types of technologies used for telerehabilitation, the various client populations, and their need for rehabilitation services. Having no framework that incorporates these factors seems to be the main cause for the existing usability and access issues in telerehabilitation.

To make telerehabilitation successful and useful for all individuals with disabilities and all rehabilitation professionals, an overarching structure needs to be in place that defines the boundaries of telerehabilitation. Information and resources need to be available to rehabilitation professionals, patients, and caregivers. Moreover, nationwide policies need to be put in place describing the requirements and responsibilities of rehabilitation professionals when providing telerehabilitation services in- or outside the state in which they are licensed.

It is also of great importance to have a framework in place that shows potential telerehabilitation services, related telerehabilitation technologies, and potential target client populations. Because technology is always changing, this framework needs to be constantly updated. To make this framework reliable, it needs to be based on outcome-based research in the area of telerehabilitation and supported by best practices of acknowledged rehabilitation professionals.

Future research and development activities will focus on a model that can function as a resource for clinicians and other stakeholders. Such a model can educate and assist clinicians in matching consumer needs with the variety of technologies based on "best practice methods." Additionally, it should be based on current literature and outcome studies that are or have been conducted in the field.

In order for telerehabilitation to become an accepted part of the rehabilitation, a conceptual model that is scientifically based on theory and empirical findings should be developed that verifies the improved outcomes of telerehabilitation.

Winters and Winters [17] recently developed a conceptual framework which is derived from three areas interfacing with each other: rehabilitative bio-systems, human-technology interfaces, and behavioral compliance. They state that "telecommunications technologies are reviewed from the perspective of systems models of the telerehabilitation process, with a focus on human-technology interface design and a special emphasis on emerging home and mobile technologies." A proposed framework within telerehabilitation can help to analyze, understand, and optimize important components of the telerehabilitative process [17].

Previous research done by Winters and Winters [17] will guide the development of a best practice model to be developed at the University of Pittsburgh's RERC. The model will provide clinicians and rehabilitation professionals with a framework to fit telerehabilitation technology to people with disabilities who are in need of rehabilitation services. The result, an online tool, will be a resource to rehabilitation professionals; Figure 29.1 outlines a framework. Besides being an educational tool on telerehabilitation, the tool will provide a framework of best practices designed to assist clinicians in making quality decisions when providing a variety of rehabilitation services. The tool will guide clinicians to structurally evaluate a variety of individuals with disabilities and provide them with services using suitable telerehabilitation technology. Additionally, it will function as an infrastructure to collect data that will shape health care policy on the use of telerehabilitation across multiple environments, purposes, and disability types.

By integrating user and client needs early on into the delivery of remote rehabilitation services, usability and accessibility of rehabilitation services will result for all clients, and the consistency and quality of telerehabilitation services will be improved.

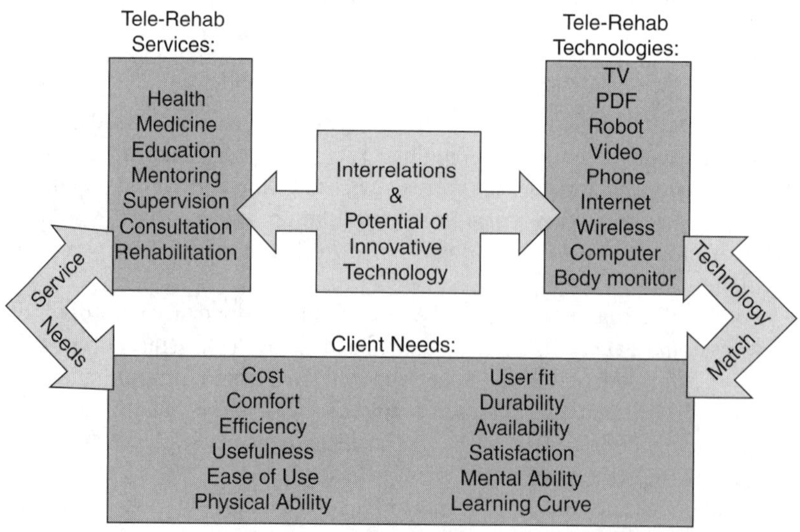

FIGURE 29.1 Telerehabilitation model including services, technologies, and end users.

29.4 DISCUSSION

Therapists who provide rehabilitation services at outpatient clinics can benefit from telerehabilitation, as can people with a variety of disabilities. Although telerehabilitation may often require some type of technical expertise and will likely decrease face-to-face contact with the clinician, benefits in the form of remote service availability and reduced cost look promising. However, additional research is needed to show how usability and access issues can be minimized and the benefits maximized. In addition, research efforts need to quantify how reliability, performance, availability, and cost of the technologies that support telerehabilitation can be optimized.

Additionally, a decrease in face-to-face contact may make more time available for clinicians to spend with their clients. A telerehabilitation consult is less time consuming than a face-to-face consult. Clients can benefit from more frequent service and can feel more confident that they receive quality treatment. However, if the time that becomes available by providing remote services is not used for the client, it may result in less contact and increased isolation of clients as well as an increased uncertainty of the patient's condition.

More research is needed to address these usability and access issues for medical devices used in telerehabilitation as well as for technology used for communication and data transfer related to telerehabilitation. Furthermore, technology is constantly changing, and each change of technology will likely result in new access and usability issues. It is therefore important that therapists who practice telerehabilitation have ongoing training or technical staff available to provide assistance on technology needed for telerehabilitation services. With improvement of technology, it will likely become more cost effective, and its availability and quality will improve.

REFERENCES

1. Vesmarovich, S., Walker, T. et al., Use of telerehabilitation to manage pressure ulcers in persons with spinal cord injuries, *Adv Wound Care*, 12(5), 264, 1999.
2. Russell, T.G., Jull, G.A. et al., The diagnostic reliability of Internet-based observational kinematic gait analysis, *Telemed Telecare,* 9(Suppl. 2), S48, 2003.
3. Rintala, D.H., Krouskop, T.A. et al., Telerehabilitation for veterans with a lower-limb amputation or ulcer: Technical acceptability of data, *Rehabil Res Dev*, 41(3B), 481, 2004.
4. Sanford, J.A., Jones, M. et al., Using telerehabilitation to identify home modification needs, *Assistive Technol*, 16(1), 43, 2004.
5. Wallace, P., Barber, J. et al., Virtual outreach: a randomised controlled trial and economic evaluation of joint teleconferenced medical consultations, *Health Technol Assess*, 8(50), 1, 2004.
6. Holden, M. K., Virtual environments for motor rehabilitation: review, *Cyberpsychol Behav*, 8(3), 187, 2005.
7. Reinkensmeyer, D.J., Pang, C.T. et al., Web-based telerehabilitation for the upper extremity after stroke, *IEEE Trans Neural Syst Rehabil Eng*, 10(2), 102, 2002.
8. Ricker, J.H., Rosenthal, M. et al., Telerehabilitation needs: a survey of persons with acquired brain injury, *J Head Trauma Rehabil*, 17(3), 242, 2002.
9. Baron, C., Hatfield, B. et al., Management of communication disorders using family member input, group treatment, and telerehabilitation, *Top Stroke Rehabil*, 12(2), 49, 2005.
10. Eze, N., Lo, S. et al., The use of camera mobile phone to assess emergency ENT radiological investigations, *Clin Otolaryngol*, 30(3), 230, 2005.
11. Hauber, R.P., Vesmarovich, S. et al., The use of computers and the Internet as a source of health information for people with disabilities, *Rehabil Nurs*, 27(4), 142, 2002.
12. Guilfoyle, C., Wootton, R. et al., User satisfaction with allied health services delivered to residential facilities via videoconferencing, *Telemed Telecare*, 9(Suppl. 1), S52, 2003.
13. Burdea, G.C., Virtual rehabilitation — benefits and challenges, *Methods Inf Med*, 42(5), 519, 2003.
14. Burk, J., Bates, J.F., Demuth, B., and Muncert, E., "Mobile telerehabilitation evaluation: increased access to telerehabilitative services in rural area," American Telemedicine Association, Tampa, FL, 2004.

15. Palmer, K. and Love, G., "Telespeech language pathology: Increasing access to quality care and education," American Telemedicine Association, Tampa, FL, 2004.
16. Palsbo, S.E. and Bauer, D., Telerehabilitation: managed care's new opportunity, *Managed Care*, 8(4), 56, 2000.
17. Winters, J.M. and Winters, J.M., A telehomecare model for optimizing rehabilitation outcomes, *J Telemed E Health*, 10(2), 200, 2004.

30 Applications and Issues with Wireless Technology in Medical Care

John W. Peifer and Michael L. Jones

CONTENTS

ABSTRACT

Wireless technologies are already in use or are rapidly being deployed in medical care for emergency communication, remote health monitoring, medication management, inventory control, data entry at the point of care, and immediate access to electronic medical records from anywhere. Although the potential benefits are great, wireless technology also introduces new concerns about security, privacy, and interference that must be addressed. In the future, wireless technologies can be expected to play a larger role in managing medical information and to enable context-aware applications that simplify user access to care.

30.1 INTRODUCTION

Wireless networks are already widely used in medical facilities for clinical documentation, nurse call systems, and remote monitoring with medical telemetry. Emerging wireless technologies make it possible to continuously monitor and communicate with patients anywhere in the hospital, at home, or throughout the community. This anytime-and-anywhere connectivity could change health management and allow greater mobility and independence in populations with fragile medical conditions. Wireless technologies can also be used to track usage of medication and therapeutic instrumentation used in patient care. Wireless sensors and location-tracking technologies are also enabling smarter applications that can exploit situational context to simplify the user interface for medical instrumentation and add another layer of safety verification for prevention of medication errors. Although the potential benefits are great, wireless technology also introduces concerns about security, privacy, and interference. Current and future applications of wireless technology in health care will be discussed as well as the potential problems and risks.

Information technology has been implemented more slowly in medicine than in other industries, but this is now changing. Mobile wireless technology may be helping to accelerate this trend. Delivering medical services is a complicated process of diagnosis, treatment, and care management that occurs in multiple venues over extended periods of time. There are extensive documentation — storage and retrieval — requirements that challenge the most advanced information systems today. However, massive low-cost digital storage, high-performance computers, and extensive networking resources are finally enabling implementation of the elusive electronic medical record that links patient history, physician assessments, lab studies, medical images, and data. Wireless technologies complement this emerging electronic record with untethered data entry at the point of care, continuous patient monitoring everywhere, and immediate remote medical assessment.

This chapter begins with an overview of wireless issues in medicine, then presents some practical issues of clinical implementation, and concludes with a discussion of emerging trends and future potential for smarter and simpler interfaces to medical instrumentation that may be enabled by mobile wireless technology.

30.2 WIRELESS OVERVIEW

Voice, text, and e-mail communications over wireless networks are becoming a regular part of medical care. Notification pagers to contact health care providers on call are being replaced by cell phones that provide more immediate access. Emerging wireless network connections introduce the potential for access to integrated electronic medical records from any place at any time. Context-aware applications — incorporating sensors to monitor environmental and biomedical status — introduce the possibility of smarter and simpler interfaces that anticipate needs and efficiently present the most important and relevant clinical decision-making information. How did the technology evolve? What is currently possible, and where are things likely to be headed? In this section, a brief overview of wireless technology is provided.

30.2.1 Progression of Wireless History

The explosive growth of wireless technology has shifted the world of communications and computing from the desktop to the pocket. By mid-2005, there were over 194 million wireless subscribers in the U.S. (Cellular Telecommunications and Internet Association estimates) and more than 1.4 billion wireless subscribers worldwide (International Telecommunication Union estimates). These cell phones are mobile computing platforms that are capable of running information management and entertainment applications previously reserved for personal, mid level, or mainframe computers. This sea change to mobile computing power will significantly impact work flow in many industries, including health care. There are more cell phones (mobile computing platforms) now being sold than desktop computers and televisions combined. Some history of how this occurred may help our understanding of where this trend may be headed.

30.2.1.1 Wireless from Marconi's Days in Late 19th Century

Today's popular cell phone and wireless Internet technologies were born over one hundred years ago, with the early research by Guglielmo Marconi and others exploring ways to transmit and receive radio signals [1]. This led to tremendous advances in ship-to-shore communications in which wireless telegraphy could be used to send important messages from far away. In the early 1900s, methods were developed to encode audio in this new wireless communication medium, and radio broadcasting became a commercial success by the early 1920s. Radio communications slowly began to be used in motor vehicles by police and emergency dispatchers as size and cost decreased. In the 1940s and 1950s, mobile phone systems were under development, and the FCC began plans for allocating bands of radio frequency spectrum for mobile phones long before the current demand emerged. All of these early phones were based upon analog technology, and the rapid acceleration of consumer adoption has followed closely with the advances of digital computing and digital signal processing.

30.2.1.2 Generations of Cell Phone Advances

The progression of cell phone technology is often described in terms of generations. The first generation cell phones (1G) began with analog technology in the 1960s and then exploded during the 1980s as cost and handset size decreased. During the 1990s, second generation (2G) cell phones emerged with digital technology that enabled better security, more efficient network management, and new data applications. Today we are at the leading edge of implementing third generation (3G) cell phone technology enabling higher speed data communications, multimedia messaging, and mobile computing applications.

30.2.1.3 Wireless Networking

Competing with cell phone networks are wireless data networks. Low-speed wireless data networks have been around for many years for pagers and, in recent years, the Blackberry two-way pager has become a popular choice for independent mobile communication. For high-speed wireless Internet access, Wi-Fi (Wireless Fidelity) technology based on IEEE standard 802.11 has spread rapidly into homes, businesses, campuses, and community facilities because it provides high-speed network access (originally up to 11 Mbps for IEEE 802.11b, now with IEEE 802.11g, up to 54 Mbps) for very low cost [2]. This technology is also attractive because it operates in one of the frequency bands (2.4 GHz) that is intended for industrial, scientific, and medical (ISM) applications and can be used without paying a license fee [3]. The main limitations are that Wi-Fi networks usually cover at most a few hundred feet, and there are security and bandwidth concerns when sharing public networks. Bluetooth technology provides short-range (up to 10 m) connections between devices, enabling unattached keyboards and wireless headsets for cell phones [4]. Similar to 802.11, Bluetooth operates in the license-free frequency band of 2.4 GHz. Although its operating range and data rates (up to 1 Mbps) are lower than 802.11, Bluetooth is attractive for its low power consumption and low implementation cost.

30.3 EMERGING TRENDS

30.3.1 Wireless Networking Technologies

In addition to widely available Wi-Fi, Bluetooth, and cellular wireless data networks, there are new emerging wide area networking technologies to bring broadband services to the home; and low-cost and low-power indoor wireless networking approaches to link appliances and sensors in homes and offices. Because there will be competing wireless networks for the foreseeable future, mobile wireless devices will support capabilities for transmitting and receiving different frequency signals, and sophisticated software radio algorithms will detect and tune to the optimal communication mode for the best currently available wireless network. Two of the more rapidly emerging networking technologies are WiMAX and ZigBee.

30.3.1.1 Wide Area Broadband Wireless

An emerging WiMAX wireless technology may solve the range and bandwidth limitations of Wi-Fi. WiMAX (short for Worldwide Interoperability for Microwave Access), based upon the IEEE 802.16 standard, is designed to provide broadband (potentially up to 134 Mbps) connectivity for long ranges (potentially up to 50 km) [5]. With the wide area broadband networking that WiMAX is designed to support, this technology may provide a wireless solution to the last mile connection problem that has required expensive and time-consuming wired installations to establish high-speed Internet access.

30.3.1.2 Low- Cost, Low- Power Wireless ZigBee

ZigBee technology offers a new wireless protocol for creating very low-cost and low-power data communications that do not require high bandwidth [6,7]. Home-monitoring and sensor-networks-linking security system, smoke alarms, and environmental control systems have been listed as potential applications for ZigBee. The advantages for health care would be that ZigBee networks can efficiently bring more sensor data to caregivers for health management and decision making.

30.3.2 Wireless Applications and Sensors

There are a variety of emerging wireless applications and sensor technologies that will support more effective communication and monitoring in medical management. If applied successfully, these technologies may produce great improvement in early detection of serious health risks. However, the transition from traditional communication technologies may create temporary problems as new network infrastructure may at first be less reliable and not universally available.

30.3.2.1 Data Networks May Accelerate Voice over Internet Protocol (VoIP)

Broadband wireless networks introduce the capability of transitioning to Voice over Internet Protocol (VoIP) services for mobile wireless voice communication. Wireless VoIP technology may facilitate integrated voice and videoconferencing for remote health assessment, but security and reliability issues must first be addressed. VoIP exemplifies the uncertain and very different directions that the communications industry could move in the next decade. Today, voice communication is still overwhelmingly provided by the telecommunications industry as voice services. Until recently, voice communications had been the primary revenue generator for the telecom industry [8]. However, data applications from e-mail, messaging, and Internet traffic are rapidly growing and generating greater demand for broadband services. If broadband wireless services can be delivered everywhere (or to enough profitable population centers), voice communications may change over to VoIP. As customers shift away from traditional voice services, the industry could face a tipping point at which it becomes more cost-effective to drop traditional voice services and move exclusively to VoIP. This may pose no problems for urban centers that will be fully covered by wired and wireless broadband services, but this could present a major problem for many rural sections of the country where broadband services have been slow and expensive to deploy.

30.3.2.2 Universal Remote Console: Alternative Wireless Interface

Another important opportunity to improve usability of medical instrumentation is through alternative wireless interface controls. Electronic products will increasingly support alternative command and control options (as additional or alternative interfaces). This is already occurring with remote control options for entertainment systems and increasingly through Bluetooth access to mobile cameras, printers, PDAs, and cell phones.

As described in Chapter 26, Chapter 27, and Chapter 28, a powerful and exciting new standard is being developed for a wireless universal remote console (URC) by the V2 subcommittee of the International Committee for Information Technology Standards (INCITS; see a V2 URC standards white paper at http://www. myurc.com/). The basic idea is that everyone will carry their own personal controller that can control any V2-compliant device. V2-compliant products will use wireless technology to automatically make their controllable functions available on the personal controller. It would be as if the TV remote control could automatically program itself to work with any new component added to the entertainment system.

Manufacturers of consumer electronic products are excited about V2 as an intelligent one-device universal remote control solution, but the standard offers additional value for people with disabilities, because it will allow them to use an alternate interface for any off-the-shelf product that adheres to the V2 standard. The key is that consumers will purchase a personal controller that is most comfortable to them. A personal controller with audio output may be preferred by someone who is visually impaired; graphical output may be preferred by someone who is deaf; and a controller with larger buttons for input may be preferred by people with limited dexterity. Whereas there will be many types and sizes of V2 personal controllers, they will all be able to interact with and control any off-the-shelf V2-compliant consumer product. This will be a tremendous advantage for people with disabilities, because it will reduce or eliminate the need to buy special-purpose assistive technology products that cost more, support fewer features, and become outdated more quickly than mainstream products. In health care, the V2 standard has great potential to support an accessible interface to medical instrumentation in the hospital, at the doctor's office, in home medical care, or for mobile health management.

30.3.2.3 Radio Frequency Identification

Radio frequency identification (RFID) is another promising technology that holds great potential for improving information management in health care. This technology is already changing the way that businesses track products and equipment. RFID tags emit a wireless signal that can be read (by a special RFID reading device) without making a physical or visual contact with the tag [9]. Some are very small, low-cost (less than 25 cents), and require no power. These are being integrated into inventory control systems by retailers and drug manufacturers for product tracking that is more accurate and efficient than bar coding.

In health care, RFID tags are being considered for inventory control, medication management, personal identification, and context-aware information systems. The full potential is just beginning to emerge. For medication management, pill containers and drug packaging are already being marked with RFID tags for inventory control, safety oversight, and controlled substance protections. This aspect of the medication management will lead to more efficient distribution of medications and will serve as a layer of protection against the growing threat of counterfeit drugs. On the consumer side, RFID technology can also improve compliance, safety, and interface simplicity. With tagged containers, it becomes possible for a smart reader to track when medications are moved. Smith describes new research that combines multiple RFID tags with mercury switches to create battery-free sensors that detect object motion [10]. Tracking which pill container has been moved and when offers a higher level of compliance monitoring. It also adds a layer of safety by indicating when the wrong medication may have been taken.

Further interface simplifications can be supported for usability. Small print on container labels and complicated medication insert materials could be replaced with individualized instructions. For example, a simple "help" button on the medicine cabinet with an RFID reader/computer built into the cabinet could initiate a voice describing the medication, what it is supposed to be doing, the dose, and most common side effects. Several groups, including the Aware Home at Georgia Tech and the RERC on Technology for Successful Aging at the University of Florida, are exploring RFID applications for this type of personal medication management. An FDA task force is promoting the use of RFID tags to track medication packing in an effort to reduce counterfeiting. Following the FDA's guidance, a variety of companies have implemented RFID tagging in selected drugs that are more likely to be abused (such as pain medication OxyContin) or counterfeited (such as Viagra or several HIV drugs) [11].

In clinical care scenarios, RFID technology could add context to simplify information management. Smith [10] explores two approaches for tracking human activity to add context: one in which the human wears an RFID reader and a second in which RFID readers are added to the environment. RFID readers have size, cost, and range limitations. However, manufacturers and retailers are pushing for this to become a standard inventory tool, so this is likely to become affordable and widely available in the future.

30.3.2.4 Motes

Tiny, battery-powered sensors called *motes* have been developed in research collaboration between Intel Research and the University of California–Berkeley [12,13]. Researchers are using motes to explore the value of monitoring and distributing information about the environment that would have previously been impractical. Lubrin et al. (2005), explore the use of remote health care monitoring with motes to help people who are aging live independently [14]. Mote technology introduces the potential of distributing tiny, inexpensive sensors that could automatically collect data on patients at home and in the hospital.

30.3.2.5 Internal and Implantable Sensors

Medical diagnostic procedures are often difficult for the patient, as well as for the care provider, because the patient must be connected to a machine, transferred to a table, or even placed inside of a scanning device. New internal and implantable sensors with wireless communication capabilities are emerging that may eliminate some of the accessibility problems by monitoring the patient from within. For example, Eggers describes implantable pressure measurement (ITPM) [15] devices that may lead to significant improvements in care by monitoring: intracranial pressure (effectiveness of shunt treatment for hydrocephalus), intraocular pressure (risks to optic nerve in glaucoma patients), and aortic aneurysm pressure (measure success of stent-graft placement).

Najafi et al. at Washington University has already demonstrated successful results (in animal studies) using miniature wireless implanted sensors to monitor pressure in the heart associated with congestive heart failure (CHF) [16]. CHF is a major health problem in the U.S. that is likely to increase with the aging population, and current monitoring is risky, expensive, and therefore only performed infrequently. Continuous pressure monitoring with implantable wireless sensors will allow physicians to more appropriately adjust medications to the patient's individual needs and reduce risks of side effects from too much or too little medication.

Wireless capsule endoscopy is a miniature telemetry system that transmits images to an external receiver as it passes through the gastrointestinal (GI) tract. It has become a preferred tool for evaluating GI bleeding in the small intestine, which cannot be fully examined by other methods [17]. Using this technology, the patient being monitored continues normal daily activities as imagery from inside is wirelessly transmitted to a small, wearable recording device. The monitoring period extends over a period of up to 8 hours, until the capsule is naturally excreted.

Webber, Loeb, and colleagues describe research in which implantable BIONs (bionic neurons) are used in an untethered wearable system to stimulate paralyzed muscles in correcting foot drop [18]. The BION is a small (diameter: 4.4 mm; length: approximately 16 mm), injectable, radiofrequency-powered, single-channel, and implantable microstimulator developed by the Alfred Mann Foundation. Implanted near a nerve or into a muscle, BIONs are being explored for use in humans to facilitate and control arm and hand movement after stroke or spinal cord injury. Webber's research found that implantable BIONs could become an effective alternative to wired surface stimulation.

30.3.3 Wireless Medical Information Systems

30.3.3.1 Wireless Alerts: Call for Help, Notify Care Providers

About one out of every seven people with disabilities requires another person's assistance. Typically, a family member fills this care provider role [19]. Alternatively, individuals receive necessary care in assistive living or institutional settings. The family frequently shoulders the burden of cost, provision of care, or both. Today, the potential exists to use available technologies so that individuals who require assistance and wish to maintain personal independence and autonomy can do so safely within their own living setting; home-based technologies can reduce costs [20]. Remote-monitoring and home automation technologies can decrease the amount of direct provider assistance needed by an individual, while at the same time maintaining safety and independence [21–24].

Remote-monitoring systems for medical emergencies already exist. Most such systems consist of a transmitter worn by the individual, a communicator connected to a telephone line or modem, and a professional monitoring center attendant. With the advancement of technology, the potential for do-it-yourself home automation, remote monitoring, and alert services is growing [22]. There are over 700 listings in the Home Automation Directory Web site including home automation devices, X-10, audio/video, security, networking, and other technologies [25]. Professional assistance (or a technical background) is usually required to design, install, network, and program user-specific applications. But this is rapidly changing as several companies are moving to networked applications that are easily installed by the do-it-yourselfer. Commercially available sensor technologies can be used for remote monitoring of activity, function, or physiological status. Remote control of various environmental systems or devices in the living setting will also be possible. These capabilities will permit minimally obtrusive monitoring of an individual to ensure safety and well-being and the ability to provide assistance to the individual through remote environmental control, local intelligent agents, or timely response to a request.

There are many potential users and applications of an easy-to-use remote-monitoring and environmental control tool kit. The parents of a young adult with cognitive impairment who is moving into his own apartment may want to be available to provide remote support as needed; an assistive technology specialist may want to configure an environmental control unit for a client with a high-level spinal cord injury. She travels to the client's home to set up the system but wants to be able to provide remote programming and support if needed.

A remote-monitoring application would permit the detection and documentation of specific events or the absence of events in the living environment. Events may include motion (or lack thereof) of occupants in the environment, activation of (or failure to de-activate) electrical devices (e.g., leaving on a stove), and manipulation of environmental features (e.g., opening/closing a door or cabinet). Various sensor devices, such as motion sensors, event recorders, and simple switches, usually wireless, could be integrated into the application. Sensor data could be transmitted via the Internet and an algorithm used to establish criteria for data processing and for triggering responses to specific events.

For example, a wireless motion sensor may be installed in the bedroom of the occupant (e.g., an aging woman) and the system programmed to trigger an alert if no movement is detected between 7:00 and 8:00 a.m., the woman's normal waking hours. At 8:00 a.m. a text message is sent to her son's two-way pager informing him that his mother has not been active. The son calls and awakens his mother. If there is no response, he phones her neighbor asking that she check on her. As another example, a switch is installed on the door of a kitchen cabinet, where medications are stored, to detect and log door opening; the system is programmed to activate a recorded message 30 min after scheduled administration time reminding the occupant to take medications.

Widespread adoption of V2 URC standard would dramatically change the landscape for remote monitoring and environmental control and would significantly enhance usability, acceptance, and implementation of these applications. For instance, common environmental appliances would become targets for URCs that through telecommunications are available for receiving and sending information using varying access systems, enabling users with differing abilities to use preferred modes of communication. Notice the clear ties to integrated universal access applications (see Chapter 25), possible personalized access to Web services (see Chapter 26 and Chapter 27), medical monitoring applications (see Chapter 28), and telerehabilitation (see Chapter 29).

30.3.3.2 Wireless Assistance for Cognitive Impairment

Wireless technology may prove useful for helping people with cognitive impairment more effectively participate in their own health management. Memory aids, reminders, and simplified information storage and retrieval could improve compliance with prescribed medication, exercise, and therapy. Szymkowiak et al. describe an approach to assist in memory that uses wireless communication; however, they describe the problems for memory-impaired persons in learning to use complicated mobile computing devices [26]. They conclude that the technology has great potential if the interface issues can be resolved.

For this population of users, context-aware applications may offer some solutions in applications that are smart enough to understand the user needs, abilities, and preferences and combine that information with time, location, and current environmental conditions to anticipate the most appropriate data and format in which to present reminders. For example, the context-aware mobile wireless application may recognize that medications, therapy, or exercise were missed.

30.3.3.3 Wireless Integration of Electronic Medical Record

As electronic medical records are being incorporated into clinical practice, wireless technologies are enabling even more efficient access to medical information. Mobile wireless workstations permit staff to document clinical information at any location, including the bedside, the exam room, the operating room, and the treatment gym. A wireless portal pointing to a clinical data repository can bring diagnostic images, lab results, and patient history to the provider wherever they are — in hospital or off site. In fact, this ubiquitous access is one of the key selling points of the electronic medical record to physicians, who are usually reluctant adopters of information technology because they perceive that it requires more effort on their part (they have to retrieve information themselves rather than have an assistant hand it to them).

In line with user buy-in, the biggest challenges to building and implementing medical information systems are not technological but, instead, have to do with the difficulty of tailoring data entry and retrieval to workflow processes in the clinical setting. In many cases, clinicians are required to change their work processes to accommodate the limitations of data entry and retrieval, or clinical documentation systems are built to emulate poorly designed workflow processes.

30.3.4 Wireless Concerns

30.3.4.1 Security and Privacy

Mobile wireless technologies facilitate access to electronic medical information, but they also demand greater precautions to safeguard security and privacy. The security and privacy of electronic medical data is protected by law through the Health Insurance Portability and Accountability Act (HIPAA). Wireless networks used for health care must implement measures to comply with HIPAA, as well as to protect from exposure to liability from unauthorized or illegal network hijackers. Wireless technology exposes networks to new threats, because the boundaries are invisible and often extend beyond the physical border of the facility or campus. In addition, mobile wireless platforms for data entry or retrieval are more easily lost or stolen than desktop systems, and measures must be taken to prevent compromise of information in this event [27,28]. Marti et al. describes the importance of new specification and implementation of security for wireless body area networks (a specialization of personal area networks) as new wearable and implantable sensors are employed to monitor health in mobile applications [29].

Although new risks are introduced with wireless networks, some unique capabilities of mobile wireless technology can be applied to improve the security and privacy of electronic medical information. Security includes protecting data from being lost, and wireless communication enables medical records to be immediately transferred to secure database servers at one or more off-site locations. Wireless sensors that provide location and context awareness can add another level of security to detect and prevent unauthorized access to medical records. For example, authorization can be made dependent upon other factors than username and password, and systems can be made smarter to automatically log out and block access after a care provider is called away to an emergency.

Bardram [30] describes a smart medical information terminal built into a patient bed. The system employs position tracking of both the care providers and the patients to simplify the interface and to add security to the system. In this scenario, as a care provider enters a patient room in the hospital, wireless sensors detect and identify the authorization level of the care provider and automatically bring up the patient records that are most likely to be involved in that care provider's visit. A nurse making a routine visit to check on vital signs may be presented with a chart of the most recent trends and a screen to add an updated note of the patient status. Another nurse bringing medications would be reminded of the dosage and warned of allergies. Patient identification bracelets in many hospitals today include bar codes that are scanned before medication is administered to confirm that the correct patient is receiving the correct medication. Wireless RFID tags on these patient bracelets could be read without waking the patient to move the wrist from under the bed covers. Simplifying patient care may further reduce medication errors.

30.3.4.2 Interference with Other Devices

With the increasing number of wireless devices and overlapping wireless networks, there is a continuing concern about electronic interference that could affect the performance of medical devices or disrupt communication. Early analog cell phones were known to create interference problems with medical instrumentation, but today's digital cell phones are less likely to cause problems.

However, a growing concern is how well the information systems and sensor networks will scale as these technologies become more popular and important in medical care. Communications failures during recent natural disasters have demonstrated that wireless networks may become overloaded and unreliable when there is unusually heavy traffic. Critical care systems cannot depend upon unreliable networks, and consideration must be given to make these technologies scale properly.

As another example, there are known interference issues with multiple RFID readers operating in close proximity [9]. Today, this is rarely an issue, because RFID is new and most implementations are designed to use one reader for inventory of many tagged products. However, a variety of innovative research and development projects are underway exploring the potential for personal or portable RFID readers (for example, in every cell phone). Similar portable RFID readers could be useful for every health care provider and staff member in the hospital, and similar interference issues arise if multiple readers are trying to access the same RFID tag at the same time.

30.4 FUTURE DIRECTIONS

30.4.1 Improved Accessibility and Usability for Caregivers

Wireless access to an integrated electronic medical record system makes it possible for caregivers to provide patient care more efficiently from anywhere. The integrated information system can support many different interface preferences that improve accessibility. For example, one physician may prefer small text displays and speech input, whereas another may prefer audio output and keyboard entry. When this customizable information system can connect to diagnostic imaging systems, access patient history, order lab studies, and control medical instrumentation, health professionals with widely varying interface preferences will be enabled to enter and continue medical practice.

30.4.2 Context Awareness Simplifies Interface

Wireless technologies enable smarter mobile devices and facilitate access to information. Eliminating the need to connect to a wired network obviously creates simpler movement and access; however, wireless sensors and position-tracking technologies make it possible for context-aware applications to anticipate user needs and preferences. For example, Bardram's concept of a context-aware hospital information system [30] could greatly reduce the burden on care providers and reduce the risk of medication or treatment errors. In this conceptual scenario, wireless RFID tags are used to identify the patient, the care providers, and medication containers. They describe a combined entertainment system and clinical information portal that is part of a smart hospital bed and wireless network. As the nurse enters the room, the system automatically detects that an authorized person is now present, immediately brings the patient's medication record up on the screen, detects that it is time for medication, and that this particular caregiver has medication dispensing and documentation responsibilities. As the nurse leaves the room, the medical record application automatically logs out and returns to the patient entertainment program. Winters (Chapter 25) discusses similar scenarios.

Managing one's own care needs can also be made simpler with RFID tagging of medications, medical devices, and home care products. People with vision or cognitive impairment can be assisted with reminders of where these objects were left, and instructions can be provided in alternative formats for the individual's preferences or abilities. Smith et al. describe new battery-free sensors combining RFID tags with accelerometers that can identify objects and detect when they are moving [10]. The additional information could be used to determine, which instrument is being picked up from a tray or when a person is sitting or moving.

Zou et al. describe mobile agents employed in a wireless medical information system to assist the caregivers in decision making and patients in self management [31]. Mobile agents are programs that automatically migrate across devices and computers on the network according to established policies. They are helpful in reducing network load and in maintaining service on mobile devices that can be carried beyond the limits of the wireless network. Session initiation protocol (SIP) management is necessary for mobile agents to establish connections automatically before sending and retrieving data or applications. Zou describes a scenario for diabetes management in which a mobile agent assists a patient at home to monitor his health status and seek advice from his physician [31].

30.4.3 Internal Sensors May Eliminate Some Diagnostic Procedures

Looking farther into the future, it is possible to imagine that internal and implantable medical diagnostic sensors will begin to replace some of the current diagnostic procedures that create accessibility problems today. Sensors may obviate the need for awkward MRI scans and mammograms. Perhaps tiny implantable sensors can even eliminate the need for many of the diagnostic information that is collected from the cold, uncomfortable, generally inaccessible, and universally disliked examination table.

REFERENCES

1. Bucci, O.M., Pelosi, G., and Selleri, S., The work of Marconi in microwave communications, *IEEE Antennas and Propagation Magazine*, 45(5), 46, 2003, Digital Object Identifier 10.1109/MAP.2003.1252809.
2. Wi-Fi Alliance, http://www.wi-fi.org/.
3. International Telecommunication Union (ITU) Description of frequency bands for industrial, scientific and medical (ISM) applications, http://www.itu.int/ITU-R/terrestrial/faq/index.html#g013.
4. Bluetooth Special Interest Group (SIG), http://www.bluetooth.com/bluetooth/.
5. WiMAX Forum, http://www.wimaxforum.org/home.
6. ZigBee Alliance, http://www.zigbee.org/en/.
7. Kinney, P., ZigBee Technology: Wireless Control that Simply Works, Kinney Consulting LLC/Chair of IEEE 802.15.4 Task Group, http://www.zigbee.org/en/resources/#WhitePapers.
8. Nicopolitidis, P., Papadimitriou, G., Obaidat, M.S., and Pomportsis, A.S., The economics of wireless networks, *Communications of the ACM*, 47(4), 83, 2004.
9. Want, R., The magic of RFID, *ACM Queue,* 2(7), 40, 2004, www.acmqueue.com.
10. Smith, J.R. et al., RFID-based techniques for human activity detection, *Communication of the ACM*, 48(9), 39, 2005.
11. FDA Embraces RFID to protect drug supply, *American Journal of Health-System Pharmacy*, 61, 2612, 2004.
12. Intel Research with Berkeley on Motes, http://www.intel.com/research/exploratory/motes.htm.
13. Polastre, J., Szewczyk, R., and Culler, D., Telos: enabling ultra-low power wireless research, *Proceedings of the Fourth International Symposium on Information Processing in Sensor Networks*, 2005, p. 364–369.
14. Lubrin, E., Lawrence, E., and Navarro, K.F., Wireless remote healthcare monitoring with Motes, *Proceedings of the International Conference on Mobile Business (ICMB)*, 2005, p. 235.
15. Eggers, T. and Wenzel, M., Implantable Telemetric Pressure Measurement, *Medical Device Technology*, 2004.
16. Najafi, N. and Ludomirsky, A., Initial animal studies of a wireless batteryless MEMS implant for cardiovascular applications, *Biomedical Microdevices*, 6(1), 61, 2004.
17. Arnott, I.R. and Lo, S.K., The clinical utility of wireless capsule endoscopy, *Digestive Diseases and Sciences*, 49(6), 893, 2004.
18. Webber, D.J. et al., Functional Electrical Stimulation Using Microstimulators to Correct Foot Drop, *Canadian Journal of Physiology and Pharmacology*, 82, 784, 2004.
19. McNeil, J.M., Current Population Reports: Americans with Disabilities 1994–1995, U.S. Department of Commerce, Economics and Statistics Administration, Washington, D.C., 1997.
20. Winters, J.M., Robinson, C.L., Simpson, R.C., and Vanderheiden, G.C. (Eds.), *Emerging and Accessible Telecommunications, Information and Healthcare Technologies*, RESNA Press, Arlington, VA, 2002.
21. Mann, W.C. et al., Effectiveness of assistive technology and environmental interventions in maintaining independence and reducing home care costs for the frail elderly: a randomized controlled trial, *Archives of Family Medicine*, 8, 210, 1999.
22. Baker, S., Cahill, M., and Teeple-Low, S., Technology Assessment of the U.S. Assistive Technology Industry, U.S. Department of Commerce, Bureau of Industry and Security, Office of Strategic Industries and Economic Security, Strategic Analysis Division Washington, D.C., 2003.

23. Winters, J.M., Telerehabilitation research: emerging opportunities, *Annual Review of Biomedical Engineering*, 4, 287, 2002.
24. Winters, J.M. and Herman, W., Report on Home Care Technologies for the 21st Century, *Technical Report HCTR-10-v1.0. 96 pages,* Catholic University of America, Washington, D.C., 1–96, 1999, see also http://www.eng.mu.edu/wintersi/HCTWorkshop.
25. Home-Automation Directory© 2005, www.home-automation.org.
26. Szymkowiak, A., Morrison, K., Gregor, P., Shah, P., Evans, J.J., and Wilson, B.A., A memory aid with remote communication using distributed technology, Springer-Verlag, London, 2004, *Personal and Ubiquitous Computing,* Volume 9, Issue 1, 2005, p. 1–5.
27. Stanford, V., Pervasive health care applications face tough security challenges, *IEEE Pervasive Computing*, 8, 2002.
28. Frenzal, J.C., Data security issues arising from integration of wireless access into healthcare networks, *Journal of Medical Systems*, 27(2), 163, 2003.
29. Marti, R., Delgado, J., and Perramon, X., Security specification and implementation for mobile e-Health services, *Proceedings of the 2004 IEEE International Conference on e-Technology, e-Commerce, and e-Services*, Taipei, Taiwan.
30. Bardram, J.E., Applications of context-aware computing in hospital work — examples and design principles, 2004, *ACM Symposium on Applied Computing*, p. 1574–1579, ACM Press, New York, NY, 2004.
31. Zou, Y., Istepanian, R.S., and Bain, S.C., Policy driven mobile agents for ubiquitous medical diagnosis assistant system, *Proceedings of the IDEAS Workshop on Medical Information Systems: The Digital Hospital*, p. 3–7, IEEE Computer Society, 2004.

Part V

Outputs of the Workshop: Key Knowledge Gaps, Barriers, Recommendations

31 Report of the Workshop on Accessible Interfaces for Medical Instrumentation: Draft Guidelines and Future Directions

Jack M. Winters and Molly Follette Story

CONTENTS

ABSTRACT

This chapter contains the final report of a state-of-the-science workshop that was held over 2 days in October 2005, and serves to disseminate the results of the event. The workshop included intermittent brief plenary presentations, with the majority of the time dedicated to three breakout sessions that addressed specific questions and had targeted goals. The participants were divided into five heterogeneous theme groups that each addressed a specific aspect of accessible medical instrumentation. Each theme group generated bullet points in each of four topical areas, which are presented here. After the event, the workshop participants voted to select the most important bullet points. These results are presented and discussed in Section 31.3. At the end of the chapter, contributions of commentary from several individual workshop participants are presented.

31.1 INTRODUCTION

This chapter presents the final report of a state-of-the-science workshop organized by the Rehabilitation Engineering Research Center on Accessible Medical Instrumentation (RERC-AMI) in conjunction with the Center for Devices and Radiological Health (CRDH) of the U.S. Food and Drug Administration (FDA). It serves to disseminate the results of this event, which was held in October 2005 at the conference facility at the FDA's headquarters building in Rockville, MD, and involved 61 participants with a diversity of expertise and backgrounds. This dissemination directly responds to a requirement by the National Institute on Disability and Rehabilitation Research (NIDRR) of the U.S. Department of Education that each of its 21 RERCs sponsor such an event during the third year of a 5-year grant cycle and then disseminate the outputs of the event during the 4th year.

The aim of the RERC-AMI is to increase access to and utilization of health care instrumentation and services by individuals with disabilities, as well as access to employment in health care professions by such persons. This is the first 5-year cycle for this topic, and an interactive workshop format was selected instead of a more conventional conference because of the desire for a truly interactive exchange that could help provide guidance for this emerging field, especially in the areas of standards and guidelines development and future opportunities for integrating more accessible medical devices into society. Additionally, the unique opportunity to hold this event at the FDA reinforced the choice of format. Two other factors impacted on early planning: the decision to narrow the scope of the workshop through a focus on the human–technology interface and the desire to focus on future possibilities for guidelines and innovative interface technologies.

31.2 METHODS: ORGANIZATION AND IMPLEMENTATION OF THE WORKSHOP

Prior to the workshop, the coauthors of this chapter held a series of planning meetings, including meeting at FDA facilities in Maryland. Based on such meetings, it was decided that the majority of the time would be allocated to breakout sessions. A previous 1999 workshop that was held at the FDA facility [1], organized by Jack Winters and the FDA with support from the National Science Foundation (NSF) as well, was used as a starting base in the planning discussions.

31.2.1 Breakout Themes and Bullet Generation Process

The following five themes were identified as priority areas for the workshop:

1. Physical positioning/orienting of patient to device
2. Interfaces for monitoring devices
3. Interfaces for home health care devices
4. Interfaces for patients with disabilities
5. Interfaces for aging and disabled providers

The first three of these themes were grouped under the general title of "Guideline Development" and the latter two under the title of "Emerging Trends and Technologies."

For each of these themes, two colleagues with unique relevant expertise were recruited to cochair the theme. Two of the ten cochairs were from the RERC-AMI, and three were senior investigators with other RERCs. Other cochairs included one person from the FDA, several university faculty members with special expertise in the area of a given theme, and several highly respected human factors consultants. Each of the five themes was also allocated a staff member or student from the RERC to assist the cochairs in any way deemed helpful.

Also, in preparation for the workshop, a core group of roughly 20 experts in human factors of medical devices and in accessibility were recruited to set the stage by producing drafts of the chapters associated with this book; the RERC-AMI also contributed a number of chapters. Drafts for roughly 80% of the 30 chapters in Part 1 to Part 4 were made available through a password-protected site prior to the workshop. Also on site at the workshop were several booths that demonstrated innovative approaches for future medical device interfaces.

The workshop started with Donald Marlowe, a key organizer representing the FDA, introducing the Director of the Office for the Science and Engineering Laboratories of the FDA, Larry Kessler. Dr. Kessler welcomed the attendees and provided a presentation that helped set the stage for the content of the workshop. After Jack Winters provided an overview of the workshop, four targeted presentations were given. The first two, by William Peterson and June Isaacson Kailes, provided perspectives of professionals with long histories in the disability field who are also individuals with disabilities and who have firsthand experience with difficulties in receiving health care services. Peterson's presentation included discussion of his role in creation of the priority for the funding opportunity for the RERC-AMI; and some of the presentation by Kailes related to material presented in Chapter 1 of this book. The next presentation, by Jill Winters, summarized the results of the RERC-AMI's national survey of over 400 individuals of their experiences as medical patients with disabilities; this presentation closely tied to Chapter 2 of this book. The next presentation was by Ron Kaye from the FDA's Human Factors Branch, which provided a general perspective of the FDA on medical device regulation procedures and human factors, as well as brief coverage of some of the material on accessibility and human factors of medical devices that is covered in Chapter 17. Finally, the authors of this chapter, who also served as codirectors of the workshop, provided discussion of the five breakout session themes, group assignments, and logistics. This set the stage for the 3 breakout sessions that collectively totaled nearly 5 h that represented the heart of this workshop. Distribution of participants between the five breakout groups was by assignment. This assignment was based on each participant completing a survey prior to the workshop where they listed their top three choices for themes, plus considerations of diversity of expertise; in all cases, participants were assigned to one of their top two choices. At two stages, results were reported to the larger group, with the second of these consisting of formal presentations of bullets that served as the closing session of the workshop.

Each of the three breakout periods had targeted aims. The first breakout had a focus on the current state of the art and future vision in the area of the theme, with roughly five high-priority bullet points to be identified in the area of future vision. The second session focused on discussions and bullet creation in the areas of challenges and barriers that might impede realization of the visions, and existing knowledge gaps in the theme area and action items that should be addressed. Finally, the third session addressed overriding recommendations and opportunities, and provided time to reach consensus on all of the four areas where a prioritized list of three to five bullet points were created. Some of these bullet points had multiple parts as groups integrated similar bullets together. During each of the three breakout periods, Jack Winters served as a rover who rotated between theme groups to help keep groups on focus and occasionally share information between groups or address any logistical issues. Of note is that different groups took varying strategies to meet these ultimate aims. A subset of bullet points was reported during the final session, with each theme group allocated roughly 10 min.

31.2.1.1 Breakout Theme A: Physical Positioning/Orienting of Patient to Device

This theme was chaired by Robert Erlandson (Wayne State University) and Molly Follette Story (Human Spectrum Design, LLC, RERC-AMI staff), and involved a total of 13 participants, including

5 from the RERC-AMI, 3 from other academic institutions and 3 from the FDA (see Table 31.1). The motivation for this theme, as defined prior to the workshop, follows:

> On the RERC-AMI's national survey of patients with disabilities, a majority of respondents reported having had significant difficulties with many categories of medical equipment (e.g., exam tables, weight scales, imaging equipment). Most of these difficulties are related to physical positioning and orientation, and are part of many of the most common medical procedures.

TABLE 31.1
Theme Group Assignments for Participants at Workshop on Accessible Interfaces for Medical Instrumentation

Theme A	Physical Positioning/Orienting
Cochairs:	
Robert Erlandson, Ph.D.	Wayne State University
Molly Follette Story, M.S.	RERC-AMI staff, Human Spectrum Design, LLC
Support:	
Brenda Premo, M.S.W.	RERC-AMI staff, Western University of Health Sciences
Melissa Lemke, M.S.	RERC-AMI staff/student, Marquette University
Participants:	
Don Marlowe, M.S.	FDA/RERC-AMI advisor/Workshop Coordinator
Tom Armstrong, Ph.D.	RERC-AMI advisor/University of Michigan
Jane Dorval, M.D.	Commission on Accreditation of Rehabilitation Facilities (CARF)
Jean Hinker	Midmark Corporation
Christie MacDonald, M.P.P.	RERC-AMI staff, Western University of Health Sciences
Amanda Maisels, J.D.	U.S. Department of Justice
Rochelle Mendonca, M.S.	RERC-AMI student, University of Wisconsin–Milwaukee
Walter Scott, Ph.D.	FDA
Donna Walsh, B.B.E.	FDA
Becky Wassem, D.N.S.	RERC-AMI advisor
Theme B	**Interfaces for Monitoring Devices**
Cochairs:	
John Gosbee, Ph.D.	VA National Center for Patient Safety (NCPS)
Jay Crowley, M.S.	FDA
Support:	
John Enderle, Ph.D.	RERC-AMI staff, University of Connecticut
Megan Conrad, M.S.	RERC-AMI student, Marquette University
Participants:	
Larry Kessler, Sc.D.	FDA
Alexandra Enders, O.T.R./L.	RERC-AMI advisor/rehabilitation, University of Montana
Erik Engstrom	ANS Medical
Ann Ferriter	FDA
Libby Grohmann	ANS Medical
Michael Mendelson, D.D.S., M.S.	FDA
Michael Wiklund, M.S.	Wiklund Research and Development
Stan Yarnell, M.D.	RERC-AMI advisor, consultant
Theme C	**Interfaces for Home Health Care Devices**
Cochairs:	
Daryle Gardner-Bonneau, Ph.D.	Bonneau and Associates
Binh Tran, Ph.D.	Catholic University of America

(Continued)

TABLE 31.1
Theme Group Assignments for Participants at Workshop on Accessible Interfaces for Medical Instrumentation *(Continued)*

Support:	
Jill Winters, Ph.D., R.N.	RERC-AMI staff, Marquette University
Eli Omiatek, B.B.E.	RERC-AMI student, Marquette University
Participants:	
Sue Bogner, Ph.D.	Institute for the Study of Human Error, LLC
Jennifer Croft	FDA
William K. Durfee, Ph.D.	RERC-AMI advisor
Al Gilman	RERC on Information Technology
Judy Brewer, Ph.D.	World Wide Web Consortium, MIT
Stephen B. Wilcox, Ph.D.	Design Science
Theme D	**Interfaces for Patients with Disabilities**
Cochairs:	
June Isaacson Kailes, M.S.W.	RERC-AMI staff, Western University of Health Sciences
Michael L. Jones, Ph.D.	RERC on Mobile Wireless Technologies, Shepherd Rehabilitation Hospital
Support:	
R. Sarma Danturthi, Ph.D.	RERC-AMI staff, Marquette University
Tyre Feng, M.S.	RERC-AMI student, Marquette University
Participants:	
Pascale Carayon, Ph.D.	University of Wisconsin–Madison
Robert Jaeger, Ph.D.	NIDRR
Chris Duff	RERC-AMI advisor
Jim Leahy	RERC-AMI advisor/RERC on Technology Transfer
Joel Myklebust, Ph.D.	FDA
William Peterson, M.S.	U.S. Department of Homeland Security
Chuck Rich, Ph.D.	Mitsubishi
Bill Schutz, Ph.D., M.S.W., M.P.H.	NIDRR
Todd Schwanke, M.S.	RERC-AMI staff, University of Wisconsin–Milwaukee
Theme E	**Interfaces for Aging and Disabled Providers**
Cochairs:	
Katherine D. Seelman, Ph.D.	RERC on Telerehabilitation, University of Pittsburgh
William Mann, Ph.D.	RERC on Technology for Successful Aging, University of Florida
Support:	
Roger Smith, Ph.D.	RERC-AMI staff, University of Wisconsin–Milwaukee
Pawan Shroff, M.S.	RERC-AMI student, Marquette University
Participants:	
David Baquis	U.S. Access Board
Jim Mueller, M.S.	RERC-AMI advisor/RERC on Mobile Wireless Technologies
John Peifer, M.A.	RERC on Mobile Wireless Technologies
David Rempel, M.D., M.P.H.	RERC-AMI staff, University of California–San Francisco
Erin Schweir, O.T.D.	RERC-AMI staff, Western University of Health Sciences
Linda van Roosmalen, Ph.D.	RERCs on Telerehabilitation and Wheelchair Transportation, University of Pittsburgh

As seen in Table 31.2, Theme Group A's vision statements reflected their concern for creating a national imperative for incorporating accessibility into the design of medical devices and into standards that affect it, as well as into tools that are used in the design process. The challenges and barriers the group identified were financial, technical, social-political, attitudinal, and economic.

They identified knowledge gaps in the areas of data, models, and assessment procedures; and they suggested three action items to improve education in accessibility and universal design, develop tools for designing for greater accessibility, and discover advanced technologies. Theme Group A's recommendations addressed tools, standards, and curricula development, as well as advanced technology identification and increased consumer advocacy (see Table 31.2).

TABLE 31.2
Bullet Points for Workshop Theme A: Physical Positioning/Orienting of Patient to Device

	Vision Statements
A1	Create the national imperative for including accessibility in medical equipment design
A2	Have models and procedures that allow us to evaluate medical devices for accessibility and design systems that are accessible to all
A3	Have standards developing organizations integrate accessibility into standards for medical equipment
	Challenges/Barriers to Vision
A1	Funding and mandate to create the national imperative for including accessibility in medical equipment design
A2	Technical: Absence of technologies that render current accessibility issues irrelevant
A3	Social–political: Public awareness of right to access; and medical vs. civil rights vs. functional models of disability
A4	Attitudinal: Within health care community; disability community; academic community; acceptance of new technologies and change
A5	Economic: Cost, reimbursement, incentive policies (carrot and stick)
	Knowledge Gaps/Action Items
A1	Knowledge gap: Insufficient credible/validated disability data and projections
A2	Knowledge gaps: • Lack of models for simulating human performance • Lack of accessibility assessment procedures
A3	Action item: More education in accessible and universal design — helps address knowledge gap of accessibility and universal design
A4	Action item: Create: • Inventory of devices with accessibility features (helps address knowledge gap) • Models and procedures for evaluating accessibility • Performance-based standards for accessible design • Legal requirements and incentives for providers to buy accessible equipment
A5	Action item: Identify new and emerging technologies that will render many existing procedures obsolete and eliminate accessibility issues
	Recommendations
A1	RERCs and other research organizations should develop models and procedures for evaluating accessibility with input from consumers with disabilities
A2	RERCs, other research organizations, and industry should partner with standards developing organizations to create performance-based standards for accessible design of medical equipment • RERC-AMI should initiate steps to coalesce national imperative for including accessibility in medical equipment design
A3	RRTCs (Rehabilitation Research and Training Centers), educators, and accreditation bodies should create curricula on accessibility and universal design appropriate for a variety of disciplines
A4	Major research organizations should identify new and emerging technologies that will render many existing procedures obsolete and eliminate accessibility issues
A5	Disability advocacy groups should increase awareness of right to equal access to health care

31.2.1.2 Breakout Theme B: Interfaces for Monitoring Devices

This theme was chaired by Jay Crowley (CDRH, FDA) and John Gosbee (VA National Center for Patient Safety), and involved a total of 12 participants, including 2 from the RERC-AMI, 4 from the FDA and 3 from industry (see Table 31.1). This group focused on interfaces for monitoring devices, especially as related to use by practitioners. This topic is clearly of key interest to the FDA and its mission. The motivation for this theme, as defined prior to the workshop, follows:

> The focus is on displays and controls of interfaces that are most often operated manually, often for assessment (e.g., physiologic monitoring devices) and therapy (e.g., infusion). The primary focus is on monitoring devices used by practitioners in hospitals and clinics.

Theme Group B participants included an intriguing mix of expertise in medical device regulation, accessibility and disability research, and biomedical engineering. As such, much of the first session was spent in cross-fertilization of ideas and in sharing conceptual frameworks. As seen in Table 31.3, Theme Group B's visions included better education, development of an exemplary accessible monitor device, advanced technologies, sufficient application of standards, and development of better design guidance. The group identified challenges and barriers of economics, awareness levels, human factors concerns, job duties, and competitive marketplace issues. There was also frank discussion of the reality that there are both synergy and conflict between the aims of device regulation and maximizing device access. The knowledge gaps and action items they identified involved educating designers and industry, developing appropriate incentives and regulations, standards and guidelines, as well as design exemplars. Theme Group B's recommendations were to use existing committees to advocate for accessibility, to have the FDA endorse the concept, and develop an award for good accessible medical device design (see Table 31.3).

31.2.1.3 Breakout Theme C: Interfaces for Home Health Care Devices

This theme was chaired by Daryle Gardner-Bonneau (human factors and accessibility consultant) and Binh Q. Tran (Catholic University of America) and involved a total of ten participants with very diverse backgrounds, with half being distinguished experts with a background that included considerable consulting activities in areas that are applicable to this theme (see Table 31.1). The motivation for this theme, as defined prior to the workshop, follows:

> This represents a large category of devices, the user of which is commonly the patient or their personal attendant or family member or friend, any one of whom may have a disability. Examples include vital sign monitors, blood glucose monitors and insulin dosers, infusion pumps, exercise equipment, and home telehealth equipment.

Theme Group C had an interesting mix of human factors expertise — technologists and clinical expertise that resulted in considerable discussion of future possibilities for home-based health care (see also Appendix 1). As seen in Table 31.4, Theme Group C's visions for the year 2010 included providing effective design guidelines and strategies to designers, development of scalable, customizable platforms and "smart" systems, a connected system of health care, and changes in reimbursement policies. The challenges and barriers they identified involved limitations in knowledge among designers, in technology, in user skills, as well as a practitioner-focused health care system and a lack of focus on prevention. The group identified two key knowledge gaps to support decision-making and the process of implementing new device designs; they also identified three action items to mandate accessibility, to make devices more customizable, and increase stakeholder involvement in the standards development process. Theme Group C's recommendations were to create funding to support policy research, to develop an effective health platform, and to conduct research — on potential humanistic barriers, on best practices in accessible design, and on chronic disease prevention and management (see Table 31.4).

TABLE 31.3
Bullet Points for Workshop Theme B: Interfaces for Monitoring Devices

	Vision Statements
B1	Universal design course required by clinical engineering students
B2	Good exemplars of an "accessible monitor" to lead, teach, and test; consider: • More of a systems solution … paperless documentation • Multiplex controls for patient information, vital signs monitoring [e.g., URC] • Wireless and other sensing • More of a choice of display: from PDA to fixed monitor to computer at home
B3	Innovations into design adaptations that help all of us (e.g., enhancement of visual display with audio supplement helping sighted and unsighted clinician)
B4	Applying the human factors standard HE-74 (and soon HE-75) in a sufficient manner (especially accurate user profile, e.g., diverse abilities)
B5	Harmony and tightening of usability and universal design guidelines
B6	Standardization of displays, icons, warnings, and alarms
B7	Wireless and other sensing incorporated into devices
	Challenges/Barriers to Vision
B1	This is a commodity environment, not boutique, so change with cost can hurt
B2	Awareness factor by stakeholders in developing new versions or new medical equipment
B3	Many devices already have issues with usability and designing to true needs of providers, so with just adding another modality (e.g., sound), these issues remain
B4	Identifying the boundary of suitability of the health care provider to accomplish the job tasks (e.g., anesthesiologist with visual impairment, neurosurgeon with tremor)
B5	Acceptance from marketing that accessibility changes would be competitive (make it sell)
B6	Design culture (given that most of technology is already there) where the product is a technology driven process (CEO, design process owner)
B7	Posing mutually exclusive goals (losing proposition) that are in stark contrast
B8	Lack of expertise and personnel in company to produce accessible equipment
B9	Off-the-shelf components may not exist (given processor and display are from consumer market)
B10	Workplace congestion and footprint size (reachability)
B11	Patient privacy issues
B12	Unauthorized use (by kids, pets) if equipment is physically accessible
B13	Income status of people with disabilities may be lower
	Knowledge Gaps/Action Items
B1	Educate/influence engineers, industry, and others about universal design and accessibility: • Create the data necessary to make the marketing case; promote it to manufacturers • Improve understanding of access — both within the design process (manufacturers) and for purchasers
B2	Carrots and sticks — develop regulations (or regulatory bodies making endorsing statement) and (tax) incentives (IRS, CMS) to improve accessibility in (monitoring) devices — through collaboration with the disability (rehabilitation) community
B3	Develop HFE standards and guidelines incorporating accessibility issues (good design)
B4	Develop examples of good accessible design (as reference for manufacturers to use); and a registry of accessible components (include consumer products that incorporate accessibility, e.g., displays and controls)
B5	Study legal and regulatory issues around the "telecom model"[a] and FEC voting booth model (usability guide) — to improve accessibility in component part design
B6	ABET does not require universal design, so make it required
B7	What exactly are the major accessibilities to be addressed (sight, hearing, mobility, etc.)?
B8	Are we talking about all users, including maintenance, attaching, and setting up cables?
B9	What is the major impact point? (FDA GMP, AAMI, or ISO 60601-1-6 were the impact points for usability.) ECRI might be an influence point

(Continued)

TABLE 31.3
Bullet Points for Workshop Theme B: Interfaces for Monitoring Devices *(Continued)*

	Recommendations
B1	Use the AAMI Human Factors Committee to strongly advocate for accessibility; develop a chapter in the proposed new standard; develop a guideline for accessibility; advocate at professional meetings
B2	Create an FDA endorsement of accessibility in device design
B3	Develop an "award" (mechanism for design excellence) for good accessible design
B4	Promote industry participation in addressing accessibility issues in collaboration with disability community (e.g., use blue ribbon panels); The idea is to promote device design that addresses patient accessibility

[a]Section 255 and 508 apply to electronic and information technologies (E&IT), e.g., by 508 the Federal government can purchase only accessible E&IT products (with some exceptions).

TABLE 31.4
Bullet Points for Workshop Theme C: Interfaces for Home Health Care Devices

	Vision Statements
C1	Provide guidelines/strategies to designers for how to be more inclusive for various groups of end users
C2	Scalable, customizable platforms enabling plug-and-play devices to be added for monitoring comorbidities and for enhanced accessibility needs
C3	Connected care system — devices can be remotely accessed, monitored, controlled, and maintained via telecom
C4	Smart systems to support disease management by all users (i.e., consumers, caregivers, and clinicians)
C5	Changes in policy for reimbursement of home health care services — spurring innovation/utilization
	Challenges/Barriers to Vision
C1	For Vision #1 (Guidelines/strategies to designers): • Knowledge gap of who/how many subjects would be needed to represent [disabled] population • Gap in available specifications for design for various cohorts of end users • Lack of knowledge by designers regarding prevalence of disabilities and nature of functional deficits.
C2	For Vision #2 (Scalable Platforms): • Currently limited multimodal, multisensory communication and interface (input/output) with devices (device interoperability and standards for device communication)
C3	For Vision #2 (Scalable Platforms): • Humanistic barriers: skill levels, comfort level with technology, and user diversity (e.g., language spoken/read)
C4	For Vision #3 ("Connected Care"): • Health care model: MD-focus vs. patient empowerment • Reimbursement streams for model • Privacy vs. increased connectivity • Increased liability for clinicians
C5	For Vision #5 (Policy Changes): • Lack of focus on prevention • Resistance to change (bureaucracy) • Need for translation of knowledge: research to policy • Lack of enforcement for accessibility • Justification: reimbursement vs. abuse
C6	For Vision #4 (Smart/Decision Support): • Increased involvement of patients in self-management [of health care] • Need for knowledge translation: research to practice (best practices) • Bandwidth of interaction with users

(Continued)

TABLE 31.4
Bullet Points for Workshop Theme C: Interfaces for Home Health Care Device *(Continued)*

	Knowledge Gaps/Action Items
C1	Action item: Make accessibility a mandate for reimbursement
C2	Action item: Increased flexibility and adaptability of medical devices (customization)
C3	Action item: Increase involvement in standards process — stakeholders
C4	Knowledge gap: Develop best practices in decision support
C5	Knowledge gap: Areas for better (integrated) understanding of: • Reimbursement • Introduction of new technology • Profitability of manufacturers
C6	Need to conduct research on appropriate sample of end users — accessibility testing
C7	Need to know what patient empowerment information is needed for promoting self-management [of health care]
	Recommendations
C1	Policy-makers and granting agencies should fund research to support policy changes leading to: • Mandated and enforced accessibility in design of medical devices • Reimbursement streams for home health medical devices and care to manage chronic diseases and disabilities • Business case for proactive prevention model (vs. reactive episodic model) of health care delivery
C2	Industry should develop a common interoperable, scalable, and customizable health platform that enables: • Health information to be collected, analyzed, and transmitted • Multimodal, multisensory communication and interfaces (input/output)
C3	Further research is needed to identify and assess potential humanistic barriers (i.e., skill, comfort with technology, and user diversity) to utilization of home health technologies for self-care
C4	Granting agencies should support research to develop evidence-based best practice guidelines to guide industry regarding how to design for accessibility and to aid practitioners in purchasing and using accessible medical devices
C5	Granting agencies should support research to address knowledge gaps in chronic disease prevention and management for the purpose of developing smart routines for in-home decision support

31.2.1.4 Breakout Theme D: Emerging Interfaces for Patients with Disabilities

This theme was chaired by Michael L. Jones (RERC on Mobile Wireless Technologies, Shepherd Rehabilitation Hospital) and June Isaacson Kailes (RERC-AMI staff, Western University of Health Sciences), and involved a total of 13 participants, including 4 from the RERC-AMI, 4 from federal different federal agencies, and 2 representing other RERCs (RERC on Mobile Wireless Technologies, RERC on Technology Transfer) (see Table 31.1). This theme focused on interfaces for patients with disabilities, especially as related to use by practitioners. The motivation for this theme, as defined prior to the workshop, follows:

> The focus is on the approaches for maximizing the accessibility of instrumentation commonly used by patients. This includes consideration of alternative strategies as appropriate for certain classes of devices, such as use of universal design strategies or multimodal interfaces that enhance certain abilities while minimizing the impact of disabilities.

Theme Group D spent considerable time discussing the tradeoffs and challenges of personalized interfaces, and of relationships between technology and access. Theme Group D's visions were the adoption of new technologies (specifically the universal remote console, URC), regulations to support acquisition of accessible equipment, use of a personal profile in medical records, and better support for telehealth activities. The challenges and barriers they identified included a number of obstacles to adoption of the URC and to development of regulations. In the area of knowledge gaps and action items, Group D focused on the needs for inclusion of a personal profile in medical records and support for telehealth services. The group's recommendations were to adopt the URC in medical device design, to develop regulatory requirements for accessible medical instrumentation, and implement an accessibility/accommodation profile as part of standard health information (see Table 31.5).

31.2.1.5 Breakout Theme E: Emerging Interfaces for Aging and Disabled Providers

This theme was chaired by William Mann (RERC on Technology for Successful Aging, University of Florida) and Katherine Seelman (RERC on Telerehabilitation, University of Pittsburgh), and

TABLE 31.5
Bullet Points for Workshop Theme D: Emerging Interfaces for Patients with Disabilities

	Vision Statements
D1	Adoption of universal remote console (URC) interface capability in some medical products, equipment, or devices with patient interfaces
D2	Regulatory requirements supporting acquisition of accessible medical products, equipment, or devices by federal purchasers (i.e., VA) and nonfederal providers
D3	Personal accessibility/accommodation profile as part of standard health information collected (along with allergies, blood type, etc.)
D4	Network-based remote assistance available for medical instrumentation use, adjustment, etc.
	Challenges/Barriers to Vision
D1	Adoption of universal remote control (URC) interface capability in some medical products, equipment, or devices with patient interfaces • Resistance by manufacturers (cost, identity, control, and liability), possible resistance or concern by regulators (e.g., controlling both a consumer device and medical instrument) • There needs to be a standard that tags features/tasks that can be controlled by the patient, patient or practitioner, or practitioner • Cost burden to manufacturer, provider, patient, payor • Relationship to consumer electronics market • Maturity of technology (reliability, security, and usability concerns) • Lack of international standard (working on ISO 24752); lack of awareness
D2	Regulatory requirements supporting acquisition of accessible medical products, equipment, or devices by federal purchasers (i.e., VA) and nonfederal providers • Need to define range (limits of) medical products, equipment, and devices that need to be controllable by the patient • Federal government must get on board
	Knowledge Gaps/Action Items
D1	Personal accessibility/accommodation profile as part of standard health information (along with allergies, blood type, etc.) • Awareness — need for this information not appreciated • Lack of a profile metastructure (don't know what data is needed) • Public/private resistance; privacy/security concerns
D2	Network-based remote assistance available for medical instrumentation use, adjustment, etc. • Privacy/security; staffing, infrastructure • Lack of standards; cost

(Continued)

TABLE 31.5
Bullet Points for Workshop Theme D: Emerging Interfaces for Patients with Disabilities *(Continued)*

	Recommendations
D1	Adoption of universal remote console (URC): • The URC Consortium should spearhead a campaign — across consumer electronics and medical instrumentation industries — to publicize advantages of URC adoption • Federal funding sources (NIH, NIDRR) should establish SBIR (small business grants) invitational priority to support development of URC prototypes of accessible MI • NIDRR should continue to support RERCs in development of real-world demonstrations of URC utility
D2	Regulatory requirements for accessible medical equipment, products, and devices: • Congress should authorize the Access Board to develop accessibility/accommodation guidelines for medical instrumentation: RERC-AMI should define the range of medical instrumentation to be included, and Department of Justice (DOJ) should quickly adopt Access Board guidelines • Health care accrediting bodies (CARF and JCAHO) should adopt standards requiring accessible medical instrumentation
D3	Accessibility/accommodation profile as part of standard health information: • RERC-AMI should form a task force to develop the accessibility/accommodation profile metastructure • Entities responsible for health information data sets should be mandated to adopt accessibility profile metastructure to the data set (RERC-AMI should identify entities) • Demonstration projects should be initiated by the VA

involved a total of 11 participants, including 4 from the RERC-AMI, 3 representing other RERCs (on Technology for Successful Aging, Telerehabilitation, and Mobile Wireless Technologies), and several from strategic bodies involved in technical implementation of accessibility standards (see Table 31.1). This group focused on interfaces for aging and disabled health care providers, especially as related to use by practitioners. The motivation for this theme, as defined prior to the workshop, follows:

> Some medical practitioners have congenital or acquired disabilities and others, as they age, may experience diminishing sensory and/or motor abilities. Ideally, medical devices should be designed to accommodate a range of abilities and (as appropriate) enable practitioners to pursue or continue in their selected profession.

Theme Group E was unique in its focus on providers. There was considerable early discussion about whether to include lay caregivers as providers within the theme, with an eventual decision that the primary focus should be on professional providers with disabilities as part of the motivation for the topic related to the RERC-AMI's focus on employment of persons with disabilities in health care professions. As seen in Table 31.5, Theme Group E's visions were that medical devices be designed to accommodate greater diversity among health care providers and that training activities do the same. They identified challenges and barriers of negative attitudes on the part of health care administrators, providers, and patients as well as manufacturers and legislators, and a number of technological challenges. The group identified knowledge gaps about disability among health care practitioners, about the need for accessibility among industry and regulators, and about how and why to design for accessibility. Theme Group E's developed three research and development recommendations, about evaluation methods, new interface technologies, and "zero-lift" solutions, one recommendation about education and training of stakeholders, and one policy recommendation about development of standards (see Table 31.6).

TABLE 31.6
Bullet Points for Workshop Theme E: Emerging Interfaces for Aging and Disabled Providers

	Vision Statements
E1	Medical instruments must address differences in abilities of providers, that is, they must address the broadest range of function in the design • Provider needs should be considered early on in the design process
E2	In designing medical instruments and applying principles of universal design, there must be consideration of "hooks" that permit individual personalization of interfaces
E3	Instruction, training, information, and discovery: • Instruction and training for use of medical devices should be multimodal and follow the principles of universal design • Accessibility and usability information and information about accessibility of technology should be available in product (medical instrument) documentation • Controls on medical devices should be easily discoverable (e.g., "stop" button is always round and red)
E4	Health care work environment for providers: • Must be modified to reduce musculoskeletal, visual, and auditory stress (e.g., sustained awkward postures, heavy lifting, high grip forces, and noise) • Should be transparent and responsive to the changes related to aging (including physical environment as well as management)
E5	Medical device companies integrate provider needs earlier on in the design process (e.g., devices should be safe, usable, accessible, desirable, and comfortable)
E6	Job position descriptions in health related professions should become more function-based rather than physiology-based
	Challenges/Barriers to Vision
E1	Communicating the technical and social issues related to accessibility and availability of medical devices to decision makers in government regulation and industry including manufacturers
E2	Prejudices and attitudes in the health care profession (management and patients) against employees and students with disabilities (if you are disabled you are viewed as a patient and not an employee)
E3	A belief that accessibility is expensive and difficult
E4	New technologies are introduced without considering accessibility, replacing older devices that may have been [more] accessible
E5	Technology challenges: • Wireless interference (e.g., with information systems, security and medical devices) • RF-ID for medication tracking • Smaller devices present challenges for interfaces (e.g., visual displays are smaller) • Robotics/mechatronics and product design to assist with fine motor tasks • Assistive robotics development for health providers and patients lags far behind industrial robotic/mechatronic development • A need to increase the intellectual investment and development of automation strategies in health care delivery
E6	Lack of standards and inadequate enforcement of accessibility
E7	Bridging the aging and disability communities (i.e., Aging and disability researchers and advocates and different funding streams and agencies for serving younger people with disabilities and older persons)
E8	FDA currently does not evaluate low-risk devices (e.g., Class I and Class II) for usability and safety
E9	Need to develop testing protocols (e.g., usability, accessibility, safety, desirability, and comfort)
E10	Assistive technologies almost by definition focus on a single impairment, often being inaccessible to [people with] other impairments or multiple impairments
E11	Disability issues are [often] addressed through accommodation rather than accessibility (not understanding what accessibility is)

(Continued)

TABLE 31.6
Bullet Points for Workshop Theme E: Emerging Interfaces for Aging and Disabled Providers *(Continued)*

E12	Privacy and security related to Electronic Medical Records (EMRs) and other electronically transmitted information can be compromised; EMRs should be accessible within the HIPAA framework
E13	A need to research and identify design strategies to improve cognitive access (e.g., E-information, consistency of interface, scalability/scaffold ability, and personalized interfaces)
E14	Things like patient acceptance, safety, liability, reliability could be barriers to implementation of these technologies
	Knowledge Gaps/Action Items
E1	Lack of knowledge about: • Causes of disability and disability retirement among health care professions (e.g., vision, hearing, dexterity, and/or lack of environmental accessibility) • Hidden disabilities and their influence on retirement or avoidance of entering the profession
E2	Assure the awareness of industry and regulators related to accessibility needs: • Keeps pace with technology development • Collaboration on development of standards (include participation by the FDA, consumer community, research community, industry, and government agencies) • Regulatory encouragement for developing an accreditation program for laboratory testing of accessibility and other factors of medical devices
E3	Need for targeted research studies about the medical device field: • Decision studies related to medical device procurement • Organization analysis or studies of the culture of various industries
E4	More knowledge transfer about: • Accessibility standards and guidelines among related technology fields (e.g., designers and manufacturers of medical devices adapting E&IT standards to blood pressure monitor design) • Capturing business and design experiences and best practices related to benefits and design of medical devices
E5	Research on technology/environmental solutions to achieving zero lift and zero handling policies (with usability testing from perspective of both patient and provider)
E6	Need for assessment protocols to identify individual interface needs for health professionals using medical devices
E7	Lack of knowledge of barriers for health professionals to successfully complete job tasks
E8	Facilitate collaboration between the assistive technology industry and the mainstream technology industry to ensure interoperability
E9	Lack of the knowledge of benefits and lack of skills for implementing universal design strategies among designers
E10	The scalability and reliability of wireless networks
E11	Study of things like patient/provider acceptance, safety, liability, and reliability that could be barriers to implementation of automation of these technologies
	Recommendations
E1	Under research and development: Investigate and develop testing methodologies for evaluating the accessibility, usability, desirability, comfort, and safety of medical equipment used by medical providers
E2	Under research and development: Find and/or develop new interface methods and strategies relevant to accessibility of medical devices and information systems for health care providers • Employ sensors and context-aware algorithms to produce secure and accessible interfaces to medical devices and data in the emerging integrated electronic medical records (EMR) • Study, develop, and implement methods and guidelines for accessible EMR systems • Research and identify design strategies to improve cognitive access (e.g., E-Information, consistency of interface, scalability/scaffold ability, and personalized interfaces)

(Continued)

TABLE 31.6
Bullet Points for Workshop Theme E: Emerging Interfaces for Aging and Disabled Providers *(Continued)*

E3	Under research and development: Study and develop technology and environmental solutions to achieve zero lift and zero handling policies (with usability testing from perspective of both the patient and the provider)
E4	Under education and training: Provide education and training to health care management, educational settings and industry (R&D) on accessibility issues/standards related to medical devices, disability incidence, issues, and effect on workforce of health care providers
E5	Under policy: Collaboration for development of medical device standards that include participation by the FDA, consumer community, research community, industry, and government agencies; FDA is also encouraged to develop an accreditation program for laboratory testing to the standards of medical devices
E6	Under research and development: Perform research to identify barriers for aging health care professionals and health professionals with disabilities to successfully complete job tasks
E7	Under research and development: Perform outcome-based studies that show the benefit of accessible medical devices by providers in health care settings
E8	Under research and development: Conduct decision studies related to medical device procurement by hospitals, VA, and DOD
E9	Under education and training: Implement more knowledge transfer (standards and guidelines) among related technology fields (e.g., designers and manufacturers of medical devices adapting E&IT standards to blood pressure monitor design)
E10	Under education and training: Implement more knowledge transfer capturing business and design experiences and best practices related to benefits and design of medical devices
E11	Under policy: Promote science agency practices related to inclusion of people with disabilities in research and development (e.g., randomized clinical trials)

31.2.2 Ranking of Bullet Points and Integration of Data

After the meeting, the bullet points generated by each group were assembled and disseminated for voting to all participants of the workshop. From each of the 4 lists of 23 bullets, each rater was asked to select 1 top choice and up to 4 other high-priority choices. The return rate was 45%, which was reasonable, considering that most participants from government agencies felt that it was not appropriate for them to participate in the voting. In assembling results, the top choice was given double the weight of the other selections. The results were tallied and the bullets were ranked. Bullets with a score of at least three are included in the tables (see Tables 31.7 to 31.10). Additionally, it was recognized that in many cases, different theme groups had bullets that overlapped. This was expected and indeed such overlap suggests areas of special importance. Raters had the option of identifying the best of a certain class of bullets, or if they really felt it was an especially important area to mark several similar bullets. Thus, in addition to absolute ranking of bullets, the authors clustered similar bullets from workshop participants to identify overriding themes.

31.3 RESULTS

Each of the 5 theme groups was allowed up to provide up to 5 final bullets in each of 4 areas, and thus up to 20 total. The actual number averaged 18.4 per group, with a range of 17 to 19. The final bullets, all of which required some degree of refining or reduction in number by the coauthors and organizers after the workshop, were previously presented in Table 31.2 to Table 31.6. Although these are numbered, they do not reflect a preferred order.

In this section, the emphasis is on integrating results across groups, using the rating process as a tool for helping prioritize and synthesize these bullets. Table 31.7 to Table 31.10 present the results of the ranking process. This is the focus of the remainder of this chapter, with an emphasis on each of the four focal discussion areas in which bullet points were generated. Of note in interpreting results is that often more general, sweeping statements scored higher than more specific statements or ones with more detail; this doesn't imply that these are less important, but simply that more raters chose them. Also, there is no guarantee that more specific bullets were fully understood by participants, as each participant was part of only one group. Nevertheless, as will be seen this process does provide guidance regarding priorities and insights of the collective group.

TABLE 31.7
Top-Rated Vision Statements, in Rank Order

Number	Description	Total	First Choices
A1	Create the national imperative for including accessibility in medical equipment design	22	10
A3	Have standards-developing organizations integrate accessibility into standards for medical equipment	22	6
D2	Regulatory requirements supporting acquisition of accessible medical products, equipment, or devices by federal purchasers (i.e., VA) and nonfederal providers	14	3
A2	Have models and procedures that allow us to evaluate medical devices for accessibility, and design systems that are accessible to all	12	2
D1	Adoption of universal remote console (URC) interface capability in some medical products, equipment, or devices with patient interfaces	10	1
C1	Provide guidelines/strategies to designers for how to be "more inclusive" for various groups of end users	8	1
D3	Personal accessibility/accommodation profile as part of standard health information (along with allergies, blood type, etc.)	8	1
E3	Instruction, training, information, and discovery: • Instruction and training for use of medical devices should be multimodal and follow the principles of universal design. • Accessibility and usability information and information about accessibility of technology should be available in product (medical instrument) documentation • Controls on medical devices should be easily discoverable (e.g., stop button is always round and red)	7	
E2	In designing medical instruments and applying principles of universal design, there must be consideration of "hooks" that permit individual personalization of interfaces	6	
E1	Medical instruments must address differences in abilities of providers, that is, they must or address the broadest range of function in the design	6	1
E4	Health care work environment for providers: • Must be modified to reduce musculoskeletal, visual, and auditory stress (e.g., sustained awkward postures, heavy lifting, high grip forces, and noise) • Should be transparent and responsive to the changes related to aging (including physical environment as well as management)	5	
E5	Medical device companies integrate provider needs earlier on in the design process (e.g., safe, usable, accessible, desirable, and comfortable)	5	

(Continued)

TABLE 31.7
Top-Rated Vision Statements, in Rank Order *(Continued)*

Number	Description	Total	First Choices
C5	Changes in policy for reimbursement of home health care services — spurring innovation/utilization	4	
B2	Good exemplars of an "accessible monitor" to lead, teach, test. Consider: • More of a systems solution ... paperless documentation • Multiplex controls for patient information, vital signs monitoring [e.g., URC] • Wireless and other sensing • More of a choice of display: from PDA, to fixed monitor, to computer at home	3	
C2	Scalable, customizable platforms enabling plug-and-play devices to be added for monitoring comorbidities and for enhanced accessibility needs	3	
C3	Connected care system — devices can be remotely accessed, monitored, controlled, maintained via telecom	3	

31.3.1 Vision 2010 Statements

Vision statements that were less specific tended to score better. Thus, the top two statements, A1 and A3 (see Table 31.7), both very general statements, would be expected to fare well with this group of experts, many of whom are invested stakeholders who were interested in participating in the workshop and had an inherent desire for greater inclusion of accessibility into medical equipment (A1) and into standards that affect such equipment (A3). The third statement, D2, on regulatory requirements that support acquisition of accessible medical products by purchasers, directly relates to the FDA and to expansion of language such as in Section 508 of the Rehab Act (see Chapter 25) and would clearly require new legislation. The fourth statement, A2, targets evaluation of devices for accessibility. (An example of such effort by the RERC-AMI is the MedAUDIT project described in Chapter 22). Interestingly, the latter two bullet points are related in that effective evaluation of accessibility seems a key step for effective regulatory action to occur.

The fifth-ranked bullet, D1, specifically addressed the URC national standard that the RERC-AMI and three other RERCs, plus partners in industry, are working on that was demonstrated at a booth at the meeting, and is discussed in Chapter 25 to Chapter 28. This trend towards personalized interfaces for access was also described in bullet points submitted by three other groups that made this top list, including E2 (hooks for personalized interfaces), B2 (exemplars of an accessible monitor included paperless and wireless monitors and interface choices such as URC and PDA), and C2 (scalable, customizable platforms with plug-and-play monitoring devices). Of note is that two of the bullets from Theme Group E that made the top ten list addressed the need for solutions that apply the principles of universal design but also specifically address the need for multimodal hooks for personalized interfaces; this is consistent with insights provided in Chapter 9, as well as concepts explicitly raised in Chapter 8, Chapter 18, and Chapter 25.

Another theme that made the top ten list was the need to provide guidelines/strategies for more inclusive design (C1); a related bullet on the top list is E5, which emphasized a process that integrates user needs earlier into the design process. Together with the highly ranked A3, these point to the recognized importance of involving intended users with a diversity of abilities in the early stages of the interface development process.

Two other bullets that made the top ten list deserve special mention: the suggestion of including a personal accessibility/accommodation profile as part of health information collected (D3) and the need for educational resources and training materials (E3). The former would clearly benefit the development of personalized interfaces such as with the URC standard, whereas the latter noted that even instructional materials should be both multimodal and universally designed.

In summary, two, broad sweeping visions on accessible equipment were strongly affirmed by participants. Four additional clear visions emerged: regulatory action, effective evaluation of accessibility, personalized interfaces, and involving users with disabilities early in the design process. In addition, many useful, more targeted visions and insights emerged that are also of great value.

31.3.2 Challenges and Barriers to Achieving Vision

As might be expected, the challenges and barriers identified by the groups tied to the visions. Also, as with the vision bullets, the top-ranked bullet, A5, was a very general statement that resounded with raters: economic realities (see Table 31.8). The clear choice for second-ranking,

TABLE 31.8
Top-Rated Challenges/Barriers Statements, in Rank Order

Number	Description	Total	First Choices
A5	Economic: Cost, reimbursement, incentive policies (carrot and stick)	21	8
D2	Regulatory requirements supporting acquisition of accessible medical products, equipment, or devices by federal purchasers (i.e., VA) and nonfederal providers • Need to define range (limits of) medical products, equipment, and devices that need to be controllable by the patient • Federal government must get on board	16	4
C1	For Vision #1 (Guidelines/strategies to designers): Lack of knowledge by designers regarding prevalence of disabilities and nature of functional deficits	12	3
A1	Funding and mandate to create the national imperative for including accessibility in medical equipment design	11	2
D1	Adoption of universal remote control (URC) interface capability in some medical products, equipment, or devices with patient interface • Resistance by manufacturers (cost, identity, control, and liability), possible resistance or concern by regulators (e.g., controlling both a consumer device and medical instrument) • There needs to be a standard that tags features/tasks that can be controlled by the patient, patient or practitioner, or practitioner • Cost burden to manufacturer, provider, patient, payor • Relationship to consumer electronics market • Maturity of technology (reliability, security, and usability concerns) • Lack of international standard (working on ISO 24752) • Lack of awareness	10	1
E3	A belief that accessibility is expensive and difficult	10	1
A4	Attitudinal: health care community; disability community; academic community; acceptance of new technologies and change	9	1
C2	For Vision #2 (Scalable Platforms): Currently limited multimodal, multisensory communication and interface (input/output) with devices	7	2

(Continued)

TABLE 31.8
Top-Rated Challenges/Barriers Statements, in Rank Order *(Continued)*

Number	Description	Total	First Choices
E5	Technology challenges: • Wireless interference (e.g., with information systems, security, and medical devices) • RF-ID for medication tracking • Smaller devices present challenges for interfaces (e.g., visual displays are smaller) • Robotics/mechatronics and product design to assist with fine motor tasks • Assistive robotics development for health providers and patients lags far behind in industrial robotic/mechatronic development • A need to increase the intellectual investment and development of automation strategies in health care delivery	7	1
A3	Social–political: Public awareness of right to access; and medical vs. civil rights vs. functional models of disability	6	1
B5	Acceptance from marketing that accessibility changes would be competitive (make it sell)	6	
E1	Communicating the technical and social issues related to accessibility and availability of medical devices to decision makers in government regulation and industry including manufacturers	6	
A2	Technical: Absence of technologies that render current accessibility issues irrelevant	5	1
B2	Awareness factor by stakeholders in developing new or new versions of medical equipment	3	
E2	Prejudices and attitudes in the health care profession (management and patients) against employees and students with disabilities (if you are disabled, you are viewed as a patient and not an employee)	3	
E4	New technologies are introduced without considering accessibility, replacing older devices that may have been accessible	3	

D2, was quite specific: the regulatory environment and specific challenges in setting the stage for the acquisition of accessible medical products, including both the challenges of addressing better information and evaluation capabilities and getting the federal government fully on board. This was followed by statement C1, the insight identifying a lack of knowledge regarding the prevalence and nature of disabilities, a barrier that clearly is something that the RERC-AMI could help address.

Two of the next three top-ranked bullets shared a common theme: funding. However, one (A1) emphasized a national funding mandate for accessible products, whereas the other (E3) emphasized the commonly perceived belief that accessibility is expensive and difficult when this may not always be the case; in one sense these are opposite perspectives, but perhaps this depends on the type of product.

The fifth bullet, D1, related directly to the adoption of URC interface capability for some strategic lines of medical products; interestingly, despite a list of six rather prescriptive subbullets, this still ranked high. Importantly, this list of six bullets under statement D1, collectively produced by Theme D, provide a sort of roadmap for the URC/personalized design community, including the RERC-AMI project described in Chapter 28. Also of interest is that this relates very closely to the barrier of scalable, multimodal platforms that was also in the top ten (C1). Two other bullets on the top list (E5 and A2) also explicitly address the lack of innovative technologies as a key barrier to accessible medical products. Thus, it is interesting that although cost and regulatory barriers appear as the top two themes for challenges/barriers, a significant subset of participants placed technical barriers high on their list.

Interestingly, most of the remaining bullets can be clustered under the theme of attitudinal barriers, expressed explicitly in statement A4. Others that fall under this umbrella include social–political awareness (A3), stakeholder awareness (B2), prejudices and attitudes within the health care profession (E2), and as mentioned in the earlier paragraph in another context, the attitudinal belief that accessibility is expensive (E3).

In summary, six overriding challenges/barriers are identified: economic, regulatory, knowledge of disability (as related to product use), URC adoption, low availability of accessible technologies, and attitudinal. For each theme, specific bullet points provide insightful details.

31.3.3 Knowledge Gaps and Action Items

The motivation behind this priority is that research activities can help address knowledge gaps, and a consensus process including diverse expertise can help refine and prioritize research activities. However, there was also a recognition that some research and development (R&D) activities are not driven by the aim of generating new knowledge, and that certain challenges/barriers may require directed activities that are beyond R&D or that need R&D activities that help support a broad scope; hence identifying specific action items is also appropriate. Of the 17 top-ranked bullet points, 13 were knowledge gaps and 4 were action items. Interestingly, however, three of the top seven in terms of ranking were action items (see Table 31.9).

TABLE 31.9
Top-Rated Knowledge Gaps/Action Items Statements, in Rank Order

Number	Description	Total	First Choices
A4	Action item: Create • Inventory of devices with accessibility features (helps address knowledge gap) • Models and procedures for evaluating accessibility • Performance-based standards for accessible design • Legal requirements and incentives for providers to buy accessible equipment	16	3
B1	Educate/influence engineers, industry, and others about universal design and accessibility: • Create the data necessary to make the marketing case; promote it to manufacturers • Improve understanding of "access" — both within the design process (manufacturers) and for purchasers	14	3
B2	Carrots and sticks — develop regulations (or "regulatory" bodies making "endorsing" statements) and (tax) incentives (IRS, CMS) to improve accessibility in (monitoring) devices — through collaboration with the disability (rehabilitation) community	13	4
D1	Personal accessibility/accommodation profile as part of standard health information (along with allergies, blood type, etc.) • Awareness — need for this information not appreciated • Lack of a profile metastructure (don't know what data is needed) • Public/private resistance; privacy/security concerns	13	1
A3	Action item: More education in accessible and universal design — helps address knowledge gap of accessibility and universal design	9	3

(Continued)

TABLE 31.9
Top-Rated Knowledge Gaps/Action Items Statements, in Rank Order *(Continued)*

Number	Description	Total	First Choices
B4	Develop examples of good accessible design (as reference for manufacturers to use); and a registry of accessible components (include consumer products that incorporate accessibility, e.g., displays and controls)	9	1
C1	Action item: Make accessibility a mandate for reimbursement	9	2
A2	Knowledge gaps: • Lack of models for simulating human performance • Lack of accessibility assessment procedures	8	2
E1	Lack of knowledge about: • Causes of disability and disability retirement among health care professions (e.g. vision, hearing, dexterity, and/or lack of environmental accessibility) • Hidden disabilities and their influence on retirement or avoidance of entering the profession	8	1
B3	Develop HFE standards and guidelines incorporating accessibility issues (good design)	7	1
E2	Assure the awareness of industry and regulators related to accessibility needs • Keeps pace with technology development • Collaboration on development of standards • Regulatory encouragement for developing an accreditation program for laboratory testing of accessibility and other factors of medical devices	7	2
E4	More knowledge transfer about: • Accessibility standards and guidelines among related technology fields (e.g., designers and manufacturers of medical devices adapting E&IT standards to blood pressure monitor design) • Capturing business and design experiences and best practices related to benefits and design of medical devices	5	
E5	Research on technology/environmental solutions to achieving zero lift and zero handling policies (with usability testing from perspective of both patient and provider)	5	
C3	Action item: Increase involvement in standards process — stakeholders	4	
E3	Need for targeted research studies about the medical device field: • Decision studies related to medical device procurement • Organization analysis or studies of the culture of various industries	4	2
B5	Study legal and regulatory issues around the "telecom model"[a] and FEC voting booth model (usability guide) — to improve accessibility in component part design	3	
C5	Knowledge gap: Areas for better (integrated) understanding: (a) reimbursement; (b) introduction of new technology; (c) profitability of manufacturers	3	

[a] Section 255 and 508 apply to electronic and information technologies (E&IT), e.g., by 508 the Federal government can purchase only accessible E&IT products (some exceptions).

The top bullet in this category, A4, was an action item: create an all-inclusive resource that includes a product inventory, approaches for evaluating accessibility, standards and legal requirements, and incentives. Given that the RERC-AMI is currently involved in the early stages of all of these activities and that Theme Group A had heavy participation by RERC-AMI staff, it is perhaps not surprising that this item was generated and it subsequently scored well; nontheless, it does provide affirmation for this strategy and its importance. Also of note is that all three of the other action items on this top list had similar themes, specifically of developing regulations and incentives (B2), mandating accessibility for reimbursement (C1), and involving stakeholders in the standards process (C3).

The highest-ranked statements of knowledge gaps, which in different forms scored second (B1) and tied for fifth (A3), related to educational approaches that would help address knowledge gaps about accessibility and universal design. Although each of the knowledge gaps is unique, they cluster into several general themes. One is the need for R&D that addresses the knowledge gap of good design for accessibility: statement B4 addresses the need for R&D that produces good examples of accessible design, A2 addresses the lack of knowledge of models for simulating performance and effective assessment procedures, B3 targets using insights from good designs to help develop standards and guidelines that incorporate accessibility issues, E4 addresses similar knowledge transfer themes, and E5 addresses the need for research that yields solutions that achieve zero lift and handling policies.

Another collection of knowledge gaps can be classified under disability and policy research, with three of four statements generated by Theme Group E. Of note is that this theme had four RERCs represented and also had a special focus on providers with disabilities. Although not ranked as high overall, the fact that four of their bullet points made the top list reflects their importance, especially for understanding barriers to employment in the health care profession. These knowledge gaps included better understanding of the causes of disability and retirement among health care professionals, together with the impact of hidden disabilities (E1); the need for broad awareness of accessibility needs (E2); the need for targeted research about the practices and culture of the medical device field (E3); and the need to study legal and regulatory issues in the context of accessibility guidelines (E4).

31.3.4 Recommendations and Opportunities

Recommendations represent the key aims of the workshop, with the previous three sets of bullets designed to help set the stage for determining, refining, and prioritizing recommendations. Six recommendation bullets were scored considerably higher than all others. Five key classes of recommendations emerged, each with specifics that were identified under two or more recommendation bullets.

By far, the top recommendation of the workshop related to collaboration on standards that tie accessibility with medical device design (see Table 31.10). Indeed, the top recommendations, statements D2, A2, and E5, from three different groups, were all variants on this theme, and a fourth group had a version of this (C1) that was not quite as highly scored. The top recommendation of the workshop (D2) explicitly tied standards to regulatory requirements and suggested a process that also included various federal agencies. The next two (A2 and E5) emphasized partnership and collaboration that involved research, industry, and governmental entities, including the sponsors of this workshop, the RERC program, and the FDA. One of these recommendations (A2) suggested that the RERC-AMI should help initiate this effort; the other (E5) mentioned a key role for the FDA in implementing a laboratory testing program, similar to the type of evaluation capability that was identified as a key knowledge gap. Two other recommendations support this, including one from Theme Group B, which focused on medical monitors and had the largest representation from the FDA, that recommended the creation of an FDA endorsement of accessibility in device design (B2). This same group also recommended that the AAMI Human Factors Committee strongly advocate for accessibility in their work on the new guidelines (B1); as an aside, the RERC-AMI has now taken the lead in working with this committee to add a strong accessibility component to the emerging HE-75 standard (see Chapter 15 and Chapter 16).

TABLE 31.10
Top-Rated Recommendations Statements, in Rank Order

Number	Description	Total	First Choices
D2	Regulatory requirements for accessible medical equipment, products, and devices: • Congress should authorize the Access Board to develop accessibility/accommodation guidelines for medical instrumentation: RERC-AMI should define the range of medical instrumentation to be included, and DOJ should quickly adopt Access Board guidelines • Health care accrediting bodies (CARF and JCAHO) should adopt standards requiring accessible medical instrumentation	19	5
A2	RERCs, other research organizations, and industry should partner with standards developing organizations to create performance-based standards for accessible design of medical equipment • RERC-AMI should initiate steps to coalesce national imperative for including accessibility in medical equipment design	16	5
E5	Under policy: Collaboration for development of medical device standards that include participation by the FDA, consumer community, research community, industry, and government agencies; FDA is also encouraged to develop an accreditation program for laboratory testing to the standards of medical devices	12	
D1	Adoption of universal remote console (URC): • The URC Consortium should spearhead a campaign — across consumer electronics and medical instrumentation industries — to publicize advantages of URC adoption. • Federal funding sources (NIH, NIDRR) should establish SBIR (small business grants) invitational priority to support development of URC prototypes of accessible MI • NIDRR should continue to support RERCs in development of real-world demonstrations of URC utility	11	1
E1	Under research and development: Investigate and develop testing methodologies for evaluating the accessibility, usability, desirability, comfort, and safety of medical equipment used by medical providers.	11	2
C1	Policy-makers and granting agencies should fund research to support policy changes leading to • Mandated and enforced accessibility in design of medical devices • Reimbursement streams for home health medical devices and care to manage chronic diseases and disabilities • Business case for proactive "prevention" model (vs. reactive episodic model) of health care delivery	10	2
A1	RERCs and other research organizations should develop models and procedures for evaluating accessibility with input from consumers with disabilities	7	3
A3	RRTCs (Rehabilitation Research and Training Centers), educators, and accreditation bodies should create curricula on accessibility and universal design appropriate for a variety of disciplines	7	1
A5	Disability advocacy groups should increase awareness of right to equal access to health care	7	2
B2	Create an FDA endorsement of accessibility in device design	6	1
E4	Under education and training: Provide education and training to healthcare management, educational settings and industry (R&D) on accessibility issues/standards related to medical devices, disability incidence, issues, and effect on workforce of health care providers.	6	1

(Continued)

TABLE 31.10
Top-Rated Recommendations Statements, in Rank Order *(Continued)*

Number	Description	Total	First Choices
B3	Develop an award (mechanism for design excellence) for good accessible design	5	
D3	Accessibility/accommodation profile as part of standard health information: • RERC-AMI should form a task force to develop the accessibility/accommodation profile metastructure • Entities responsible for health information data sets should be mandated to adopt accessibility profile metastructure to the data set (RERC-AMI should identify entities) • Demonstration projects should be initiated by the VA	5	
B1	Use the AAMI Human Factors Committee to strongly advocate for accessibility; develop a chapter in the proposed new standard; develop a guideline for accessibility; advocate at professional meetings	4	
C3	Further research is needed to identify and assess potential humanistic barriers (i.e., skill, comfort with technology and user diversity) to utilization of home health technologies for self-care	4	
B4	Promote industry participation in addressing accessibility issues — collaboration with disability community (e.g., blue ribbon panels); promote device design that addresses patient accessibility	3	
C5	Granting agencies should support research to address knowledge gaps in chronic disease prevention and management for the purpose of developing smart routines for in-home decision support	3	1
E3	Under research and development: Study and develop technology and environmental solutions to achieve zero lift and zero handling policies (with usability testing from perspective of both the patient and the provider)	3	

Another of the top five recommendations was D1, the adoption of the URC standard and its implementation for strategic classes of medical devices, including the importance of identifying funding sources for this activity. The theme group responsible for this recommendation, Emerging Trends and Technologies (Theme D), also promoted the need for an accessibility/accommodation profile as part of the standard health information, with the RERC-AMI recommended as an appropriate entity for coordinating a task force to develop a profile metastructure (D3). This is an insightful approach, since for the URC standard to be used for personalized interfaces, such user profile data is critical. This also affirms the approaches described in Chapter 27 and Chapter 28.

Another of the top five recommendations, E1, addressed the need for testing methodologies for evaluating the accessibility (plus usability, desirability, comfort, and safety) of medical devices. This bullet ties to another recommendation that mentions the importance of involving input from consumers with disabilities (A1).

The sixth-ranked recommendation, C1, targets the need for granting agencies and policy-makers to fund targeted disability-related research that could support policy changes. Although this was the only recommendation of this type that made the top group of six bullets, also supporting this were recommendations for research to identify and access the humanistic barriers to utilization of home health care technologies for self-care (C3), research that addresses chronic disease prevention and management for developing smart in-home decision support (C5), and approaches that promote collaboration between industry and the disability community (B4).

The final core recommendation did not make the top six overriding bullets, but represents the theme of two bullets that made the top ten: the need for educational and training materials and programs. This included the creation of curricula (A3) and the provision of educational and training infrastructure (E4). Chapter 8 of this book directly addresses this issue and of note is that the process of addressing this issue has begun, with two ongoing activities: a textbook that is being written by Erlandson on universal and accessible design that will also be published by CRC Press, and a planned expansion of educational resources through the RERC-AMI's Web pages that goes well beyond the current training materials associated with the RERC-AMI's annual student design competition that is also described in Chapter 8.

31.4 DISCUSSION AND FUTURE DIRECTIONS

Perhaps the overriding take-home message of this workshop is that there is much work to be done. There is much to be done to achieve the consensus vision statements (described in Subsection 31.3.1) to overcome the challenges and barriers identified in Subsection 31.3.2, to implement the R&D activities associated with the knowledge gaps of Subsection 31.3.3, and to implement the recommendations of Subsection 31.3.4. All of these stand on their own merit. This section briefly summarizes some of the key outputs of the workshop, and then briefly discusses some of the intangible outputs of the workshop that are not necessarily captured by bullets. Of note is that the cochairs for Theme Group A and Theme Group C briefly disseminate, in Appendix 1 highlights of the internal discussions for their groups. Other insights are reflected in commentaries in the Appendices written after the workshop by individual attendees in response to the event, and in the fact that a number of chapter authors made modifications to their chapters after the workshop that in many cases were directly based on observations or insights from the workshop.

As planned, there were two sweeping themes from this workshop, one related to standards and guidelines that comprised of Theme A, Theme B, and Theme C, and the other on emerging trends and technologies that related to Theme D and Theme E. At least that was our original intent. It is interesting, however, that two of the top three recommendations of the entire workshop, both related to standards, came from groups D and E. Clearly, there is a tight relationship between guidelines/standards, especially ones with enforcement support, and emerging technologies. Through the assembled bullet points related to standards, the RERC-AMI and other stakeholder entities have a clearer vision of paths to take to address the challenges and opportunities in this area.

An advantage of having the type of melting pot of expertise that was assembled at this state-of-the-science workshop is that ideas can be distilled and refined in a way that can compress or redirect the evolutionary process. Of note is that participants to the workshop included, by invitation, leaders in the practice of human factors and the development of disability/accessibility standards; interestingly, in many cases, these individuals were meeting each other for the first time, despite decades of work in standards that in principle should already have had overlap. This is the type of value-added intangible that cannot be captured on paper but can have an impact over time. In relation to existing standards that cut across these areas, Chapter 15 is of especial value; Chapter 19 provides a practical sense of the challenges associated with standards implementation.

Theme D and Theme E did take leadership in the area of emerging trends and technologies, and of all of their discussions, the concept of personalized interfaces that build on the URC standard seems to resonate the most. This is an intriguing development and points out the reality, at least in the eyes of many (e.g., Chapter 25), that both personalized design and universal design will have key roles in the future as strategies for achieving accessible medical instrumentation. The challenge is in the details; for example, determining which product lines should emphasize which approaches, and why.

Both personalized design and universal design relate tightly to another overriding theme, and that is the need for solid methods of evaluating accessibility of specific products. This theme, although never at the top of any bullet list, was a recurring theme for all four focal area lists. It is the motivation behind the RERC-AMI's MedAUDIT approach (Chapter 22), which is still at a sufficiently early stage that it can be impacted by insights from the workshop, but a large number of other chapters in this book provide hints at other approaches (e.g., Chapter 6, Chapter 7, Chapter 9, Chapter 13, Chapter 14, Chapter 16, Chapter 17, Chapter 18, Chapter 20, and Chapter 21).

In summary, much work remains to be done to achieve the top two general visions of creating a national imperative for including accessibility in medical equipment design, and having accessibility integrated into standards that are effective and enforceable. But this was to be expected. This workshop helped define, refine, and prioritize the future directions for this area, and the organizers are grateful to the participants for their involvement, enthusiasm, and ideas.

ACKNOWLEDGMENT

This work is supported by the RERC-AMI, funded by the National Institute on Disability and Rehabilitation Research (NIDRR) of the U.S. Department of Education under grant number H133E020729. All opinions are those of the authors. The authors also thank the Office of Science and Engineering Laboratories, which is under the Center for Devices and Radiological Health of the U.S. Food and Drug Administration, with special thanks to the leadership of Larry Kessler and Don Marlowe. The authors also thank the theme cochairs (Robert Erlandson, Jay Crowley, John Gosbee, Daryle Gardner-Bonneau, Binh Tran, Mike Jones, June Issacson Kailes, Kate Seelman, and William Mann) for their hard work in coordinating theme sessions. Finally, although many members of the RERC-AMI staff and students were involved in this project, three stand out, without whose work this event would not have been possible: Brenda Premo, Melissa Lemke, and Erin Schwier.

APPENDIX: SPECIAL WORKSHOP CONTRIBUTIONS: PARTICIPANT COMMENTARIES

Workshop cochairs and participants were invited to provide targeted commentary on topics related to the workshop. This appendix presents perspectives by the cochairs for Theme C, plus by a few individual workshop participants who accepted the opportunity to provide specific commentary after the event. The editors appreciate their taking the time to document their thoughts. Five appendices follow.

Appendix 1

Chairs' Perspectives on Workshop Breakout Theme C: Interfaces for Home Health Care Devices

Daryle Gardner-Bonneau and Binh Q. Tran

CONTENTS

This section summarizes the activity of the breakout theme of the Workshop on Accessible Interfaces for Medical Instrumentation that focused on interfaces for home health care devices (Theme C). It is authored by the cochairs for this theme.

A1.1 STATUS AND TRENDS

Theme Group C cochairs Daryle Gardner-Bonneau and Binh Tran gave short presentations summarizing the current status of standards work and medical technology user interfaces, respectively. With respect to standards, Dr. Gardner-Bonneau briefly described the lack of consistency in definitions of accessibility vs. usability, along with the differences in the way accessibility is defined in the U.S. and internationally. She also described the status of ongoing medical device and accessibility standards efforts (see Chapter 15).

Dr. Tran discussed the state of the technology in the home health care area and noted the chronic diseases that are the best candidates for management through home health care, the top four being diabetes, hypertension, congestive heart failure, and asthma. He showed a number of examples of the technologies being used to manage illnesses at home and pointed out the increasing trend toward the design of small, compact or handheld devices for monitoring and medication dosing. Dr. Tran also noted the increasing use of integrated telehealth systems for monitoring patients.

A1.2 VISION STATEMENTS

There was no complete agreement about the status of all aspects of medical instrumentation user interface design among the participants. Some felt designers were addressing many usability and accessibility issues, whereas others felt that, currently, there were many challenges still to be addressed. Table 31.4 outlines the vision statements of this group, which reflect some of the challenges still to be met in the design of medical instrumentation for home health care. Most participants agreed that designers need additional guidelines and strategies for how to be more inclusive in designing for various end users. Designers probably need to know more about the prevalence of disabilities and the nature of the functional deficits involved. The second vision statement reflects the need for adaptability and simplicity in devices designed for the home health care environment, emphasizing customizability, scalability, ease of operation, and interoperability of devices. Device designers also need to consider the variation in user skill levels, comfort with the technology, language issues, and variations in sensory and information processing capabilities that suggest the use of multimodal, multisensory user interfaces.

The third vision statement reflects a longstanding need, not only in home care, but in the health care system generally, for connected, or integrated, care systems. There are too many individual and incompatible devices, and devices that do not "talk" to each other. A worthy goal in home health care is to have integrated systems that can be remotely accessed, monitored, controlled, and maintained. Inherent in the discussion of this vision statement was the need to empower patients, as components of the system, to take greater responsibility and control of their care (as opposed to perpetuating the medical model of care). Medical equipment could also be "smarter," not only in applying appropriate context-specific interpretations to data, but in adapting its interaction to the specific user (patient, lay caregiver, and clinician). The need to consider not only clinicians, but also patients and lay caregivers, in the development of decision support systems, was highlighted. Finally, more and more health care is moving out of the hospital and into the home, but the reimbursement for home health care services, particularly telehealth services, needs to be modified in light of the capabilities of the technology that we have now, and which will become, no doubt, the norm in the future. New reimbursement policies should have a greater focus on preventive care.

A1.3 CHALLENGES AND BARRIERS TO VISION

Medical device designers have been fairly far removed from the home health care equipment user. Devices have generally been designed for hospital use by trained professionals, and the movement of this equipment into the home environment reveals a gap in the knowledge of the home care environment among designers. In order to design appropriately, they need to understand that home environment, as well as the capabilities and limitations of this new user population. The first barrier listed in Table 31.4 identifies the narrowing of this knowledge gap as a significant challenge to be met in order to meet the goal of inclusive design. The second challenge reflects the limitations of current medical technology. Most devices and instrumentation rely on the visual user interface and manual control of devices. To meet the needs of users with disabilities, devices will need to have more flexible user interfaces with multimodal and multisensory input and output options. The third challenge is similar: to meet the vision goal of scalable platforms, devices will need to address the requirement for flexibility and adaptability to different skills and ability levels of users, different comfort levels of users with the technology, and diversity of languages understood by users.

One of the barriers to having a connected care system is the current medical health care model. Connected care will not be achieved until patients are empowered and have a specific and active role to play in the health care process. This concern is reflected in the fourth challenge listed in Table 31.4. Similarly, the final challenge in the table — the lack of focus on prevention — also implies that patients are not sufficiently involved in the process. The medical model has always involved acute care — dealing with the current crisis, not preventing future crises from occurring.

A1.4 KNOWLEDGE GAPS AND ACTION ITEMS

The knowledge gaps and action items created by Theme Group C are also shown in Table 31.4, and relate closely to the vision statements and challenges/barriers statements. Many of the action items related to increasing the involvement of various stakeholders — mainly users and designers — in the tasks that must be carried out to make medical instrumentation accessible. Designers and manufacturers should become more actively involved in the standards process, to help establish both process and design guidance for achieving the accessibility goal for medical instrumentation. Similarly, designers should be at the forefront of work to be done in enhancing the decision support capabilities of medical instrumentation for all expected users, as well as in increasing the flexibility and adaptability of medical device user interfaces to meet the needs of users in the home health care environment. This work will require research to ensure that the end results do, indeed, have the desired effect; in other words, the resulting designs should be tested for accessibility with appropriate samples of end users. Ways to enhance patient empowerment towards self-management should be explored and validated. Finally, the complex relationships that exist among reimbursement, policies introduction of new technologies, and manufacturer profitability need to be better understood in order to meet accessibility goals in a way that is both feasible and financially sound.

A1.5 RECOMMENDATIONS

The recommendations of Theme Group C (see Table 31.4) again relate closely to the original vision statements but refer specifically to the roles that policymakers and granting agencies can play in the process of achieving accessibility goals for medical instrumentation used in the home health care arena. Policymakers and granting agencies can be key "cheerleaders" for accessibility by making changes and/or establishing programs that would mandate and enforce accessibility in the design of devices, provide reimbursement options for home health care that take advantage of telehealth technology for the management of chronic diseases, and by seriously promoting the prevention model of health care delivery. Granting agencies are encouraged to establish and support research programs that will help to fill the knowledge gaps that exist with respect to designing for accessibility, appropriately managing chronic disease through telehealth, and designing flexible and smart decision support systems for medical equipment. Research should also be supported that would better describe home health care clients in terms of their likely skills and abilities and their comfort with technology, and identify and ameliorate barriers to self-management. Finally, the medical instrumentation industry is encouraged to work towards the goals of interoperability, scalability, and customizability of systems and equipment designed for the home health market.

A1.6 DISCUSSION

Many of the user interfaces and accessibility problems in medical instrumentation stem from issues that plague the health care system as a whole. In fact, many would say that, in the U.S., at least, health care is fragmented and inefficient, and not really a system at all. The lack of a systems approach has, no doubt, created many of the problems we face in health care. We do not have a connected system of care, generally; therefore, a lack of technology integration is an expected byproduct of the fragmented care system itself.

Historically, the medical device industry has been a "cottage" industry; therefore, it is not surprising that there are interoperability problems and a lack of integrated systems. In addition, as an industry that is regulated by the federal government through the FDA, the medical device industry places its priority where the government does — on the safety and effectiveness of individual medical devices. Only during the last 10 years has the FDA emphasized usability as an additional goal, and the goal of accessibility is only now being placed on the table.

Further, much medical equipment that was designed for use by highly trained clinicians in the hospital environment has migrated to the home environment and into the hands of lay caregivers — a much more variable population of users across many dimensions. More medical devices are becoming, in effect, consumer products, and the same levels of usability and accessibility we have come to expect from other consumer products should be applicable to these devices.

If we truly believe in patient empowerment and patient self-management of chronic illnesses, then we must also believe in and support usability and accessibility goals. Unless medical instrumentation is accessible and usable, patients cannot be empowered or manage their own care. It is as simple as that. The vision statements of Theme Group C — with words like *scalable*, *customizable platforms*, *smart systems*, a *connected care* system, strategies and guidelines for *inclusive design*, and *reimbursement models* that support telehealth and preventive care — will, if met, increase both the accessibility and usability of medical instrumentation and empower patients.

Appendix 2

Commentary on Distinguishing Accessibility from Accommodation

David Baquis

Fundamental to designing and procuring accessible technology is an understanding of what accessibility actually means. This is important because patients, guests, and staff with disabilities may be offered an accommodation as a way of adapting to an environment that was not designed with accessibility in mind. For example, people with low vision may need caregiver assistance with taking their blood pressure if they cannot see the display of portable blood pressure measuring devices. Such "work-arounds" hinder independence.

There are two ways to design for accessibility. One is to build the accessible solution into the technology. For example, some glucometers offer an option to "speak out" the blood sugar level in addition to displaying it visually. Accessibility is often provided through such redundancy, also referred to as multimodal functionality. In the case of closed, self-contained medical instrumentation, this may be the preferred method.

The other accessibility strategy is to design for compatibility. For example, a web site with health information could be developed to conform with the Section 508 web accessibility standards so that users with assistive technologies can read the information. This "open architecture" model allows people with disabilities to access technology with their preferred adaptive equipment (e.g., screen readers or refreshable Braille displays).

Accessibility is "technology centered," whereas accommodation is "person centered." That means that people with a range of abilities would be considered at the time of design and procurement of technology, before the occasion of someone complaining or requesting help. Sometimes it is said that "accessibility occurs before the fact," whereas "accommodations are provided after the fact."

Accessibility focuses on how to design mainstream technology so that assistive technology may not even be necessary. For example, software installed in wireless PCs, which clinicians may use to enter patient information during office or hospital room visits, could provide display options to enable magnification and adjust contrast. Also referred to as *universal design*, accessibility can increase usability for many people and reduce the incidence of marginalizing people with disabilities as "special."

Until those who manufacture, finance, and request electronic and information technology transform their approach up-front to include the needs of people with a wide range of abilities, we can expect individuals with less apparent (invisible) disabilities to function less effectively because they may not ask for help. In addition, as the number of older people increases (both patients as well as employees), the impact of barriers to medical instrumentation can be expected to increase dramatically.

Appendix 3

Commentary on Data, Models, and Procedures for Design of Accessible Medical Instrumentation

Thomas J. Armstrong

Gaps between demands imposed on an individual by a task and an individual's capabilities are often identified after the system has been designed and a user is unable to successfully perform the task, becomes injured, or develops a health problem. In some cases, user trials, in which the equipment is tested by a wide range of users before it is produced, are conducted so that the final design can be modified in ways that enable all users to achieve the goals of the system. However, a wide range of users often are not available to try the equipment and procedures. Data, models, and procedures for applying them are needed that can be used to evaluate equipment and procedures before they are produced [1]. Models should consider physical demands and capacities, such as users' ability to see, reach, grasp, and exert necessary forces without becoming injured. It also should consider sensory and cognitive abilities, such as users' ability to detect and process information about the equipment and environment.

The evaluation and design of an examining table illustrates how models and analysis tools can be used to identify physical barriers to persons with conditions that restrict their reach and strength. An analysis of the task and equipment show that users must reach and grasp something on the opposite side of the table to pull themselves into position and to stabilize their body. Using three-dimensional biomechanical models, it can be shown that persons with spinal cord injuries (SCIs) have reduced reach capacities compared to persons without SCIs [2]. Designers can use these models to locate handles that will enable patients with SCI to complete the transfer. In addition to reaching, it is necessary to grasp a solid object to pull against. Often this solid object is the side of the table. Figure A3.1a shows a hand posture predicted for gripping the edge of a table using a three-dimensional biomechanical hand model [3]. All of the force must be exerted with the fingertips, which only have about 15% as much strength as the hand in a power grip posture. Figure A3.1b shows that the predicted posture for gripping a 3.5 cm diameter rail is a power grip — a position of maximum hand strength. Additionally, the rail can be mounted in such a way that it can be moved closer to the opposite side of the bed for a patient with a reduced reach or limitation, and it can be positioned as a guard rail to prevent persons who cannot control their posture from falling over the edge.

The use of models can proactively increase the number of persons who will be able to use the medical equipment and reduce their risk of injuries and illnesses. Basic biomechanical models have been developed, but additional research including population studies are necessary to develop models for evaluating and designing all medical devices.

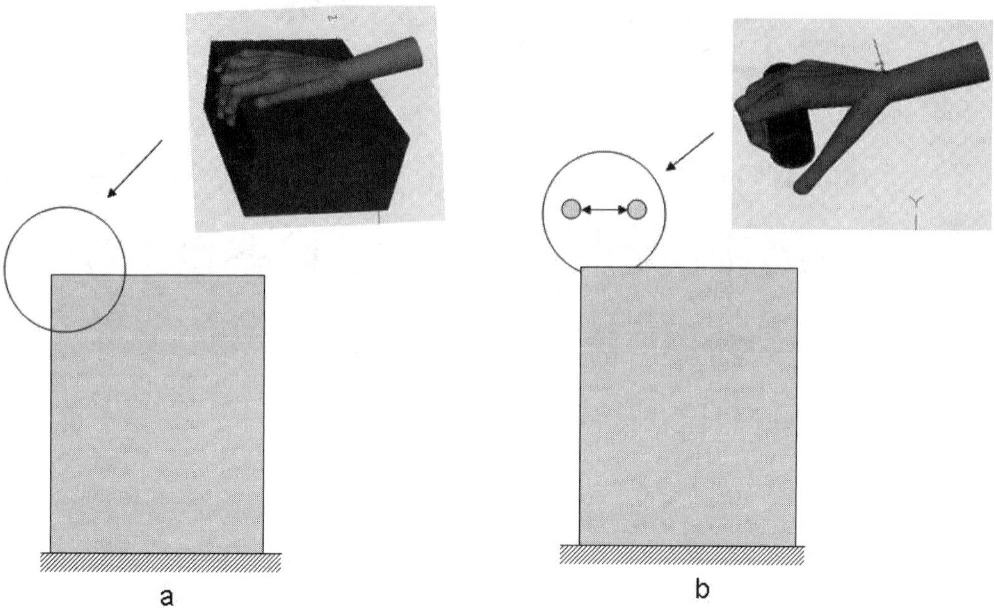

FIGURE A3.1 (a) Biomechanical hand model shows that fingertips must support transfer loads. (b) Model also shows that adjustable handle can be used to eliminate barriers due to reach and hand strength limitations.

REFERENCES

1. Brandt, E. and Pope, A., Ed., *Enabling America: Assessing the Role of Rehabilitation Science and Engineering,* Washington, D.C., National Academy of Press, 1997.
2. Chaffin, D., Woolley, C., Martin, B., Womack, N., and Dickerson, C., Reaching and Object Movement Capability in Spinal Cord Injured Population, NIDRR Workshop on Anthropometrics, Buffalo, New York, 2001.
3. Choi, J. and Armstrong, T., 3-Dimensional Kinematic Model for Predicting Hand Posture during Certain Gripping Tasks, International Society of Biomechanics, Cleveland, OH, 2005.

Appendix 4

Commentary on What Is Accessibility? And What Does It Have to Do with Medical Device Design?

Ron Kaye and Jay Crowley

Having spent the past 15 years working to better identify, understand, and resolve problems with use of medical devices, we understand many of the issues and problems associated with improving the usability of medical device design for the intended user. But what is meant by *accessibility*, and how can it successfully be incorporated into device design?

The medical device manufacturing industry in the U.S. is large and diverse, with several large manufacturers and many specialized small ones. The majority of device manufacturers are small, with fewer than 20 employees. FDA currently lists over 80,000 different brands and models of medical devices manufactured by more than 10,000 device companies.

Medical devices include a wide range of products — from expensive, complex equipment (such as x-ray machines) to simple items (such as bandages). These vary dramatically in complexity, packaging, and application. The industry is constantly producing new innovations, which causes relatively short life cycles for many products as well as intense competition among manufacturers.

Stimulating the medical device industry to consistently follow human factors engineering design principles has been difficult and only been partially successful. FDA's Quality System Regulation of 1996 provided a mandate for manufacturers to design devices, which met the needs of the intended users. And in 2000, CDRH published specific guidance to further help manufacturers address hazards related to medical device use during device design and development. Although both were widely published and promoted, only limited progress has been made in establishing human factors engineering as a consistent and visible component of device design.

For accessible interfaces in medical device design to be successfully encouraged, the first step will be to clearly articulate the need. Device designers typically work within constraints established by the company's business plan. They must balance competing priorities to bring about the most cost-effective and marketable device design, including its user interface. The accessibility community must therefore help the medical device design and development community by succinctly describing accessibility both in general as well as for different types of disadvantaged users and specific devices. The following questions would help define these issues:

- Who are these disabled users for which accessible designs could be helpful?
- What could disabled users accomplish with accessible devices?
- How do disabilities currently affect use of medical devices?
- What modifications would address the existing accessibility issues?
- How have accessibility solutions been successfully applied to other domains?

Appendix 5

Commentary on the Difference between "Usability" and "Accessibility," Which May Be the End Users

Molly Follette Story

The distinction between the terms *usable* and *accessible* may be no more than the identification and definition of who the end user is: if a device is *usable* by someone who has a disability, then it becomes labeled *accessible*. The two terms lie on a continuum of design accommodation.

Figure A5.1 shows relationships among mainstream design, assistive technology, and expert systems. Most people in the population have abilities that lie in the middle portion of normal distribution curves and mainstream design suits them fine. But either in place of or in conjunction with mainstream designs, people whose abilities fall on the lower end of the curve may benefit from assistive technologies, and people whose abilities fall on the upper end of the curve may benefit from expert systems. Note the large "gray zones" between the categories, where some mainstream designs may not extend (in fact, there may be a gap between categories), or depending on context and perspective, a device may be considered to fall into either zone.

Small changes in design of a mainstream device can have a large effect on usability and accessibility. We will always need assistive technologies because no design will ever be usable by all people in all circumstances; and beyond the extent of or along with assistive technologies, we will always need personal assistance. But making a device that is more accommodating of a broader diversity of user abilities also makes it suit a variety of user preferences (e.g., learning or operational mode) and circumstances (e.g., dark hallway, noisy emergency department, or occupied hands), and may reduce the need for assistive technologies (and/or expert systems).

The concepts of usability and accessibility are not mutually exclusive. Because improving the interactions between people and medical devices can increase health care access and safety, optimizing usability for *all* users should be accepted as a beneficial design challenge, not condemned as an unnecessary burden.

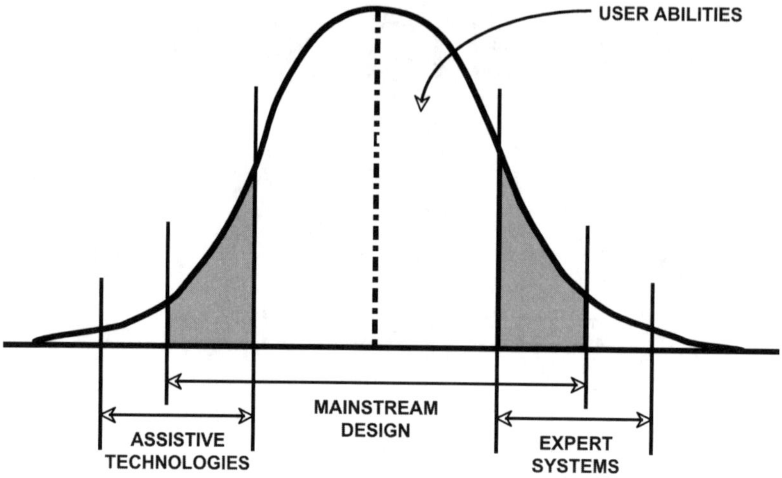

FIGURE A5.1 Relationship between mainstream design, assistive technologies, and expert systems.

Glossary of Terms

Ability A basic trait that a person brings to a new task.

Access Board An independent Federal agency devoted to accessibility for people with disabilities. Created in 1973 (as the Architectural and Transportation Barriers Compliance Board, or ATBCB) to ensure access to federally funded facilities, the Access Board is now a leading source of information on accessible design. The Board develops and maintains design criteria for the built environment, transit vehicles, telecommunications equipment, and for electronic and information technology. It also provides technical assistance and training on these requirements and on accessible design and enforces accessibility standards that cover federally funded facilities.

Accessibility (Chapter 25) Ability to access the intended use of a product or environment or service for which there is a possibility of benefit.

Accessibility (ISO 9241-171, Definition 3.2) Usability of a product, service, environment, or facility by people with the widest range of capabilities.

Accessibility (Carmona) The degree to which an environment (physical, social, or attitudinal) makes appropriate accommodations to eliminate barriers or other impediments to equality of access to facilities, services, and the like, for persons with disabilities.

Degrees of Accessibility There are degrees of ability to access a product or service, potentially both at the level of the individual and the level of the total population. Proposed scales include degree of difficulty (up to *impossible*), and degree of handicap (up to *fully handicapped*). The former is commonly used in accessibility guidelines and the latter is used in an draft standard (ISO/IEC 24756, 2005).

Accessibility Guidelines Typically a sequence of stated guidelines and standards, each of which is followed by a list of checkpoints, with each checkpoint given a priority level (e.g., "must" because otherwise some users will find use impossible; "should" because some will find use difficult; "may" because some will find use somewhat difficult). In this context, these guidelines are part of a formalized, consensus process coordinated by a standards body or an agency of the government.

Accessibility Metric Measures or scores aimed at estimating the degree of accessibility of a product, typically as a collection of scores that represent accessibility for different general categories of activity limitation, impairment, or disability. The metric typically takes into account both design features and anticipated task procedures.

Accessibility Features Design features that enhance the accessibility of a product or environment or service.

Accessible Design (Legal Perspective, U.S.) The design of entities (products, environments, or services) that satisfy specific legal mandates, guidelines, or code requirements with the intent of providing accessibility to the entities for individuals with disabilities.

Accessible Design (General) Accessible design strives to maximize accessibility and minimize barriers that prevent individuals from participating in the use of an entity. There are two basic design strategies for enhancing access: *direct access* (direct adaptations to designs that significantly improve their accessibility) and *assistive access* (interfaces that enable an add-on assistive technology to provide the user with access).

Accessible Product or Environment or Service — A product or environment or service is accessible if the intended use or benefit can be realized effectively by people with disabilities.

Activity (International Classification of Function, Disability, and Health) — Execution of a task or action by an individual.

Activity — The process of doing something, representing the functional result of human performance. Activities often can be broken down into smaller tasks.

Activities of Daily Living (ADL) (National Center for Health Statistics) — Activities of daily living are activities related to personal care and include bathing or showering, dressing, getting in or out of bed or a chair, using the toilet, and eating. In the National Health Interview Survey respondents were asked about needing the help of another person with personal care needs because of a physical, mental, or emotional problem. Persons are considered to have an ADL limitation if any causal condition is chronic.

Activity Limitations (ICF) — Difficulties an individual may have in executing activities.

Alternate/Alternative Formats (Legal, Section 508) — Alternate formats include, but are not limited to, Braille, large print, disks, audio formats, and electronic formats.

Alternate/Alternative Methods (Legal, Section 508) — Different means of providing information, including product documentation, to people with disabilities. Alternate methods may include, but are not limited to, voice, fax, relay service, TTY, Internet posting, captioning, text-to-speech synthesis, and audio description.

Assistive Technology (Legal, Section 508) — Any item, piece of equipment, or system, whether acquired commercially, modified, or customized, that is commonly used to increase, maintain, or improve functional capabilities of individuals with disabilities.

Assistive Technology — An extrinsic enabler that is the basis by which human performance is improved in the presence of disability.

Assistive Technology — A means of reducing handicap.

Assistive Technology Service (Legal, U.S.) — Any service that directly assists an individual with a disability in the selection, acquisition, or use of an assistive technology device.

Auxiliary Aides and Services (June Isaacson Kailes) — These may include: Qualified interpreters, qualified readers, note takers, computer-aided transcription, 1:1 facilitators (for people with learning and understanding disabilities), telephone handset amplifiers, assistive listening systems, telephones compatible with hearing aids, open and closed captioning, e-mail or other electronic communications; use of telecommunications devices (TTYs) for people who are deaf, hard of hearing, or have speech disabilities, video text displays, and other effective methods of making aurally delivered materials available to individuals with hearing impairments; audio recordings, Braille materials, large print materials, and other effective methods of making visually delivered materials available to individuals with visual disabilities.

Body Functions (ICF) — Physiological functions of body systems (including psychological functions).

Body Structures (ICF) — Anatomical parts of the body such as organs, limbs, and their components.

Cognitive Walkthrough (U.S. Dept. of Health and Human Services, HHS) — An inspection method for evaluating the design of a user interface, with special attention to how well the interface supports "exploratory learning," i.e., first-time use without formal training. The evaluation is done by having a group of evaluators go step-by-step through commonly used tasks. It can be performed by evaluators in the early stages of design, before performance testing is possible.

Communication Access Providing content in methods that are understandable and usable by people with reduced or no ability to speak, see, and hear and limitations in learning and understanding.

Cross-Disability Access Accessibility across groups of people with different disabilities.

Design for All (European Institute for Design and Disability, EIDD) Intervention in environments, products, and services with the aim that everybody, including future generations, and without regard to age, capabilities, or cultural origin, can enjoy participating in our societies. To achieve this broad goal, we must follow two basic principles: facilitate the use of products and services [and] ensure that users take part in the product design and evaluation processes.

Device Class A set, collection, or group of medical devices that have certain attributes or traits in common.

Disability (Older ICF, ICIDH-2) Restriction or lack of ability to perform an activity in a manner considered normal, manifested in the performance of daily tasks; the functional consequences of impairments.

Disability Reduced ability or lack of ability of an individual to perform an activity in daily life. A loss, absence, or impairment of physical or mental fitness that can be seen or measured.

Electronic and Information Technology (Legal, U.S. Access Board, Section 508) Includes information technology and any equipment or interconnected system or subsystem of equipment that is used in the creation, conversion, or duplication of data or information. The term electronic and information technology includes, but is not limited to, telecommunications products (such as telephones), information kiosks, and transaction machines, World Wide Web sites, multimedia, and office equipment such as copiers and fax machines. The term does not include any equipment that contains embedded information technology that is used as an integral part of the product, but the principal function of which is not the acquisition, storage, manipulation, management, movement, control, display, switching, interchange, transmission, or reception of data or information.

Environmental Factors (ICF) The physical, social, and attitudinal environment in which people live and conduct their lives.

Ergonomics The science of work. Ergonomics removes barriers to quality, productivity, and safe human performance by fitting products, tasks and environments to people.

Ergonomics (International Ergonomics Association, IEA) Ergonomics (or human factors) is the scientific discipline concerned with the understanding of interactions among humans and other elements of a system, and the profession that applies theory, principles, data, and methods to design in order to optimize human well-being and overall system performance.

Ergonomics (Legal Dictionary) An engineering science concerned with the physical and psychological relationship between machines and people who use them.

Handicap (Older Definition) A disadvantage resulting from an impairment or disability that limits or prevents fulfillment of a role that is normal for the affected individual.

Handicap (June Isaacson Kailes) Barriers that people with disabilities encounter in environment. The gap between a person's capabilities and demands of environment. People are not handicapped by their disability all the time. Wheelchair users are not handicapped in an environment where there are accessible routes and pathways.

Handicap (ISO-IEC 24756 Draft Document, 2005) Anything that may interfere with the accessibility of interactions between users and systems.

Heuristic Evaluation (HHS) An inspection method for finding certain types of usability problems in a user interface design. Heuristic evaluation involves having one or more usability specialists individually examine the interface and judge its compliance with recognized usability principles. These usability principles are the "heuristics" from which the method takes its name.

Human Factors A multidisciplinary science that studies and applies information about human behavior, capabilities, limitations, and other characteristics to the design and evaluation of tools, machines, tasks, jobs, systems, and environments for productive, effective, and safe human use. This term is often viewed as synonymous with "ergonomics" — in comparison, ergonomics tends to have a stronger focus on biomechanics, and human factors on cognitive performance.

Human Factors Engineering (ANSI/AAMI HE74:2001) Application of knowledge about human behavior, abilities, limitations, and other characteristics to the design of tools, machines, equipment, devices, systems, tasks, jobs, and environments to achieve productive, safe, comfortable, and effective human use.

Human Performance (Bailey) The result of a pattern of actions carried out to satisfy an objective according to some standard.

IADL (Instrumental Activities of Daily Living, Centers for Disease Control and Prevention, CDC) Activities related to independent living and including preparing meals, managing money, shopping for groceries or personal items, performing light or heavy housework, and using a telephone.

Impairment (Older ICF, ICIDH-2) A loss or abnormality of structure or function at the organ level. We commonly speak of "functional impairments" or "dysfunction" of a part of (or system within) the body.

Impairment (ICF) Problems in body function or structure such as a significant deviation or loss.

Inclusive Design (Royal Society for the Encouragement of Arts, Manufactures and Commerce, RSA, U.K.) Inclusive design is a process whereby designers, manufacturers, and service providers ensure that their products and environments address the widest possible audience, irrespective of age or ability. It aims to include the needs of people who are currently excluded or marginalized [sic] by mainstream design practices and links directly to the concept of an inclusive society.

Information Technology (Legal, U.S. Access Board, Section 508) Any equipment or interconnected system or subsystem of equipment that is used in the automatic acquisition, storage, manipulation, management, movement, control, display, switching, interchange, transmission, or reception of data or information. The term information technology includes computers, ancillary equipment, software, firmware and similar procedures, services (including support services), and related resources.

Labeling (ANSI/AAMI HE74:2001) (1) Act of describing the nature or contents of some device with respect to the name of the product, the manufacturer, the amount present, indications and instructions for use, or warnings associated with its use; (2) act of identifying display or control elements of a system with text or pictorial designators.

Labeling (U.S. Food and Drug Administration) " … All labels and written, printed, or graphic matter: (1) on the device or any of its containers, or (2) accompanying the device … " (in Section 201(m) of the Food, Drugs, and Cosmetics Act, 21 CFR Part 801, Labeling).

Multimodal Multiple sensory and motor modes for an interface channel (e.g., between text and speech), such that more than one modality is available to access content or operate a product, and support for transformations among them. Multimodal interfaces are often necessary for a product or service to be accessible.

Operator (IEC 60601-1)	Person handling a device for the purposes for which the device was intended.
Operable Controls	A component of a product that requires physical contact for usual operation. Operable controls include, but are not limited to, mechanically operated controls, input and output trays, card slots, keyboards, or keypads.
Participation	Involvement in a life situation.
Participation Restrictions (ICF)	Limitations that an individual may experience in involvement in life situations.
Pathology	The interruption of, or interference with, normal bodily processes or structures by a disease process.
Reasonable Accommodation	A modification or adjustment to a job, the work environment, or the way things usually are done that enables a qualified individual with a disability to enjoy an equal employment or access opportunity. Reasonable accommodation is a key nondiscrimination requirement of the ADA.
Risk Analysis (ANSI/AAMI HE74:2001)	Structured review of a system to identify undesirable events that can occur because of that system's use (including maintenance, etc.) and estimation of the likelihood and potential severity of those events. This term is often used synonymously with the term hazard analysis.
Self-Contained, Closed Products (Legal, Section 508)	Products that generally have embedded software and are commonly designed in such a fashion that a user cannot easily attach or install assistive technology. These products include, but are not limited to, information kiosks and information transaction machines, copiers, printers, calculators, fax machines, and other similar types of products.
Telecommunications	The transmission, between or among points specified by the user, of information of the user's choosing, without significant change in the form or content of the information as sent and received.
TTY	An abbreviation for teletypewriter, or text telephone; machinery or equipment that employs interactive text-based communications through the transmission of coded signals across the telephone network. TTYs may include, for example, devices known as TDDs (telecommunication display devices or telecommunication devices for deaf persons) or computers with special modems.
Transgenerational Design (James J. Pirkl)	The practice of making products and environments compatible with those physical and sensory impairments associated with human aging and which limit major activities of daily living.
Undue Burden (Legal, Section 508)	Undue burden means significant difficulty or expense. In determining whether an action would result in an undue burden, an agency shall consider all agency resources available to the program or component for which the product is being developed, procured, maintained, or used.
Universal Access (Chapter 25)	Ability of all persons to fully access the intended uses of a product or service for which there is potential benefit. Universal access is rarely fully achievable, and barriers include the dimensions of interface design, distance, and cost.
Universal Design (Synonyms)	Inclusive design. Lifespan design. Transgenerational design. Design for All (Europe). Barrier-free design (old term).
Universal Design (Center for Universal Design, North Carolina State University)	The design of products and environments to be usable by all people, to the greatest extent possible, without adaptation or specialized design.

Universal Design (Council of Europe Committee of Ministers, 2001)
Universal design is a strategy, which aims to make the design and composition of different environments and products accessible and understandable to as well as usable by everyone, to the greatest extent in the most independent and natural manner possible, without the need for adaptation or specialized design solutions.

Universal Design/Usability (Gregg C. Vanderheiden)
Process of designing products so that they are usable by the widest range of people operating in the widest range of situations as is commercially practical.

Usability (Short)
Ability to use.

Usability (ISO 9241-11, Definition 3.1)
Extent to which a product can be used by specified users to achieve specified goals with effectiveness, efficiency, and satisfaction in a specified context of use.

Usability Testing (CDC)
Usability testing includes a range of test and evaluation methods that include automated evaluations, inspection evaluations, operational evaluations, and human performance testing. In a typical performance test, users perform a variety of tasks with a prototype (or an operational system) while observers note what each user does and says while performance data are recorded. One of the main purposes of usability testing is to identify issues that keep users from meeting the usability goals.

Use Error (ANSI/AAMI HE74:2001)
Act or omission of an act that results in a different outcome than that intended by the manufacturer or expected by the user, which may result from a mismatch between user, man–machine interface, task, and environment.

User Profile (ANSI/AAMI HE74:2001)
Summary of the mental, physical, and demographic traits of the end-user population as well as any special characteristics such as occupational skills and job requirements that may have a bearing on design decisions.

Web Accessibility (WAI, W3C)
Web accessibility means that people with disabilities can use the Web. More specifically, Web accessibility means that people with disabilities can perceive, understand, navigate, and interact with the Web, and that they can contribute to the Web. Web accessibility also benefits others, including older people with changing abilities due to aging.

Index

A

B

C

D

E

F

G

H

I

K

L

M

V

W

X

Y

Z

RELATED TITLES

Designing Usability into Medical Products
Michael E. Wiklund and Stephen B. Wilcox
ISBN: 0849328438

Reliable Design of Medical Devices, Second Edition
Richard Fries
ISBN: 0824723759

The Medical Device R & D Handbook
Theodore R. Kucklick
ISBN: 0849327172